# Dr. J. Stephan Jellinek
## Formulation and Function of Cosmetics

DR. J. STEPHAN JELLINEK

# FORMULATION
# AND FUNCTION
# OF COSMETICS

Translated from the German by G. L. Fenton

WILEY–INTERSCIENCE

a Division of John Wiley & Sons, Inc.

New York . London . Sydney . Toronto

TO MY DEAR WIFE

# Preface to the English Language Edition

The approach and purpose of this book are different from those of the several excellent English-language books currently in print on the formulation of cosmetics. It is not intended primarily to inform the reader of the most up-to-date types of cosmetic preparations or of the most modern raw materials, although these preparations and raw materials are fully discussed. Rather the book attempts to explain why these preparations are compounded as they are and to treat the function of the various raw materials.

Most important of all, it is intended to stimulate consideration of different and better ways to solve the problems that cosmetics are designed to overcome.

Features of this book directly related to its central purpose are the following:

. The grouping of cosmetics in terms of their basic functions—cleansing, protecting, and beautifying. This introduces some unorthodox bedfellows such as shampoos, dentifrices, and nail polish removers into the chapter on cleansing preparations. It is hoped that juxtapositions such as these will be found not only surprising but also meaningful and thought provoking.

. Some formulations of little current commercial interest (e.g., metallic hair dyes) or products that are not normally classified as cosmetics (e.g., industrial protective creams) are treated because they present interesting alternative approaches to cosmetic problems.

. The book draws on the experience of many experts from different countries, both recent and not so recent, and represents an outlook that is, in some areas, different from that currently prevailing in the English-speaking world.

It is hoped that these features will give the book a special usefulness as a stimulator of new ideas.

It is a pleasure to thank Mrs. L. Fenton for the excellent way in which she turned a translation into an improvement of the book and to express my appreciation to Dr. Alfred Hüthig and Wiley–Interscience, without whose cooperation it would not have come into being.

Irvington, New York                                                    J. Stephan Jellinek
January 1970

# Preface to the Second Edition

The German humorist Wilhelm Busch was hardly thinking of technical and scientific books and their authors when he coined his wise saying about the ease of becoming a father and the problems of being one; but I have, with quite a few of my colleagues, come to the conclusion that it is not so simple to be the father of such a book as you might imagine in the first flush of relief when the book at long last appears in print. You are then likely to believe that the end of all toil and trouble has come. Not so: you no sooner get used to basking in the sun of paternal pride than the publisher starts hinting at a new edition, soon to be required, and you realize that you have created not just a book but an obligation, an obligation to revise it from time to time with a critical eye, to bring it up to date with the latest scientific results.

I am much obliged to Mr. Paul Piep for consenting to collaborate in this work. I should also like to thank all critics of the first edition, not only for the appreciation they have shown but in particular because they gave me many valuable ideas for altering the new edition.

Many of the reviewers were of the opinion that this book reflects a field of knowledge that in the course of the last 10 years has developed from empiricism to science. If my book can contribute to this development in some degree, it will be ample reward for the labors of becoming and being a father.

Irvington, New York, Autumn 1966

# Preface to the First Edition

If all the people with a professional interest in cosmetics were convened at a meeting, it would be a very mixed gathering. We should find, in the medical profession, dermatologists who see in cosmetic products both a means of preventing skin lesions and a possible cause for them; there would be plastic surgeons, biologists, and physiologists who make a study of the structure of skin, hair, and teeth as well as the processes occurring in them and their immediate environment. There would also be organic chemists who would develop new basic and active substances for the cosmetic industry, physical chemists who study the behavior of emulsions and surfactants, and microbiologists who deal with problems of preservation. We should certainly meet hairdressers and makeup specialists whose job is actually to apply cosmetic products and processes to the satisfaction of their individual customers and, finally, cosmetic chemists who are responsible for the industrial preparation of cosmetics and the development of new products.

If we were to ask all these groups what they understand by "cosmetics," the replies would vary widely. Just because the word is used by so many different professional groups, cosmetics has acquired a broad and ill-defined significance.

The term "cosmetology"* has been in use for about 10 years now, first in English and French and lately also in German. This word as well will not mean the same to everyone who uses it; nevertheless I think it is generally accepted that cosmetology does not deal with cosmetic methods but with cosmetic products, not with specific properties or "tricks of the trade" in preparing or applying them but with fundamental problems. Taking this as a basis, I suggest the following definition:

"Cosmetology is the science that deals with the laws governing the production, storage, and application of cosmetic products, whether they be chemical, physical, biological, or microbiological." This science is of interest to all who are concerned with cosmetics, but in particular to the cosmetic chemist. For him it is the point of departure for his work.

Like all technical terms, the word cosmetology has not been coined at random, but has risen out of a need. That it has been circulating during the last 10 years is no accident for it follows logically from the evolution of the cosmetic industry.

For about 20 years cosmetics have been developing rapidly. The chemical industry has placed at the disposal of the cosmetic industry innumerable new basic and active substances and every year further developments appear. The quantity and quality of biological materials which are made available for application are also steadily improving. The medical profession is concerning itself more and more with cosmetics—not critically or disapprovingly —but rather in the spirit of fruitful collaboration with the cosmetician.

The standing of the expert who develops new products has changed radically. Formerly, the nucleus of his knowledge consisted of formulations he had developed himself or inherited from his predecessors. He knew how to

* The German title of this book is *Kosmetologie*.

prepare lotions, powders, and cream bases according to the properties required (greasy or drying, soft or viscous), and he knew which substances would achieve specific effects. Today such "static" knowledge (i.e., being conversant with a formulary) is no longer sufficient. A formula for a cream that may well be acceptable today may no longer be the best next year if a new synthetic fat or a new emulsifier has in the meantime been introduced. A substance tested with satisfactory results last year may be superseded by one more effective or with less undesirable side effects.

If he wants to make creative use of the many suggestions he obtains from medicine, biology, and the chemical industry and to meet the ever-new demands of beauty treatment, today's cosmetic expert must know more than just formulations. He must be aware of the properties of the skin surface and hair and he must know how his preparations affect these tissues. He must know the microscopic structure of his creams, how he can affect it by his selection of raw materials and emulsifiers, and how changes in the microscopic structure in turn affect the macroscopically discernible properties. He must know, in the light of the latest findings, the effect achieved when various synthetic and biological substances are employed and how the value of these substances can be tested usefully. Finally, he must also have some "historical" knowledge: he must know how earlier cosmetic chemists solved their problems, for on entering new territory he will want to utilize the experience of his predecessors.

To summarize: although yesterday's experts could be content with a knowledge of formulations and raw materials, the work of the modern cosmetic chemist requires a knowledge of cosmetology in an ever-increasing degree.

This book is no encyclopedia. It makes no pretense of mentioning every basic material and preparation that occurs in the cosmetic industry. I have tried to cover the most important features and connections in this large and confusing field and therefore have had to refrain in many instances from going into detail.

Nor is the book meant to be a formulary, although in the second part numerous formulations are given. These should not be used as tried and proved prescriptions but rather as suggestions and examples of how cosmetic chemists have tried to solve their problems. I have endeavored to deal with different solutions of a given problem side by side or in sequence. Face lotions, cleansing creams, and face masks, for instance, appear in the same chapter, although these products have little in common as far as their structure and production are concerned, but all are attempts to deal with one problem: the best way of removing impurities from the skin surface.

Even if the dermatological, biochemical, and physical-chemical aspects of cosmetics are dealt with in broad outline, I definitely do not want to give the impression that no further collaboration with physicians, biologists, and chemists is required by the cosmetic chemist who is fully conversant with the contents of this book. On the contrary: I hope that they will encourage just such collaboration. The idea that the future development of cosmetics depends largely on a cross fertilization of cosmetics, medicine, and natural sciences is one "leitmotiv" of this work.

In conclusion I want to thank all who have helped in the preparation of this book; in particular my father Dr. Paul Jellinek, who not only gave me the original impetus to begin but also provided many pointers and hints during the writing, and Dr. Gerhard Everts who, in rare altruism, critically worked through the whole manuscript. My thanks are due also to Messrs. O. Birman, J. Bossina, H. D. Daute and to Dr. G. H. Carrière, Dr. H. Fiedler, and Dr. C. Fuchs for the critical reading of individual chapters and their valuable observations.

Amersfoort, Summer 1959                         J. Stephan Jellinek

# Contents

## Part I

*Chapter 1   Skin and Hair* . . . . . . . . . . . . . . . . . . . . . .   3

Anatomy of the Skin. . . . . . . . . . . . . . . . . . . . . . .   4
  The Surface. . . . . . . . . . . . . . . . . . . . . . . . . . .   4
  The Deeper Layers . . . . . . . . . . . . . . . . . . . . . .   6
Physiology of the Skin . . . . . . . . . . . . . . . . . . . . .   10
  The Hydroregulatory System . . . . . . . . . . . . . . . .   10
  Breathing of the Skin . . . . . . . . . . . . . . . . . . . .   12
  The Acid Mantle . . . . . . . . . . . . . . . . . . . . . . .   12
The Exterior Appearance of the Skin. . . . . . . . . . . . .   14
  Color . . . . . . . . . . . . . . . . . . . . . . . . . . . . .   14
  Luster . . . . . . . . . . . . . . . . . . . . . . . . . . . . .   16
  Relief . . . . . . . . . . . . . . . . . . . . . . . . . . . . .   16
Anatomy of the Hair. . . . . . . . . . . . . . . . . . . . . . .   17
Hair Growth . . . . . . . . . . . . . . . . . . . . . . . . . . .   18
Color and Gloss of the Hair . . . . . . . . . . . . . . . . . .   18
The Chemistry of Skin and Keratin . . . . . . . . . . . . .   19
Compatibility of Skin and Cosmetic Preparations . . . . . . .   24
  Toxic Reaction and Intolerance . . . . . . . . . . . . . . .   25
  Precautions in the Production of Cosmetic Preparations . . . .   26
  Experimental Determination of Skin Compatibility. . . . . . .   27


*Chapter 2   Surfactants in Cosmetics* . . . . . . . . . . . . . . . .   32

Principle of Effectiveness . . . . . . . . . . . . . . . . . . . .   32
  General Structure . . . . . . . . . . . . . . . . . . . . . . .   33
  Polar and Nonpolar Atom Groups . . . . . . . . . . . . . .   34

Reduction of Surface Tension . . . . . . . . . . . . . . . . 40
Micell Formation . . . . . . . . . . . . . . . . . . . . . 41
Surface and Interface Films . . . . . . . . . . . . . . . . . 43
The Functions of Surfactants in Cosmetics . . . . . . . . . . 44
The Wetting Effect . . . . . . . . . . . . . . . . . . . . . 44
The Foaming Effect . . . . . . . . . . . . . . . . . . . . 46
The Solubilizing Effect . . . . . . . . . . . . . . . . . . . 48
The Emulsifying Effect . . . . . . . . . . . . . . . . . . . 48
The Dispersing Effect . . . . . . . . . . . . . . . . . . . 58
The Cleansing Effect . . . . . . . . . . . . . . . . . . . . 60
Further Practical Requirements . . . . . . . . . . . . . . . 61
Chemical Classification . . . . . . . . . . . . . . . . . . . 66

Chapter 3   Microbiological Aspects of Cosmetics . . . . . . . . . 75

Bacteria and Molds . . . . . . . . . . . . . . . . . . . . . 75
Microbiology of the Skin Surface . . . . . . . . . . . . . . 77
Skin Flora . . . . . . . . . . . . . . . . . . . . . . . . . 77
Defense Methods of the Skin . . . . . . . . . . . . . . . . 79
Disinfectants . . . . . . . . . . . . . . . . . . . . . . . . 80
Significance in Cosmetics . . . . . . . . . . . . . . . . . . 80
Principle of Effectiveness . . . . . . . . . . . . . . . . . . 80
Factors Determining Effectiveness . . . . . . . . . . . . . . 81
Experimental Determination of the Effect . . . . . . . . . . 82
Selection of a Disinfectant . . . . . . . . . . . . . . . . . 83
Specific Disinfectants . . . . . . . . . . . . . . . . . . . . 84
Microbiological Contamination of Cosmetics . . . . . . . . . 97
Extent and Significance of the Problem . . . . . . . . . . . 97
Microflora of Cosmetic Preparations . . . . . . . . . . . . 98
Cosmetic Preservatives . . . . . . . . . . . . . . . . . . . 98
Phenols . . . . . . . . . . . . . . . . . . . . . . . . . . . 98
Application . . . . . . . . . . . . . . . . . . . . . . . . . 103

Chapter 4   The Composition of Cosmetic Preparations . . . . . . . 108

Oils and Anhydrous Creams . . . . . . . . . . . . . . . . . 108
Mineral Oils, Petrolatum, and Mineral Waxes . . . . . . . . 108
Vegetable and Animal Oils and Fats . . . . . . . . . . . . . 114
Oil and Fat Derivatives . . . . . . . . . . . . . . . . . . . 115
Vegetable and Animal Waxes and Their Derivatives . . . . . . 116
Synthetic Waxes . . . . . . . . . . . . . . . . . . . . . . . 119
Fatty Alcohols and Sterols . . . . . . . . . . . . . . . . . 119

Phospholipids and Synthetic Phosphoric Acid Esters . . . . . . 120
Silicone Oils and Waxes . . . . . . . . . . . . . . . . . . 120
Dispersed Solids. . . . . . . . . . . . . . . . . . . . . . 124
Antioxidants . . . . . . . . . . . . . . . . . . . . . . . 125
Preservatives . . . . . . . . . . . . . . . . . . . . . . . 130
Composition . . . . . . . . . . . . . . . . . . . . . . . . 130
Thixotropic Creams . . . . . . . . . . . . . . . . . . . . 131
Nongreasy Products . . . . . . . . . . . . . . . . . . . . 131
Protective Preparations. . . . . . . . . . . . . . . . . . . 132
Pastes . . . . . . . . . . . . . . . . . . . . . . . . . . 132
Preparation . . . . . . . . . . . . . . . . . . . . . . . . 132
Water-in-Oil Emulsions . . . . . . . . . . . . . . . . . . . 133
Raw Materials . . . . . . . . . . . . . . . . . . . . . . . . 133
The Raw Materials of the Oil Phase . . . . . . . . . . . . 133
The Raw Materials of the Aqueous Phase . . . . . . . . . 133
Emulsifying Agents . . . . . . . . . . . . . . . . . . . . 133
Preservatives . . . . . . . . . . . . . . . . . . . . . . . 136
General Remarks . . . . . . . . . . . . . . . . . . . . . . 136
Preparation . . . . . . . . . . . . . . . . . . . . . . . . 138
Dual Emulsions . . . . . . . . . . . . . . . . . . . . . . . 138
Comparison with W/O and O/W Emulsions . . . . . . . . 140
Preparation . . . . . . . . . . . . . . . . . . . . . . . . 140
Oil-in-Water Emulsions . . . . . . . . . . . . . . . . . . . 141
The Raw Materials for the Oil Phase. . . . . . . . . . . . . 141
The Raw Materials of the Aqueous Phase . . . . . . . . . 142
Emulsifying Agents . . . . . . . . . . . . . . . . . . . . 152
Insoluble Solids . . . . . . . . . . . . . . . . . . . . . . 159
Cosmetic Preparations without Oil. . . . . . . . . . . . . . 161
Raw Materials . . . . . . . . . . . . . . . . . . . . . . . 161
Water and Low Molecular Alcohols . . . . . . . . . . . . 161
Emollients . . . . . . . . . . . . . . . . . . . . . . . . 163
Thickening Agents. . . . . . . . . . . . . . . . . . . . . 163
Film-Forming Substances. . . . . . . . . . . . . . . . . . 164
Suspended Solids . . . . . . . . . . . . . . . . . . . . . 165
Solubilizers . . . . . . . . . . . . . . . . . . . . . . . . 165
Powders . . . . . . . . . . . . . . . . . . . . . . . . . . 166
Raw Materials . . . . . . . . . . . . . . . . . . . . . . . 166
Materials which impart Softness and Slip . . . . . . . . . . 167
Materials which impart Adhesion . . . . . . . . . . . . . 168
Materials which impart Covering Power . . . . . . . . . . 168
Materials which impart Absorbency . . . . . . . . . . . . 169
Preparation . . . . . . . . . . . . . . . . . . . . . . . . 171

Aerosol Preparations. . . . . . . . . . . . . . . . . . . . . . . . .   171
   History  . . . . . . . . . . . . . . . . . . . . . . . . . . . . .   171
   Advantages and Disadvantages . . . . . . . . . . . . . . . . .   172
Principles of Action . . . . . . . . . . . . . . . . . . . . . . . .   173
   Two-Phase Aerosols . . . . . . . . . . . . . . . . . . . . . . .   173
   Three-Phase Aerosols  . . . . . . . . . . . . . . . . . . . . . .   174
   Aerosols with Inorganic Propellants . . . . . . . . . . . . . .   177
   Powder Aerosols  . . . . . . . . . . . . . . . . . . . . . . . .   179
Raw Materials  . . . . . . . . . . . . . . . . . . . . . . . . . . .   179
   Propellants . . . . . . . . . . . . . . . . . . . . . . . . . . .   179
   Active Ingredients . . . . . . . . . . . . . . . . . . . . . . . .   185
   Solvents . . . . . . . . . . . . . . . . . . . . . . . . . . . . .   185
   Emulsifying Agents . . . . . . . . . . . . . . . . . . . . . . .   186
Containers . . . . . . . . . . . . . . . . . . . . . . . . . . . . .   186
   Glass Bottles . . . . . . . . . . . . . . . . . . . . . . . . . .   186
   Metal Containers . . . . . . . . . . . . . . . . . . . . . . . .   187
   Plastic Containers . . . . . . . . . . . . . . . . . . . . . . . .   188
   Valves . . . . . . . . . . . . . . . . . . . . . . . . . . . . . .   188
   Protective Caps . . . . . . . . . . . . . . . . . . . . . . . . .   188
Formulation of Aerosol Products . . . . . . . . . . . . . . . . .   188
   Preparation . . . . . . . . . . . . . . . . . . . . . . . . . . .   193
Testing of Aerosol Products  . . . . . . . . . . . . . . . . . . .   194
   Spraying Tests  . . . . . . . . . . . . . . . . . . . . . . . . .   194
   Storage Tests . . . . . . . . . . . . . . . . . . . . . . . . . .   195

# Part II

*Chapter 5   Cleansing Preparations*

Cleansing of the Skin  . . . . . . . . . . . . . . . . . . . . . . .   206
   Water-Based Skin Cleansers. . . . . . . . . . . . . . . . . . .   206
   Oil-Based Skin Cleansers . . . . . . . . . . . . . . . . . . . .   226
   Solid Cleansing, Soil Adsorbing Preparations . . . . . . . . .   234
   Rolling Creams . . . . . . . . . . . . . . . . . . . . . . . . .   235
Cleansing of the Hair and Scalp . . . . . . . . . . . . . . . . . .   236
   Active Ingredients . . . . . . . . . . . . . . . . . . . . . . . .   241
   Preparations  . . . . . . . . . . . . . . . . . . . . . . . . . .   247
Cleansing of the Teeth . . . . . . . . . . . . . . . . . . . . . . .   260
Anatomy of the Teeth and Physiology of the Oral Cavity . . . . .   260
   Preparations  . . . . . . . . . . . . . . . . . . . . . . . . . .   263
Cleansing of the Nails . . . . . . . . . . . . . . . . . . . . . . .   281

Raw Materials . . . . . . . . . . . . . . . . . . . . . . . . 282
Preparation . . . . . . . . . . . . . . . . . . . . . . . . 282


*Chapter 6    Deodorant and Anti-perspirant Preparations*

Body Deodorants . . . . . . . . . . . . . . . . . . . . . . . 288
Physiology of Sweat . . . . . . . . . . . . . . . . . . . . . 288
Principle of Effectiveness . . . . . . . . . . . . . . . . . . 290
    Active Ingredients . . . . . . . . . . . . . . . . . . . . . 291
    Preparations . . . . . . . . . . . . . . . . . . . . . . . . 295
Evaluation . . . . . . . . . . . . . . . . . . . . . . . . . . 302
    Effectiveness . . . . . . . . . . . . . . . . . . . . . . . . 302
    Skin Compatibility . . . . . . . . . . . . . . . . . . . . . 303
    Fabric Compatibility . . . . . . . . . . . . . . . . . . . . 304
    Shelf Life . . . . . . . . . . . . . . . . . . . . . . . . . . 304
Other Deodorants . . . . . . . . . . . . . . . . . . . . . . . 304
    Foot Deodorants . . . . . . . . . . . . . . . . . . . . . . 305
    Mouthwashes . . . . . . . . . . . . . . . . . . . . . . . . 306


*Chapter 7    Protective Preparations*

Preparations with Protective Action Against Chemical Agents . . . 311
    Preparations with Protective Action Against Aqueous Solutions . 312
    Preparations with Protective Action against Organic Solutions and
      Solvents . . . . . . . . . . . . . . . . . . . . . . . . . . 318
Testing Chemically Protective Preparations . . . . . . . . . . . 320
Preparations with Protective Action Against Dry Soils . . . . . . 320
Preparations with Protective Action Against Ultraviolet Radiation . 323
    Physiological Effects of Ultraviolet Rays . . . . . . . . . . . 323
    Effect of Ultraviolet Rays on Epidermal Tissue . . . . . . . . 324
Principle of Effectiveness of Sunscreens . . . . . . . . . . . . 325
    Active Ingredients . . . . . . . . . . . . . . . . . . . . . 326
    Preparations . . . . . . . . . . . . . . . . . . . . . . . . 332
Evaluation of Sunburn Preventives . . . . . . . . . . . . . . . 338
Perfuming of Sunburn Preventives . . . . . . . . . . . . . . . 340
Preparations with Protective Action Against Mechanical Stress . . 340
    Skin Oils and Fats . . . . . . . . . . . . . . . . . . . . . 341
    Body and Baby Powders . . . . . . . . . . . . . . . . . . . 343
    Massage Creams . . . . . . . . . . . . . . . . . . . . . . 345
Insect-Repellent Preparations . . . . . . . . . . . . . . . . . 345

*Chapter 8   Emollients*

Physiological Principles. . . . . . . . . . . . . . . . . . . .   351
   Degreasing of the *Stratum Corneum* . . . . . . . . . . . .   351
   Dehydration of the *Stratum Corneum* . . . . . . . . . . .   352
The Anatomic Picture of Dry Skin. . . . . . . . . . . . . . .   354
Preparations . . . . . . . . . . . . . . . . . . . . . . . . .   355
   Preparations Based on Fat . . . . . . . . . . . . . . . . .   358
   Preparations Based on Glycerol and Similar Active Ingredients  .  361

*Chapter 9   Preparations with Depth Effect*

Problems . . . . . . . . . . . . . . . . . . . . . . . . . . .   365
   Senescence and Degeneration of the Skin . . . . . . . . . .   365
   Disorders in Scalp Physiology. . . . . . . . . . . . . . .   366
Function of Cosmetics . . . . . . . . . . . . . . . . . . . .   368
   Active Ingredients . . . . . . . . . . . . . . . . . . . . .   369
   Individual Ingredients . . . . . . . . . . . . . . . . . . .   372
   Complexes of Active Ingredients. . . . . . . . . . . . . . .   387
Preparations . . . . . . . . . . . . . . . . . . . . . . . . .   394

*Chapter 10   Decorative Preparations: Preparations with Surface Effect*

Preparations for Coloring Skin and Nails. . . . . . . . . . . .   415
   Coloring Agents in Cosmetics . . . . . . . . . . . . . . . .   416
   Rouges. . . . . . . . . . . . . . . . . . . . . . . . . . .   420
   Eye Shadow . . . . . . . . . . . . . . . . . . . . . . . . .   424
   Mascara . . . . . . . . . . . . . . . . . . . . . . . . . .   425
   Eyebrow Pencils and Crayons . . . . . . . . . . . . . . . .   427
   Lip Makeup . . . . . . . . . . . . . . . . . . . . . . . . .   428
   Nail Lacquer . . . . . . . . . . . . . . . . . . . . . . . .   437
Preparations for Masking Skin Imperfections and Shininess . . . .   443
   Face Powders . . . . . . . . . . . . . . . . . . . . . . . .   444
   Foundation Creams . . . . . . . . . . . . . . . . . . . . .   448
   Foundation Makeup . . . . . . . . . . . . . . . . . . . . .   450
   Wrinkle Concealers . . . . . . . . . . . . . . . . . . . . .   457
Hairgrooming Aids . . . . . . . . . . . . . . . . . . . . . .   457
   Anhydrous Brilliantines, Pomades, and Hair Oils . . . . . . .   458
   Hair Creams (Water-in-Oil and Dual Emulsions) . . . . . . .   461
   Hair Creams (Oil-in-Water Emulsions) . . . . . . . . . . . .   462
   Gum-Based Hair Dressings . . . . . . . . . . . . . . . . . .   465
   Hair Lacquers. . . . . . . . . . . . . . . . . . . . . . . .   466
   Alcohol-Based Hair Lotions . . . . . . . . . . . . . . . . .   468
   Two-Phase Lotions . . . . . . . . . . . . . . . . . . . . .   469

*Chapter 11   Decorative Preparations: Preparations with Lasting Effect*

Hair Dyes and Bleaches . . . . . . . . . . . . . . . . . . 472
  Temporary Coloring . . . . . . . . . . . . . . . . . . . 473
  Permanent Dyes . . . . . . . . . . . . . . . . . . . . . 474
  Bleaches . . . . . . . . . . . . . . . . . . . . . . . . 484
  Dye Removers . . . . . . . . . . . . . . . . . . . . . . 486
Skin-Bleaching Preparations . . . . . . . . . . . . . . . 487
Preparations that Change the Configuration of the Hair . . . . . 489
  Principle of Action . . . . . . . . . . . . . . . . . . . 490
Preparations . . . . . . . . . . . . . . . . . . . . . . . 496
  Waveset Preparations . . . . . . . . . . . . . . . . . . 496
  Hot-Wave Preparations . . . . . . . . . . . . . . . . . 497
  Cold-Wave Preparations . . . . . . . . . . . . . . . . . 499
  Neutralizing Agents . . . . . . . . . . . . . . . . . . . 503
  Determination of the Efficacy of Cold-Wave Preparations. . . . 503
  Damage to Hair, Scalp, and Health by Permament-Wave Prep-
    arations . . . . . . . . . . . . . . . . . . . . . . . 504
Cosmetics Used in the Removal of Hair . . . . . . . . . . . 504
  Methods . . . . . . . . . . . . . . . . . . . . . . . . 505
Preparations . . . . . . . . . . . . . . . . . . . . . . . 506
  Chemical Depilatories . . . . . . . . . . . . . . . . . . 506
  Powders . . . . . . . . . . . . . . . . . . . . . . . . 510
  Liquid Depilatories . . . . . . . . . . . . . . . . . . . 511
  Pastes . . . . . . . . . . . . . . . . . . . . . . . . . 512
Preparations for Mechanical Hair Removal . . . . . . . . . . 513

*Chapter 12   Preparations for Enjoyment*

Bath Preparations . . . . . . . . . . . . . . . . . . . . 531
  Bath Salts . . . . . . . . . . . . . . . . . . . . . . . 531
  Bath Tablets . . . . . . . . . . . . . . . . . . . . . . 533
  Bubble Bath Powders . . . . . . . . . . . . . . . . . . 534
  Bath Oils . . . . . . . . . . . . . . . . . . . . . . . 535
  Solutions of Perfume Oils in Solubilizers . . . . . . . . . . 536
  Bubble Bath Oils . . . . . . . . . . . . . . . . . . . . 536
  Bath Milks . . . . . . . . . . . . . . . . . . . . . . . 536

*Postscript   Perfuming and Coloring Cosmetic Preparations* . . . . . 538

*Table of Incompatibilities* . . . . . . . . . . . . . . . . . . 545

*Author Index* . . . . . . . . . . . . . . . . . . . . . . . 549

*Subject Index* . . . . . . . . . . . . . . . . . . . . . . . 559

Dr. J. Stephan Jellinek
Formulation and Function of Cosmetics

# PART 1

# CHAPTER 1

# Skin and Hair

The raison d'être for all cosmetic preparations is their application, for long or short periods, to skin, hair, teeth, and nails. The "active life" of any cosmetic preparation begins the moment it is brought in contact with the skin (it would be awkward to repeat "hair, teeth, and nails" in every instance, but all remarks apply to them as well) and ends when it is removed or has evaporated. During this active life the skin and cosmetic share an intimate reciprocal relationship. The cosmetic may protect the skin from noxious external influences, prevent its outermost layers from drying out, penetrate below the external layer and introduce active substances into deeper lying strata, or adhere only superficially to change the color or luster of definite areas. It is hardly necessary to enumerate all the possible functions of cosmetic preparations to demonstrate that they are always concerned with the skin.

The close contact between skin and cosmetic, on which the effectiveness of the latter is based, carries the inherent risk of undesirable side effects. Any cosmetic, always a substance alien to the skin, may at times inhibit important physiological processes, chemically modify certain skin constituents or contribute toward their removal, and even give rise to allergic reactions.

For these reasons a knowledge of certain aspects of the anatomy, physiology, and pathology of the skin is as essential to the cosmetic chemist who aims at developing effective preparations as is an awareness of the character and applicability of the basic materials of cosmetics.

My intention here is not to present an all-embracing treatise on dermatology and therefore I have confined myself to those aspects that are essential to the modern cosmetic chemist. In this chapter I deal briefly with those properties of skin and hair that are of general interest. Other important facets of the physiology of skin and hair as well as the anatomy of teeth and nails are treated in later chapters.

## ANATOMY OF THE SKIN

### The Surface

The skin, like all organs of the human body, is not a uniform tissue: it is composed of cellular strata of different kinds which lie one under the other parallel to the surface. The majority of all cosmetic skin preparations comes into contact with the outermost layer only, the *stratum corneum*, and therefore we deal with this layer first.

The *stratum corneum* consists of the corneal or horny cells which are flat and colorless. They lie almost parallel to the skin surface and are arranged in "roof tile" layers. They have no nucleus, a very low moisture content, and are "dead" in the sense that no metabolic processes occur in them. They are completely cut off from the body circulation and are unable to absorb nutrients from externally applied preparations. It is nevertheless possible to preserve or reconstitute the elasticity of the corneal layer by preparations applied to the skin surface (see Chapter 8).

The corneal cells consist mostly of keratin, a protein insoluble in water, which is characterized by its high resistance to chemical action. This chemical resistance, which differentiates keratin from other body proteins, is, of course, of great importance to the function of the stratum corneum, that is, the protection of the body from external influences.

Although keratin is insoluble in pure water, dilute acid, or alkali, the horny cells can, particularly in an alkaline environment, absorb a certain amount of water. In this swollen state they are softer and chemically less resistant than when their water content is normally low. These cells are not linked to one another. If a sliver of the stratum corneum is introduced into an organic solvent, the cells break apart like fine sand. In living skin the cells are bonded together by a waxlike substance that acts like glue. This substance is frequently called "skin fat," a term that is confusing because it is also applied to various other substances occurring in the skin, all of which have a fatty consistency but vary considerably in origin, function, and chemical composition.

The waxlike substance between the horny cells derives from the degradation of components of the cytoplasm and nuclei in the course of the cornification process. Apart from free and esterified cholesterol, fatty acids (partly free, partly esterified with higher fatty alcohols), amino acids, polypeptides, purine derivatives, and pentoses (ribose and desoxyribose, the degradation products of the nucleotides) have been observed in this substance. Although Rothman [1] states that lecithin and other phosphatides, which occur frequently in the deeper skin layers, are not present in the cement substance, Flesch [2] reports the isolation of lipoglycoproteins, which contain amino sugar and phospholipids, from the stratum corneum. Furthermore, this waxy substance contains a certain amount of water whose presence is of the greatest importance to the elasticity of the corneal layer (see Chapter 8). Certain components of the "wax" (amino acids, purines, choline, and possibly others) are hygroscopic and regulate the moisture content.

On its surface the stratum corneum is covered by another fatty substance which is also often referred to as skin fat. This surface fat probably occurs in the form of an emulsion. It consists of sweat, an aqueous component produced by the sweat glands (the physiology of sweat is discussed in Chapter 6), sebum, a fatty substance secreted by the sebaceous glands, and waste products of the cellular proteins.

Wheatley [3] lists the following constituents of sebum: free fatty acids ($C_7$-$C_{18}$, mostly palmitic and oleic acids), 28%; triglycerides, 32%; waxes (esters of normal and branched $C_{14}$-$C_{24}$ aliphatic alcohols), 14%; cholesterol (approximately half of which is esterified), 4%; squalene, 5%; other hydrocarbons, 8%; dihydrocholesterol and other steroids (provitamin D, oxidation products of squalene, 17-ketosteroids, and estrogens), 9%. Traces of vitamin E and other fat-soluble vitamins (but not A or K) are also present.

Reports of other authors differ, sometimes considerably, from those quoted above; in particular, it is usual to find a much higher cholesterol content. The reason for these differences is probably the difficulty in isolating sebum without including a certain amount of skin wax, a waste product of the epidermal cell substances.

A comparison of the composition of skin surface fat and the secretions of the sebaceous glands, according to Nicolaides and Wells [4], is most interesting:

TABLE 1-1

| | Content of Sebaceous-Gland Cysts (%) | Skin Surface Fat (88 hr, %) |
|---|---|---|
| Free fatty acids | Trace | 34.0 |
| Esterified fatty acids | 61.5 | 29.6 |
| Unsaponifiable matter | 33.0 | 33.8 |
| Total extraction | 94.5 | 97.5 |
| Analysis of the unsaponifiables: | | |
| Squalene | 11.7 | 12.0 |
| Wax alcohols | 15.0 | 11.6 |
| Sterols | 2.7 | 3.4 |
| Unidentifiable | 1.5 | 3.6 |

"This indicates that sebum, on its way to the skin surface, is subjected to hydrolysis, possibly through the presence of enzymes. (Hermann and collaborators, Griesemer). Hoff and Winkler are of the opinion that it is the presence of free fatty acids which explains the surface activity of skin fat, demonstrable by spreading tests" [4].

It is the function of the surface fat to keep the skin surface supple and to regulate the moisture content of the deeper lying strata. It also acts as a barrier against solids penetrating from the outside; in many instances these solids do not penetrate into normal, untreated skin but are absorbed by it once the surface has been removed by rubbing with alcohol or fat solvent. Kligman [5], however, denies that sebum can fulfill the above-mentioned function in the small amounts in which it occurs on the skin and regards the sebaceous glands as rudimentary organs.

The smooth surface of the skin is disrupted by the mouths of the hair follicles. (In common parlance these mouths are referred to as "pores." The general assumption that pores have something to do with the breathing of the skin is not correct.) The follicles are slanting tubular invaginations of the epidermis; the hair sprouts from their lower ends. The sebaceous glands which secrete the sebum also terminate in the hair follicles so that the sebum reaches the skin surface by way of the follicle mouths. If these mouths are obstructed by cosmetic products (coarse powder, impermeable ointments), the sebum becomes congested in the hair follicles and this may lead to "blackheads" or inflammations. Apart from the follicle mouths, the much finer mouths of the sweat glands are also on the skin surface (see Chapter 6).

Most parts of the body are covered with very fine almost colorless hair (lanugo hair); on the scalp, above the eyes, and in the axillary and pubic regions it is more strongly colored and textured.

### The Deeper Layers

The skin is divided, primarily, into three layers: the epidermis, the corium, and the hypodermis (see Table 1-2).

TABLE 1-2    THE SKIN LAYERS

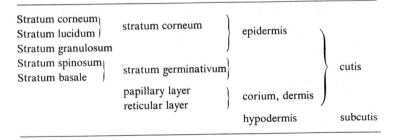

**The Epidermis.** The corneal layer, discussed in the preceding paragraph is the outermost layer of the epidermis. Below it lie a number of other layers which, like the corneal layer, vary in thickness at different locations of the body. We differentiate here, starting from the surface:

The *stratum lucidum*, which is immediately below the corneal layer (and frequently regarded as part of it): inside as well as outside the cells it contains droplets of an oily liquid (eleidin). This layer is particularly well developed at the palms and soles, where the corneal layer is also thick.

Between the *stratum lucidum* and the *stratum granulosum*, which lies below it, there is a thin continuous keratin membrane, the co-called Rein's barrier, which was first isolated and described by Szakall [6]. The effect of this membrane is probably due to the existence of a charge differential: the pH value on the outside is about 5, whereas on the inside it is higher (less acid reaction). Therefore the outside of the membrane carries a positive charge as against the inside; a membrane charged in this way cannot be penetrated by either negatively or positively charged ions.

Rein [7] in the 1920s had already deduced the existence of a membrane which (as proved correct later) would have to be a barrier against the diffusion of moisture and electrolytes (salts).

Rein's barrier acts as a sharp demarcation between the corneal layer and the deeper lying skin tissues. Above the membrane there is no flow of tissue fluids. The fluids in the corneal layer constitute a reducing medium, those in the lower layers an oxidizing medium. Above the membrane fatty substances are present outside the cells; below the membrane they are inside.

The *stratum granulosum*, in which the cell nuclei are just barely distinguishable, contains granules in the protoplasm of a solid substance (keratohyalin) which act as light reflectors and thus give the skin its opaque appearance. This layer, one to four cells thick, according to the part of the body on which it occurs (thickest again on the hands and feet) is completely absent in the red parts of the lips and underneath the finger nails.

The *stratum spinosum* (prickle-cell layer) or *stratum malpighii* (Malpighian layer) is also thickest wherever the corneal layer is thick. Cytoplasm threads (called epithelic fibers or tonofibrils), which act as intercellular bridges, radiate from the cells of this layer. In these cells the nucleus is still easily visible. The deeper cells contain granules of the brown pigment melanin.

The cells of the *stratum basale* or *stratum cylindricum* are also linked with one another and the cells of the spinous layer by tonofibrils. This layer is only one cell deep; the cells are cylindrical and have well developed oval nuclei. In this layer, and to a lesser degree in the stratum spinosum, there is active cell division; hence these two layers are sometimes referred to as the *stratum germinativum*. The constant cellular division in the stratum germinativum causes the cells above to be continuously displaced toward the skin surface. At the same time essential modifications in the inner structure of the cells lead to the metamorphosis of the germinal cells to corneal cells, a process called keratinization or cornification. This process is thoroughly discussed, for example, in Rothman [8]. The part played by glycogen, present in the stratum spinosum, as a source of energy and of phosphorylase enzymes in the cornification process is discussed in detail by Wegemann, Hewitt, Guignon, and Guha [9].

The skin layers described, which in a microscopic preparation can actually be seen to lie underneath one another, may be regarded alternatively as stages in the development of epidermal cells.

The cylindrical cells on their way through the spinous layer become first polyhedral and then increasingly flat. Cellular division nearly ceases and chemical modifications occur in which the proteins of the cytoplasm gradually change to keratin. The keratinization process starts in the epithelic fibers and at the walls of the prickle cells. The components of the nucleus are degraded and ejected from the cells. It is likely that the enzymes ribonuclease and desoxyribonuclease play an important part in this process [10]. Changes in keratinization, either pathological or caused by drugs such as vitamin A, are at least occasionally accompanied by changes in the activity of these enzymes. Probably the keratohyalin granules of the granular layer, the eleidin of the stratum lucidum, and the cement of the corneal layer consist of degradation products of the cell content in the prickle-cell layer. The cells also lose the major part of their moisture content, partly through evaporation; the remainder is bound in the substance between the corneal cells. The corneal cells migrate farther upward until they desquamate as microscopically small scales at the skin surface and are finally removed by rubbing or washing. The life span of an individual cell is about 30 days. This constant process of keratinization is of fundamental significance because it determines the character of the epidermis. Some consequences, important to the cosmetic chemist, become immediately apparent. The constant migration of cells directed outward causes a regeneration of the skin by replacing old dead cells, in which foreign bodies may have lodged, with fresh corneal cells. (The renewal time of the outermost corneal layer differs considerably in much or little used parts of the body and amounts, for example, to 100 days at the forearm bend, to 20 days at the knee and only about 10 days at the elbow.) The intercellular wax is constantly renewed as well.

Another result of the dynamic character of the epidermis is that many internal diseases, vitamin deficiencies, and so on, first become apparent in skin symptoms. In order to keep up cell proliferation, the stratum germinativum requires an uninterrupted flow of all necessary nutrients—vitamins, etc.—through the blood; furthermore the keratinization process requires the presence of substances that provide energy (glycogen) and nutrients (amino acid containing sulfur). Changes in the blood level of the substances required soon become apparent in various pathological skin symptoms.

**The Corium.** Below the basal cell layer, and probably separated from it by a membrane [11], lies the corium. Although the cell layers of the epidermis gradually merge into one another in time and structure, the corium is a tissue completely separated from the epidermis. It consists mostly of bundles of intertwined fibers of the fibrillary and collagenous connective tissue; skin tension is caused by these fiber bundles. The so-called elastic fibers entwined among the collagenous fiber bundles probably serve as supports for the collagenous connective tissue. We also find reticular formations that do not appear to fulfill any specific function. The space between the fiber bundles is filled by an aqueous gel-like matrix that contains hyaluronic acid and chondroitin sulfate (both probably linked to proteins). This matrix serves as a lubricant between the connective tissue fibers, possibly plays a part as moisture reserve, and inhibits the spread of infections.

Two layers are distinguished in the corium: at the borderline of the epidermis lies the papillary layer which has fine fiber bundles at right angles to the skin surface. The borderline is not smooth. Epidermis and corium are firmly interconnected by the papillary bodies. In aging skin, in which cell division decreases in the basal layer, the papillary bodies flatten out. The contact between epidermis and corium loosens and the epidermis loses its elasticity. At the borderline with the epidermis the finest collagenous and elastic fibers intertwine with epithelic fibers radiating downward from the basal cells. The papillary layer gradually merges into the reticular layer below in which the fiber bundles are in a coarser arrangement and lie tangentially to the surface. The fine blood vessels which nourish the skin and carry off its waste products, the nerve endings which transmit sensations of touch, heat, cold, and pain, and the sweat and sebaceous glands are in the corium. The hair follicles go as far as the corium, and here lie the roots of the hair.

Table 1-3 gives an idea of the number and distribution of the sense organs for touch and temperature sensations embedded in the corium, starting at the outer surface.

TABLE 1-3

| | |
|---|---|
| Free nerve endings (pain) | $200/cm^2$ |
| Merkel corpuscles (receptors for mechanical sensations) | $3000/cm^2$ |
| Meissner corpuscles (pressure) | $25/cm^2$ |
| Krause end bulbs (cold) | $12/cm^2$ |
| Ruffini cylinders (heat) | $2/cm^2$ |
| Pacinian corpuscles (mechanical) | $2/cm^2$ |
| Sebaceous glands | about 15 (none in palms or soles) |

The sebaceous glands occur wherever there is growth of hair and their ducts terminate in the hair follicles. An exception are the lips and eyelids where sebaceous glands alone are present. The connection of sebaceous glands and hair follicles is most important in certain skin diseases or irritations (seborrhea or acne).

The sweat glands lie in the deeper layer of the corium (see Chapter 6), their ducts following a spiral course through the epidermis.

**The Hypodermis.**  The corium gradually merges into the hypodermis, a loose fiber tissue that contains a great number of adipose cells. The hypodermis protects the organs underneath from mechanical shocks or changes and serves also as a fat reservoir. Many histologists still regard this tissue as part of the corium.

In conclusion, let us look at a few facts and figures that will interest the cosmetologist because they contribute to the understanding of the biological conditions of the human skin.

The area of the skin surface differs according to race and a number of other factors. The average European has a skin surface of about 12–16 ft². The thickness of the skin also fluctuates not only according to race and climatic conditions but in each individual at different localities of the body, according to use and protective or biological functions. The thinnest skin is at the eyelids, which have only about 0.2–0.6 mm, but at the palms and soles there is 2–4 mm. The skin can absorb a third of the total blood content of the body (skin capillaries). The germinal layer itself is filled only with lymph, a light-colored fluid, which is why quite shallow cuts do not bleed. They excrete lymph: they wet. Only a cut that reaches the corium will bleed. A skin blister (caused by long pressure, friction, or slight burning) is a hollow space formed when the epidermis separates from the corium and fills with lymph.


## PHYSIOLOGY OF THE SKIN

### The Hydroregulatory System

The skin has very limited water permeability. The barrier that controls the escape of moisture from and penetration into the body does not lie immediately on the skin surface but below the corneal layer and is called Rein's barrier [12].

The tissues below this membrane are connected with the blood capillaries of the skin, and there is a normal flow of blood; the moisture content of the cells is about 70–80%. The moisture content of the corneal layer lying above the membrane is considerably lower, about 10%. This dryness of the outermost skin layer is physiologically significant: skin keratin owes its mechanical and chemical resistance to it. Moreover, the low moisture content of the skin surface inhibits the growth of bacteria and fungi.

The drying out of the corneal layer should, however, not go too far, for, as tests by Blank and Shappirio [13] have shown, the elasticity of the corneal layer depends on the presence of a certain quantity of moisture. If the corneal layer dries out, it becomes brittle and will not regain its elasticity through fatty substances but only through a supply of water.

The moisture content of the corneal layer is determined by the rate at which it is supplied with water and the rate with which it loses water. Rein's barrier below, although impermeable to liquid water, does permit water vapor to permeate, and sweat may penetrate from above. The loss in moisture depends primarily on the humidity of the immediately adjacent air. Buettner [14] has observed that the resistance of the skin to vapor diffusion is not constant but adjusts to the humidity of the air or osmolarity of solutions with which it is in contact. The skin therefore does not behave passively toward vapor diffusion. This also explains why anhydrous glycerol accelerates water evaporation from the skin, as observed by Powers and Fox [15].

It is because of its content of hydrophilic substances and the presence of the sebaceous coating on its surface that the corneal layer does not dry out even in an atmosphere with very low humidity. According to Flesch [16], the corneal layer consists of about 20% water-soluble substances, part of which are highly hygroscopic. Free amino acids play an important part here: riboses, desoxyriboses, and purines, which result from the waste of nuclear cell material, are also present. Many years ago Jacobi recognized the presence of hydrophilic substances in the corneal layer and designated them as "X bodies"; Fox, Tassoff, Rieger, and Deem [17] examined their effect in the presence of externally applied moisturizers (glycerol, propylene glycol, and sorbitol).

Although sebum is not completely water-impermeable, it holds water, probably as a water-in-oil emulsion, and therefore delays its evaporation. By covering projecting edges of the corneal scales with a smooth layer it also reduces the surface for evaporation.

Many cosmetic preparations affect the moisture content of the corneal layer and, in this way, its elasticity or stability and chemical resistance. Many have an adverse effect: soaps and detergents, for example, may remove the skin fat, subsequently extract some of the hydrophilic components of the corneal layer, and foster the drying out of this layer. If cosmetic creams leave a closed film on the skin that is quite impermeable to water, sweat congestion may possibly result in the swelling and weakening of the keratin.

On the other hand, it is one of the functions of some cosmetic preparations to prevent or counteract disturbances in the hydroregulatory system of the corneal layer. Hand lotions and hand jellies supply the required moisture to dry skin. Night creams take over the function of lost skin fat, that is, the conservation of the moisture content of facial skin. Absorbent powders which are used in situations in which heavy perspiration is coupled with inhibited sweat evaporation (bedridden patients or the feet during long marches) aim at preventing swelling and weakening of the corneal layer by blocked sweat.

### Breathing of the Skin

Like any living animal tissue, the skin consumes oxygen and emits carbon dioxide. By far the largest portion of the required oxygen is taken from the blood stream, but a small part comes directly from the surrounding air [18]. The disposal of carbon dioxide also occurs mostly through the blood and only to a small degree into the surrounding atmosphere. Although the "direct breathing" of the skin is restricted in comparison to pulmonary breathing, Shaw and Messer [19] state that the skin not only needs the oxygen absorbed from the blood stream but also a certain amount taken directly from the air.

Water permeability of various cosmetic and pharmaceutical preparations and their effect on the health of the skin has been studied thoroughly during the last few years but little attention has been given so far to their gas permeability.

Goldschmiedt [20] reports that breathing of the skin in humans is strongest up to the age of 20 and decreases markedly after about 50.

Zenisek [21] suggests using the intensity of skin breathing as a method of evaluating the effectiveness of biologically active skin preparations and quotes a list of substances that increase or inhibit skin breathing or leave it unaffected.

### The Acid Mantle

The surface of healthy human skin has a weakly acid reaction. Measurements taken by many researchers on different continents show that the pH value of the fluid surrounding the skin surface (the pH value of the solid keratin, of course, cannot be measured) lies generally between 4 and 6. The pH value, determined at a specific spot on the skin, varies from individual to individual. In each the reaction differs from area to area (e.g., under the arms and between the toes, where sweat cannot freely evaporate, it is particularly high and can rise to about pH 7) and is also subject to temporal fluctuations.

The fact that human skin normally has an acid reaction has been known since the beginning of the century, but only since the twenties has any notice been taken. Marchionini, in particular, who has made a thorough investigation in this field and is responsible for the term "acid mantle," pointed again and again to the significance of this skin characteristic. In his opinion the function of the acid mantle lies primarily in inhibiting the growth of bacteria and fungi. He bases this view on observations that showed that most normal skin bacteria exhibit optimal growth on an artificial culture medium with pH 6–7.5, and that bacterial and fungus infections are particularly common in those areas of the human body that have comparatively high pH values. According to Marchionini [22] the acid reaction in itself is the important factor and it is irrelevant how this reaction is caused. In accordance with this opinion it has even been suggested that fungus infections be treated with diluted hydrochloric acid.

Later Peck and his collaborators [23] found that a number of fatty acids occurring in sweat act as growth inhibitors on bacteria as well as fungi. Propionic, capronic, and caprylic acids were particularly effective. Peck came to the conclusion that the significance of the acid mantle does not lie in the pH value itself but in the specific substances that produce it.

This opinion was supported by later findings that showed that skin fat also contains acids with fungicidal ($C_9$–$C_{15}$ saturated acids) [24] and bactericidal ($C_{14}$–$C_{22}$ unsaturated acids) [25] effects. Harry (26) suggests a further possibility: the acid mantle might be conserving a still unknown protective agent that would be ineffective at a higher pH value.

Apart from the pH value of the surface, the buffer capacity of the skin and the regenerative ability of the acid mantle play important parts. A temporary treatment of the skin with alkaline reagents results in only slight shift of the pH value. As soon as the alkaline reagent is removed, the normal pH value of the skin is quickly re-established. Szakall, for example, demonstrated with pH tests on living skin that after washing with soap the pH of the surface rose to about 7 and sometimes even into the alkaline range. This alkali shock, however, is neutralized by normal skin (provided it is thoroughly rinsed) within half an hour [27]. With some people it takes longer for the skin to revert to its original pH value. According to Burkhardt [28], it is these persons who are prone to suffer from professional dermatoses and skin diseases of various kinds. One explanation may be that longer duration of the almost neutral reaction of the skin surface gives the germs a better opportunity to grow. In our opinion the noxious effect of a continually increased pH value lies rather in the diminishing of the chemical resistance of the skin keratin.

There is still no agreement as to which acid substances occurring on the skin are the most important originators of the acid reactions and the buffer sheath. (This description was coined by Szakall. It may be confusing because acid substances present in the deeper layers of the skin may also participate in its neutralization capacity [29].) The lower fatty acids ($C_2$–$C_7$) are probably primarily responsible. Higher fatty acids are also present but are not sufficiently water-soluble to cause an acid reaction; they may have a buffering effect. Lactic acid, amino acids, and other protein degradation products, derivatives of phosphoric acid and carbonic acid, also occur on the skin surface. Probably most or all of these substances play a certain part, together with the skin keratin, in achieving the acid reaction and the buffering effect.

Summarizing, we may say that healthy skin has an acid reaction on its surface (pH 4–6), that an alkalinization of the skin for longer periods is damaging, and that there is a close relation between the acid mantle and the bacteriological and chemical resistance of the skin.

## THE EXTERIOR APPEARANCE OF THE SKIN

One of the main purposes of cosmetics is the improvement of the skin's appearance by suitable external means. In this section we discuss briefly the most important anatomical and physiological characteristics that determine the appearance of clean, cosmetically untreated skin.

### Color

The color of the skin is primarily determined by oxyhemoglobin, which is red, reduced hemoglobin, which is bluish-red, melanin, which is brown, melanoid, similar in color to melanin, keratohyalin, which gives the skin its white opaque appearance, and the corneal layer, which has a faintly yellow or greyish tinge. Less important are carotene, a yellow pigment that occurs in very small concentrations and has little effect, and the eleidin of the stratum lucidum, which is visible only in the thickened skin of the heel.

The red or bluish-red of the blood pigments becomes more apparent in the color of the skin the closer the blood capillaries are to the surface (this is related to the thickness of the epidermis) and the smaller the amount of melanin present. High color indicates good circulation and creates an impression of freshness and well-being, although too much red or unattractive red spots are symptomatic of pathological changes such as inflammation or distended capillaries. A bluish-red caste of the skin indicates a lack of oxygen in the blood. It is linked to faulty circulation in the corium and creates the impression of an "unhealthy," "frail," or "delicate" condition. Rothman [30] remarks that blue light is more strongly diffused than the red by the fine particles that occur in the epidermal tissue and therefore the skin pigments appear the more intensely blue, the deeper they lie in the skin. A weak development of the red and bluish-red shades is unattractive and unhealthy if no predominant brown pigment is present.

**The Biosynthesis of Melanin.** Since Bloch described the mechanism of this process in broad outline in the twenties [31], many researchers, particularly in the United States, have been engaged in its clarification. Studies of the formation of melanin constitute an extensive literature [32].

The histology of skin pigmentation is discussed by Gates [33]. There is still no agreement on many details. We cannot enter into these arguments here, however, and therefore we only sketch the subject. The basic substance in the formation of melanin is the amino acid tyrosine which is found in the body protein (bound) and probably reaches the skin tissue from the bloodstream. First, tyrosine is oxidized enzymatically to dioxy-

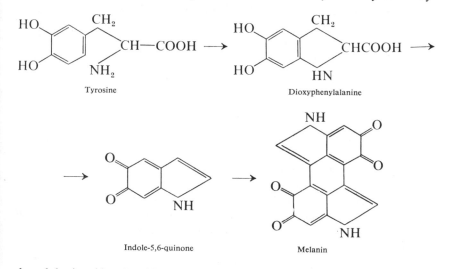

Tyrosine

Dioxyphenylalanine

Indole-5,6-quinone

Melanin

phenylalanine (dopa). This substance is further oxidized in several stages to indole-5,6-quinone (in this oxidation, the enzyme dopa-oxidase probably plays an important part) from which melanin, which is present in the tissue as a protein complex, is formed by oxidative polymerization. Melanin occurs only in cells of the germinal layer; apparently the required enzymes exist only in these cells. The formation is stimulated and intensified by light but can also be engendered by nonspecific irritation in the absence of light.

The enzymes that cause oxidation can be inhibited—"poisoned"—by a number of substances. For practical cosmetics mercury salts are the most important (see Chapter 11); hydroquinonebenzylether acts in the same way. Other substances, in particular 8-methoxypsoralene, appear to encourage the formation of melanin. In the white race melanin is present mainly in the form of a colorless precursor. The action of sunlight causes this precursor to change to brown melanin and stimulates the formation of new melanin. Tanning of the skin therefore is more prevalent among the inhabitants of southern regions—people who spend much time in the open air for recreational or professional reasons, who live in the mountains, or who have been exposed to the sun for relatively short periods, for example, while on vacation. Among "temporarily" brown people of the latter kind tanning is usually accompanied by increased blood circulation in the skin, and the result is a reddish-brown. People exposed to intensive radiation for considerable periods of time experience a thickening of the corneal layer. The skin then acquires a yellowish-brown or pale brown tinge. In the dark races the brown of melanin completely predominates over all other shades.

How important "white" keratohyalin is to the skin color of the Caucasian race (the other layers also contribute, but to a lesser degree, to the opacity of the skin) can easily be seen by mixing white, red, blue, brown, and possibly yellow to obtain a natural skin tone; white is the main ingredient. The yellowish or grayish tinge of the corneal layer may predominate in people who have bad blood circulation of the skin or a particularly thick epidermis with weakly developed melanin.

## Luster

Luster is determined by the activity of the sweat and sebaceous glands and by the lanugo hair. According to the activity of the sebaceous glands, we differentiate between people with dry, normal, or fatty skins.

The lanugo hair imparts to the skin a mat velvetlike appearance; for this reason the facial parts that are least covered by hair, for example, the forehead and nose, tend most to shine. Finally, the character of the skin surface also plays a part: a rough and broken skin does not shine, even if it is oily.

## Relief

The coarse folds of the skin are caused by the underlying organs and adipose tissue. Fine wrinkles are caused by skin movements; they are particularly well developed on hands and feet and sometimes the face. With every bend, every contraction, every stretch of any part of the body, the skin shifts a little and folds and lines develop. Normally the elasticity of the corium allows these folds and wrinkles to disappear as soon as the part returns to its normal position; but if the same movement is repeated often, every day, the constantly forming folds leave traces on the skin and finally develop into fine lines. The development of these lines increases with diminishing skin elasticity. This elasticity is due mostly to the collagenous fiber tissue and decreases with age as tension of these fibrous bundles decreases and as the papillary bodies that link epidermis and corium flatten out, thus loosening the linkage between these two layers so that the epidermis can no longer utilize the elasticity still present in the corium. The appearance of fine wrinkles and lines is therefore a sign of age and their removal (or, rather, delaying their onset) is one of the most important objectives of cosmetics (see Chapter 9).

An even closer examination of the skin reveals the hair-follicle mouths (pores) and the fine lines that divide almost all of the skin surface into small triangular and rhombic fields. The fine lines do not present a cosmetic problem, but the pores are another matter when they distend (frequently as the unwelcome result of the application of the wrong kind of cosmetic) and become visible to the naked eye.

Finally, the skin relief is determined by the character of the corneal layer. If it is healthy, it is usually a completely smooth surface. A rough and grooved skin surface always carries the risk of infection and inflammation and is unattractive in appearance. To keep the surface smooth is the purpose of the preparations discussed in Chapter 8.

An examination of the finger tips immediately discloses the characteristic ridge formation which imparts to every individual his unique fingerprints. This ridge formation is caused by the peculiar interconnection of epidermis and corium. The ducts of the sweat glands invariably terminate on the ridges and are absent from the intervening sulci. In warm weather fine droplets of fluid are easily observed at the mouths of these glands. In contrast to this ridge formation on completely hairless parts of the skin, other areas, for example, the backs of the hand, show a field pattern.

## ANATOMY OF THE HAIR

The hair is an appendage that consists of one part embedded in the skin (the root) and one part projecting from the skin (the hair shaft). Starting at the outside, a cross section of the hair is seen to contain three layers [34]:

1. The cuticle consists of interlocking flat keratine cells and serves as a protection against drying out and the penetration of foreign substances. The cuticle may become damaged by mechanical stress.

2. The cortex consists of longitudinally arranged fibers closely bound together. According to Astbury [35], these fibers occur normally in the folded alpha shape. If the hair is moistened and stretched, it can be pulled into the elongated beta shape, and if this is done slowly a fiber can be extended to 1.5 times its original length. This layer contains the major part of hair pigment and air spaces. The cortex represents the main body of the hair; its structure determines its type (smooth, wavy, or crinkled).

3. The medulla is composed of three or four layers of cubelike cells that contain keratohyalin, fat granules, and air spaces. Thin hair has no medulla.

According to Stoves [36], the hair also contains small quantities of urea, uric acid, xanthine, creatine, glycogene, citric and lactic acids, and several mineral salts and enzymes. These substances are probably mostly contained in the medulla. If the hair is washed repeatedly with water at 35°C, these substances are at least partly removed.

The hair root lies in the follicle. The lower part, the hair bulb, like the germinal layer of the epidermis, consists of almost round soft cells (some of which develop the hair melanin) and rests on the hair papillary which is richly supplied with blood and nerves. The hair is formed in the papillary, and here the constantly proliferating cells gradually push the progressively keratinizing cells above them out of the follicle. Human scalp hair has a diameter of about 1/15 mm; beard and pubic hair is thicker.

## HAIR GROWTH

Hair grows at the rate of about 0.2–0.3 mm a day, regardless of whether it is being cut. The growth of scalp hair is not uniform over its life duration. For a time the new hair grows actively. Then there is a period of rest and finally the hair is displaced by another new one coming from the same hair papillary. The life duration of one scalp hair is about 2.5 years on the average and that of eyelashes only about 100 to 150 days. Although in many animals every hair of the pelt is more or less in the same stage of the growth/rest cycle, the individual human hair papillaries are completely independent of one another, and each hair can therefore be said to have its own stage of growth and rest. It is important to take this difference into account when interpreting animal tests (rats, rabbits, etc.); the effect of hair-growth-stimulating agents on animals does not permit any conclusions regarding their action on humans.

## COLOR AND GLOSS OF THE HAIR

Hair contains two pigments: brownish black melanin and an iron-containing red pigment. The color of human hair can be divided into two ranges: the drab range (platinum blond, ash blond, grayish brown, and deep black) and the red range (light blond, gold blond, brown blond, and blackish-brown). In the drab range melanin is predominant; in the red range the red pigment plays an important part. The depth of color depends on the amount and size of the pigment granules and the absence or presence of air bubbles in the cortex [37].

Not every hair on the head of an individual has the same color. Blond people may also have grey and medium brown hairs. When the hair has been dyed too deeply and has assumed an even color, the effect is quite unnatural.

A great many sebaceous glands are distributed over the scalp. When the hair is brushed or the scalp is massaged, sebum spreads over the surface of the hair and makes it glossy and supple. Complete removal of the hair fat, for example, by washing with a strongly degreasing shampoo, makes the hair lusterless, brittle, and difficult to arrange. If the sebaceous glands in the scalp are overactive (seborrhoea capillitii), the hair becomes sticky and has an oily gloss.

## THE CHEMISTRY OF SKIN AND KERATIN

The chemical structure of human epidermal cells has the following composition: proteins 27%, fats 2%, mineral salts 0.5%, water and traces of water-soluble substances, 70.5%. The most important structural proteins are albumin, globulin, mucin, elastin, collagen, and the keratins. Roughly 40% of the water-soluble matter consists of free amino acids (Weber, Lustig, Gohlke, Benk). According to researches by Leonhardi, Glasenapp, and Brühl, 22 amino acids are found in skin extracts, namely, aspartic acid, glutamic acid, serine, glycocoll, threonine, alanine, tyrosine, tryptophane, valine, phenylalanine, leucine, lysine, arginine, glutamine, citrulline, histidine, ornithine, taurine, cystine, oxyproline, proline, and α-aminobutyric acid. In addition, α-pyrrolidone carboxylic acid, a dehydration product of glutamic acid, is found in the water-soluble components. The presence of lactic acid, hydrochloric acid as well as formic acid, citric and phosphoric acids has also been established. If glutamine and methionine are present in sufficient quantities, tryptophane can be synthetized within the cell. The evolution of living skin cells (not the horny dead cells) also requires the presence in the water-soluble matter of citrate, formiate, lactate, chloride, sodium, potassium, ammonium, urea, calcium, magnesium, and uric and gluconic acids.

The cells of the corneal layer consist mostly of the protein keratin. The same substance is the main constituent of human hair and nails. It would take too long to discuss its complicated chemistry in detail, but certain particulars must be mentioned in connection with the effect of cosmetic preparations on skin, hair, and nails.

We can imagine that every protein molecule is composed of many amino acid molecules which are chemically linked with one another through the reaction of the amino group (—NH₂) of one molecule with the carboxyl group (—COOH) of another by forming an amide group (—CONH—).

At present about 50 amino acids which differ in the structure of their "R" groups are known. About 30 of them have definitely been identified in natural proteins.

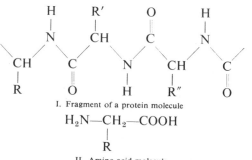

I. Fragment of a protein molecule

$$H_2N—CH_2—COOH$$
$$\overset{|}{R}$$

II. Amino acid molecule

The properties of every protein are determined partly by the size and shape of its molecules and partly by the characteristics of the amino acids it contains. The "R" groups of some amino acids are quite unreactive; for example, R = H (glycerol), R = $CH_2CH(CH_3)_2$ (leucine), R = $CH_2(C_6H_5)$ (phenylalanine). Sometimes the "R" group is phenolic as in tyrosine, R = $CH_2(C_6H_4)OH$, sometimes acid, as in glutamic acid, R = $CH_2CH_2COOH$, or basic, as in lysine, R = $(CH_2)_4NH_2$, or arginine,

$$R = (CH_2)_3NH{-}\underset{\underset{NH}{\|}}{C}{-}NH_2.$$

Keratin is built up of neutral as well as acid and basic groups.

In their X-ray analytical studies Astbury and collaborators throw some light on the structure of keratin [38]. According to Astbury, the amino acid groups in keratin are linked in long chains which may occur in the so-called folded alpha shape or the elongated beta shape. The chains are linked to one another by various connections ("bridges"). Although degradation of individual chains leads to a more or less complete destruction of keratin, the bridges may be partly broken (this may occur under very mild conditions) without causing any permanent damage to the keratin.

Many of the bridges consist of the so-called salt linkages which develop through the close approach of basic and acid end groups of the side chains ("R" groups) [39].

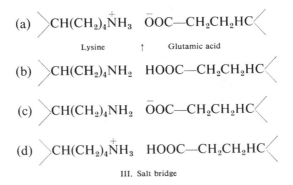

III. Salt bridge

Salt linkages can develop only if both basic and acid end groups occur in ionized (a) or nonionized (b) form. If only the carboxyl group (c) or only the basic group (d) is ionized, no salt linkages can develop. The structure of the keratin then loosens, and water molecules may penetrate between the individual chains, pressing them apart: the keratin swells. The degree of ionization of the basic and acid groups depends on the prevailing pH value; in a strongly acid environment only amino groups are ionized; in an alkaline environment, only the carboxyl groups. With a definite pH value, which differs for each protein molecule, there is an equal amount of negative and positive charges, the molecule may be said to neutralize itself. At this particular pH, the "isoelectric point," conditions for the formation of salt bridges are most favorable. The internal structure of the substance is particularly strong at this pH; the readiness to react with substances coming from the outside is particularly low because the major part of the reactive polar substances is bound in the molecule and not free for reaction with alien substances.

According to Marchionini and Schade [40], the isoelectric point of keratin lies at pH 4.1. It follows that keratin is most resistant to external influences at a pH of about 4 and is most subject to swelling by aqueous solutions with a pH farthest removed from this value.

In the same way that positive and negative ions are firmly linked in a dry salt crystal but move freely in an aqueous solution the connection between positive and negative end groups of the keratin side chains is also loosened in the presence of water. Keratin in a swollen state is therefore softer and less resistant to mechanical shocks.

Keratin differs chemically from most of the other proteins by its high content of the amino acid cystine, and the two types of keratin are again differentiated by their cystine content: hard keratin, which occurs in nails and hair, contains 16.6–18% cystine; soft keratin, the substance of the horny cells of the epidermis, contains only 2.3–3.8%.

Cystine (IV) is actually a di-amino acid because it consists of two amino

$$HOOC-CH-CH_2-S-S-CH_2-CH-COOH$$
$$\underset{NH_2}{|} \qquad\qquad \underset{NH_2}{|}$$

IV. Cystine

and two carboxyl groups. It accounts for the presence of the disulfide bridges in keratin (V). Although these bridges can also be disrupted by alkali

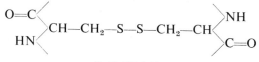

V. Disulfide bridge

$(-S-S- + H_2O \rightarrow SOH + HS-)$, their stability does not depend primarily on the prevailing pH but on the equilibrium of oxidation/reduction, or the redox potential. The bridges are broken down by reducing agents to

$$>-CH-CH_2-SH + HS-CH_2-CH<$$

but can be reconstituted by mild oxidants.

The cold-wave process utilizes the properties of the two types of bridge: first, the salt and disulfide bridges are broken with alkaline reducing solutions and subsequently reconstituted with acidic oxidizing solutions.

Still another type of linkage plays an important part in the structure of keratin: the hydrogen bridge. Bridges of this kind originate in the mutual attraction between the imido and carbonyl groups, present in the protein molecule, when they approach one another. As can be seen in VI, the hydrogen

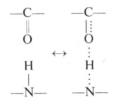

VI. The hydrogen bridge

atom is weakly linked to the nitrogen and oxygen atoms and thus forms a bridge between them. If, in many tissues, keratin does not occur in the elongated beta shape but in the folded alpha shape, it is probably due to the presence of hydrogen bridges.

Hydrogen chains may also contribute to the linkage between different keratin chains (VII) and may form between carbonyl groups of the main and

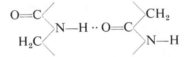

VII. Hydrogen bridge between two keratin chains

side chains and hydroxyl groups of the side chains. Salt bridges may actually be regarded as special cases of hydrogen bridges.

The side chains of two polypeptide chains may be linked by amide bridges (VIII).

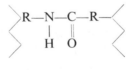

VIII. Amide bridge

According to Astbury, the structure of keratin may be described in the following way: keratin chains are connected by salt and disulfide bridges to form flat two-dimensional nets, all of which lie in the same plane. Hydrogen bridges then connect these nets to a three-dimensional tissue. Alexander [41] postulates a somewhat different structure, but it applies mostly to hair keratin. According to Alexander, the keratin chains are arranged parallel to one another, not, however, in the form of a flat net but as a closed cylinder. The chains are linked by hydrogen and disulfide bridges. The tensile strength of dry hair is attributable to hydrogen bridges, whereas both hydrogen and disulfide bridges contribute to the elasticity of wet hair. The side chains are arranged in such a way that the nonpolar ones (alkyl, alkylaryl) project inside the cylinder, whereas the polar groups (acid, amine, phenol groups etc.) are directed outward.

In any case, every theory of keratin structure must take into account that there is available at the surface of the keratin tissue (hair, corneal cells, etc.) a number of polar side chains, for only in this way can the adsorption of surfactants or dyestuffs by keratin be explained.

Let us summarize the four types of linkage in keratin:

1. The amide or peptide linkage (—CO—NH—) that connects individual amino acids to polypeptide chains and may also occur as a cross linkage. This connection may be broken by the action of concentrated aqueous solutions of strong acids or bases. Certain enzymes can break the amide linkage in an almost neutral environment at body temperature. These enzymes are used in certain special cleansing preparations and face masks which are intended to destroy old keratin and uncover new fresh layers.

2. The salt linkage (e.g., —COO$^-$ $^+$NH$_3$—), which probably plays an important part in the connection of the keratin chains, is most strongly pronounced in a weakly acid environment (pH about 4) and occurs less frequently in alkaline or strongly acid environment; keratin then swells and loses its mechanical and chemical resistance. Swelling and softening of the keratin by alkaline solutions is utilized in a number of cosmetic preparations: shaving soaps and creams, cold-wave solutions, and depilatory creams. Various skin and hair cleansing agents (in particular, all products based on soap) cause a softening of the keratin by their alkaline reaction in an aqueous solution. This effect is undesirable and is counteracted by acid face lotions and hair rinses.

3. The hydrogen linkage (—CO · · · HN$^-$ or —CO · · · HO—) fixes keratin chains in a folded state and also contributes to the interconnection of the chains. Water (swelling) weakens hydrogen bridges and concentrated solutions of certain salts break them. Lithium bromide is especially well suited to this purpose. Rothman and his collaborators have used it in the treatment of fungus infections in the hair shaft [42] and on the inside of the nails [43].

4. The disulfide linkage (—S—S—) is important also in the cementing of keratin chains and, in contrast to the salt linkage, is retained in wet hair. It

can be broken by reducing chemicals and enzymes. In cosmetics sulfides (in particular, thioglycolates) are used to break the disulfide links of the hair keratin in cold-wave processes and to remove hair in depilatory creams. The disulfide linkage can also be broken by alkaline hydrolysis.

## COMPATIBILITY OF SKIN AND COSMETIC PREPARATIONS

In his *Modern Cosmetocology* [44] Harry puts forward the opinion that undoubtedly no producer of cosmetic preparations has ever been lucky enough never to have received a complaint that his product had caused someone some skin irritation.

As a matter of fact, strictest quality control during production can achieve an absence of claims on both appearance and packing. Should such claims be made after all, it is usually quite easy to determine whether they are justified and remove the reasons.

It is not quite so easy to deal with skin irritations. Different investigators have different opinions about the frequency of irritations caused by cosmetic preparations. Good surveys of the relative literature are given by Friedrich [45] and Kinmont [46].

According to Tzanck [47], 7% of all cases of hypersensitivity to exterior damage in patients of a Paris clinic could be traced to cosmetic preparations. In 1956 Sidi [48] estimated this proportion to be 20% for the whole of France. Schulz [49] found that in Hamburg about 10% of all contact dermatitis (skin lesions caused by surface contact with skin irritants) originated from cosmetic preparations, and Appy [50] estimates about 5%.

The striking differences in these percentages may be attributed to a number of factors, the most important being the following:

1. Personal hygiene of the population tested.
2. Consumption of cosmetic preparations at the different locations.
3. The quality of cosmetic preparations most frequently used locally.

The proportion of skin-care products to decorative products used varies considerably from one region to another. In addition, the quality control of finished products is not equally stringent in different countries nor at different periods in the same country.

4. The economic structure of the tested area is also of importance; in industrial districts skin damage in the main is accounted for by industrial dermatoses; compared with them, cosmetic dermatoses are far less important.

5. The statistician himself may also be biased; his results may be influenced by his own attitude toward cosmetic preparations.

In any case, every producer of cosmetics must see to it that the risk of skin damage is kept as low as possible by carefully selecting the raw materials and controlling the finished product. This is not only an ethical responsibility but also a practical requirement, because every instance of damage to the skin reduces the public's confidence in this product and, indirectly, in the whole cosmetic industry.

## Toxic Reaction and Intolerance

Fundamentally, there are two different types of incompatibility: toxic reaction and intolerance. According to Sidi [51], "toxic reaction is a passive damage to the organism caused by the action of some poison." Substances that have a toxic effect when applied to the skin are called "caustic" or "primary irritants" and the effect, a "primary irritation." The symptoms of a primary irritation depend on the nature of the irritating substance, the strength of its concentration, and the duration of its action. With any given preparation, the effect is more or less identical in all persons, although the character of the skin, its present condition, and the general health of the subject all play a certain part. "Primary irritants," in this sense, are the soaps of the low fatty acids (caprylic and lauric acids), quaternary ammonium salts, and certain ingredients of perfumes (aliphatic aldehydes). Intolerance differs fundamentally from toxic reaction. The type and intensity of the skin reaction does not depend so much on the character and concentration of the noxious product as on the individual disposition of the person. The individual character of intolerance is clearly expressed in Tzanck's definition [Sidi, 52]: "Intolerance is the appearance of incompatibility symptoms in a certain person, caused by substances which do not cause any such symptoms in all other individuals." The manifestations of intolerance are often described as "allergic" reactions. With an intolerance, the noxious product is not the "primary active element; it rather appears as the triggering factor and discloses, through its effect, the individual disposition" [Sidi, 53]. Substances acting in this way are called "sensitizers": a one-time application sensitizes some people and makes them susceptible to the continued use of the product. It is a characteristic of intolerance that it does not become apparent immediately after application of the damaging product but only somewhat later. At times the skin lesion develops after 24 to 48 hours, and sometimes a product is used without any apparent reaction for weeks and months; only then do acute symptoms of intolerance suddenly appear. It follows from the character of intolerance that it is impossible to list "sensitizers" in the same way as caustic substances. Which particular substances will act as sensitizers depends on the individual disposition. The Austrian dermatologist Professor Oppenheim states that there is probably no substance that does not cause someone a skin inflammation. Caustic substances as well may act as sensitizers; the affected person would produce symptoms of incompatibility even with very low concentrations and after short periods of contact that normally would be acceptable.

## Precautions in the Production of Cosmetic Preparations

It is comparatively easy to avoid a primary irritant effect because it is known which of the basic substances used in cosmetics are irritants. Should one particular substance be doubtful, its effect can easily be established with patch tests. An irritant action of the finished product is best prevented by avoiding as much as possible all materials that cause primary irritant reactions; if any of these substances are required to achieve a specific effect, they must be used in such small amounts that a normal application of the finished product will be innocuous.

It is considerably more difficult to produce a preparation in a way that will eliminate all possibility of the occurrence of intolerance, for, contrary to toxic reactions, the appearance of intolerance is unpredictable. A product may be acceptable in a usage test for 100 persons and still, when marketed, produce symptoms of allergy. It is therefore never possible to guarantee that any product will be "free of allergenous effects."

Even so, the manufacturer of cosmetics is not completely helpless as far as intolerance is concerned. Experience has shown that many substances give rise more frequently than others to allergic reactions. Antibiotics, quinine salts (in hair lotions), phenyl mercury salts (in bleaching and antiseptic preparations), certain perfumery materials or pigments to mention but a few examples, are known in this connection. Lanolin, generally a valuable raw material, is not always tolerated, whereas no intolerance has ever been reported regarding the lanolin derivatives, acetylated wool-grease alcohols. With some hair dyes (p-phenylene and p-toluylene diamine and their derivatives) allergic reactions are so frequent that a patch test is generally made before they are applied. The manufacturer can reduce the probability of intolerance to his preparations as far as possible by avoiding the use of raw materials that are known to be occasionally unacceptable and by submitting his finished product to rigid tests.

It does happen that certain preparations which contain neither primary irritants nor sensitizers are still not tolerated. A typical example is soap and certain cleansing creams when used by persons with dry skin. A degreasing of the skin makes it more susceptible to the action of real irritants, but the public is often inclined to ascribe the damage to the sensitizing preparation (soap in this instance) and not to the actual irritant.

Products that are generally tolerated without reaction lead to skin lesions in some people if the skin is exposed to sunlight after application. This condition is called "photodermatitis." Certain medicinal substances (e.g., sulfonamide), pigments (e.g., eosine), and perfume materials (e.g., oil of bergamot and oil of angelica) are known to result in photodermatitis. In these cases irritation is caused by certain chemical substances that do not normally act as irritants but are activated if they absorb ultraviolet rays of a certain wavelength.

The toxicity of certain substances in cosmetic preparations must not be underestimated if there is a chance that they will be constantly resorbed by cumulative use of the preparation, even if only small quantities are involved. Professional use of hair shampoos containing the antidandruff agents selenium and selenium disulfite may become dangerous by precipitation of amorphous selenium in the body [54].

### Experimental Determination of Skin Compatibility

An extensive survey of the pharmacological-toxicological and dermatological test methods has been made by Dorr-Lux and Lietz [55]. A minimum of 200 persons should use the product normally for at least three or four weeks under clinical supervision. If at the end of this test period the test subjects show no skin irritations, the preparation may be considered safe to use. The possibility of individual intolerances at a later date can, of course, not be altogether excluded, but this chance is reduced the more persons are included in the test. (The apparently large number of subjects is required because of the incalculable character of intolerance. The greater the number of individuals tested, the higher the chance of including persons who will not tolerate the preparation. If, for example, a usage test were made with only 50 persons, the probability of there being some among them who would react allergically to the product would be so slight that the absence of reactions in the test would have no significance.)

Even if a preparation has been made with nothing but basic materials of "proved compatibility," it cannot necessarily be assumed that the finished product will be completely harmless; there is always a possibility that two substances, both of which are innocuous in the concentrations used, can cause an irritation when combined. One substance may open the way to irritation by the second (cross sensitization). Sidi [56] describes the case of a hair dressing in which the presence of a petroleum derivative caused the user to react to a pigment. Furthermore, it may depend on the vehicle whether a certain agent, pigment, or perfume ingredient will act as an irritant in a preparation. A pigment that may well be tolerated as part of a powder can cause irritations in a cream, which brings it into much closer contact with the skin.

These observations should not be taken to imply that the clinical results quoted in the professional literature regarding caustic and sensitizing effects of basic and active cosmetic materials may be disregarded because their effects differ individually anyway. Such reports are valuable but are not sufficiently comprehensive to predict the total effect of the finished product, which still needs to be tested in use.

If a test shows that the product is not always tolerated without reaction, the ingredient or ingredients causing the irritation must be identified.

First, it must be determined whether the skin reactions are due to toxic reaction or intolerance. This is comparatively easy because in toxic reaction all subjects react more or less alike, whereas an intolerance occurs only in a few persons. Subsequently each ingredient of the preparation must be tested individually for its skin compatibility. If it is a matter of primary irritation by the finished product, it is sufficient to apply each ingredient to the healthy skin of 20 or 30 subjects and to examine these treated areas after a short time. It is important that the concentration of the tested substances and the time of contact in the test correspond to those prevailing during the actual application of the finished product. A primary irritation becomes apparent by a more or less strong reddening (erythema), accumulated watery fluid in the sub-cutaneous tissue (edema) or blistering, and sometimes a shriveling of the skin at the point of contact [57]. If it is a matter of intolerance, the raw materials contained in the preparation must be checked in patch tests. This is done by applying each of them to sound skin in a dilution to exclude the possibility of a primary irritation. The substance is removed after 24 to 48 hours; the area is examined immediately after removal of the substance, again after 48 hours, and then after 6 to 10 days. (Because of the length of the test period, the contact area must be protected by a plaster or bandage. "Aerosol plasters," in which a protective layer is sprayed on, are also suitable.) If the reaction is positive, the skin changes may be characterized by edema formation, dry or wet eczema, or some pigmentation and are accompanied by strong itching, a characteristic symptom of every contact intolerance.

Frequently a small piece of cotton is soaked in a dilute solution of the substance and then fastened to the skin; hence the term "patch test." Some-times the suspected substance is not applied to sound skin but to a spot that has been scratched with a sharp instrument; this provides a direct contact between the substance and the blood circulation of the corium. Some allergies are detected in this way. It may be that a patch test which has been negative will turn positive if it is repeated after about 10 days, in which case the first test would have sensitized the subject. In order to exclude any chance of this sensitizing effect, the patch should never be left in contact with the skin for longer than 48 hours.

If it is found that none of the ingredients, taken individually, causes the damage observed when using the finished product, the possibility of cross sensitization, photodermatitis, or the vehicle affecting the skin action of the reactant must be considered. Although the patch test is basically simple to apply and diagnose, it should nevertheless be carried out only by experienced specialists, preferably dermatologists, because error or incorrect interpretation could have most unpleasant results for the subject. If we have gone into some detail regarding test methods, it is because the patch test is doubly important to the cosmetics manufacturer: first, as previously mentioned, because each new cosmetic preparation should be tested before it is offered to the public and, second, because this test should be carried out in all cases in which a cosmetic preparation is suspected of having caused some intolerance. Not infrequently a patch test has proved to be negative, but it was ultimately found that after the simultaneous use of two otherwise compatible preparations a certain dietary factor or possibly even an emotional crisis was the cause of the reported skin irritation and that no blame attached to the cosmetic product itself.

Skin rashes caused by contact dermatitis are also often erroneously attributed to the use of cosmetics, whereas the real cause can be traced to modern textiles. Professor P. V. Marcussen wrote in this connection:

"Within the last decades, the incidence of rashes caused by dress and shirt fabrics has quadrupled. They are due to the no-iron, crease-resistant textile finishes based on formaldehyde urea and formaldehyde melanin resins. Allergies of this type occur on face, neck, hands, arms, armpits, crotch, legs, and feet." [58]

Hence, when dealing with complaints about cosmetic preparations, many facts outside the actual field of cosmetics should be taken into consideration.

The patch test is also important in any determination of the skin compatibility of new raw materials. The first stage is usually animal testing (mostly rabbits and guinea pigs), and only if these tests are completely negative are they extended to humans. Modern test methods have been described by Davidow [59] and Rubenkönig and Quisero [60]. Vonkennel [61] describes the acanthosis test, a method that permits conclusions regarding the human skin compatibility of cream bases to be drawn from animal tests.

A review of topical testing which outlines the nature of topical toxicities and the principal test methods is given by Idson [62].

## REFERENCES

[1] Rothman, *Physiology and Biochemistry of the Skin*, University of Chicago Press, 1954, p. 309 ff.

[2] Flesch, *J. Soc. cosmet. Chem.*, **13**, 113 (1962).

[3] Wheatley, *Soap Perfum. Cosm.*, **29**, 181 (1956); *Am. Perfumer*, 37 (October 1956).

[4] Manneck, Die Haut und ihre Waschmittel, *SÖFW*, **9** (1961).

[5] Kligman, *Brit. J. Derm.*, **75**, 307 (1963).

[6] Szakall, *Fette Seifen*, **53**, 399 (1951); *Archs. Derm. Syph.*, **194**, 376 (1952); *Arch. klin. exp. Derm.*, **201**, 331 (1955).

[7] Rein, *Z. Biol.*, **81**, 125 (1924); **84**, 41 (1925).

[8] Rothman, *op. cit.*

[9] Wegemann, Hewitt, Guignon, and Guha, *Annls. Histochim.*, **7**, 45, 89 (1962); *Parfum. Kosmet.*, **44**, 301 (1963).

[10] Santoioanni and Rothman, *J. invest. Derm.*, **37**, 489 (1961); Steigleder and Raab, *ibid.*, **38**, 209 (1962).

[11] Ochoa, Smith, and Sweralow, *Archs. Derm.*, **15**, 70 (1957).

[12] Blank, *J. invest. Derm.*, **21**, 259 (1953).

[13] Blank and Shappirio, *J. invest. Derm.*, **18**, 433 (1952); **25**, 391 (1955); see also Peck and Glick, *J. Soc. cosmet. Chem.*, **7**, 530 (1956).

[14] Buettner, *Proc. scient. Sect.*, *Toilet Goods Ass.*, **40**, 8 (1963).

[15] Powers and Fox, *Drug Cosmet. Ind.*, **82**, 32 (1958).

[16] Flesch, 3rd Annual Cosmetics Seminar, Society of cosmetic Chemists, New York, October 1956.

[17] Fox, Tassoff, Rieger, and Deem, *J. Soc. cosmet. Chem.*, **13**, 263 (1962).

[18] Rothman and Schlaf, in Jadassohn, *Handbuch der Haut- und Geschlechtskrankh*, 1/2 p. 161 ff., Springer Verlag, Berlin, 1929.

[19] Shaw and Messer, *Am. J. Physiol.*, **98**, 93 (1931); Adams, *Am. Perfumer*, 134 (February 1949).

[20] Goldschmiedt, *Drug Cosmet. Ind.*, **84** (1) 40 (1959); *Am. Perfumer*, **75** (11), 41 (1960).

[21] Zenisek, Fiser, Kris, Spanlangova, and Paroulkova, *Parfum. Kosmet.*, **46**, 226 (1956); Ruckbusch, *Fette Seifen, Anstr-Mittel*, **65**, 228 (1963).

[22] Marchionini, *Arch. Derm. Syph.*, **158**, 290 (1929).

[23] Peck et al., *J. invest. Derm.*, **1**, 237 (1938); *Archs. Derm. Syph.*, **39**, 126 (1939); *ibid.*, **56**, 601 (1947).

[24] Rothman, Smiljanic, Shapiro, and Weitkamp, *J. invest. Derm.*, **8**, 81 (1947).

[25] Burtenshaw, *J. Hyg. Camb.*, **42**, 184 (1942).

[26] Harry, *Modern Cosmetocology*, 4th ed. L. Leonard Hill, London, 1955, p. 19.

[27] Szakall, *Fette Seifen*, **52**, 3, 171 (1950); **53**, 5, 284 (1951).
Tronnier and Bussius, *Arch. klin. exp. Derm.*, **205**, 586 (1958).

[28] *Dermatologica*, Basle, **81**, 3 (1940); **94**, 73 (1947); **102**, 294 (1951).

[29] Tronnier and Bussius, *Z. Haut-u. Geschl. Krankh.*, **30**, 177 (1961); Schoenherr, *Arch. klin. exp. Derm.*, **214**, 157 (1961).

[30] Rothman, *op. cit.* p. 515.

[31] Bloch, "Das Pigment," in J. Jadassohn, *Handbuch der Haut- und Geschlechtskrankh*, Springer Verlag, Berlin 1927, Vol. I, Part 1.

[32] Peck and Michelfelder, in Sagarin, *Cosmetics, Science, and Technology*, Interscience, New York, 1957, p. 1113 ff; Fitzpatrick, *J. Soc. cosmet. Chem.*, **15**, 297 (1964).

[33] Gates, *Jl. R. microsc. Soc.*, **80**, 121 (1961).

[34] Randenbrock, *J. Soc. cosmet. Chem.*, **13**, 404 (1962); **15**, 595 (1964).

[35] Astbury, in Savill, *The Hair and Scalp*, 4th ed., Baltimore 1952, p. 65 ff.

[36] Stoves, *J. Soc. cosmet. Chem.*, **2**, 158 (1951).

[37] Schopping and van Sluis, *Perfum. essent. Oil Rec.*, **51**, 181 (1960).

[38] Astbury and Woods, *Phil. Trans. Roy. Soc. (London)*, **A232**, 333 (1933).

[39] Speakman et al., *Trans. Faraday Soc.*, **29**, 148 (1933); **30**, 539 (1934); **32**, 897 (1936).

[40] Marchionini and Schade, *Münch. med. Wschr.*, **74**, 1435 (1927).

[41] Alexander, *Kolloidzeitschrift.*, **122**, 8 (1951).

[42] *J. invest. Derm.*, **17**, 9 (1951).

[43] *Archs. Derm. Syph.*, **67**, 239, 259 (1953).

[44] Harry, *Modern Cosmetocology*, 4th ed., L. Leonard Hill, London, 1955, p. 45.

[45] Friedrich, *Parfum. Kosmet.*, **37**, 551 (1956).

[46] Kinmont, *J. Soc. cosmet. Chem.*, **15**, 3 (1964).

[47] Tzanck (1953), by Molin, *Industrie Parfum.*, **10**, 30 (1955).

[48] Sidi, *Tolérance et intolérance aux produits cosmétiques*, Paris, 1956. German translation published by Dr. A. Hüthig Verlag, Heidelberg, *Verträglichkeit von kosmetischen Präparaten*. Pages quoted refer to the German translation.

[49] Schulz, *J. Kosm.*, 42 (1954).

[50] Appy, Inaug.-Diss., Tuebingen, 1955.

[51] Sidi, *op. cit.*, 9.

[52] Sidi, *ibid.*

[53] Sidi, *op. cit.*, 10.

[54] Tornow, *Pharm. Zentralhalle Dtl*, **100**, 511 (1961); *Kosmetik-Parf.-Drog.* **11/12** (1962).

[55] Dorr-Lux and Lietz, *Parfum. Kosmet.*, **46**, 256, 289 (1965).

[56] Sidi, *op. cit.*, 26.

[57] Sidi, *op. cit.*, 11–12.

[58] P. V. Marcussen, *Ugeskrift for Laeger, Kosmetik-Parf.-Drog.* 7/8 (1962).

[59] Davidow, *Drug Cosmet. Ind.*, **80**, 608 (1957).

[60] Rubenkönig and Quisero [*Am. Perfumer*, **71** (1), 33 (January 1958)]; *SÖFW*, **84**, 184 (1958).

[61] Vonkennel, *Parfum. Kosmet.*, **37**, 249 (1956).

[62] Idson, Topical Toxicity and Testing, *J. Pharm. Sci.*, **57** (1), 1–11 (1967).

# CHAPTER 2

# Surfactants in Cosmetics

Surfactants are among the most important basic materials used in cosmetics. In creams they appear as emulsifiers; in soaps and shampoos they increase the washing intensity of the water; in shaving products they act as wetting and foaming agents; in lipsticks they facilitate the dispersion of the insoluble pigments in the fat vehicle; in bath oils they make the perfume water-soluble; in deodorants cationic surfactants are used as bactericides. It is no exaggeration to say that only very rarely do cosmetic preparations lack a surfactant as an important constituent.

Until recent times only a limited number of surfactants had any practical significance, but in the last 20 years, in particular in the United States, innumerable new substances with surface activity have appeared on the market. Published lists [1] contain hundreds of these materials. This abundance may appear confusing, particularly since manufacturers offer different products for the same purpose (e.g., wetting agents) which makes it difficult for the user to decide which product is most suitable for his purpose; on the other hand, a certain material is sometimes recommended for different purposes (as a wetting, washing, or emulsifying agent). In addition, the trade literature often seems to convey the impression that, for example, foaming, wetting, and washing agents and emulsifiers are completely different products. (If this were so, a wetting agent with washing and emulsifying effects would indeed be a miraculous material!) In other instances all surfactants are summarized under the heading of "wetting agents" or "detergents." (The reader might therefore be misled into arbitrarily selecting any emulsifier or foaming agent to improve the wetting properties of his product.)

It is the purpose of this chapter to bring some order into the confusion in the field of surfactants. First, we consider the general principle underlying the effect of these substances; we then deal with the individual functions that surfactants fulfill in cosmetics and ultimately discuss the main properties of the most important types. Because of the great number of existing materials, we cannot and do not claim complete coverage in the last section.

## PRINCIPLE OF EFFECTIVENESS

### General Structure

We define surfactants as those substances that, when dissolved in a liquid, tend to concentrate on its surface.

This property permits even comparatively small amounts of surfactant to cause strong modifications in the surface character of a solvent and consequently in its reaction to air, other liquids, or solids. The ability to accumulate at the surface of a solvent is due to a certain duality in the chemical-physical character of surface-active agents. On the one hand, surfactants must be soluble or dispersible in a solvent (otherwise they would accumulate as a separate layer or in drops or crystallize and remain ineffective); on the other hand, their molecules must contain groups that, speaking qualitatively, are not "at home" in the solvent. Under the influence of these contradictory trends the molecules move in the interior or on the surface of the solvent and finally come to rest in a position that is the most favorable, energetically speaking; in this case it would be where the lyophilic part of the molecules (i.e., the part with high affinity to the solvent) is still in the solvent but the lyophobic part projects from it, that is, onto the surface of the solvent. The molecule of a surfactant is always composed of a lyophilic and a lyophobic part. Its surface-active properties depend primarily on the potency ratio of these two parts.

A practical example is usually much clearer than a theoretical explanation; let us consider the effect of surfactants in an oil-in-water emulsion.

The energetically most favorable position for a molecule containing a hydrophilic and a lipophilic (hydrophobic) part in which the hydrophilic predominates is right in the middle of the aqueous phase. A substance consisting of such molecules would therefore not be surface-active. An example is sodium butyrate

$$\underbrace{CH_3CH_2CH_2}_{L}\underbrace{COO^-Na^+}_{H}$$

where $H$ stands for the hydrophilic and $L$, for the lipophilic part of the molecule. If, however, the hydrophilic part is less strongly pronounced than the lipophilic, the substance easily dissolves in the oil phase and once again would not be surface-active. Such a type is ethyl palmitate

$$\underbrace{CH_3(CH_2)_{14}}_{L}\underbrace{COOC_2H_5}_{H}$$

Only in cases in which the hydrophilic and lipophilic parts are more or less evenly matched would the substance be surface-active. The molecules then form a layer on the oil/water interface, with the lipophilic part in the oil and the hydrophilic part in the water.

The potency ratio of the hydrophilic and lipophilic parts must therefore be within certain limits; otherwise the substance will not act as a surfactant. Within these limits are still a number of possibilities; variations within this range result in variations in the type of activity of the surfactant. In this way a substance whose lipophilic part is stronger than the hydrophilic will be mostly in the oil phase at the surface. Such a substance acts as a water-in-oil emulsifier and tends to cause a state of emulsion in which the water is dispersed in fine droplets in the continuous oil phase. On the other hand, a surfactant whose hydrophilic part is more effective than the lipophilic will act as an oil-in-water emulsifier; that is, it usually leads to the formation of an emulsion in which the continuous phase is aqueous. An example of the first type of surfactant is cetyl alcohol:

$$CH_3(CH_2)_{14}CH_2OH.$$

An example of the second type is sodium palmitate:

$$CH_3(CH_2)_{14}COO^-Na^+.$$

A comparison of the formulas for sodium palmitate, cetyl alcohol, and ethyl palmitate shows that the lipophilic group in these materials is the same. The strength of the hydrophilic group in these three substances, however, differs to such an extent that in the first instance the result is an oil-in-water (O/W) emulsifier (sodium palmitate) and in the second, a water-in-oil (W/O) emulsifier (cetyl alcohol); finally, ethyl palmitate is no longer a surface-active agent because it is completely oil-soluble.

### Polar and Nonpolar Atom Groups

How, then, is the strength of the hydrophilic or lipophilic character of any atom group (or of a molecule or parts thereof) determined? The affinity of molecules to one another is based on electrostatic attraction. Without elaborating on the quantitative aspects of this point, we can say that the strength of attraction between two molecules depends on the distribution of the electrons and, consequently, on the distribution of the electrical charge inside the molecules. From this point of view molecules and atom groups can be divided into two types: polar and nonpolar. The nonpolar type is characterized by an even distribution of the electric charge over the total molecule or atom group. Typical examples of this group are the saturated hydrocarbons; for example, hexadecane,

$$CH_3(CH_2)_{14}CH_3.$$

The polar type, on the other hand, is characterized by an uneven distribution of the electrons throughout the molecule or atom group so that more or less strong electron-rich (negative) or electron-poor (positive) centers are formed within. An example of strongly polar atom groups is found in the salts of organic acids, in which the oxygen atoms of the carboxyl group are rich in electrons and carry a negative charge, whereas the electron-poor metal carries a positive charge:

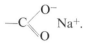

A group of less polar character is found in alcohols, in which the hydrogen and carbon atoms bound to oxygen have a weak positive charge and the oxygen atom itself, a negative one.

$$\overset{(+)\ (-)\ (+)}{-C-O-H}.$$

It is of great significance—certainly to cosmetics—that water is also a polar substance. The negative center again lies in the oxygen atoms; the hydrogen atoms are weakly positive

$$\overset{(+)\ (-)\ (+)}{H-O-H}.$$

As far as the reciprocal attraction of molecules is concerned a simplified rule may be formulated from the known fact that polar molecules or atom groups have a stronger affinity for other polar substances than for nonpolar atom groups. In systems containing substances of different polarity the most polar materials will therefore tend to associate, leaving, as it were by default, the nonpolar materials to group together. Most substances that are used in cosmetic emulsions in the oil (lipid) phase have a more or less nonpolar character, whereas water represents a polar solvent. The nonpolar part in surfactants is therefore obviously lipophilic, and the polar group or groups, hydrophilic; that is, they have an affinity with the aqueous phase.

It is remarkable that the same hydrophilic or lipophilic group will impart to the molecule not only an emulsifying effect but also wetting and foaming. A prerequisite of foam formation is that the surfactant molecules gather at the surface of the solvent. In an aqueous solution of sodium laurate the laurate ion does indeed migrate to the surface and places itself in such a way that the carboxyl group remains in the water but the lipophilic hydrocarbon chain projects from it. The reason for this behavior is not the attraction between the lipophilic group and air nor the repellent effect of water on the lipophilic group; what actually happens is that a stronger attraction exists between the water molecules than between water molecules and the hydrocarbon chain and that the latter is constantly replaced by water molecules until it finally comes to rest at the surface. (This "coming to rest" should not be taken too literally. In most cases the molecules of surfactants continually move very quickly over the surface of the liquid but return only comparatively rarely to the interior of the solvent.) As we have seen, the behavior of the surfactant is largely determined by the potency ratio between the hydrophilic and lipophilic groups contained in its molecules. It would be useful therefore to be able to express this potency quantitatively to calculate the behavior of the material. Although the present state of science permits the fairly exact calculation of the attraction between two molecules or atom groups, it has not much bearing on cosmetics because the systems here are so complicated (both phases, oil and water, as well as the emulsifier usually consist of mixtures) that they cannot be defined with quantitative calculations.

Based on experience, we can, however, establish certain facts regarding the comparative strength of polar and nonpolar groups which occur in the most commonly used surfactants.

1. *The nonpolar groups.* In practice these groups always consist of saturated or unsaturated, straight or branched hydrocarbon chains, saturated, unsaturated, or aromatic hydrocarbon rings, or of a combination of these atom groups. The following rule usually applies: the strength of the nonpolar part of a molecule is directly proportional to its content of carbon atoms. Saturated carbon chains have a slightly more pronounced nonpolar character than the unsaturated, and alicyclical (nonaromatic ring) groups act more strongly nonpolar than the aromatic. The following substances contain different types of lipophilic groups which may serve as examples for the nonpolar groups occurring in surfactants.

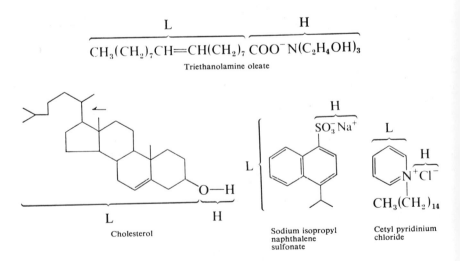

$$\overbrace{\hspace{3cm}}^{L} \quad \overbrace{\hspace{3cm}}^{H}$$
$$CH_3(CH_2)_7CH{=}CH(CH_2)_7\,COO^-\,N(C_2H_4OH)_3$$

Triethanolamine oleate

Cholesterol

Sodium isopropyl
naphthalene
sulfonate

Cetyl pyridinium
chloride

2. *The polar groups.* Although size or molecular weight is the most important factor in determining strength in the nonpolar group, there are considerable differences in effectiveness in polar groups with roughly the same molecular weight. Here the decisive factor is the distribution of electrons; the polar effect of the atom group will be all the higher, the more strongly pronounced the positive and negative centers. The strongest polar groups found in organic surfactants are the end groups of salts:

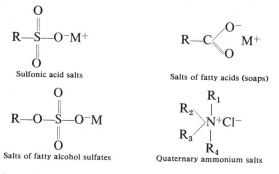

Sulfonic acid salts                    Salts of fatty acids (soaps)

Salts of fatty alcohol sulfates        Quaternary ammonium salts

Free fatty acids are less polar:

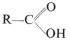

(Free sulfonic acid or alkyl sulfuric acid groups would be strongly polar, but they cannot be considered for use in cosmetics because of their highly acid character.)

Free hydroxyl groups, as they occur in alcohols and glycols, have an even weaker polar effect; free amino groups fall into the same category:

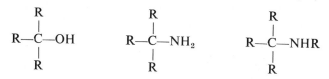

(Tertiary amino groups would have a stronger polarity but are out of the question in a free state because of their strong alkalinity.)

Ether, ester, and amide groups belong to the weakest polar groups used in practice:

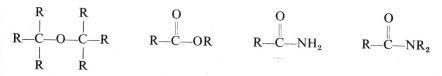

The weakest polar groups are probably the oxyethylene groups:

$$-CH_2CH_2O- \qquad\qquad -CH_2CH_2CH_2O-$$

Oxyethylene group  Oxypropylene group

Here the nonpolar tendency of the ethylene ($-CH_2CH_2-$) group is just overshadowed by the polar tendency of the oxygen atoms so that the total effect of the oxyethylene group is weakly hydrophilic (polar). The weakness of the hydrophilic effect of the oxyethylene is evident in the fact that sodium oleate (HLB value 18) is much more hydrophilic than polyethylene glycol 400 mono-oleate (HLB value 11.4), so that a single carboxyl ion behaves more strongly hydrophilic than a chain of about eight oxyethylene groups.

$$CH_3(CH_2)_7=CH(CH_2)_7-COO^-Na$$

Sodium oleate

$$CH_3(CH_2)_7CH=CH(CH_2)_7-COO(CH_2CHO_2)_nH$$

Polyethylene glycol 400 mono-oleate ($n$ = about 8).

In the oxypropylene group, which contains three methylene groups for each oxygen atom, the hydrophobic effect of the latter is already predominant. In this connection the structure of Pluronic surfactants (Wyandotte Chemical Co.) is interesting: it consists of an oxypropylene polymer to which oxyethylene chains are linked on both sides:

$$HO(CH_2O)_a(CH_2CH_2CH_2O)_b(CH_2CH_2O)_cH$$

Here the polypropylene oxide represents the hydrophobic and the polyethylene oxide groups the hydrophilic parts of the molecule. In certain cases practical conclusions may be drawn from the rules given; we can predict, for example, that in sodium butyrate the hydrophilic (polar) part will predominate more than in sodium palmitate or that sodium palmitate, cetyl alcohol, and ethyl palmitate will, in that order, show an increasingly lipophilic character. These rules, however, are not sufficient to predict the behavior of a new substance that contains both hydrophilic and lipophilic groups, except when it is closely related to already known surfactants. A system that can really predict the behavior of some surfactants was developed by Griffin [2]. Griffin suggested the so-called HLB value (HLB = hydrophilic/lipophilic balance) as a measure of hydrophilic or lipophilic character. For fatty acid esters of polyhydric alcohols the formula

$$HLB = 20\left(1 - \frac{SV}{AV}\right)$$

applies ($SV$ = saponification value of the emulsifier, $AV$ = acid value of the fatty acid). For esters for which it is impossible to determine the saponification value accurately, such as rosin acid esters, lanolin esters, the equation

$$HLB = \frac{E + P}{5}$$

applies ($E$ = oxyethylene content in weight percent, $P$ = polyhydric alcohol content in weight percent).

The second equation may be simplified for substances whose hydrophilic constituent consists only of oxyethylene groups (e.g., polyethylene glycol ester or fatty alcohol ethylene oxide condensation products):

$$\text{HLB} = \frac{E}{5}.$$

An alternate and more general formula for the calculation of HLB values was developed by Davies [38]:

$$\text{HLB} = 7 + \text{(hydrophilic group numbers)} - m \times 0.475.$$

In this formula $m$ is the number of carbon atoms in the lipophilic group. The sum of the hydrophilic group numbers is calculated from Table 2-1.

TABLE 2-1   HLB HYDROPHILIC GROUP NUMBERS

| Group | Group Number |
| --- | --- |
| $-SO_4^- Na^+$ | 38.7 |
| $-COO^- K^+$ | 21.1 |
| $-COO^- Na^+$ | 19.1 |
| Sulfonate | About 11 |
| Ester (sorbitan ring) | 6.8 |
| Ester (free) | 2.4 |
| $-COOH$ | 2.1 |
| Hydroxyl (free) | 1.9 |
| $-O-$ | 1.3 |
| Hydroxyl (sorbitan ring) | 0.5 |
| $-(CH_2CH_2O)-$ | 0.33 |

The HLB value of a surfactant mixture may be calculated by adding the values of its components. A mixture consisting of 60% surfactant with HLB 20 and 40% surfactant with HLB 8 would have a HLB value of $0.6 \times 20 + 0.4 \times 8 = 15.2$.

Originally Griffin determined HLB values not by calculation but by emulsification tests. This method was not only laborious and time consuming but also, as proved by Riegelman and Pichon [3], theoretically unsound. The "required HLB values" as well, which Griffin and his collaborators established on the strength of tests on oils and waxes used in cosmetics, have only a restricted validity. Griffin's original intention had been to establish a system to calculate the suitability of emulsifiers or emulsifier mixtures for any one emulsion. Even though this did not materialize altogether, the HLB value has proved a very useful tool for expressing the hydrophilic or lipophilic affinity of surfactants and surfactant mixtures. Substances with low HLB values (roughly below 10) are generally good water-in-oil emulsifiers, whereas the more hydrophilic surfactants with higher HLB values act as oil-in-water emulsifiers. According to Griffin, the best wetting effect for surfactants is in the range of HLB 7–9, the best solubilizing effect at HLB 15–18, and the best detergent effect at HLB 13–25.

## Reduction of Surface Tension

The effectiveness of a surfactant is due directly to the tendency of its molecules to accumulate at the surface of a solvent: it thereby reduces the surface tension between solvent and liquids or insoluble solids. As previously mentioned, surface tension of a pure liquid is caused by the electrostatic attraction between adjacent molecules. Let us consider one individual molecule of a liquid, for example, water, and assume that this molecule is somewhere in the middle of a body of water. It is exposed to attraction exercised by surrounding water molecules. The attraction, which is equal on all sides, cancels itself out, and the molecule is not drawn in any one direction. If, however, we look at a water molecule on the surface of a body of water, we find other water molecules on all sides, on the surface and also below it (in the liquid); above the surface, in the gaseous phase, the concentration of water molecules is considerably smaller than in the liquid. Thus a surface molecule is exposed to much stronger attraction by others below the surface because of their greater number than by the smaller number of water molecules in the gaseous phase. The surface molecule is therefore not balanced; it is subject to an attraction that pulls it down into the middle of the solution. As each molecule is continually drawn inward, the smallest possible number of molecules will be at the surface, which means that any body of liquid will assume the form that gives it the smallest possible surface and will oppose any effort to enlarge it. This condition is known as "surface tension." Similar conditions account for interfacial tension: a molecule at the interface is generally more strongly attracted by similar surrounding molecules than by those of an alien substance and consequently is drawn away from this substance. The liquid opposes the enlargement of the interface, and the result is interfacial tension. This image can be elaborated. The more the two substances forming the interface differ in their polarity, the greater the imbalance of the forces acting on the polar molecules at the interface (and, to a lesser extent, on the nonpolar molecules) and the greater the interfacial tension. On the other hand, if two substances under consideration are similar in their polar characteristics, they become intersoluble and interface tension is nil (see Figure 1).

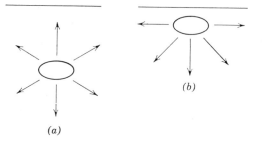

FIGURE 1    FORCES THAT ACT ON A MOLECULE IN A LIQUID (a) AND AT THE SURFACE OF
A LIQUID (b).

In view of the foregoing we may say that surface and interface tension in a liquid is caused by a surface molecule being in an unfavorable position energetically and therefore drawn away. As previously mentioned, conditions for a surfactant molecule in solution are exactly the opposite: for such a molecule the position at the surface is favorable energetically. Obviously the energy associated with surface formation is smaller if at least some of the molecules present in this plane feel "at home"; and the surface tension of a pure liquid will therefore be reduced by a surfactant. The surfactant, even if it is present only in small quantities, can have a surprisingly strong effect on the character of the surface because this is the position in which it accumulates.

## Micell Formation

The following discussion of this phenomenon is based on a theory by MacBain (4). This theory is not entirely in accord with current knowledge of the subject, but it offers a plausible and easy explanation for many effects in colloidal chemistry.

As we have seen, surfactant molecules migrate to the solvent surface as the result of the mutual attraction solvent molecules have for one another and the lesser attraction between them and the lyophobic parts of the surfactant molecules. Yet another factor assumes importance in surfactant solutions which are not too strongly diluted: the mutual attraction of the lyophobic parts of the surfactant molecules. Because of this attraction, these molecules tend to nestle together. In this way they form surfactant aggregates or "micells" in the solvent; the micells are stable, particularly if their structure permits them to turn only their lyophilic parts toward the solvent, whereas the lyophobic parts accumulate in their interior. In aqueous solutions of surfactants with ionized hydrophilic groups (e.g., soap), micell colloids are formed in this manner; the micells, like colloidal particles, are charged on their surface. From the point of view of the surfactant this is a favorable situation energetically, and for this reason micell formation occurs with most surfactants. It is also remarkable that it invariably occurs at a definite and reproducible concentration of the surfactant, the so-called "critical concentration," which differs for different surfactants and also, for any given substance, depends on the temperature and (for aqueous solutions) electrolyte concentration of the solvent.

A number of theories exist in regard to the shape of micells. Probably the most important shapes are spherical or elongated (Figures 2 and 3). The ease of micell formation obviously depends on the structure of surfactant molecules. If, for example, the hydrophobic component of a water-soluble surfactant consists of a long straight hydrocarbon chain, conditions for the nestling of several molecules are favorable. If, on the other hand, the hydrocarbon chain has many branches, the hydrophobic component of the molecule contains large rings (as in naphthalene), or the hydrophilic group is not placed at one end of the molecule but closer to the center, conditions for the formation of micells are much less favorable. This immediately becomes apparent in the study of models of these molecules and can also be established by experiments: the critical concentration, that is, the concentration at which micell formation begins, lies considerably higher for surfactants with hydrocarbon chains with pronounced branching (e.g., sodium-1-ethyl-2-methylundecyl-(4)-sulfate, "Tergitol 4"), with large ring systems (e.g., the alkylnaphthalene sulfates), or with the hydrophilic group nearer the center of the molecule (e.g., sodium-dioctylsulfosuccinate) than for soaps of the higher fatty acids and straight-chain hydrocarbons [5].

With these soaps the tendency to form micells also depends on structural factors, particularly the length of the hydrocarbon chain. It has been established that the affinity between hydrocarbon chains of different molecules (hence the tendency toward micell formation) is less pronounced in soaps of shorter hydrocarbon chains (caprylic and lauric acid soaps) than with higher molecular soaps. Nor must the hydrocarbon chains be too long or the molecules become water-insoluble.

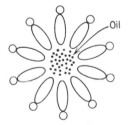

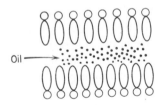

FIGURE 2   SPHERICAL MICELL.                    FIGURE 3   ELONGATED OR LINEAR MICELL.

The optimum length of a hydrocarbon chain for micell formation in soaps lies at $C_{16}$ to $C_{18}$. If several different surfactants are present in a solution, mixed micells may be formed.

## Surface and Interface Films

We now come to the last factor that plays an important part in many applications of surface-active agents: the character of the film they form on surfaces and interfaces. The cohesion of the lyophobic parts of the molecules is not only responsible for micell formation, it also affects the stability of the surface film. When molecules (or ions of a surfactant) accumulate on a surface, they assume a position in which hydrocarbon chains of different molecules (or ions) lie parallel to one another. This position maximizes the attraction between hydrocarbon chains lying side by side, and these forces of attraction stabilize the surfactant film.

We differentiate between three types of surface and interface film:

1. Gaseous films occur when the attraction between surfactant molecules is small and they move freely and independently at the surface. These films have little cohesion and no mechanical resistance.

2. In solid films surfactant molecules cohere rigidly in a fixed arrangement similar to a crystal. These films are firm and hard. When they are exposed to strong mechanical impact (heating or freezing of the water), they disintegrate and completely lose their effect.

3. In liquid films surfactant molecules cohere but not so strongly that they are completely immobile, as in solid films. They return to their original state of stability after mechanical disturbances. They behave elastically and are highly resistant.

The terms "gaseous," "solid," and "liquid" do not refer to the surfactant itself but to the kind of surface film it forms. In this way sodium myristinate, a solid, forms liquid or gaseous films on the surface of water; butyl alcohol, a liquid, forms gaseous films on water.

It depends on different factors whether in any given circumstances a surfactant will form gaseous, solid, or liquid films; the decisive ones are the concentration of the surfactant and the shape of its molecules.

If the concentration is so low that not enough molecules are present to form a connected film, it will be gaseous. In this case the surfactant molecules are not close enough to one another to exercise enough attraction to form a resistant film. The shape of the molecules has a similar effect on film as on micell formation; these two phenomena are closely linked. Long straight hydrocarbon chains are favorable for liquid film formation with strong cohesion. In short hydrocarbon chains (predominantly hydrophilic) cohesive properties are not pronounced, and gaseous films result. Molecules with very long hydrocarbon chains tend to form solid films. It is remarkable and most important in practice that mixed films formed by molecules from two different surfactants show higher stability in many instances than simple films from only one substance. The greatest stability in films is achieved by two surfactants when hydrophilic properties predominate in one (e.g., sodium lauryl sulfate) and lipophilic in the other (e.g., cholesterol).

## THE FUNCTIONS OF SURFACTANTS IN COSMETICS

### The Wetting Effect

**Practical Significance.** Only very rarely does the wetting effect of a surfactant alone play an important part; more often it occurs as part of the cleansing action or as part of the dispersing property because solids must be wetted before they can be dispersed in the surrounding liquid. In a few cases, however, the wetting effect, as such, is desired; for example, in shaving soaps or creams, hair dyes, or cold-wave preparations. In bath oils, which should spread quickly over the bath water, oil-soluble wetting agents are used. The effect of additives such as lanolin and cholesterol to hair and skin oils is also based to a large extent on an increased oil wetting of the keratin. On the basis of the theory just sketched, we can now explain how these substances can increase the wetting properties of a liquid.

**Principle.** It will make matters clearer if we consider an example, say the case of a water-insoluble substance being wetted by water. What happens is that the interface between solid and air disappears and two new interfaces develop: solid/water and water/air. The energy required for this wetting equals the energy required by formation of the new interfaces, less the energy associated with the original interface. Put differently, the following equation may be applied to every surface unit:

$$\text{required energy} = t_{\text{s/water}} + t_{\text{water/air}} - t_{\text{s/air}},$$

where $t_{\text{s/water}}$ is the interfacial tension between solid and water, and so on. What would happen if pure water were replaced by an aqueous solution of a surfactant? The interfacial tension solid/air (which, incidentally, is difficult to gauge) remains unchanged. The interfacial tensions solid/water and water/air are reduced (as shown above) by the addition of a surfactant. The preceding equation shows that the addition of a surfactant to the water definitely reduces the amount of required energy. This is the phenomenon we call "wetting effect." The extent of interfacial tension reduction depends on the concentration of the surfactant. Starting with low concentrations, the wetting effect will be seen to increase as the concentration increases. However, this applies only up to a given strength; if this is exceeded, the wetting effect will be affected only very slightly by any further additions of the surfactant. This concentration coincides with the critical concentration of the surfactant: as soon as micell formation is initiated, further additions will no longer lead to an increased concentration of the wetting agent on the surface but rather to further micell formation in the aqueous solution.

Because the wetting effect depends on the presence of surfactants on the surface of the wetting liquid and is not favored by micells contained in it, conditions delaying micell formation until the highest possible surfactant concentration has been reached would heighten the wetting effect. As a matter of fact, all good wetting agents have structures that do not favor micell formation (alkyl benzene sulfonates, alkyl naphthalene sulfonates, Na-dioctylsulfosuccinate, polyoxyethylene-2-butyloctanol) [6].

It is an interesting but not fully explained phenomenon that the wetting effect of aqueous solutions of some surfactants is increased by the addition of small quantities of insoluble organic substances. The wetting effect of an aqueous solution of sodium-dibutylnaphthalene sulfonate, for example, is increased by the addition of diamyl phenol, tert. octyl phenol, aliphatic ketones (such as methylhexyl ketone), or ethers. Davidson [7] quotes a sinking time of 14–17 seconds for a 0.1% solution of teepol in the Draves test; when 0.02% pine oil is added, the sinking time is reduced to 3–4 sec. Pine oil shows a synergistic effect with soap and Turkey red oil.

**Experimental Determination.**    The most commonly used test method for the wetting effect was developed by Draves and Clarkson [8]. A 5-g skein of cotton yarn, standard quality (gray, 40 s/2), weighted at the lower end, is introduced into the solution. (Unfortunately different investigators have used different weights so that their results are not comparable.) Initially the skein floats because of entrapped air but it sinks after the skein has become thoroughly wetted. (The air spaces within the skein are comparatively large, and wetting is not due to capillary action. The penetration of a liquid into capillaries cannot be accelerated by wetting agents.) The time required to make the skein sink is the measure of the wetting effect of the solution. A few typical values, taken with 0.05% solutions of wetting agents in distilled water at 30°C, with a load of 1.5 g [9], follow:

| | |
|---|---|
| Aerosol OT (Na · dioctyl sulfosuccinate) | 7 sec |
| Igepon T (Na · N-methyl oleyl taurine) | 45 sec |
| Duponol WA (Na · lauryl sulfate) | 118 sec |
| Potassium coconut oil soap | more than 180 sec |
| Pure water | more than  8 hr |

Unfortunately the test is not really reproducible and completely fails if "Draves sinking time" is less than 4 seconds and more than 180 seconds [10].

A similar test is described by Seyfert and Morgan [11] in which a canvas disk is floated below the surface of the solution and the time it requires to sink by its own weight is measured.

Although these tests are simple and easy enough to carry out, they nevertheless necessitate cotton skeins or canvas disks to meet the standardized requirements of the testing methods. Sometimes quick laboratory tests of the wetting effect of some preparations are needed when no Draves cotton skeins happen to be available. We suggest the following test as a simple rough method of comparing the wetting effects of different surfactants:

Prepare a solution of the surfactant, say 1 % in water or in the liquid in which it is to be applied, and allow a number of drops, say 10–20, to drip slowly into a beaker. The total weight of these drops is determined. If this test is repeated with different surfactants in the same way and with the same pipet the substance whose solution has the smallest drop weight is usually the best wetting agent.

Actually this method measures surface tension rather than wetting action. Hartley and Brown have even worked out an accurate method of determining surface tension on the basis of drop size. Generally, however, the reduction of the surface tension and the wetting effect are directly related, as demonstrated by Fischer and Gans [12]. In a similar way the interfacial tension between two liquids can be determined by filling a beaker with the lighter liquid and the pipet with the denser liquid and positioning the pipet in the beaker so that its tip is below the surface of the liquid. A definite number of drops is then allowed to fall and their total weight established. In this test the surfactant may be in the denser, in the lighter, or in both phases.

It is absolutely essential in these tests that the pipet, and in particular its tip, is perfectly clean before starting each test.

## The Foaming Effect

**Practical Significance.**    Foam development that occurs during the application of cleansing agents is actually an unimportant side effect and probably has little to do with the cleansing process. However, the public has long been accustomed to associating ample lathering with good cleansing action and a nonfoaming detergent appears somehow to be unnatural and unsatisfactory. This attitude may well go back to the position that soap has enjoyed for centuries. It is quite true that if the water is not too hard soap will lather as long as it is active and failure to do so means that it has been used up; that is, the major part of the soap ions have been bound to fat and dirt particles. With many of the new synthetic detergents, foam development and cleansing action are no longer identical, but as long as the public retains this prejudice manufacturers of cosmetic cleansing agents will be forced to include the foaming effect in their preparations. Moreover, foaming in some cosmetic preparations does not serve simply to indicate cleansing action. In shaving soaps a firm fine bubble lather helps to keep the beard erect. In bubble baths the foam is actually the main purpose.

**Principle.**  The mechanism of foam development and stability and the part surfactants play in these processes are complicated and even today not completely understood. Darvichian [13] and De Vries [14] give good accounts of the present state of knowledge. In any case, an important part is played by the reduction of surface tension and the formation of liquid "crystals" of the surfactant molecules (similar in structure to elongated micells) in the foam bubble wall. The formation of a "liquid surface layer" of surfactant molecules is essential; hence only substances capable of forming such films will be good foam producers. Mixtures of two surfactants in some cases achieve quicker lathering as well as greater foam stability than either surfactant by itself (e.g., sodium lauryl sulfate and caprylic acid diethanol-amide); in other instances lathering is reduced (e.g., sodium lauryl sulfate and soap). As in nearly all surface phenomena, foam development is often affected by the salt concentration in the solvent. Again, there are no general rules: in some surfactants foam development increases if the salt concentration is increased (e.g., the esters of sulfosuccinic acid); in others it is hardly affected (e.g., many of the nonionic surfactants); again in others foam formation fails if the water contains a small amount of salt, a condition well known of soaps of higher fatty acids.

**Experimental Determination of the Foaming Effect.**  The most commonly used method of measuring the foaming effect is the Ross-Miles test [15]: 50 ml of the test solution are poured into a glass column (100 cm high, ID 5.0 cm). A 200-ml pipet is positioned so that its lower end lies exactly 90 cm above the liquid surface in the glass. The orifice of the pipet has an ID of 2.9 mm and breaks up the liquid flowing through it into drops. Fill the pipet with the test solution. If the liquid in the pipet is allowed to fall by its own weight into the liquid in the glass, foam develops, and its volume is reproducible under test conditions (the temperature during the test must remain constant; Ross and Miles chose 120°F = 49°C). The height of the foam is read immediately and again after 5 minutes so that foam stability can also be gauged at the same time.

Although the results of this test are reproducible, by itself it permits no conclusions to be reached regarding the foam development of any substance in practical applications. Sanders [16] tested a number of surfactants by washing dirty plates that carried definite amounts of edible fat remnants in 0.1% solutions of these substances and established how many plates could be washed until foaming stopped. He found that with sodium lauryl sulfate 16 plates could be washed, whereas with Igepon T foaming stopped after eight plates. In the Ross-Miles test both had shown an equally good foaming effect, and in hard water Igepon T was even superior. Bromley [17] describes a method of measuring foam viscosity and foam volume that is based on a gradual dilution of surfactant solutions.

If a chemist wants to get a quick idea, under laboratory conditions, which of a number of surfactants will impart the best foaming effect to his preparation or how the addition of a certain ingredient will affect its foaming properties, he can do so without the special equipment required by the Ross-Miles test. Even quite primitive methods will yield comparable results; here is one of them: 25 ml of the test solution are introduced into a 100-ml glass column. Shake by turning the vessel over 5 times, read the height of the foam immediately and again after 5 minutes. If the solution is too viscous, it must be diluted with water in definite proportion.

### The Solubilizing Effect

Cosmetics occasionally require a dispersion of water-insoluble substances in an aqueous medium without clouding. The most important example is the perfuming of aqueous cosmetic preparations (e.g., cold-wave preparations) or those with very low alcohol content (e.g., face and shaving lotions). In so-called water-soluble bath oils the main ingredient in addition to perfume is a solubilizing surfactant. Actually the "solubilizing" effect has nothing to do with surface action but is purely a function of micell formation. The water-insoluble oils are built into the spheric or linear micells of the surfactant and in this way dispersed in the water (see Figures 2 and 3). For many years Turkey red oil (sulfonated castor oil) was being used for this purpose. Recently nonionic surfactants (in particular Tween 20) have replaced Turkey red oil to a considerable extent. The quantity of surfactant required for solubilizing an oil depends on the character of the oil. Perfume oils that do not contain too many terpenes usually yield a clear water-soluble preparation if 1 part by weight of perfume oil is mixed with 3 to 5 parts of Tween 20.

The solubilizing effect is important also in the cleansing action of concentrated surfactant solutions: the removal of oils and fats is achieved partly by solubilizing these substances in water.

### The Emulsifying Effect

**Practical Significance.** The most important application of surfactants in cosmetics is as emulsifying agents. There is no need to enumerate all the preparations that are emulsions; such a list would comprise a considerable part of all cosmetics. From the cosmetic point of view emulsions have many advantages:

1. They are easily spread on skin and hair.

2. They are economical because they often contain much water, yet, after having been rubbed on, leave an adequate concentration of active substances on the skin.

3. They make possible the simultaneous use of oil-soluble and water-soluble substances in the same preparation.

4. Emulsions usually break down after being applied to the skin and the emulsifying agent then becomes active as a wetting agent, thus facilitating the penetration of other components.

5. Almost any consistency can be achieved with emulsions, which are more likely to retain stability in spite of temperature fluctuations than anhydrous creams or aqueous gels.

6. The appearance and consistency of emulsified products is generally very satisfactory; they avoid the sticky, greasy feeling that anhydrous products often leave on the skin and the "insubstantial" thin sensation of pure aqueous products.

**Origin, Form, and Stability of Emulsions.**    Emulsions are systems in which minute globules of a liquid (the "dispersed phase") are held in suspension in another liquid (the "continuous phase"). In principle, therefore, emulsions consist of two immiscible liquid phases. Usually in cosmetics one phase called the "aqueous phase" is mostly water. The other phase which may contain oils, fats, waxes of animal or vegetable origin, mineral oils and waxes, and oil-soluble synthetic materials (glycerol monostearate, isopropyl myristate, silicone oil, etc.) is called the "oil phase." If water is the continuous phase, we speak of oil-in-water (O/W) emulsions; if oil is the continuous phase, we speak of water-in-oil (W/O) emulsions. In so-called dual or mixed emulsions O/W and W/O structures are found side by side in the same system. A number of other complicated emulsion systems also exist, but they have little importance in practical cosmetics.

The diameter of the droplets in the dispersed phase may range from 0.2 to 50 $\mu$ but lies mostly between 1 and 5 $\mu$ (1 $\mu = 0.001$ mm). These droplets therefore cannot be seen with the naked eye; under the microscope they can be observed at 200 to 1000 X.

Let us consider the processes that lead to the production and maintenance of emulsified systems and discuss the part surfactants have to play here.

To make an emulsion oil and water phases can be stirred together or ultrasonic energy may be applied to a vessel containing both phases. In both instances the emulsification effect is achieved by breaking the phases into droplets, and droplets of the one phase disperse to a certain extent in the other. If, for argument's sake, pure water is stirred together with pure mineral oil, this emulsionlike system will break down again as soon as stirring is discontinued, and the two phases will soon separate into two distinct layers.

This is not really surprising. If one liquid is dispersed in another in fine drops, it means an enormous increase in interfaces for both liquids in comparison with the situation in which the layers are clearly separated. As previously explained, an interface molecule is in an unfavorable position energetically, and this fact is reflected in interfacial tension, that is, the tendency to minimize interfaces between the two immiscible liquids. In view of the foregoing, interfacial tension obviously opposes the production and stability of an emulsionlike system: the greater the interfacial tension, the less stable the emulsion obtained by stirring two immiscible liquids together.

As we have also seen, one aspect of the surfactant effect is the reduction of interfacial tension between two immiscible liquids. Part of the effect of surfactants acting as emulsifiers is based on the reduction of the interfacial tension between the two phases of the emulsion. This facilitates the dispersion in small droplets of one phase in the other.

The emulsifier may reduce the interfacial tension but cannot eliminate it altogether. As long as there is any interfacial tension left at all, the system will be the more stable, the smaller the interfaces between the two phases. If such a system is left to itself, the small droplets will tend to coalesce into larger units on collision, because this means a reduction in the total surface. The larger drops will continue to combine until finally the system appears in two clear layers, distinctly separated, one above the other: this is the most stable form.

In spite of the theoretical instability of emulsions, they can be left standing for years without separating. This unexpected stability is due to surfactants or, more accurately, to the presence of a resistant film of such substances at the oil/water interfaces which prevents the coalescence of the droplets even when they do collide.

Let us look first at oil-in-water emulsions. The molecules lodge at the interface, with the hydrophobic hydrocarbon chains in the oil phase and the hydrophilic groups in the aqueous phase. In principle, all three types of film—gaseous, liquid, and solid—would be possible here. For the production of a stable O/W emulsion it is essential, however, that the interfacial film be liquid and consequently resistant and elastic.

Strong liquid films are often produced by the simultaneous use of two emulsifiers: one with the hydrophilic part predominating and therefore mostly in the aqueous phase and one in which the lipophilic part is stronger and therefore mostly in the oil phase. Since the preparation of stable O/W emulsions is also feasible with the exclusive use of predominantly hydrophilic emulsifiers (but not with predominantly hydrophobic emulsifiers) we classify surfactants of this type as the principal emulsifying agents in an O/W system. The more lipophilic surfactants with supporting action are described as "auxiliary emulsifying agents" in this connection.

The image of an emulsion being stabilized by the presence of a mono-molecular liquid film at the interface explains the effect of emulsifiers in a simplified way. In reality the situation is complicated by more or less organized layers of emulsifier molecules collecting around the interface in the aqueous phase and the incorporation of water molecules in the spaces between these layers. If an excess of emulsifier is present, such hydrated multilayered structures are responsible for the stability of the emulsion. The development of hydrated layers around the individual drops can also be achieved by adding a substance that tends to form hydrophilic colloids. Such "protective colloids" can be formed by the addition of mucins (gum tragacanth or gum arabic), inorganic substances, such as certain silicates, cellulose derivatives, proteins, lecithin, or polysaccharides. These additives, which need not be surface-active themselves but help to stabilize completed emulsions, are classified as "stabilizers." If a sufficient amount of emulsifier and colloid-forming stabilizer is present, the stabilizing layers surrounding the individual oil droplets may merge into one another. A continuous net of resistant filmlike structures then develops in the aqueous phase which imparts a gel-like con-sistency to the whole system and stabilizes the emulsion to a considerable extent.

Another important factor is added if ionic emulsifiers are used: the electro-static repulsion between the drops of the dispersed phase. In an O/W emulsion with, for example, sodium stearate as the emulsifier the carboxyl ions of the emulsifying agent project from the surface of the oil droplets and this surface is therefore negatively charged. The positive sodium ions which were formed by the dissociation of the soap molecules are in the aqueous phase. These ions accumulate in a cloud around the negatively charged oil droplets. If two oil droplets approach each other, the clouds of $Na^+$ ions also come close. The proximity of these uniformly charged clouds then produces a repulsion force that opposes a collision of the droplets.

An emulsifier for an O/W emulsion will therefore have to meet the following requirements: it should form a liquid film at the interface and it should be ionized. The second point is not essential because nonionic emulsifiers also have the capacity to make stable emulsions.

In W/O emulsions the ion clouds are formed inside the droplets. No ions or electrostatic forces can develop in the continuous oil phase; therefore there is no electrostatic repulsion as a stabilizing factor in W/O emulsions. Here the surfactant molecules often form an interfacial film of the solid type.

It may be accepted as a general rule that preponderantly hydrophilic sur-factants produce O/W type emulsions, whereas preponderantly hydrophobic surfactants act as W/O emulsifiers. A number of theories have been advanced to explain this point; these theories can be found in any work on emulsions and surfactants; see, for example, Perry and Schwarz [18].

If both water-soluble and oil-soluble emulsifiers are present in an emulsion in roughly equimolecular quantities, stable O/W emulsions are sometimes formed (e.g., with both sodium lauryl sulfate and cholesterol, or sodium stearate and stearic acid). In other instances the stability of O/W emulsions is reduced by the oil-soluble emulsifier (e.g., sodium cetyl sulfate and oleic alcohol).

If an excess of oil-soluble emulsifier occurs with a small quantity of water-soluble emulsifier, the result frequently shows a higher stability than a pure W/O emulsion; beeswax/borax creams are examples of this type.

**Separation of Emulsions.**   A perfect emulsion is a system that is completely homogeneous in appearance and consistency and in which the presence of two immiscible phases can be discerned only microscopically.

In practice, an emulsion may appear quite homogeneous on completion but will separate partly or completely in storage. If separation is complete, both phases form drops which may be large enough to be visible to the naked eye; the extreme case of complete demulsification would be separation of the emulsion into two distinct layers. In a partial separation ("creaming") the fine dispersion of the internal phase is retained but the particles settle at the top or bottom of the system; for example, fat floating to the surface of milk.

*Complete Separation: Breaking.*   Complete separation of an emulsion is caused by the coalescence of droplets of the internal phase. As we have seen, this coalescence always produces a reduction of the interfaces between the two phases and is therefore favored energetically. In stable emulsions coalescence is inhibited by the film of emulsifier molecules which surrounds each droplet of the dispersed phase. All factors that lead to a weakening of the surfactant film will therefore obviously endanger the stability of the emulsion. Apart from inadequate emulsifier dosage, these factors are the following:

1. *Chemical reactions.*   If one of the phases contains substances that react with the emulsifier, this may lead to breaking of the emulsion. A few well-known examples of this type of reaction are given:

(a) In an emulsion that has been stabilized with a fatty acid salt (soap) the anions ($RCOO^-$) play an important part. If calcium or magnesium salts are added to this emulsion, insoluble calcium or magnesium soaps are formed and the anions are lost to the system.

$$2RCOO^- + Ca^{2+} \rightarrow (RCOO)_2Ca$$

If acids are added, insoluble fatty acids

$$RCOO^- + H^+ \rightarrow RCOOH$$

are formed. A similar case is the precipitation of polypeptides, the protective colloids that act as emulsion stabilizers.

Calcium as well as magnesium salts and free fatty acids as emulsifiers are capable of stabilizing the other emulsion type, W/O. These W/O emulsions however, do not form spontaneously but can be prepared only under special conditions. If, therefore, an excess of calcium, magnesium, or hydrogen ions is added to an O/W emulsion stabilized by soap, the result is usually not the inversion of the emulsion type but rather complete separation.

(b) If the aqueous phase contains bases or acids in too high a concentration, glycerol monostearate and other esters acting as surfactants are hydrolized and lose their effectiveness.

(c) If an emulsion contains anion-active as well as cation-active emulsifiers, the differently charged ions interact to form high molecular, often insoluble, combinations which have no emulsifying effect.

2. *The precipitation of water-soluble emulsifiers.* We have already seen that an O/W emulsifier must have a certain, though not necessarily very high, water solubility. It may occur in ionic O/W emulsifiers with very low water solubility that the addition of electrolytes (salts, acids, or bases) to the aqueous phase further reduces their solubility; the emulsifiers then precipitate and lose their effectiveness. A well-known example of this symptom is the ineffectiveness of higher fatty acid soaps (tallow soaps, etc.) in salt or hard water, even when its calcium or magnesium content is low.

3. *Microbiological effects.* Some emulsifying agents, for example, polypeptides, carbohydrates, and other mucins, may be attacked and decomposed by bacteria and molds. In other instances the microbiological decomposition of some other component of the emulsion generates substances, for example, acids, which render the emulsifier ineffective by chemical reaction.

4. *Dehydration of the protective mantle.* In many, perhaps even in all O/W emulsions the droplets are not surrounded by a simple layer of emulsifier molecules but by a complicated system which may also contain protective colloids and water molecules apart from the emulsifier molecules. If water is extracted from this system, the "protective mantle" around the oil droplets is weakened. This dehydration may be caused by the addition of electrolytes to the aqueous phase, probably also by heating or freezing the emulsion.

As already mentioned, complete separation consists in the coalescence of the individual droplets of the dispersed phase; to prevent this coalescence it is essential that there be a stable and resistant surfactant film around each droplet. As coalescence of two droplets is, of necessity, preceded by their collision, we may also say that all factors favoring such collision generally affect the stability of the emulsion adversely.

First there is the viscosity of the external phase: the lower it is, the faster the dispersed droplets will move, and the more frequently a collision will occur. Moreover, this collision will increase in strength if the droplets move faster under the influence of thermal currents in the emulsion; the lower the viscosity of the external phase, the faster the movement. This is one of the reasons for using additives to increase the viscosity of the external phase. With W/O emulsions, these additives are mostly waxes, fats, or high-viscosity oils; with O/W emulsions they are usually mucins (gum tragacanth, quince mucilage, alginates, silicates, or pectines) or cellulose derivatives (cellulose ethers or carboxymethylcellulose). One of the reasons for the reduced stability of emulsions in tropical or summer weather is probably the lowering of the viscosity or higher temperatures. Another factor contributing to the stability of emulsions is the ratio of the dispersed and continuous phases. If the concentration of the internal (dispersed) phase is very high (there are emulsions whose internal phase accounts for more than 90% of the whole system!), its droplets are densely packed, separated by only a very thin layer of the continuous phase. This may easily lead to the collision and coalescence of the droplets.

On the other hand, the viscosity of an emulsion depends to a large extent on the ratio of the phases. The viscosity of diluted emulsions (with a low concentration of the dispersed phase) is generally low unless thickening agents have been added to the external phase; and as a low viscosity reduces the stability of an emulsion, a very low concentration of the dispersed phase also endangers its stability.

*Partial Separation: Creaming.*   This type of breakdown may occur with homogeneous emulsions and is known as "creaming." It is not caused by coalescence of the internal phase droplets which results in larger drops but by another phenomenon: the droplets of the dispersed phase move up or down depending on whether the specific gravity of the dispersed phase is lower or higher than that of the continuous phase. A well-known example is the migration of emulsified fat droplets to the surface of milk, where the fat-rich cream layer is formed. Creaming is not desirable in cosmetic preparations because they lose their homogeneity: after partial separation the top layers of cream in a jar would differ in quality from the lower layers. The most important factors related to this problem are the following:

1. *The specific gravity of the phases.*   If the specific gravity of the two phases differs widely, the risk of creaming is increased.

2. *The size of the dispersed phase droplets.*   With a decrease in size, the force of gravity diminishes in favor of other forces in the system and the tendency of the droplets to collect at the top or bottom of the system also lessens. It has therefore become common practice to homogenize cosmetic creams by subjecting them to a process that tears the internal phase into the smallest possible droplets which disperse evenly in the system [19].

3. *The viscosity of the external phase.*   A low viscosity of the external phase not only increases the probability of collision of the internal phase particles, it also accelerates their tendency to follow the force of gravity and migrate either up or down. Any factors that reduce the viscosity of the emulsion will therefore promote creaming. Measures that increase the viscosity will also increase stability.

**Experimental Classification of the Emulsion Type.**   The type of an emulsion (O/W, W/O, or mixed) can be determined by different experimental methods.

*Microscopical Methods.*   (a) If the aqueous phase of an emulsion is tinted with a water-soluble dye or an oil-soluble dye is used to color the oil phase, the emulsion can easily be studied under a normal microscope at 200–1000 X.

(b) Blanck [20] developed a method of coloring the emulsion with fluorochromes (acridine orange and fluoroscein) for observation under a fluorescence microscope.

(c) A method developed by Simmonite [21] does not require coloring of the phases and thus avoids any possible modification of the emulsion pattern by the addition of dyes. The probability that such modification will occur may be very slight but it remains a fundamental objection to any method that requires the addition of an indicator. According to Simmonite, the microscope is sharply focused on the edge of the droplets. When the lens is raised, O/W type droplets show a light rim and a light spot in the middle, whereas the picture becomes cloudy and blurred when the lens is lowered. W/O emulsions behave in exactly the opposite way. This behavior of emulsions is due to the different light refraction of the individual phases.

(d) Carrière's method [22] is based on the same principle. The iris diaphragm of a standard microscope is replaced by a crescent-shaped one which allows light rays to penetrate from only one side (e.g., the right). The emulsion pattern on the glass slide is therefore lighted only on one side from below. If the light shines from the right and the dispersed phase droplets show a light spot on the right and a dark rim on the left, an O/W emulsion is indicated. With a W/O emulsion, on the other hand, the water drops show a dark rim on the right and a light spot on the left. In this pattern air bubbles look similar to water droplets, but the dark rim is much stronger and can still be discerned when the diaphragm has been opened to such an extent that the remaining emulsion pattern is no longer visible. Given sufficiently strong magnification and an adequate screening of light, finer emulsion patterns (oil droplets within the water drops of a W/O emulsion, etc.) can also be observed.

Generally speaking, the main disadvantage of microscopic methods is that good microscopes are not necessarily available to every cosmetic chemist.

Furthermore, the preparation and study of microscopic slides requires some practice. Microscopic methods have the important advantage that not only the type of emulsion can be identified but an estimate of the particle size can also be made, which again permits conclusions to be drawn regarding the probable stability of the emulsion.

*Macroscopic Methods.*   There is a convenient rule of thumb to differentiate between types of cosmetic emulsion: they generally behave in accordance with their external phases. This rule is the basis for all macroscopic testing methods that identify the different types.

(a) *The indicator method* is based on the principle that water-soluble dyes will spread in an emulsion only if the external phase is aqueous, whereas oil-soluble dyes are absorbed by W/O emulsions. Macroscopic tinting tests may be carried out in different ways. The easiest method to determine the type of emulsion is the following:

Prepare two small samples of the emulsion. Sprinkle a few crystals of an oil-soluble dye on one (e.g., Sudan III, scarlet) and a few crystals of a water-soluble dye on the other (e.g., methylene or nile blue). If the dyes disperse, a colored halo will form around each crystal within a few minutes. If the dye does not spread, this halo will not form at all or do so only very slowly. If only the water-soluble dye spreads, the emulsion is the O/W type; if only the oil-soluble dye spreads, it is a W/O emulsion. In mixed emulsions there will be halos around the crystals of both samples.

This test can also be carried out in a different manner: prepare two samples of the test emulsion in two flat bowls and pour an aqueous solution of a water-soluble dye over one and an oil solution of an oil-soluble dye over the other; after a few minutes decant the dye solutions and rinse with the respective solvent. If the surface of the emulsion appears tinted after this treatment, the dye will have spread.

Using the indicator method, double check with both water- and oil-soluble dyes; it must not be assumed that the emulsion belongs to the O/W type if, for example, the water-soluble dye test is positive. The oil-soluble dye test must also be made; if it is positive also, the emulsion will not be O/W but mixed.

(b) *The dilution method* is based on the fact that O/W emulsions can be freely diluted with water and do not mix with oil, whereas W/O emulsions behave in the opposite way. Any liquid may be used that is immiscible with water but mixes with the standard ingredients of the oil phase of cosmetic emulsions without itself having any emulsifying properties (e.g., mineral oil, hydrogenated or nonhydrogenated peanut oil, isopropyl myristinate). Dual emulsions may be diluted to a certain extent with both water and oil. It is advisable to use different samples of the emulsion for the water- and oil-dilution tests because a dual emulsion might invert to an O/W emulsion and would then no longer be miscible with oil if, for example, an excess of water were added. The lower the viscosity of the emulsions, the easier the dilution method. O/W emulsions whose aqueous phase has been thickened to a considerable degree with mucins are often not easily diluted with water. A fundamental objection to the dilution test is that, similar to the indicator test, the addition of water and oil may change the emulsion pattern.

(c) *The washing test* is closely related to the dilution test. W/O emulsions cannot be removed from the skin with pure water, and O/W emulsions are easily washed off. It is usually difficult, and occasionally impossible, to remove dual emulsions by washing. The washing test may be of great practical significance because it is essential to know how cosmetic preparations will react to water. Application to the skin may cause inversion of the emulsion type in certain preparations (an O/W emulsion may invert to W/O after the loss of water, an emulsifier may be adsorbed to the skin keratin and consequently lose its effectiveness, or the cholesterol in the skin fat may affect the emulsion pattern) and the behavior of the emulsion will not be the same in the washing test as could be assumed after tests *in vitro*.

(d) Since water is a polar liquid and therefore a conductor of electricity, but nonpolar fats have almost no conductivity, W/O and O/W emulsions can be differentiated by their *electrical conductivity*. The conductivity of O/W emulsions is considerably higher than that of W/O emulsions because water is the continuous phase. Generally, dual emulsions also show good conductivity which makes it difficult to differentiate between them and O/W emulsions.

Kleine-Nathrop [23] found that the various types of emulsion also differ in heat conductivity, but a comparatively complicated apparatus is required for tests of this property. Moreover, the difference between types is not sufficiently distinct to make the method practical.

(e) *The filter method*, according to Ehrlich, is easy to carry out. A sample of an O/W emulsion spread on a filter paper will soon develop a broad wet rim around the treated surface: the water easily diffuses through the filter. W/O emulsions at best will show a narrow rim, but dual emulsions behave similarly to O/W emulsions and are therefore hard to classify with this test.

**Experimental Determination of the Emulsifying Action.**   Basically there is only one way to determine whether a substance is an efficient emulsifier: an emulsion must be prepared and tested for its stability. The effectiveness of various emulsifiers may be shown by using them in identical systems and comparing the emulsions that result. It is important to use the emulsifier in small doses (about 0.5% of the total), for with the commonly used higher concentrations the major part of the emulsifier does not lie at the surface but within the external phase, where it does not affect the stability by its surface active properties but by a modification of the rheological character of the external phase [24].

A great number of such tests were carried out in the laboratories of the Atlas Chemical Company under the supervision of W. C. Griffin [25/26]. It was found that the ability of a surface-active substance to act as an emulsifier in a given system depends on the ratio of its hydrophilic and lipophilic components. Oleic acid, for example, is not a suitable emulsifier for emulsions from mineral oil and water (O/W type). The best measure of the stability of an emulsion is the particle size (or, more accurately, the dispersion of the particle sizes) of the internal phase. As long as this size does not change, the emulsion may be regarded as stable, even if creaming occurs, because creaming without coalescence of the droplets can be reversed by light stirring or shaking. Once the average particle size begins to increase, this is a sure sign of impending separation of the emulsion. The particle-size distribution is best determined microscopically by tinting the dispersed phase. Lloyd [27] describes a method in which the average particle size of the dispersed phase is determined at the emulsion surface by measuring the reflection.

Storage tests of emulsions may be accelerated by alternate freezing and thawing, gentle heating, or centrifuging, but accelerated tests are generally not conclusive in regard to the behavior of emulsions under standard conditions.

## The Dispersing Effect

**Practical Significance.** Dispersions are systems in which small particles of a solid are held in suspension in a liquid. Dispersions therefore resemble emulsions in many respects but differ in that the dispersed phase is a solid. In cosmetics dispersions are comparatively unimportant. They occur in liquid and creamy make-up which are powder dispersions in an aqueous vehicle. Lipsticks, in which an insoluble dye has been dispersed in a fatty substance, are also dispersions. Dispersing agents are frequently added to soap shampoos to prevent the precipitation of calcium soaps, present in hard washing or rinsing water, on the hair.

**Principle.** The part played by surfactants in dispersions is similar to that in emulsions. Between a liquid and a solid (insoluble in the liquid) a certain interfacial tension always exists which causes the system to be the more stable, the smaller the interfaces. The situation therefore becomes energetically more unfavorable as the number of interfaces increases, that is, with an increasingly fine dispersion of the solid in the surrounding liquid. Surfactants facilitate fine dispersion by reducing interfacial tension.

Because interfacial tension may be small in the presence of a surfactant but never entirely absent, there is always a tendency for the small solid particles to coalesce to larger granules. The surfactant inhibits the coalescence of the solid particles by (a) forming a film around each particle, which mechanically prevents contact between the individual particles, and (b), in the presence of ionic substances and an aqueous dispersion, by imparting to all dispersed particles the same electrostatic charge, which results in mutual repulsion.

Partial or complete separation may also occur with dispersions. In both instances the solids precipitate, usually in a visible layer at the top or bottom of the system. To avoid creaming it is essential that they occur in very fine particles. Furthermore, the stability of dispersions increases with the viscosity of the liquid phase. In many respects the situation is the same as that in emulsions.

In addition, it should be emphasized that to achieve a stable dispersion the solid particles must be completely wetted by the liquid. Air bubbles adhering to the solid particles adversely affect stability.

**Experimental Determination of Dispersing Action.** The dispersing properties of surfactants can easily be demonstrated experimentally. If a suspension of animal charcoal in water is filtered through filter paper (not too coarse), the charcoal, or at least the major part of it, will be left on the filter. If a surfactant (e.g., soap) is added to the water, little or no charcoal at all will be left. In pure water the fine particles of charcoal coalesce to larger units which are then retained by the paper. In the presence of a surfactant this coalescence does not occur and the individual particles are sufficiently fine to be filtered through.

This experiment unfortunately provides only a qualitative but not a quantitative picture of the dispersing property.

The ability of calcium-resistant surfactants to disperse calcium soaps may be taken as a measure of their dispersing effect in water. Baird [28] has developed a quantitative method for this purpose. Prepare a series of solutions of surfactant and sodium oleate in distilled water with different ratios of surfactant: sodium oleate not exceeding a total concentration of abt. 10%; 5 ml of each of these solutions are then added to 45 ml of hard water with a calcium content of about 200 mg CaO/l; 5 ml of this "first dilution" are then added to another 45 ml of hard water. Although the first dilution will usually be cloudy but well dispersed, the second dilution will show mostly flocculation. More than enough calcium soaps are present here to precipitate the soap completely, and the total soap and surfactant concentration is about 0.1%. The dispersing effect of a surfactant is expressed as the amount required in the original soap/surfactant mixture to prevent flocculation in the second dilution. Igepales and Igepon T have been found to be active dispersing agents. Igepon T (100 %) already acts in additions of 8 %; there are then 0.008 % Igepon T and 0.092 % soap in the second dilution. Coconut fatty alcohol sulfates are active in additions of about 40 %, whereas 70–90 % are required for alkyl benzene sulfonates and alkyl naphthalene sulfonates.

## The Cleansing Effect

We have left an examination of the cleansing or detergent effect of surfactants to the end because this effect is really a combination of all those previously discussed. Let us consider an example of the washing process; namely, the washing of a skin area carrying various impurities: water-insoluble solids (dust, sand, and soot), water-insoluble oily substances (skin fat or remnants of creams, etc.), and water-soluble dirt (dried perspiration). If water alone is the washing agent, the water-soluble dirt will simply dissolve and be removed by the water. Skin and water-insoluble impurities will be more or less wetted by the water, brushing or rubbing will dislodge them with the upper layers of skin fat, and rinsing off with clean water will remove them mechanically. If, instead of pure water, an aqueous solution of a cleansing agent is used, water still remains the actual washing medium: water-soluble impurities will be dissolved and skin and insoluble impurities wetted, mechanically loosened, and finally rinsed off with clean water. This fact is often overlooked when cleansing agents are discussed. So-called cleansing agents, more properly described as cleansing aids, act only by heightening the property of water to wet skin and dirt and to hold the latter in suspension.

The first step in the washing process consists in wetting skin and dirt. The cleansing agent (a surfactant) here acts as a wetting agent. Adam [29] microscopically examined the removal of a fat layer from a single wool fiber. The fat, originally present in a continuous layer, first contracted into comparatively large drops which could be detached from the fiber by mild rubbing. A certain amount of mechanical agitation is always required to dislodge dirt but it need not be strong if skin and dirt are completely wetted.

The second important function of the cleansing agent is to keep the dirt particles in the water in suspension so that they cannot readhere to the skin before being rinsed off. Here the cleansing agent acts in different ways: it keeps water-insoluble dirt (dust, sand, and soot) in suspension. If dirt is very finely dispersed, it will be retained less easily than are larger solids by the uneven surfaces of hair and skin. Water-insoluble oily dirt (and this includes skin fat in which a major part of the dirt is embedded) is partially kept in suspension by emulsification; that is, the cleansing agent also acts as an emulsifier. Finally, particularly in concentrated detergent solutions, some of the insoluble oils are incorporated into the detergent micells; that is, they are being solubilized. There is an indication that solubilization may be more important than emulsification because the HLB value of nonionic cleansing agents comes closer to that of typical solubilizers than to the HLB value of O/W emulsifiers. By surrounding the individual dirt particles and oil droplets with a film ionized cleansing agents give them an electric charge. This charge not only prevents collision and coalescence with other dirt particles but also the return of the dirt to the skin, because skin will also absorb surfactant molecules and will thereby acquire the same charge as the dirt particles and oil droplets. This results in repulsion between skin and dirt.

The preceding summary shows how surfactants promote the washing process; the same considerations apply to skin and hair, but the very effectiveness of surfactants also implies some inherent risks in their use.

1. These materials strongly increase the effectiveness of water in the removal of oily matter. However, skin and hair fat also belong to such oily matter; therefore repeated contact with cleansing agents will result in drying the skin and hair (see Chapter 5).

2. Skin and hair adsorb cleansing-agent molecules and in many instances rinsing does not completely remove them. Hence the washing process does not return skin and hair to their original state; adsorbed foreign matter remains. According to Jaeger [30], this adsorbed detergent film may cut off the epidermal corneal cells from their natural fat supply and in this way lead to drying of the skin (see Chapter 5); adsorbed detergents in the hair could result in brittleness and difficulty in shaping and setting.

**The Experimental Determination of the Cleansing Effect** of surfactants has become an almost independent branch of technology, and there are laboratories that deal exclusively with tests of this kind. Although the effectiveness of the different cleansing agents, the conditions for their optimum application, etc., are of great importance to the textile industry, they do not play a major part in cosmetics. Skin, hair and teeth have surfaces from which dirt is quite easily removed and, in comparison with textiles, the amount of dirt on them is rather small. Even the mildest detergents are strong enough for bodily cleanliness. The only problem is to find products that affect the substrate (skin, hair, teeth) as little as possible while performing the cleansing action. This aspect is considered in Chapter 5.

# FURTHER PRACTICAL REQUIREMENTS

So far, surfactants have been considered from the point of view of their effectiveness. In practice, all other properties must be taken into account. A product with excellent foaming and detergent effect will still not be suitable as a base for shampoos if it has an unpleasant odor or a strong irritant action on the eyes. If an otherwise perfectly good emulsifier is unstable in an alkaline environment, it will certainly be unsuitable in emulsified cold-wave preparations. Good nonionic emulsifiers are excluded from certain preparations because they suppress the effectiveness of bactericides. The "secondary requirements" a surfactant must meet may be summarized as follows:

1. The surfactant must remain stable in the medium in which it will be used and develop its full effect. The prevailing pH and salt concentration must not restrict its effectiveness and it must not react with any of the other ingredients present.

2. In the concentration in which the surfactant will be used it must not cause skin lesions, irritations, or sensitization. In preparations that are expected to come in contact with the eyes (shampoos) or to be absorbed orally (lipsticks, toothpastes) the effect on the eyes or the oral toxicity of the surfactant are important factors [31].

3. The surfactant must have no undesirable side effects on the preparation in which it is to be used. In aerosol products, for example, metal corrosion caused by certain surfactants may be important, and in disinfectants any possible inhibition of their effectiveness must be considered.

4. The surfactant must not affect the color and odor of the preparation.

Consider each point separately:

**Effect of pH.**    Soaps are the classical example of surfactants in which the effect depends on the prevailing pH value. As previously mentioned, the surface-active properties of soap are based on their dissociation in water:

$$RCOONa \rightarrow RCOO^- + Na^+$$

The anions ($RCOO^-$) represent the actual surface-active species, but because they are anions of weak acids we must also take into account the following equilibrium:

$$RCOO^- + H^+ \rightleftharpoons RCOOH$$

In the presence of hydrogen ions ($H^+$) some of the soap anions are modified into free fatty acids. From the point of view of surface activity this means that the polar group is weakened considerably and that the HLB value is strongly lowered. (According to Griffin [32] sodium oleate has an HLB value of 18, and oleic acid of about 1.)

With an increasing concentration of hydrogen ions (and a lowering of the pH) the quantity of $RCOO^-$ anions becomes correspondingly smaller; hence the frequent observation that soaps are ineffective in an acid environment. It would be better to say that the HLB value of any soap solution and its consequent interface activity depends on its pH. According to Rhodes and collaborators [33], the cleansing effect under standard textile-washing conditions is best at pH 10.5 and 11, and this result has been confirmed by many other investigators.

Soaps are by far the most important representatives of the class of surfactants whose effect is subject to the prevailing pH. One of the most important advantages of fatty alcohol sulfates and alkylaryl sulfonates is that, compared with soap, their effectiveness depends much less on the pH value because they are salts of strong acids (i.e., acids that are completely or almost completely ionized even at higher hydrogen ion concentrations).

The most important cationic surfactants are salts of strong organic bases with strong inorganic acids. Here, as well, the degree of ionization is largely independent of the pH.

The effect of nonionic surfactants is not based on ionization, and these substances are therefore completely unaffected by the pH. The fact that many nonionic substances nevertheless cannot be used in strongly alkaline solutions, is due to different reasons (see below).

Amphoteric surfactants such as N-alkyl-$\beta$-aminopropionates are at the same time weak organic acids and weak organic bases and therefore completely dependent on the pH value. Actually, however, they are active over a wider pH range than soaps. If, for example, a solution of such a substance is acidified so that the ionization of the acid group is reduced, the ionization of the amino group rises simultaneously. This results in little change in the HLB value of the substance. With a certain pH value at which the carboxyl group (to $RCOO^-$) and the amino group (to $NH_3^+$) are equally strongly ionized some amphoteric substances become insoluble. This pH value is called the "isoelectric point." With both higher and lower pH values such substances develop surface activity.

Some substances used as stabilizers in emulsions or as protective agents in cleansing preparations (gelatin and other proteins and degradation products) also have an amphoteric character and therefore become ineffective at a certain pH (their isoelectric point) through precipitation.

As indicated above, many nonionic substances cannot be used in strong alkaline or acid solutions, although theoretically their action is quite independent of the pH, but in substances containing ester or amide groups (polyoxyethylene ester, sorbitan ester, etc.) hydrolysis may occur in acid or alkaline solutions.

Lecithins, protein degradation products, and other anionic compounds (e.g., sulfosuccinic acid ester) are also unstable in strong acid or alkaline solutions: quaternary ammonium salts may break down in strong alkaline solutions. An important difference between this type of acid or alkali sensitivity and the acid sensitivity of soap is that in soap the reaction with acid occurs quickly (a stearate cream breaks down within a short time if acid is added), whereas the hydrolysis of esters and particularly amides occurs very slowly so that an emulsion that is quite stable initially may start bleeding only after weeks or months (bleeding is caused by water precipitating in visible drops and is a sign of separation).

**Effect of Ion Concentration.**   Here again soaps are considered first, since they are the most important products affected by the prevailing ion activity. The physical-chemical processes involved here are too complicated to be discussed thoroughly at this point. One factor is the importance of water molecules in the formation of micells and surfactant films. The addition of electrolytes (salts, acids, and bases) to the aqueous phase withdraws water from these micells and films and thus reduces their stability which has an adverse effect on the emulsifying, dispersing, and foaming capacity of the surfactant. Flocculation will occur in such instances with substances with strong colloidal properties for example, soaps of higher molecular acids, pectines, proteins, and protein degradation products.

The effect of the addition of electrolytes may be described in the following way: as we have seen, the "required HLB value" in emulsions depends on the composition of the oil phase. This may be an oversimplification; the composition of the aqueous phase may conceivably also play a part. The addition of electrolytes increases the required HLB value of the aqueous phase; in order to develop a stable emulsion, an emulsifier system with a higher HLB value than that for pure water would be required. In the same way the optimum HLB value for wetting and cleansing action would probably also be increased. In these processes the ion concentration is the determining factor. Here it is immaterial whether the ions are derived from dissolved salts or from strong (hence completely ionized) acids and bases. It may occur that substances not actually affected by the prevailing pH may nevertheless be precipitated by the addition of acids and bases. In such instances it is not the specific effect of hydrogen or hydroxyl ions that matters but the ion concentration as such. Generally, polyvalent ions (e.g., $Ca^{2+}$, $SO_4^{2-}$, $Al^{3+}$, $PO_4^{3-}$) have a much stronger effect than monovalent ions such as $Na^+$ or $Cl^-$.

**Incompatibility Between Surfactants.**   In many instances in cosmetics better results are obtained with a combination of surfactants than with only one surfactant. On the other hand, the effectiveness of one surfactant may well be reduced by the presence of another in the same system. Here two situations are possible:

1. If anionic as well as cationic substances are present in the same preparation, they will have a reciprocal weakening effect. The active anions and cations will combine to high molecular salts which are usually insoluble,

hence ineffective. Occasionally, however, anionic and cationic substances may be combined with good results.

2. There are instances also in which, for example, anionic substances behave antagonistically toward one another or anionic and nonionic surfactants mutually reduce their effectiveness. We discuss these chemical effects throughout the book but here we give only one example: although small additions of sodium lauryl sulfate to soaps may be useful, larger additions restrict its foaming effect; obversely, the foaming effect of lauryl sulfates may be suppressed by soaps.

**Various Chemical Reactions.** Apart from the various chemical effects on surfactants discussed here, certain other reactions may also occur between the surfactant and other ingredients of the preparations. These are discussed in detail in connection with individual preparations and only a few examples are given at this point:

Soaps are sensitive to the presence of calcium, magnesium, mercury, and other heavy metal ions. For this reason a stearate cream (with sodium stearate as the emulsifier) would be an unsuitable base for a freckle cream that contains mercury nitrate.

Unsaturated compounds such as oleic acid soaps are unstable in the presence of oxidants (e.g., iodine and hydrogen peroxide).

**Irritating and Sensitizing Effects of Surfactants.** It is absolutely essential that no cosmetic preparation be permitted to cause any irritation (possibly with the exception of hypersensitive persons) or sensitization (see Chapter 5). Each ingredient intended for use in cosmetic preparations must therefore be tested for possible irritating action. When testing surfactants, particular attention must be paid to preparations with high surfactant concentrations (e.g., skin cleansers or shampoos) or those that might come into contact with the eyes (eye baths, shampoos).

Since this question concerns cleansing preparations, the irritation, sensitization, and toxic effects of various surfactants are discussed in Chapter 5.

**Metal Corrosion through Aqueous Solutions of Surfactants.** Corrosion becomes a problem in the preparation of aerosol shampoos, but because it is not a matter of general interest to cosmetic chemists it is dealt with in Chapter 5.

**Antagonism of Surfactants Against Bactericides.** According to Bouchardy and Mirimanoff [34], nonionic surfactants reduce the effectiveness of certain antiseptic materials. Bailey and de Navarre [35] have demonstrated that in the presence of nonionic emulsifiers standard preservatives for cosmetic creams lose their effectiveness at least partially. Quaternary ammonium salts are precipitated by anionic surfactants and thereby lose their bactericide action. An extensive and confusing literature has appeared in recent years about the alleged antagonism between soap and the antiseptic effect of phenols. These problems are discussed in Chapter 4.

**Odor and Discoloration.** In some instances discoloration and undesirable odors in cosmetic preparations are due to the emulsifier used. The strong smell of shampoos based on Teepol is well known; equally well known is the discoloration of creams that contain triethanolamine salts as the emulsifier. In general color and odor depend more on the degree of purity of the surfactant than on its chemical composition. Certain technical grades of sodium lauryl sulfate, for example, are brown and have a pronounced odor, but some sodium salts of secondary fatty alcohol sulfates (chemically resembling Teepol) are colorless and odorless. Triethanolamine pretreated with sulfur dioxide causes no discoloration in emulsions [36].

In view of the importance of the irritating action on skin and conjunctiva, toxicity, pH in aqueous solutions, effect of pH, ion concentration, and metal concentration on the Action of surfactants, especially in cleansing preparations, a listing of these properties for a number of surfactants is included in Chapter 5.

## CHEMICAL CLASSIFICATION

Having considered the effects and behavior of surfactants in general, we now turn to the chemical structure of the most important types. After due consideration I am omitting a list of the most important surfactants commercially available today. If such a list were really comprehensive, it would take up too much space. It would also be of no practical value if nothing were said about the effectiveness (cleansing, foaming effect, etc.) of the product. This is unfortunately not possible for two reasons: first because testing methods are not sufficiently standardized to compare the results produced by different laboratories and, second, because in practice effectiveness depends to a high degree on the conditions of application.

Chemically, surfactants can be divided into two major types: ionic and nonionic. Nonionic substances do not dissociate in aqueous solutions; the ionic dissociate and form ions, one of which then becomes the actual surface-active agent. The accumulation of identically charged ions at the surface results in charges that play an important part in the effectiveness of ionic surfactants.

Ionic surfactants are divided into three groups: anionic (in which the anion is surface-active), cationic (in which the cation is surface-active), and

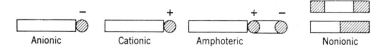

Anionic     Cationic     Amphoteric     Nonionic

FIGURE 4   THE STRUCTURES OF SURFACTANTS.

amphoteric in which the effectiveness of the substance as an anion or cation or both (hybrid ion) depends on the pH. The different types are schematically presented in Figure 4, according to Velde [37].

The individual types can be subdivided further, according to their chemical characteristics. A survey of the most important chemical groups appears in Table 2.2.

A relatively recent problem is that of the biodegradability of detergents in natural effluvia, and most industrialized countries have passed, or are passing, laws in this connection. This involves not only the manufacturers of detergents but in time will also affect the producers of bath preparations, shampoos, cleansing lotions based on detergents, and so on. So far, only detergents used in laundries and cleaning establishments seem to be affected.

The old popular cleansing agent "soap" and all products of simple sulfonation are precipitated and made insoluble by the heavy metal ions, particularly calcium and magnesium, that occur in all water and sewage systems, and render them ineffective by destroying their foaming action. Should soap nevertheless still reach a water-treatment plant it would be broken down according to its chemical composition (i.e., an anionic substance with a straight carbon chain, uninterrupted by substituents) by biological treatment through decomposition by microorganisms. In a similar way no disturbance in the purification process is caused by other surfactants with a chemical composition resembling that of the soap molecule (e.g., alkyl sulfates, fatty-acid condensation products, alkyl sulfonates, and even alkyl benzene sulfonates with only few branch chains) because they are subject to biological degradation and can then no longer cause foaming in sewers, rivers, and canals.

Detergents such as tripropylene-phenyl-polyglycolethers with pronounced branching in their chains or a quaternary carbon atom show a strong resistance to biological attack by microorganisms: they are only partly or even completely undegradable and are therefore classified as "biologically hard" surfactants. The situation is more complicated in the case of nonionic agents; apart from the degree of branching, their length and degree of hydroxy-ethylization are also important. Easily water-soluble ethylene oxide adducts of fatty alcohols, fatty acids, and fatty-acid amides appear to be readily biodegradable.

68

TABLE 2-2  CHEMICAL CLASSIFICATION OF SURFACTANTS

| Chemical Type | Examples, Formulas | Remarks |
|---|---|---|
| ANIONIC | | |
| Salts of carboxylic acids "soaps" | $CH_3(CH_2)_{10}COO^-Na^+$ <br> Sodium laurate <br><br> $CH_3(CH_2)_7CH=CH(CH_2)_7COO^-N(C_2H_4OH)_3^+$ <br> Triethanolamine oleate | "Soaps," until recently the most important surface-active substances, are inexpensive and versatile but acid-, electrolyte-, and calcium-sensitive |
| Protein-fatty acid condensation products [39] | $C_{17}H_{13}CONHR(CONHR)_yCOO^-Na^+$ <br> Maypon | Insensitive to weak acids $Ca^{2+}$ and $Mg^{2+}$ ions; less electrolyte-sensitive than soaps: good emulsifiers; strongly degreasing as detergents |
| Salts of fatty alcohol sulfuric acid esters "fatty alcohol sulfates" [40] | $CH_3(CH_2)_{11}OSO_3^-Na^+$ <br> Sodium lauryl sulfate <br><br> $(CH_3CH_2)_2CHCH_2CH_2CHCH_2CH_2CH(CH_2)_3CH_3$ <br> $\qquad\qquad OSO_3^-Na \quad C_2H_5$ <br> Tergitol 7 | Good detergent and foaming effect; low electrolyte sensitivity |
| Salts of polyoxyethylene monoalkyl mono-sulfates [41] | $CH_3(CH_2)_{11}(OCH_2CH_2)_nOSO_3^-Na^+$ <br> Sipon ES | Good detergent and foaming effect |
| Salts of monosulfate monoesters of polyhydric alcohols | $CH_2OOC-(CH_2)_{16}CH_3$ <br> $\vert$ <br> $CHOH$ <br> $\vert$ <br> $CH_2O-SO_3^-Na^+$ <br> Sodium glyceryl monostearate monosulfate | Good detergent and solubilizing effect; weak foaming effect |
| Salts of sulfated oils [42] | OR  OR  OR <br> $\vert \quad \vert \quad \vert$ <br> $CH_2-CH-CH_2$ <br> $R=CH_3(CH_2)_5CHCH_2CH=CH(CH_2)_7CO$ <br> $\qquad\quad OSO_3^-Na^+$  The $-OSO_3Na$ group may also add across the double bond <br> Sulfated castor oil, Turkey red oil | |

| | | |
|---|---|---|
| Salts of organic sulfonic acids from amides | $CH_3(CH_2)_7CH=CH(CH_2)_7CO-N-CH_2CH_2SO_3Na$ <br> $\quad\quad\quad\quad\quad\quad\quad\quad\quad\quad\overset{\displaystyle CH_3}{\underset{}{\mid}}$ <br> Igepon T | Good detergent, excellent dispersing effect |
| from esters of dibasic acids [43] | $CH_3(CH_2)_7OOC-CH_2$ <br> $CH_3(CH_2)_7OOC-CHSO_3^-Na^+$ <br> Sodium dioctyl sulfosuccinate <br> $Na^+ \ ^-OOC-CH_2$ <br> $\quad\quad ROOC-CH-SO_3^-Na^+$ <br> Sulfosuccinate half (Na salt) [46] | Excellent wetting agent <br><br> Detergent, emulsifiers |
| from alkylaryl compounds [44] | $R-Ar-SO_3Na$    R = Alkyl residue <br> Ar = Benzene or Naphthalene ring | Inexpensive detergent, raw materials from petroleum High skin affinity, colloid-forming |
| Phosphates, sulfamates | $[CH_3(CH_2)_{10}O]_2=P=O$ <br> $\quad\quad\quad\quad\quad\overset{\displaystyle}{\underset{\displaystyle O^-Na^+}{\mid}}$ <br> Sodium dilauryl phosphate | |
| CATIONIC [45] | | |
| Amine salts | $C_{17}H_{33}CONH-CH_2CH_2\overset{+}{N}(C_2H_5)_2Cl^-$ <br> $\quad\quad\quad\quad\quad\quad\quad\quad\quad\quad\overset{\displaystyle}{\underset{\displaystyle H}{\mid}}$ <br> Sapamin hydrochloride | Good wetting and emulsifying agents, poor detergent |
| Quaternary ammonium salts | $R-\overset{\displaystyle R'}{\underset{\displaystyle R'}{\overset{+}{N}(CH_3)_2}}A^-$   A⁻ = chloride or bromide <br> R = alkyl ($C_8-C_8$) may also contain aryloxy groups <br> R' = methyl, ethyl, or benzyl | Wetting and emulsifying agents, but used mostly as disinfectants |
| Morpholinium compounds |   R = alkyl ($C_{12}-C_{18}$) <br> ⁻OSO₂OR'   R' = methyl or ethyl | Used mainly as disinfectants |

TABLE 2-2  *(Continued)*

| Chemical Type | Examples, Formulas | Remarks |
|---|---|---|
| Pyridinium salts<br>Phosphonium, sulfonium compounds | 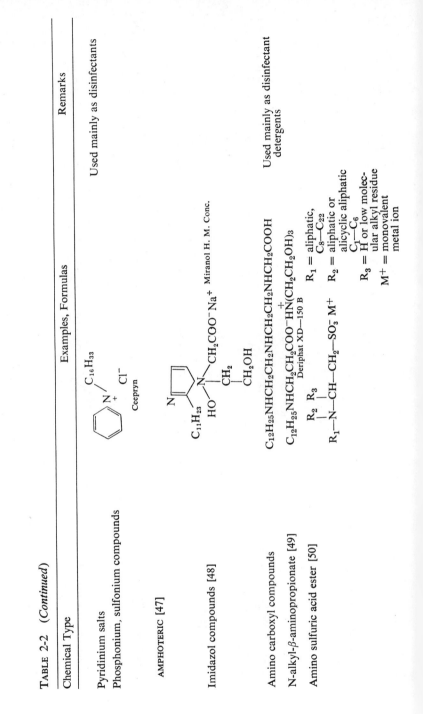 | Used mainly as disinfectants |
| AMPHOTERIC [47] | | |
| Imidazol compounds [48] | | |
| Amino carboxyl compounds<br>N-alkyl-$\beta$-aminopropionate [49] | $C_{12}H_{25}NHCH_2CH_2NHCH_2CH_2NHCH_2COOH$<br>Deriphat XD—150 B | Used mainly as disinfectant detergents |
| Amino sulfuric acid ester [50] | | |

Ceepryn

Miranol H. M. Conc.

$C_{12}H_{25}NHCH_2CH_2COO^- HN(CH_2CH_2OH)_3$

$R_1$—N—CH—CH$_2$—SO$_3^-$ M$^+$

$R_1$ = aliphatic, $C_8$—$C_{22}$

$R_2$ = aliphatic or alicyclic aliphatic $C_1$—$C_6$

$R_3$ = H or low molecular alkyl residue

$M^+$ = monovalent metal ion

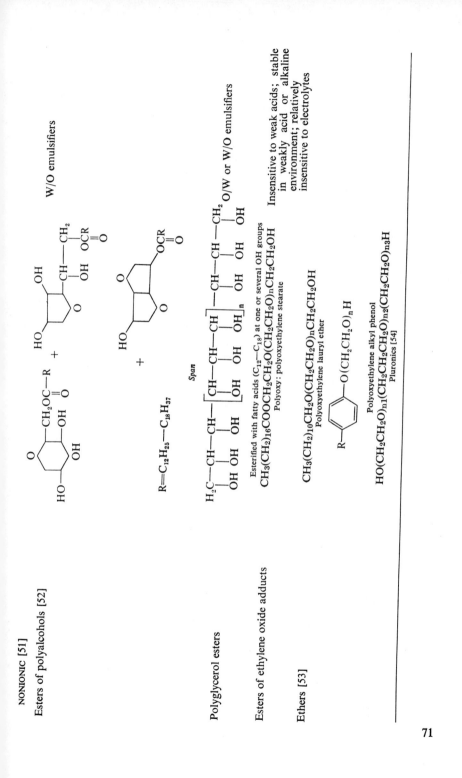

NONIONIC [51]

Esters of polyalcohols [52]

W/O emulsifiers

*Span*

$R=C_{12}H_{25}—C_{18}H_{37}$

Polyglycerol esters

O/W or W/O emulsifiers

Esters of ethylene oxide adducts

Esterified with fatty acids ($C_{12}$—$C_{18}$) at one or several OH groups

Polyoxy: polyoxyethylene stearate

Insensitive to weak acids; stable in weakly acid or alkaline environment; relatively insensitive to electrolytes

Ethers [53]

Polyoxyethylene lauryl ether

Polyoxyethylene alkyl phenol

Pluronics [54]

TABLE 2-2 (Continued)

| Chemical Type | Examples, Formulas | Remarks |
| --- | --- | --- |
| Ester ethers | 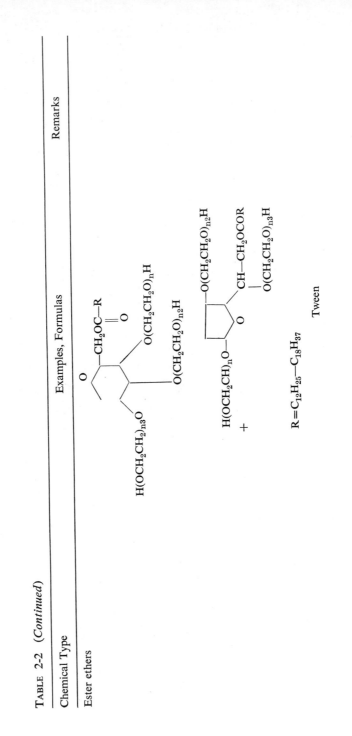 | |

$$R = C_{12}H_{25} - C_{18}H_{37}$$

Tween

## REFERENCES

[1] *Chem. Eng.*, **34**, 4665 (1956).
[2] *J. Soc. cosmet. Chem.*, **1**, 311 (1949); **5**, 249 (1954). Davies, *Proc. 2nd Intern. Congr. Surface Activity* CT 409, London (1957); Kanig, Chavkin, and Lerea, *Drug Cosmet. Ind.*, **75**, 180 (1954); Becher, *Am. Perfumer*, **76**, (9) 33 (1961).
[3] *Am. Perfumer*, **77**, (2), 31 (1962).
[4] Alexander, *Colloid Chemistry*, Vol. V, Reinhold, New York, 1945.
[5] Hartley, *Trans. Faraday Soc.*, **37**, 130 (1941).
[6] Hartley, *Trans. Faraday Soc.*, **37**, 130 (1941).
[7] *SÖFW*, **82**, 461 (1956).
[8] *Am. Dyestuff Rptr.*, **20**, 201 (1931); Draves, *ibid.*, **28**, 421 (1939).
[9] Sanders, in Harry, *Modern Cosmetocology*, Leonard Hill, London 1955. 4th ed., p. 398.
[10] Personal Communication, Dr. G. Carrière.
[11] *Am. Dyestuff Rptr.*, **27**, 525 (1938).
[12] *Ann. N.Y. Acad. Sci.*, **46**, 389 (1946).
[13] *Bull. Soc. chim. Fr.* 15 (1956).
[14] *Revue Trav. chim. Pays-Bas*, **77**, 81, 209 (1958).
[15] *Oil Soap*, **18**, 99 (1941), also U.S. Pat. 2,315,983; Gohlke, *Parfum. Kosmet.*, **45**, 59 (1964).
[16] *Soap, N.Y.* (December 1951) in Harry, *op. cit.*, 400.
[17] *J. Soc. cosmet. Chem.*, **15**, 631 (1964).
[18] Perry and Schwarz, *Surface Active Agents*, Reinhold, New York, 1949.
[19] Janistyn, *Riechstoffe-Seifen-Kosmetika*, **II**, Hüthig Verlag, Heidelberg, 1950, p. 58.
[20] Banck, Inaug. Diss. Kiel, 1954, in *Kleine Nathrop Parf. Kosmet.*, **37**, 547 (1956).
[21] *Pharm. J.*, **163**, 386 (1949).
[22] *Chem. Weekbl.*, **26**, 413 (1929).
[23] *Parfum. Kosmet.*, **37**, 547 (1956).
[24] Riegelman and Pichon, *Am. Perfumer*, **77**, (2) 31 (1962).
[25] *J. Soc. cosmet. Chem.*, **1**, 311 (1949).
[26] Becher, *Am. Perfumer*, **76**, (9) 33 (1961).
[27] *J. Colloid Sci.*, **14**, 441 (1959).
[28] PB 32565, Office of Technical Services, Dept. of Commerce, Washington D.C.
[29] *J. Soc. Dyers Colour.*, **53**, 121 (1937).
[30] Quoted in Czetsch-Lindenwald and Schmidt-La Baume, *Salben, Puder, Externa*, 3rd ed., Springer Verlag, 1950, p. 457 ff.
[31] IV. Report of GKC: "Tenside in der Kosmetik," G. Lietz, Ed. *Parfum. Kosmet.*, **45**, 249 (1964).
[32] *J. Soc. cosmet. Chem.*, **1**, 321 (1949).
[33] *Ind. Engng. Chem.*, **23**, 778 (1931); **29**, 55 (1937).
[34] *Pharm. Acta Helv.*, **26**, 69 (1951).

[35] *Soc. Am. Perf.*, 34 (June 1956).

[36] Wolff, *Fette Seifen*, 142 (1952).

[37] *SÖFW*, **82,** 747 (1956).

[38] Davies, *2nd Intern. Congr. Surface Activity*, **1,** 426, Butterworths, London (1957).

[39] Schuster and Modde, *Parfum. Kosmet.*, **45,** 337 (1964); **46,** 1 (1965).

[40] Goette and Meinhard, *Am. Perfumer*, **72** (4), 90 (October 1958); Felletschin, *J. Soc. cosmet. Chem.*, **15,** 245 (1964).

[41] Felletschin, *ibid.*

[42] Levy, *Am. Perfumer*, **72** (4), 62 (October 1958).

[43] Faust, *Am. Perfumer*, **79** (1), 23 (January 1962).

[44] Harris, *Am. Perfumer*, **72** (4), 62 (October 1958).

[45] Dubrow, *Am. Perfumer*, **72** (4), 95 (October 1958).

[46] Hoffmann, *J. Soc. cosmet. Chem.*, **14,** 591 (1963).

[47] Andersen, *Am. Perfumer*, **72** (4), 59 (October 1958); Mannheimer, S.P.C., 62 (January 1962).

[48] Mannheimer, *Am. Perfumer*, **72** (4), 69 (October 1958).

[49] Freese and Andersen, *Am. Perfumer*, **67** (3), 37 (March 1956).

[50] DAS 1.188.236.

[51] Passedouet, *Parfum. Cosmét. Savons*, **1,** 23 (1958).

[52] Babayan, Kaufmann, Lehman, and Tkaczuk, *J. Soc. cosmet. Chem.*, **15,** 473 (1963).

[53] Milling, *Am. Perfumer*, **72** (4), 39 (October 1958).

[54] Mayhew and Cleney, *Am. Perfumer*, **72** (4), 82 (October 1958).

[55] Santon, *Am. Perfumer*, **72** (4), 54 (October 1958).

CHAPTER 3

# Microbiological Aspects of Cosmetics

There are two reasons why cosmetic chemists must have some knowledge of the behavior of bacteria and fungi: first, because many of the commonest skin diseases as well as unpleasant body odors are caused by these organisms; second, because cosmetic preparations themselves may well become useless when affected by bacteria or molds and will be safe for storage only if preservatives are added. In this chapter we describe bacteria, yeasts, and molds and then discuss the two problems: the formulation of disinfectant cosmetics and the preservation of cosmetics in general.

## BACTERIA AND MOLDS

Bacteria are microscopically small unicellular organisms. In spite of the simplicity of these organisms, bacteriology recognizes thousands of different species. They are classified into three large groups according to their shape: spheres (cocci), slender or plump rodlets (bacilli), and spirals (spirillae). From the cosmetic chemist's point of view the most important function of bacteria is their metabolism because this determines the chemical modifications they cause in their environment. During this process many bacteria induce the degradation of certain components of the skin tissue or of cosmetics and form substances that have an unpleasant odor, an irritant, or a toxic effect on the skin. Although in some industries it has been possible to utilize the metabolism of bacteria (and of yeast to an even larger extent), the cosmetic chemist is no friend of microorganisms; at best, they may be expected to be innocuous but never to have any beneficial effect.

The various types of bacterium can exist under varying conditions and have widely differing requirements for subsistence (some feed on inorganic salts, others require complicated organic compounds); however, each type of bacterium is confined to comparatively narrow limits of survival conditions. A certain type of bacterium will be able to exist only if its environment is correctly adjusted with respect to moisture, absence or presence of air, pH, osmotic pressure, temperature, concentration of nutrients and of damaging substances. In an environment that meets all requirements of any one bacterium it may develop unbelievably rapidly. This development does not consist in the growth of the organism (i.e., the individual cells) but in a proliferation during which many thousands of cells may develop from one cell within an hour. Such conditions occur only in the laboratory, however; in practice the individual types must compete against others also present. It also occurs that one type of bacterium may, by the modifications it causes in its own environment, render this environment increasingly unfavorable to itself until it can no longer survive in it.

If one environment does not meet all the requirements of a given type of bacterium, this does not mean that this type cannot live there but only that its growth is inhibited by less than optimum conditions. Most normal skin bacteria thrive at a pH between 6 and 8 and a temperature between 35 and 40°C. Since, in practice, the temperature of the skin is usually lower and the pH value at about 5, the bacteria "grow" less well than under ideal conditions. In addition, because there is never only one type of bacterium present on the skin, but several species always in competition with one another, the result is a balance in which none of the types present spreads at the expense of the others.

Some bacteria are able to encapsulate themselves if conditions are too unfavorable and form so-called spores that are much more resistant to all external influences than the mother cells and may well develop to reproductive cells if once again they find a favorable environment even after many years.

The fact that germs may in certain instances show a much higher virulence than in others is also partly related to the environment and the absence or presence of competing types. Other factors probably also contribute because there does certainly appear to be a strain of streptococci that is more virulent than others.

*Yeasts* are, in many respects, similar to bacteria; they are also unicellular organisms. The difference most important in practice is the fact that, contrary to bacteria, yeasts all play a part in the fermentation of sugar to alcohol. Although some also appear to be present on the skin, they are not of interest to the cosmetic chemist.

*Fungi* are a large and diverse class of organisms that includes simple unicellular organisms such as yeasts and molds as well as larger plants such as mushrooms. Unicellular fungi are as ubiquitous as bacteria. Generally the following conditions must be met for fungi to grow well:

1. High degree of moisture in the environment.
2. Presence of carbon and nitrogen compounds.
3. Presence of oxygen.
4. Moderate temperatures, the optimum being 20–40°C.

On living skin the moisture content is usually too low for the effective development of fungi. (The skin of the axillaries and between the toes is occasionally an exception.) Many cosmetic preparations, however, constitute an almost ideal culture medium. Spores of fungus molds exist almost everywhere, including the air, and under favorable conditions a few of them may well engender large colonies of molds that can coat the surface of a cosmetic preparation with a black, gray, or green layer; the inhibition of mold growth therefore becomes an important and often difficult problem of cosmetic manufacture.

## MICROBIOLOGY OF THE SKIN SURFACE

### Skin Flora

Normal human skin is always the carrier of numerous germs. Some, always present, are the "resident flora" of the skin; others reach it by accident, from the air or from contact with germ-containing solids or liquids, and are not always present. It has not yet been fully agreed which types of bacterium can be considered the "resident flora." In any case, the presence on the human skin of the following types has been confirmed by various investigators:

*Staphylococcus aureus* (also *staphylococcus pyogenes aureus, micrococcus aureus*) are spherical bacteria (cocci) and have a diameter of 0.7 to 0.9 $\mu$; they can easily be colored with the usual aniline dyes and are gram positive.

The bacteriologist Christian Gram discovered in 1884 that in some bacterial preparations, which had first been colored with the aniline dye crystal violet, then treated with an iodine solution, and finally rinsed with alcohol, certain bacterium cells had absorbed the dye and others had not. It was found that this test made possible a division of bacteria into two groups: gram positive—those that absorb the dye—and gram negative—those that do not. The different reactions in the gram test correspond to other differences in the physiology of the organisms, for example, in their reaction to many disinfectants; therefore this classification into gram-positive and gram-negative organisms has been retained until now. Apart from the gram-positive and gram-negative organisms, those that are "acid resistant" are also known. It is extremely difficult to color them with normal dyes but, contrary to most other bacteria, they retain the dye once they have absorbed it even after being rinsed with acid alcohol. Acid-resistant bacteria (e.g., *myobacterium tuberculosis*) are highly resistant to most disinfectants.

Staphylococci can live in an environment with a pH value between 2.6 and 10; a pH 6.8–8.2 is the optimum. They occur regularly on skin and hair of man and animals and are also encountered in the mouth, the intestines, and occasionally in dust. Their virulence is usually slight, but if they penetrate open wounds or macerated or otherwise irritated skin areas they can cause suppuration, abscesses, or tumors. If they reach the bloodstream, they may cause organic damage.

*Staphylococcus albus* (*staphylococcus pyogenes albus, micrococcus albus*) resembles the *staphylococcus aureus* in many respects, both in character and behavior. Various *streptococci* also occur regularly on the skin. Several types are summarized under the name *streptococcus pyogenes,* one of which is *streptococcus haemolyticus.* Streptococci are, like staphylococci, spherical (diameter of about 1 $\mu$) and easily colored. They live only in the pH range of 5.5–8 and their virulence varies greatly. Strains often appear without any pathogenic effect; then, again suppuration, inflammation, abscesses, tumors, and (if the streptococci reach the blood stream) severe internal disturbances may be caused by the same germ. It must be borne in mind that individual resistance to bacteria fluctuates and probably also depends on the general health.

*Bacillus subtilis* and various *sarzins* are spread by air, water, and soil and are consequently frequently encountered on the skin; they are not pathogenic. In the presence of air *bacillus subtilis* may cause degeneration of proteins; generally, unpleasant odors do not develop. This organism forms spores that are capable of germinating in fats and oils, including paraffin oil, even after two years.

Some bacteria whose culture medium is human or animal feces also occur on the skin, in particular on the hands. The most important type in this group is *escherichia coli,* a gram-negative rodshaped organism that is only rarely pathogenic. The fermentation *bacterium proteus vulgaris* is also rod shaped and gram-negative. It can cause saccharose to ferment under formation of gas and acids and can decompose casein; it is also the cause of the objectionable odor of putrefaction.

On the body areas that are almost always moist and greasy (e.g., the armpits) *myobacterium smegmatis* is reported to be present; this is a gram-positive organism related to typhogenic germs and difficult to color.

The formation of dandruff on the scalp has been attributed to the organism *pityosporum ovale,* although it also occurs on the scalps of most healthy people.

We mention only a few of these bacteria that do not actually belong to the resident flora of the skin of healthy humans but are occasionally found on it: *ebertella typhosa,* the typhus germ, is gram-negative, easily colored, and has the shape of plump rodlets that move with the aid of flagellae. *Clostridium botulinum,* the cause of meat poisoning, grows best in the absence of air (anaerobic). *Pseudonoma aeruginosa* (moving rods, gram-negative, capable of decomposing protein) occasionally occur in wounds.

Apart from the bacteria mentioned, various yeasts also occur on normal skin [1]. Fungi are extremely rare on healthy skin. The molds *trichophyton purpureum* and *trychophyton gypseum* have been held to be responsible for the often occurring inflammations of the skin between the toes which are usually connected with the formation of scales, erythema, and pruritus. Recent results [2], however, show that bacteria and not molds were the cause of these inflammations.

*Trichophyton tonsaurus* causes a similar inflammation of the skin of the scalp, with formation of dandruff and often loss of hair.

## Defense Methods of the Skin

One of the main functions of human and animal skin is to protect the deeper lying organs from noxious external influences. Certainly an attack by bacteria and molds belongs in this category. In fact, the skin does provide an effective shield against attack by such organisms; a microorganism coming from outside is almost entirely unable to penetrate healthy skin.

The following skin properties play an important part in this connection:

1. The continuous stream of epidermal cells directed outward transports organisms, which may have penetrated the skin to a minor degree, back to the surface.

2. The comparatively low moisture content of the corneal layer (keratin contains only about 15% water) is not favorable to the growth of molds and some bacteria.

3. The basic substance of the corium acts as an effective barrier to the penetration of bacteria. The white blood corpuscles, which, in the corium, are partly outside the capillaries, are often capable of destroying invading microorganisms.

4. The always present and normally harmless resident flora of the skin makes it difficult for newly arrived germs to develop, either because it is already using the existing nutrients or destroying the alien germs. Koechel reports on experiments in which staphylococci with penicillin resistance were applied in turn to hands treated with penicillin and untreated; they could no longer be traced on the untreated hands after several hours, whereas on the treated hands they could still be found in large quantities. The penicillin had destroyed the resident flora [3].

5. The acid reaction of healthy skin, the "acid mantle of the skin," probably also restricts the growth of bacteria. One theory explains the fact that the growth of many species of bacteria is restricted in an acid environment because the carbon-dioxide content in any system decreases with an increase of its acidity, and carbon dioxide plays a very important part in the metabolism of bacteria [4].

## DISINFECTANTS

### Significance in Cosmetics

It may appear paradoxical that the skin, the body's natural protection against microbiological attacks, should itself have to be protected against such attacks. It is obvious that in the case of wounds or skin diseases microorganisms should be fought, but the use of antiseptic substances on healthy skin seems redundant, hence undesirable. The partisans of "natural" care of the skin often reproach modern cosmetic chemists, not always without justification, that in their endeavor to help or correct nature they often cause more damage than good.

It is evident, however, that not everything can be left to the natural defensive mechanisms of the skin if we consider just how unnatural in many respects our mode of life has become. Day in and day out we compress our feet into shoes that restrict air circulation and evaporation; men daily scrape their facial skin with a sharp blade, during which process small cuts and nicks are almost impossible to avoid. Furthermore, the result of natural processes is not always desirable from a cosmetic point of view—think only of the odor of axillaries and breath. Allegedly, such odors would not occur in a completely natural way of life in which only natural food were eaten, even if no soap were ever used and the mouth rinsed only with water. It is difficult, however, to check this assertion in present-day civilized society. In any case, the use of antiseptic substances in certain preparations is definitely justified. Disinfectants are today encountered in nearly all preparations used for cleansing or protecting the skin, hair, and nails. They are found in soaps, shampoos, hand cleaners, certain toothpastes and denture cleaners, shaving creams and lotions, mouth washes, body and foot deodorants, hand creams, and barrier creams. Even in lipsticks and nail polishes the use of disinfectants has been suggested.

### Principle of Effectiveness

In spite of the great number of bactericides and fungicides known today and the steadily growing literature about their effectiveness, we still do not know exactly in what way these active substances actually affect microorganisms. In broad outline we may imagine two ways of action [5].

1. The cells of the microorganisms are enveloped by a thin membrane. On the one hand, this membrane prevents the spreading of the cell contents and the penetration of water or foreign bodies from the environment. It also imparts shape to the cell because it is impermeable to many substances of the cell content and the outside world. On the other hand, the membrane acts

as receiver of nutrients for the organism from the environment, and waste products are excreted through it. A very fine balance between permeability and impermeability, an essential prerequisite for the existence of microorganisms, is maintained. Many disinfectants act by being absorbed on the outside of the membrane and by modifying it through a physical or chemical reaction to such an extent that it can no longer be effective.

2. Although it is part of the function of the cell membrane to act as a barrier to substances that are harmful to the microorganism, some are nevertheless able to penetrate the membrane and subsequently to cause toxic effects within the cell by, for example, blocking enzymatic systems.

### Factors Determining Effectiveness

Let us now consider some of the many factors that determine the effects of disinfectants on microorganisms.

**Characteristics of the Active Substance.** As long as we do not know exactly on which reaction between agent and organism the effectiveness of the agent is based, we cannot predict which particular substances will have the best effect. Proteins make up an important part of the cell membranes of microorganisms; hence many substances act as bactericides which react with proteins or precipitate them (phenols, alcohols, and cationic surfactants). The first phase of the action of a disinfectant is its adsorption onto the cell surface. For this reason substances that tend to be adsorbed onto the cell wall from aqueous solutions become active even in small concentrations. Surfactants, in particular the cationic, belong to this group of substances, some of which act as bactericides even in dilutions of 1:1,000,000. The fact that the effectiveness of phenolic substances is increased, the smaller their water solubility, is probably due to a similar reason.

**Concentration of the Agent.** The effectiveness of a disinfectant also always depends on its concentration. Some substances that act as bactericides in certain concentrations may in much lower concentrations (e.g., at $\frac{1}{10}$ of the minimum bactericide dosage) even promote the growth of the identical microorganisms. Above the range of concentration that promotes the growth lies a margin in which the substance does not kill the bacteria or fungi but inhibits their growth that is, it acts bacteriostatically. At a higher concentration the organisms are then killed. Which concentration is required for each of the different effects depends very much on the properties of the agent. Ethanol, for example, acts as a bacteriostat on *streptococcus pyogenes* only in concentrations above 15%, whereas penicillin has this effect even in dilutions of 1:1,000,000,000. Davis, Bloch, and Stonehill [6] describe a method that can be used to determine the effectiveness of a substance in different concentrations.

In this connection it is important to note that the *duration* of the influence also affects the effectiveness. A solution of an agent which acts as a growth inhibitor after short contact may well destroy the respective organism if contact is extended.

The *presence of other substances* may well affect the disinfectant drastically. There are cases in which a disinfectant becomes ineffective because of some chemical reaction with other compounds (e.g., organic mercury salts in the presence of thio or mercapto compounds; penicillin and other antibiotics in the presence of bases, acids, oxidizing substances, or metal ions). Anionic and cationic surfactants do not inactivate each other by chemical reactions but by mutual precipitation because the particles of the two substances carry opposing charges.

In other cases complexes may be formed between phenols and poly-oxyethylene compounds or phenols and serum proteins in which the disinfectant loses its effectiveness.

Disinfectants may be inactivated in the presence of finely dispersed solids by adsorption to their surfaces (e.g., quaternary ammonium compounds with talcum or kaolin powder).

Finally, antiseptic substances may lose their effectiveness by displacement if they have been used in a preparation containing substances that will be even more absorbed by the microorganisms without affecting them adversely; this is the same effect as that of certain skin-protecting soap additives.

*The type of the microorganism* is an important factor because all antiseptic agents have a different effect on the various microorganisms. Some are more effective against staphylococci and streptococci, others against coli bacteria; others, again, are most effective against fungi. Generally speaking, no conclusions can be drawn from the effect of a substance on one microorganism to that on another.

*The environment* also plays an important part because microorganisms show a much higher resistance in a favorable environment (sufficient nourishment, optimum pH and moisture, favorable temperature) than in an unfavorable one. In view of this rather incomplete list of factors on which the effect of a disinfectant depends, it is hardly surprising that it is difficult to express the strength of such a substance in numbers.

### Experimental Determination of the Effect

Rideal and Walker (1903) developed a testing method in which the concentration of the tested substance in aqueous solution which kills *bacterium typhosum* within a fixed period is determined. Phenol is used as a basis of comparison and the tests with phenol and the test substance must be carried out under identical strictly controlled conditions. The "phenol value" then indicates the effectiveness of the test substance in comparison to phenol;

if a 0.1 % solution of the test substance is as effective as a 1 % phenol solution, the phenol value of the substance is 10.

Although the phenol value is still used frequently to indicate the effectiveness of a substance, it should not be forgotten that it has many shortcomings as a gauge of the practical applicability of the substance. Test conditions are quite often completely different from the conditions of practical application. The phenol value which has been established on the basis of tests with *bacterium typhosum* can be used only with the greatest caution as an indication of the effectiveness of a substance on other microorganisms. This testing method is valid only as long as substances that closely resemble phenol in their characteristics and can therefore be tested under identical conditions are examined; for substances that strongly deviate from phenol, for example, in their water solubility, it has been observed time and again that different investigators find different phenol values.

The only reliable test method is therefore an examination of the effect of the finished preparation on microorganisms whose reaction is of interest, under conditions that should be as close as possible to those of practical application. Here it is not only the bactericidal effect that must be checked but also the effect on the human skin.

Testing the effectiveness of disinfectants is a specialized craft that belongs to the bacteriologist's scope of activities and can be discussed here only briefly. A more detailed description will be found in Theile and Pease [7].

1. The preparation (or an aqueous solution of it) is mixed into a culture medium onto which cells of a living bacteria culture are then transferred. In a parallel test cells of the same culture are applied on an identical medium which does not contain the test preparation. A comparison of the growth of the two new cultures will indicate the disinfectant effect of the preparation. If the culture containing the preparation develops much less than the other, it should be determined whether destruction or inhibition of growth has occurred by transferring the cells of this culture to a new medium and checking whether growth recurs.

2. A drop, or a small piece, of the disinfectant is placed on a fresh bacteria culture. A halo will develop around the area of application within which the growth of bacteria will be inhibited. The degree of effectiveness can be measured by the diameter of this halo. The same test may be made with fungus cultures.

### Selection of a Disinfectant

When choosing a disinfectant for a cosmetic preparation, care must of course be taken that it is compatible with the other ingredients of the preparation. The substance must, on the one hand, retain its effectiveness even after prolonged periods of storage; on the other hand, it must not cause undesirable modifications in the preparation. It must not reduce the foaming effect of a shampoo, cloud a hair or shaving lotion, discolor creams and soaps, or have an unpleasant odor.

Substances that are fatal to microorganisms are usually not completely harmless to macroorganisms, including man; they are often toxic, irritating or sensitizing. An antiseptic must be used only in a cosmetic preparation after it has been tested for safety to the consumer in the proposed dosage. At the same time, the dosage must be large enough to achieve a bactericide or at least bacteriostatic effect under standard conditions. The degree of skin substantivity is an important criterion in the selection of ingredients for soaps, shampoos, and other preparations. One method of measurement is sited by McNamara and collaborators [8].

It should finally be borne in mind that every disinfectant will have different degrees of effectiveness against different kind of microorganisms; therefore the particular kind (gram positive or gram negative) of bacteria or fungi to be attacked should be considered; then the agent that can attack this particular group of organisms specifically can be selected.

### Specific Disinfectants

**Ethyl and Propyl Alcohols.**   Ethyl alcohol is the only antiseptic ingredient in many hair and before-and-after-shave preparations. In recent years isopropyl alcohol and n-propyl alcohol have also been used increasingly. With these substances the disinfectant capacity depends largely on their concentration. The maximum effectiveness for ethyl alcohol lies at about 70% concentration, for isopropyl alcohol at about 50%, and n-propyl alcohol at about 30–35%. With lower and higher concentrations the disinfectant effect diminishes strongly. If it is only a matter of protecting a lotion from molds and bacteria (preservation), 15–18% ethyl or smaller amounts of the propyl alcohols are quite sufficient.

**Acids.**   Based on the physiological significance of the acid mantle, professional literature occasionally demands the adjustment of all cosmetic preparations to the pH value of the skin (i.e., about pH 5). Up to now acid preparations have not made much headway because neutral products as well (and this means the majority of all modern cosmetics) hardly affect the skin pH and only rarely have a damaging effect. There are some specialized products that are intended to reconstitute the acid mantle of the skin after alkaline treatment. Hyperacid after shave lotions belong to this category (see Chapter 11). There are other types of cosmetic preparation that contain acids, such as astringent creams and lotions, hair rinses [9] and bleaching creams.

The addition of acid in these preparations is intended neither to achieve an antiseptic effect nor to reconstitute the acid mantle.

Organic acids, such as lactic, citric, or tartaric acid, are suitable for acid mantle restoring preparations. Schneider [10] recommends phosphoric acid esters that resemble lecithin which not only regulate the pH but also have emulsifying properties.

Although the acids already mentioned only reconstitute the acid mantle, others have a specific antiseptic effect.

Boric acid [11] occupies an important place in this category. In medical practice it is used extensively as an antiseptic in treating wounds of all kinds. An inquiry among American dermatologists [12] showed that 94% of them were using boric acid and attributed a good bacteriostatic effect to it. In cosmetics it is frequently added in solid form to baby, body, and shaving powders or in solution in eye preparations. In aqueous or aqueous/alcoholic solution boric acid reacts weakly acid; in the presence of glycerol or sorbitol a very strong acid due to complex formation develops. Free boric acid (not its salts) easily penetrates the skin. Perhaps its palliative and antiseptic action is due partly to this property, but internal poisoning is also a risk if larger amounts of boric acid are applied to the skin surface. For this reason boric acid is prohibited in baby powders in the United States, although many American dermatologists consider it harmless if used normally. Undecylenic acid and its salts have fungistatic properties and are used specially in footcare preparations. The monoethanolamide of this acid is also reported to have fungicide and bacteriostatic effects. The same effects are found in the sulfo-succinic-acid ester of the amide [13] which is surface active and tends to be strongly adsorbed on the skin. This ester seems to offer interesting possibilities as a shampoo ingredient.

Several polyunsaturated fatty acids inhibit the growth of bacteria and fungi. Sorbic acid ($CH_3$—CH=CH—CH=CH—COOH) and its salts are used as preservatives not only in cosmetics but also in food [14]. Since the active component is the undissociated acid, sorbic acid is more effective in the acid than the neutral range and largely loses its effectiveness above pH 7. In neutral or alkaline products the low alkyl esters of sorbic acid may be used [15]. Sorbic acid and its esters have the advantage that they are not, like phenolic preservatives, rendered ineffective by nonionic emulsifiers in certain circumstances.

Bacteriostatic effect is also attributed to the polyunsaturated fatty acids that are present in several oils, particularly cod-liver oil. This may possibly be due to peroxides [16] which develop when thin layers of these oils are exposed to air.

Triacetin (glycerol triacetate) is in itself a neutral substance but is believed to be effective by splitting off acetic acid in low concentrations under the influence of skin enzymes [17]. It is effective as a fungicide [18]. Salicylic acid and benzoic acid are discussed in the next section, even though this is not quite justified from a chemical point of view.

**Phenols.**   The oldest known disinfectant is phenol itself; it was introduced into surgery by Sir Joseph Lister in 1867. Probably phenol owes its bactericide effect to its capacity to decompose or modify the cellular proteins of bacteria, but since it also affects the cells of the carrier it acts as a skin irritant and may also cause internal poisoning because it easily penetrates the skin. For these reasons substances that would be more effective as bactericides than phenol were sought so that they could be used in smaller concentrations and have no toxic effects on the human organism. Paul Ehrlich found (1906) that phenols containing a methyl group or halogen atoms are more effective against diphtheria bacilli than phenol itself and in many cases less toxic. Later it was established that the bactericide effect of alkyl phenols depends on the length of the alkyl group, that polyalkyl phenols also show an increased effectiveness, and, finally, that some compounds with two phenol rings have a particularly strong antibacterial effect, especially against gram-positive bacteria. During the search for highly effective substances compromises between effectiveness and solubility often become necessary; for example, with alkyl phenols whose effectiveness against *staphylococcus aureus* and other gram-positive bacteria increases with a growing alkyl chain, whereas their water solubility becomes too slight for practical purposes if the chain contains more then nine carbon atoms. The effectiveness of substances with a low solubility may be increased by solubilization [see Russell and Hoch [19]. An extensive study of the composition and effectiveness of bisphenols is given by Gump and Walter [20].

A great variety of phenolic compounds with no deleterious effect on humans in concentrations that act effectively against microorganisms is known today. Their water solubility is usually very low but small amounts can be brought into solution in the form of the sodium salt which usually has the same effectiveness as free phenol. No difficulties are encountered in incorporating low concentrations of these substances in most cosmetic products because they have a certain solubility in fats, oils, ethyl and propyl alcohols, propylene glycol, ethylene glycol monomethylether, and other cosmetic raw materials. Since they are chemically stable and also retain their effectiveness when added to cosmetic preparations, phenols are today the most commonly used preservatives and disinfectants.

The only important classes of substances with which phenols cannot be combined without losing their effectiveness are the polyoxyethylene compounds (polyglycols, polywaxes, and most of the nonionic surfactants), unsaturated acids and their esters or salts (e.g., sodium oleate), and proteins or certain protein degradation products. Phenols play a minor part in medicine because almost all of them are inactivated in the presence of blood serum and cannot therefore be used internally.

There are also a great number of phenolic compounds that are rarely used as preservatives but rather as active substances in soaps or other cosmetic preparations.

The idea of a disinfectant phenol soap is not new; this type of product has been marketed since the beginning of the century, but the question whether such products have any effect beyond the bacteria-removing property of the soap itself has always been raised. R. Heu [21] gives a historical survey of this question. The main argument against using phenols in soaps was that their effectiveness is limited to their being free (as acids) and therefore they must lose this effectiveness when they are mixed in alkaline soap. Partisans of phenolic soaps, on the other hand, stressed that low-solubility phenols increase their water solubility in combination with soaps and therby increase their effectiveness. The experimental data about the effectiveness of phenolic soaps were also contradictory, probably because of the use of different soaps and different test organisms.

Today the question has been decided completely in favor of phenolic soaps substantiated by the fact that in the United States about one third of all toilet soaps sold contains some disinfectant substance, usually a phenol. Although phenolic soaps were once used mostly by doctors, and especially surgeons, they are today bought by the general public. Regular use of these soaps can lead to deodorant (removal of axillary perspiration odor) and disinfectant (inhibition of skin infections) effects.

Agreement has been reached that phenolic compounds can develop disinfectant effects if the soap is suitably formulated (low in unsaturated acids and a small excess of lye).

There are still many conflicting opinions regarding the range of effectiveness required for a good disinfectant for soaps. On the one hand there is the opinion that substances like G-11, which are particularly effective against gram-positive staphylococci and streptococci, are most suitable for disinfectant soaps because the resident flora of the skin, which is responsible for body odors and small infections, consists for 95% of these gram-positive organisms. Other investigators object that such drastic interference with the resident flora is undesirable because it would considerably disturb the natural microbiological balance of the skin surface. They would prefer a disinfectant that acts less strongly on the gram-positive organisms but would also include in its range of effectiveness gram-negative organisms (constituting many pathogenic germs) and fungi [23]. Which of these two opinions is correct can be proved only by comparative clinical studies.

*Hexachlorophene* [G-11 or 2,2'-methylene-bis(3,4,6-trichlorophenol)] was the first bactericide that could be proved to strengthen the effect of soaps on the microbiological skin flora. Previous trials with other phenols had mostly shown unsatisfactory results, probably due to technical difficulties and loss of effectiveness in the soap. Even small additions of hexachlorophene to soap retain their effectiveness. According to Jacobsen [24], the substance still acts as a growth inhibitor on staphylococci in a 1:4,000,000 dilution.

The effect of hexachlorophene soaps *in vivo* is increased by traces of hexachlorophene retained on the skin after each application [25]. With soaps that contain 1.5–2% hexachlorophene, the skin germs are reduced to about 5% of their original number and remain on this low level as long as these disinfectant soaps are in regular use. No diminution of the skin flora has been observed when standard nondisinfectant soaps are used [26]. Studies by Killian [27] and Traub [28] show that this reduction of germs following the use of hexachlorophene soaps results in a deodorant effect and a decrease in skin infections. It should be borne in mind that these results are obtained only with regular, not with occasional, use of these soaps.

As with all disinfectants, the effectiveness of hexachlorophene varies for different germs. It is excellent against gram-positive staphylococci and streptococci but much less against gram-negative rods (coli etc.). The objections against a "one-sided" antiseptic have been mentioned above.

Hexachlorophene has also proved satisfactory in emulsified products (deodorant creams, hand creams), aqueous-alcoholic solutions (shaving lotions, deodorant sticks), fatty mixtures (antiseptic lipsticks), baby powders, and shampoos and has even been added to toothpaste.

*Dichlorophene* ["G-4," 2,2'methyl-bis-(4-chlorophenol)] is closely related to hexachlorophene, which it surpasses in fungicide effect and is therefore recommended for certain hair and foot preparations.

*Dichloro-m-xylenol* ("XX DCMX," 2,4-dichloro-3,5-dimethylphenol) is reported to have an effectiveness in soaps similar to that of hexachlorophene [29]. It is probably less effective against gram-positive and more effective against gram-negative organisms than hexachlorophene. It is also recommended as a preservative for cosmetic products.

*Actamer* (Monsanto) again resembles hexachlorophene more in its chemical composition [(2,2'-Thio-bis (4,6-dichlorophenol)] and effect, and like it acts primarily against gram-positive skin bacteria. Usage tests of Actamer in soaps showed a higher effectiveness than hexachlorophene at identical concentrations. After 12 days of regular use a soap containing 2% Actamer reduced the number of skin germs to 2.6% of the original and 1% Actamer soap to 8% of the original [30]. The greater effectiveness of Actamer compared with hexachlorophene is attributed to its closer adherence to the skin.

Closely related to Actamer is "S-7" [(bis-(2-hydroxy-5-chlorophenyl)

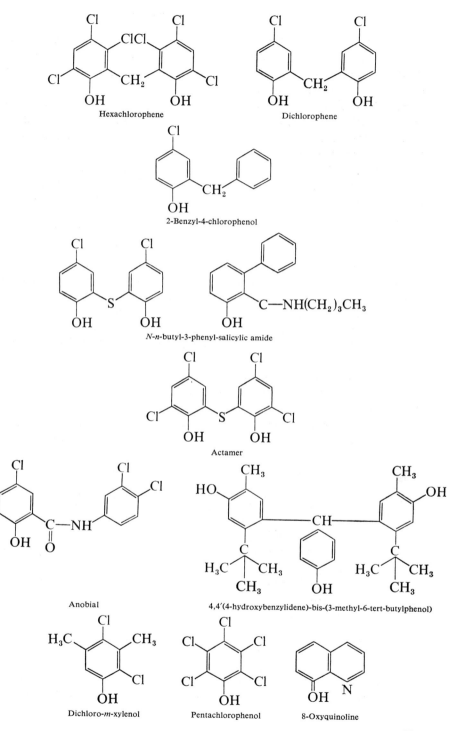

Hexachlorophene

Dichlorophene

2-Benzyl-4-chlorophenol

N-n-butyl-3-phenyl-salicylic amide

Actamer

Anobial

4,4'(4-hydroxybenzylidene)-bis-(3-methyl-6-tert-butylphenol)

Dichloro-m-xylenol

Pentachlorophenol

8-Oxyquinoline

sulfide, Norda Essential Oil and Chemical Co.], which is particularly recommended for shampoos and shaving creams. It is reported to act bacteriostatically against gram-positive and gram-negative germs, even in small concentrations, and to have no toxicity [31].

Hexachlorophene and dichlorophene are poly-substituted diphenyl methanes. It has recently been reported that a substituted triphenylmethane, 4,4'(4-hydroxybenzylidene-)bis-(3-methyl-6-tert. butylphenol), also has disinfectant properties and is effective in soaps [32].

*Anobial* (4-chlorosalicylic acid-3,4-dichloroanilide, Firmenich) is also effective against gram-positive skin bacteria [33]. After 12 days of using 1.5% Anobial soap, the skin germs are reduced to 4% of the original and after 13 days of using 2% Anobial soap, to 2%.

*N-n-butyl-3-phenylsalicylamide* is reported to be particularly effective against mold infections, only slightly toxic, and to contain no skin irritant [34].

*8-oxy-quinoline* is used as a disinfectant in some soaps and cosmetic preparations in the form of one of its salts (sulfate or benzoate). According to Zentmayer [35], its bactericide effect is due to its capacity to bind traces of heavy metals (which are essential for the survival of microorganisms) through complex formation. However, 8-oxyquinoline has been mentioned as possibly being carcinogenic [35a]; it would be important to study this point closer.

*2-benzyl-4-chlorophenol* (Ketolin H) [36] is reported to have a high bactericide capacity and to inhibit the growth of skin fungi even in 0.005% solutions. It is odorless and almost nontoxic.

*Pentachlorophenol* is used as a sodium salt. Although it has a good bactericide effect, it is not suitable for use in soaps because it does not adhere to the skin and has no lasting action [37].

Recently a number of halogenated salicylic anilides have been recommended as cosmetic and pharmaceutical preservatives [38], particularly Geigy's 3,5,4'-tetrachlorosalicylic anilide. ("Irgasan BS 200") [39] was considered as an antiseptic for soaps, but it was later established that this substance may cause photodermatites [40].

Diaphene, a synergistic mixture of 5,4-dibromo and 3,5,4'-tribromo salicylic anilides, may be used as an effective antimicrobic agent in soaps, cosmetics, and external pharmaceuticals. It is a broad-spectrum disinfectant, particularly against gram-positive bacteria. Additions of 0.01–0.2% impart effectiveness to these preparations.

**Surfactants.** In many cases the effect of disinfectant preparations is increased by ionic surfactants. They break up bacteria conglomerations and thereby facilitate the wetting of the germs by the disinfectant solution. The effect of active agents with little solubility is increased if they are incorporated into the micells of the surfactants [41] and, finally, some surfactants have a certain disinfectant action of their own.

The affinity of ionic surfactants for proteins is well known; the formation of sediments on adding a surfactant solution to an aqueous protein solution has often been observed. By attaching themselves to certain positions of the protein molecule surfactants can also modify its spatial configuration.

The first phase of the process in which a surfactant destroys bacterial cells consists in its adsorption on the cell surface. It is not known whether this is followed by the inactivation of important enzymatic systems or the destruction of the semipermeable cellular membrane, which would lead to the emptying of the cell; actually the mechanism may differ, depending on the surfactant or microorganisms involved.

*Anionic.* According to Roelcke and Reichel [42], only the $C_8$–$C_{18}$ saturated soaps are effective against *b. typhi*, the maximum effect being at $C_{12}$. According to Lhoest, Bolle, Stein, and Chodat [43], Duponol C (a commercial product based on sodium lauryl sulfate) in 0.1–0.2 % solution acts as a growth inhibitor and partly as a germicide against *E. coli, pseudomonas fluorescens, proteus vulg.*, and as a growth inhibitor only against *micrococcus pyogenes aureus* and *b. subtilis*. Kaden [44] observed growth-inhibiting effects with 0.7% solutions and germicidal action with 1.4% solutions against various skin fungi and yeasts. Cutter and Wilson [45] report growth inhibition on some yeasts by a 0.5% solution of sodium dodecylbenzene sulfonate, which, however, was canceled out by small additions of lecithin, sodium oleate or stearate, or Tween 40.

The effect of anionic surfactants is presumably also weakened by various additives; otherwise it would be hard to explain why cosmetic preparations containing a few percent of anionic substances are attacked by bacteria and mold unless they contain additional preservatives. Anionic surfactants therefore have no practical significance as disinfectants in cosmetics.

*Nonionic.* Nonionic surfactants not only have no disinfectant action of their own but even reduce that of other disinfectants and preservatives in the same preparation. This is because most nonionic surfactants contain polyoxyethylene chains in their molecules which form complexes with the phenols and often cause them to lose their disinfectant effect.

*Cationic.* The isoelectric point of most natural proteins lies in the acid range. This indicates that they have more strongly dissociated anionic than cationic centers. Consequently human skin and microorganisms whose surfaces contain proteins will have a negative charge in contact with a neutral aqueous solution. This results (according to the principle of attraction between opposing charges) in a strong affinity between cationic substances and skin or microorganisms. The cationic surfactants are adsorbed more strongly on these surfaces than are the anionic. They are therefore more toxic and irritant to the animal organism and have a stronger disinfectant action than the others. To illustrate the effect of these substances, we list (see Table 3-1) some of the data supplied by the manufacturers (Rohm & Haas Corp., Philadelphia) about "Hyamine 2389" (a preparation based on alkyl cetylmethyl trimethyl ammonium chloride and containing 50% active substance, in which "alkyl" represents a mixture of $C_9H_{19}$—$C_{15}H_{31}$ alkyl chains). Skin molds require concentrations of 0.04–0.2%.

TABLE 3-1

| Organism | Minimum Growth-Inhibiting Concentration | Minimum Germicidal Concentration |
|---|---|---|
| *Staphylococcus pyogenes* | 0.000025% | 0.0001% |
| *Streptococcus fecalis* | 0.0002% | 0.0004% |
| *Salmonella typhosa* | 0.003% | 0.003% |
| *Proteus vulgaris* | 0.025% | 0.05% |

Nearly all commercial cationic surfactants are quaternary ammonium compounds. In aqueous solutions these compounds have neutral or weakly acid reactions and are stable against not too highly concentrated acids, less stable against alkalis. They are precipitated by anionic substances and can be combined with them to only a limited extent. It does not appear that cationic surfactants completely lose their effectiveness by additions of equivalent amounts of an anionic substance; according to Botwright [46], this would require, if the anionic substance were soap, a tenfold excess. Cationic compounds are strongly adsorbed on the surface of certain solids (kaolin, talcum, cellulose, glass, etc.) whose presence therefore reduces their effectiveness, particularly if the solids are in powder form and the surfaces are consequently increased. The effectiveness of quaternary ammonium compounds is also reduced by phospholipids, proteins, magnesium, calcium, and iron salts [47].

According to their structures, the most important cationic disinfectants can be divided into four groups:

1. Aliphatic quaternary ammonium compounds of the general type

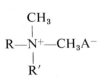

where R is a $C_8$—$C_{18}$ carbon chain and R′, a methyl, ethyl, or benzyl group.

The anion is chloride or bromide. Zephirol [48], Cetavlon, Roccal, Bradosol [49], and Hyamine 2389 belong to this group.

2. Aryloxy compounds with the well-known example of Phemerol [50]:

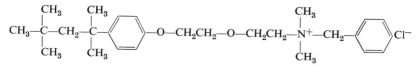

Hyamine 1622 and Hyamine 10X also belong to this group.

3. Heterocyclic compounds such as Ceepryn or Vancide 126 (lauryl pyridinium-5-mercaptobenzothiazol)

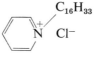

4. Morpholine derivatives of the general type

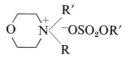

where R is a long alkyl group ($C_{12}H_{25}$—$C_{18}H_{37}$) and R' methyl or ethyl. Compounds of this group are extensively discussed by Hart, McGrea, and Niederl [51]; they are reported to have a strong disinfectant and deodorant action, with little toxicity and skin irritant effect, and high chemical stability.

Data on the skin compatibility of quaternary ammonium compounds is conflicting. As far as the medical profession has worked with these materials, it seems to be of the opinion that they are not harmful if used by experts [52]. According to Botwright [53], patch tests with 3% solutions caused no irritation after 48 hours, but erythema was observed with 10% solutions. The mucous membrane of the eyes is irritated by concentrations above 0.2%, and concentrations above 0.5–1.0% may cause permanent damage. Caution is therefore required when cationic compounds are used in shampoos. According to Woodward and Calvery [54], the $LD_{50}$ of alkyl dimethyl benzyl ammonium chloride for rats if taken orally is 0.35 g/kg.

Botwright recommends the following concentration for using these materials in various cosmetic products: antiseptic powders, 0.05–0.2%; mouth rinses, 0.02–0.04% of the solution diluted for use; toothpastes and powders, 0.25%; liquid or cream deodorants up to 2%.

*Amphoteric.* The molecules of these compounds contain both anionic and cationic groups; an example would be the hydrochloride of

$$C_{12}H_{25}—NH—CH_2CH_2NHCH_2CH_2NHCH_2COOH$$

D. A. G.

Amphoteric compounds react less strongly with proteins in aqueous solutions then cationic agents (instead of heavy sedimentation, only clouding occurs as a rule) and, compared with them, also have a good cleansing effect. They share with cationic substances the disinfectant action which is, however, less pronounced with amphoteric products.

Commercial examples of amphoteric detergents are the "Deriphats" of General Mills (N alkyl-$\beta$-aminopropionate, $RNHCH_2CH_2COO^-X^+$)[55] and "Miranols" or Miranol Co. (Imidazol compounds, e.g., Miranol HM):

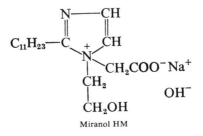

Miranol HM

**Iodine Complexes.**   For many years tincture of iodine has been standard in nearly all home medicine cabinets for use as an antiseptic for small wounds. Until a short time ago the disinfectant properties of iodine could not be utilized in cosmetics: it acts as an irritant in simple solution, its color leaves spots on textiles, and the solutions corrode metal. It has now been established that iodine-surfactant complexes have none of these disadvantages (nonionic surfactants are particularly suitable; e.g., polyethylene glycol ether of nonylphenol). These complexes are termed iodophores [56] and are recommended for various cosmetic applications, especially for disinfectant shampoos [57]. Iodine forms complexes with quaternary ammonium compounds that are highly effective bactericides and are even compatible with anionic detergents.

**Sulfur Compounds.**   We are discussing sulfur and the various sulfur compounds under the same heading merely for reasons of easier reference. This does not imply that in all cases the effect is due to the sulfur content and that these substances all act in the same way. The effectiveness of elementary sulfur, for example, is based on its effect on the oxidation state of the cells into which it penetrates; sulfonamides kill bacteria by their antagonistic action on the metabolism of $p$-aminobenzoic acid. For many of the following substances the basis of their effectiveness is not yet known.

Sulfur itself, one of the oldest materials in dermatology, is still widely used in the treatment of acne, scabies, seborrhoea, and certain fungus infections. Its action is keratolytic, keratoplastic, and disinfectant, with colloidal sulfur being the most effective. Sulfur is used in certain antiseptic hair lotions and shampoos, but it is unimportant in general cosmetics because it is not generally compatible and may, if applied to large skin areas, lead to toxic and irritation reactions.

For similar reasons *sulfonamides*, which frequently appear in dermatological powders and ointments for external use, are of no particular interest in cosmetics.

*Captan* ("Vancide 89," N-trichloromethyl thio-4-cyclohexene-1,2-dicarboximide) is mentioned by Stolz and Rogers [58] as a bactericide and fungicide of broad effectiveness. It is inexpensive and may be used in soaps and cosmetic preparations; it does not discolor white soaps. A 1% concentration in soap is reported to reduce the skin germ count considerably after regular use. The composition of the soap is, of course, important, as it is with all disinfectants and as demonstrated by results obtained by Bechtold, Lawrence, and Owen [59], who could determine no effectiveness in Captan in tests *in vitro*.

*Tetramethylthiuramide sulfide* (TMTD) is used in a number of commercial products [60].

*Zinc dimethyl dithiocarbamate* (DMDTC) acts in a similar way. It is remarkable that the two last-mentioned substances were used in the rubber industry in the vulcanization process before their disinfectant properties were known. "Actamer" also contains sulfur, but we have already discussed this material under phenolic compounds.

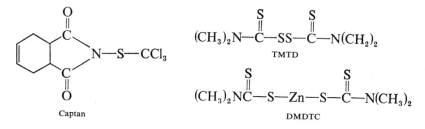

Captan                    TMTD                    DMDTC

B. Tarnoff [58] reports on the effectiveness of zinc-1-hydroxy-2-pyridin-thiol-1-oxide a white-to-cream-colored powder, insoluble in water and most of the known solvents, but easily incorporated in soaps, deodorants, and foot-care products. A zinc-5-chloro-2-mercapto-benzothiazol is marketed under the name "Vancide 30" and is reported to have excellent fungicide and bactericide properties. This product, which is neither a sensitizer nor a primary irritant of human skin, is recommended for use in shampoos, deodorants, and foot-care products. Dosage 0.5–2%, reported to be compatible over a wide pH range.

According to Meinhoff [61], 3,5-dibenzyl tetrahydro-1,3,5-thiadizin-2-thion (dibenzthion) acts antimyocotically and up to 3% is added to ointments or liquids.

**Phenylmercuric Salts.**   Phenylmercuric nitrate is strongly toxic and a skin irritant when concentrated, but in low concentrations it is harmless. Weed and Ecker [62] have pointed out the suitability of this salt as a bactericide and fungicide and De Navarre has recommended various phenylmercuric salts as preservatives for cosmetic preparations. According to De Navarre, 0.004% phenylmercuric borate is sufficient as a preservative for cosmetic creams. The related substance "thimerosal" is reported to be particularly effective [63]. Phenylmercuric acetate has also been used occasionally. Phenylmercuric salts react with certain thiols and become ineffective in their presence.

**Antibiotics.**   The highly effective antibiotics penicillin and streptomycin may seem to be suitable for cosmetic preparations at first glance because they are active in small doses, almost nontoxic, odorless, tasteless, and colorless. Nevertheless, on closer inspection they have to be excluded for this purpose because they have only a very limited stability in aqueous products, and at very low concentrations (or if they are partly decomposed) they can cause the development of immune bacteria cultures. On many people they also act as sensitizers. Recently, several antibiotics which are believed to have none of these disadvantages have been recommended [64]. They are tyrothricin (or the more active derivative gramicidin), neomycin, and bacitracin. Tyrothricin and bacitracin act in particular against gram-positive germs, neomycin (used mostly as the sulfate or palmitate), against gram-negative germs. Shelley and Cahn [65] report that neomycin is especially effective against axillary odor.

According to Pirillä and Wallenius [66], neomycin and bacitracin rarely irritate or senstize the skin. Bacitracin is not compatible with many surfactants and does not appear to be stable in aqueous products in general [67], which makes its use in cosmetics rather difficult. Not much is known so far about the stability of the two other antibiotics in different vehicles. Bech and Gardenhje [68] give a few formulations for the use of tyrothricin. Very probably these antibiotics will gain more importance in medicine and pharmaceutics than in cosmetics.

**Others.**   The substance 6-acetoxy-2,4-dimethyl-*m*-dioxane (Dioxine, Sindar Corp.) [69] is outside any of the groups discussed so far but is reported to have a wide antimicrobic range. It is not inactivated by nonionic surfactants, is adequately soluble in water and many oils, and should be used in concentrations of about 0.1%. Dioxin has a strong odor that merges well with some fragrances (rose, spike lavender, citrus) but not with others.

Although formaldehyde as such is not used in cosmetics, it is slowly split off in an acid environment by hexamethylenetetramine, which is used in body deodorants as a bactericide.

According to Marzurella [70], many of the essential oils and synthetic fragrances used in perfumery have a bactericide and particularly a fungicide effect.

# MICROBIOLOGICAL CONTAMINATION OF COSMETICS

## Extent and Significance of the Problem

The majority of cosmetic preparations provides a good breeding ground for various kinds of bacterium and fungus molds. They are almost neutral, usually contain water and organic matter and often even organic nitrogen compounds and traces of mineral salts (possibly from the water used), that is, everything many germs need for growth. Considering that germs and spores of various kinds are not only in the containers in which cosmetics are first prepared and then packed but in many raw materials, it is obvious that there is a good chance that microorganisms will get into the product and develop into colonies during storage or after the container is opened. Careful cleaning and hygienic working methods can, of course, reduce the incidence of bacterial or fungus development.

Needless to say, the consumer will reject any cosmetic product if it is covered with white, green, brown, or gray molds after being opened. Even if there were no such mold formation, an invasion of microorganisms usually becomes apparent as spotting or as changes in odor and consistency. In other cases it may lead to inactivation by degradation of active substances (vitamins, hormones, etc.). Finally, the application of bacteria-infested creams may cause skin infection; the application of spoiled products, skin irritations.

Discoloration and a slimy texture in shampoos and the swelling of tubes are due to an invasion by bacteria of the type *aerobacter aerogens*, a gram-negative, gas-forming bacillus. These bacteria are often found in shampoos based on sodium lauryl sulfate and may penetrate with the water (particularly if it is demineralized by ion exchangers). Even if no microbes can be traced in the shampoos by bacteriological methods, changes may be caused by enzymes which originate from some bacteria, for example, *pseudomonas aerugionosa* (enzyme pyocyanase). Once pyocyanases are present in the shampoo, the use of preservatives by the manufacturer is already too late; only timely preservation of the lauryl sulfates will help.

The conclusion to be drawn from the foregoing is simple: there are hardly any cosmetics that do not require preservation for stability. G. A. Nowak [82] points out that in recent years preservation problems have become more and more complicated. This is due to the increasing use of nonionic emulsifiers and biological substances; moreover, some strains of microbes seem to have developed immunity against traditional preservatives such as parasept and paraben.

## Microflora of Cosmetic Preparations

Several good reports have been published during the past few years [71]. In some points the results of various investigators differ, which is not really surprising, since the microflora varies from product to product, even from batch to batch. The following organisms seem to occur frequently:

*Bacteria. b. subtilis, E. coli, b. mycoides, aerobacter aerogens, pseudomonas, sarcina lutae, proteus vulgaris,* and staphylococci. All are widely spread in nature and can thrive well under the conditions prevailing at the surface of many cosmetic products.

*Yeasts.* Torula, manilia, and saccharomyces were identified.

*Fungi.* A common species is *penicillium,* found as a velvety green coating on rotten fruit and vegetables. This fungus can split carbohydrates, proteins, and fats. *Penicillium glaucum* also thrives on hydrocarbons. Several kinds of *aspergillus* (green, yellow, brown, or black) are also frequently found. *Aspergillus* needs higher temperatures and a higher concentration of nutrients than *penicillium. Rhizopus nigrideus* (black bread mold) and the silver grey *mucor mucedo* are also widely spread and require more moisture than *penicillium* and *aspergillus.* Nowak [72] describes the occurrence of *botrytis cinerea* in creams. Holt and Carroll [73] traced *alternaria* in creams and established that the fungus came from the inside the cover. Recently De Navarre and Bailey [74] identified *paecilomyces* in cosmetic preparations.

## COSMETIC PRESERVATIVES

### Phenols

This group constitutes the majority of cosmetic preservatives. Table 3-2 lists the main properties of the most important materials. The esters of *p*-hydroxybenzoic acid ("parabens") are of particular interest in this group. They approximate the "perfect preservative" and have received the widest use. Schneider [75] gives an extensive report on these substances; Boehme and Jones [76] report on their practical application. Combinations of two or three of these esters are often used in cosmetic formulations because they vary in their effectiveness against different microorganisms [77] and in their solubility (the methyl ester is more readily soluble in water and is dissolved in the aqueous phase; the high molecular esters are soluble in oil and dissolved in the oil phase).

Compared with free esters, the alkali salts of *p*-hydroxybenzoic acid esters are characterized by a much higher water solubility. Aqueous solutions of these salts should not be heated above 30°C because the alkalinity of the solutions will lead to a hydrolysis of the ester groups [78].

TABLE 3-2  PHENOLS AS COSMETIC PRESERVATIVES

| Name | Odor | Solubility (wt. %) | | pH Range | Recommended Dosage | Remarks |
|---|---|---|---|---|---|---|
| Benzoic acid | — | $W^{20}$: | 0.44 | a | 0.1–0.2 | |
| | | E: | 43 | | | |
| | | $W^{100}$: | 5.5 | | | |
| Salicylic acid | — | W: | 0.22 | a | 0.2 | |
| | | E: | 37 | | | |
| | | HPO: | 1.5 | | | |
| | | MO: | 0.05 | | | |
| Methyl-*p*-hydroxy-benzoate | — | $W^{25}$: | 0.25 | a,n,b | 0.1–0.2 | Particularly effective against fungus mold |
| | | $W^{80}$: | 2.0 | | | |
| | | E: | 52 | | | |
| | | Gl: | 4.5 | | | |
| | | PG: | 22 | | | |
| | | PO: | 0.5 | | | |
| Ethyl-*p*-hydroxy-benzoate | — | $W^{25}$: | 0.25 | a,n,b | 0.1–0.2 | |
| | | $W^{80}$: | 0.86 | | | |
| | | E: | 70 | | | |
| | | Gl: | 1.5 | | | |
| | | PG: | 25 | | | |
| | | PO: | 1.0 | | | |
| Propyl-*p*-hydroxy-benzoate | — | $W^{25}$: | 0.05 | a,n,b | 0.05–0.10 | Particularly effective against yeasts |
| | | $W^{80}$: | 0.11 | | | |
| | | E: | 95 | | | |
| | | Gl: | 1.0 | | | |
| | | PG: | 26 | | | |
| | | PO: | 1.4 | | | |
| *n*-Butyl-*p*-hydroxy-benzoate | — | $W^{25}$: | 0.02 | a,n,b | 0.02–0.05 | The only substance in the series that is soluble in hydrocarbons |
| | | $W^{80}$: | 0.05 | | | |
| | | E: | 210 | | | |
| | | Gl: | 1.4 | | | |
| | | PG: | 110 | | | |
| | | PO: | 5.0 | | | |
| | | MO: | abt. 0.1 | | | |
| Benzyl-*p*-hydroxy-benzoate | — | $W^{25}$: | 0.01 | a,n,b | 0.01–0.02 | Particularly effective against fungus mold |
| | | $W^{80}$: | 0.05 | | | |
| | | E: | 42 | | | |
| | | Gl: | 1.5 | | | |
| | | PG: | 12 | | | |
| | | PO: | 4.5 | | | |

TABLE 3-2    (*Continued*)

| Name | Odor | Solubility (wt. %) | pH Range | Recommended Dosage | Remarks |
|---|---|---|---|---|---|
| Phenyl-*p*-hydroxy-benzoate | — | $W^{25}$: 0.002<br>$W^{80}$: 0.01<br>E: 17<br>Gl: 0.3<br>PG: 23<br>PO: 1.5 | a,n,b | | |
| *o*-Phenylphenol | + | W: almost insol.<br>O: sol. | a,n,b | 0.05–0.1 | Also used in food in the United States |
| Oxyquinoline benzoate | — | W: sol.<br>E: sol.<br>O: slightly sol. | | 0.04 | The sulfate and other salts are also used |
| Amyl-*m*-cresol | + | W: 0.003<br>O: sol.<br>E: 0.7 | a,n,b | 0.01 | |
| *p*-Chloro-*m*-cresol | + | $W^{20}$: 0.4<br>$W^{80}$: 2.0 | a,n,b | 0.05–0.1 | |
| *p*-tert. Butyl-*m*-cresol | + | W: 0.03<br>$E_{30}$: 0.01<br>O: sol. | a,n,b | 0.1 | |
| *p*-Chloro-*m*-xylenol | | $W^{15}$: 0.03<br>$W^{100}$: 0.5 | a,b | 0.1 | |
| "Chloroxylenol," PCMX | + | E: sol.<br>O: sol. | | | |
| Dichloro-*m*-xylenol-2.4-dichloro-3,5-dimethyl phenol DCMX | — | W: 0.01<br>E: sol.<br>O: sol. | a,n,b | 0.05 | |
| *p*-tert-Amyl phenol | + | W: almost insol.<br>E: sol.<br>O: sol. | a,n,b | 0.1 | |
| Isothymol | + | W: almost insol.<br>E: sol.<br>O: sol. | a,n,b | 0.05–0.1 | |

See REMARKS on page 101.

TABLE 3-2   (*continued*)

| Name | Odor | Solubility (wt.%) | pH Range | Recom- mended Dosage | Remarks |
|------|------|------|------|------|------|
| Chlorothymol (4-Chloro-3-isopropyl 5-methylphenol) | + | W: 0.03 E: sol. O: sol. | a,n | 0.02 | |
| Chlorocavacrol (4-Chloro-3-isopropyl- 6-methyl phenol) | + | W: 0.02 E: sol. O: sol. | a,n | 0.02 | |
| *p*-Chlorophenol-α- glyceryl ether | − | W: 0.6 E: sol. | a,n,b | 0.15–0.3 | |

REMARKS

*Odor.* — The substance is odorless or its slight odor is not noticeable in the concentration used.   + The substance has a more or less strong "phenolic" odor.

*Solubility.* Unless otherwise mentioned, the concentrations given refer to room temperature (18–25°C):

W = water ($W^{80}$ = solubility in water at 80°C, etc.).
E = 95% ethyl alcohol ($E_{50}$ = 50% ethyl alcohol).
O = vegetable and animal oils and fats, essential oils.
PO = peanut oil.
HPO = hydrogenated peanut oil.
Gl = glycerol.
PG = propylene glycol.
MO = mineral oil.

Where no values have been given for the solubility, "sol" means that more than required for normal preservation is soluble in the respective solvent at room temperature. The solubility of phenolic compounds is usually much higher in alkaline aqueous solutions than in pure water.

*pH range.*  a = acid, n = neutral, b = basic (alkaline) environment.

*Recommended Dosage.* These values are based on data in De Navarre, *The Chemistry and Manufacture of Cosmetics*, Van Nostrand, New York, 1941; Harry, *Modern Cosmetocology*, 4th ed., Leonard Hill, London 1955; and Janistyn, *Riechstoffe-Seifen-Kosmetika*, Dr. Alfred Hüthig, Heidelberg, 1950.

TABLE 3-3

| Preparation Requiring Preservation | Concentration of Preservative (%) | | |
| --- | --- | --- | --- |
| | Methyl-*p*-Hydroxybenzoate | Propyl-*p*-Hydroxybenzoate | Na Salt of Propyl-*p*-Hydroxybenzoate |
| Boric acid solutions | 0.05 | + | 0.02 |
| Cream: without fat | 0.05–0.15 | | |
| 5–10% fat | 0.05 | + | 0.12 |
| 20% and more fat | | | 0.2–0.25 |
| with hormones, lecithin | 0.25 | + | 0.05 |
| Glycerol jellies and solutions | 0.15 | | |
| Lipsticks | | | 0.2 |
| Vegetable mucins | 0.1–0.2 | | or 0.15 |
| Starch solutions | 0.15 | + | 0.05 or 0.3 |
| Toothpastes | 0.1–0.2 | + | 0.02 or 0.1 |

The only important restriction in the use of *p*-hydroxybenzoates (which applies to all phenolic preservatives) is due to their tendency to form inactive complexes with some cosmetic raw materials. Raw materials that inactivate preservatives in this way are primarily the esters of polyethylene glycols, hence many nonionic emulsifiers [79], gum tragacanth [80], and reportedly polyvinyl pyrrolidone, Carbopol 934, and methylcellulose (but not hydroxyethylene cellulose) [81].

Lach et al. have demonstrated [82] that the esters of *p*-hydroxybenzoic acid form complexes with polyethylene glycol.

Today, parabens remain important part preservatives; nevertheless some substitution or additional use of nonphenolics should be considered in many cases.

Fisher pointed out as early as 1941 that nonionic emulsions react with certain chemicals, particularly phenols. Bolle and Mirimanoff reported in 1950 that a number of preservatives, including the widely used *p*-hydroxybenzoic acid, are inactivated by nonionic emulsifiers. De Navarre was able to confirm on the basis of extended tests that *p*-hydroxybenzoic acid is inactivated in nonionic emulsions; 95% of the propyl ester of *p*-hydroxybenzoic acid is bound by nonionics such as polyoxyethylene sorbitan oleate (Tween 80), whereas 80% of the methyl ester is inactivated, as demonstrated by Kostenbauer and Patel.

The incompatability of nonionic emulsifiers and phenols was recognized during the revision of the U. S. Pharmacopoeia XIII for the fourteenth edition. The calamine lotion of the USP was adjusted by replacing bentonite with a mixture of polyethylene glycol 400 monostearate and polyethylene glycol 400 in order to obtain a smoother and more homogeneous product. However, the emulsion separated when 1% phenolium liquifactum was added to arrive at the official NF "Phenolic Calamine Lotion."

According to Barr and Tice [83], sorbic acid, phenylmercuric salts, Vancides, and benzalkonium chloride are suitable preservatives for products containing nonionic emulsifiers.

**Others.** Some of the other disinfectants already mentioned in this chapter may also be used as preservatives. The main difference between typical preservatives and typical disinfectants is their application: preservatives are used primarily against molds (the main contaminants of the watery surface of a cosmetic product); disinfectants are used primarily against bacteria (which thrive on the relatively dry skin surface).

*Alcohols* are effective only as preservatives in concentrations above 10% and are hardly ever used. Obviously, preparations with a higher alcohol content need no additional preservation.

Among the acids *sorbic acid* is recommended most frequently [84] in doses of about 0.2%. De Navarre, however, mentions [85] that this substance is not very effective at pH 5.6 and higher. According to Nowak [82], sorbic acid is inactive in shampoos. Instead of the acid, the more readily soluble potassium sorbate may also be used.

Cationic substances are only rarely used as preservatives. Many, but not all, are inactivated by anionic surfactants. Occasionally phenylmercuric salts are used as preservatives [83].

Lately there has been some reference to preservatives for shampoos whose effectiveness is probably due to the splitting off of small amounts of formaldehyde: 1-methylol-5,5-dimethyl hydantoin [86] and N-hydroxymethylphthalimide (General Aniline and Film Co.) [87]. Formalin itself (0.1%) is active but causes discolorations with perfume oils containing citral and precipitations with proteins.

### Application

Microorganisms will react to antagonistic influences in one of four ways: (a) they may die; (b) they may encapsulate; (c) they may adjust (develop resistance) and continue to thrive; (d) they may continue to develop at a reduced rate. Every preparation must be preserved in such a way that all germs react according to (a) or (b).

The effectiveness of a bactericide or fungicide substance depends on its "effective concentration," that is, the concentration on the germ surface. This is not only determined by the amount of material added to the preparation but by various other factors as well.

The solubility of the preservatives in the respective medium is important here. In several types of preservative such as *p*-hydroxybenzoic acid esters the antibacterial and fungicide effectiveness increases at the same ratio as water solubility diminishes. This may be an effect similar to that known from surfactants: the agent collects at the walls of the cells (or inside the microbes). When water solubility is too slight, the substance becomes inactive because it can no longer disperse evenly throughout the whole system. Actually a substance need not be completely dissolved to be effective. It also acts, sometimes even more strongly than when completely dissolved, if it is in a colloidal state [88]. Increased effectiveness of some disinfectants by the additions of surfactants is based on this phenomenon.

In preparations that consist of more than one phase, that is, in all emulsified products, the distribution coefficient of the preservative between the two phases is certainly important [89]. No agreement has yet been reached about the necessity of preserving the oil phase as well as the aqueous phase in emulsions. According to Galloway [90], fungi can be combated only by the part of the fungicide that is water-soluble, whereas Deakers [91] and Nowak [92] maintain that the presence of preservatives in both oil and aqueous phases is required and recommend the addition of two preservatives, one to be more water-soluble, the other, more oil-soluble.

The prevailing pH plays an important part in preservatives that dissociate into ions (i.e., all acids and phenols). Generally only undissociated acids and phenols are effective [93]; ions are not absorbed by microorganisms (see also the ability to permeate human skin, Chapter 9). The higher the pH of a preparation, the lower the concentration of undissociated acid or phenol molecules. The concentration of undissociated acid or undissociated phenol in both phases of the emulsion can be calculated from the pH of the aqueous phase, the dissociation constants of the acid (or phenol), the distribution coefficient of acid/phenol between the phases, and the ratio of the phases [94].

Nowak [82] recommends the following measures, to be observed in order to obtain stable preparations:

1. *Selection of raw materials.* Raw materials and agents that might turn the emulsion into a culture medium for fungi and bacteria are dangerous. Use sterile raw materials and an aseptic working method. Pay particular attention to the water to be used.

2. *Suitable containers and covers.* Do not use cork disk liners. If possible, sterilize or disinfect containers and covers before packing. Tubes are suitable for long storage of products.

3. Pay particular attention to O/W emulsions, especially if they contain nonionic emulsifiers.

As Czetsch-Lindenwald [95] remarks, the demands made on the preservative are largely dependent on the nature of the ingredients of a cosmetic. Gels containing gelatin or preparations containing organ extracts such as placenta extract, are, for example, extremely prone to microbial attack.

REFERENCES 105

Hjorth and Trolle Lassen [96] have written about skin reactions to preservatives: primary irritations and sensitizations to preservatives in creams
are rare because these substances are used in low concentrations, but if the
users have been exposed to high concentrations of these products in other
forms skin reactions may occur because of previous sensitization. Such
reactions have been observed, for example, with paraben esters, sorbic acid,
and organic mercury compounds.

## REFERENCES

[1] Rieth, *Arch. klin. exp. Derm.*, **207**, 413 (1958); Roia, Vanderwyk, and Beal, *J. Soc. cosmet. Chem.*, **14**, 81 (1963).

[2] Sarkany, Taplin, and Blank, *J. Am. med. Ass.* (June 15, 1961).

[3] *Dt. Apothekerztg.*, **30**, 542 (1952).

[4] Wiame, Rosenblum, and Bourgeois, *Biochim. biophys. Acta*, **20**, 43 (1956).

[5] Weinberg, *J. Soc. cosmet. Chem.*, **13**, 89 (1962).

[6] *Bull. natn. Formul. Comm.*, **41**, 69 (1948), in Harry, *Modern Cosmetocology* 4th ed., p. 696.

[7] Theile and Pease, *J. Soc. cosmet. Chem.*, **15**, 745 (1964).

[8] McNamara, Steinbach, Schwartz, *J. Soc. cosmet. Chem.*, **16**, 499 (1965).

[9] Czetsch-Lindenwald and Schmidt-La Baume, *Die äusseren Heilmittel*, 1950–1955, p. 35.

[10] *Hautarzt*, **4**, 12, 460 (1953); **5**, 1, 29 (1954).

[11] Pfeiffer, *J. Am. med. Ass.*, **128**, 266 (1945).

[12] Fisher, *Archs. Derm.*, **73**, 336 (1956).

[13] Hoffmann, *SÖFW*, **88**, 613 (1962); DAS 1.192.786.

[14] Lueck, *Parfum. Kosmet.*, **45**, 123 (1964).

[15] Nowak, German Pat. DAS 1.139.610; Czetsch-Lindenwald, *Pharmaz. Ztg. Apotheker-ztg.*, **107**, 856 (1962).

[16] Sabalitschka, *Therapie Gegenw.*, 297 (1950); Fiedler, *Fette Seifen*, **52**, 12 (1950).

[17] Knight, *Antibiotics Chemother.*, **7**, 172, (1957); Draize, Wazeter, Kelley, and Zwickley, *Proc. scient. Sect. Toilet Goods Ass.*, **27**, 12 (1957).

[18] Johnson and Tuura, *Archs. Derm.*, **74**, 73 (1956).

[19] Russell and Hoch, *J. Soc. cosmet. Chem.*, **16**, 169 (1965).

[20] Gump and Walter, *ibid.*, **11**, 307 (1960).

[21] R. Heu, *SÖFW.*, **81**, 479, 503, 530 (1955).

[23] Hausam, *SÖFW.*, **81**, 675 (1955).

[24] Jacobsen, *Pharm. Weekbl.*, **86**, 733 (1951).

[25] Fahlberg, Swan, and Seastone, *J. Bact.*, **56**, 323 (1948); Shemano, Irving et al., *Fedn. Proc.*, **13**, 305 (1954).

[26] G. Meyer, *Riechstoffe-Parf-Seifen*, 1 (April 1956).

[27] Killian, *J. Soc. cosmet. Chem.*, **3**, 30 (1952).

[28] Traub, *ibid.*, **1**, 251 (1949).

[29] Gemmell, *Soap Perfum. Cosm.*, **25**, 1158, 1160 (November 1952).

[30] Shumard, Beaver, and Hunter, *Soap sanit. Chem.* **29**, 34 (1953).

[31] *Perfume essent. Oil Rec.*, **49**, 112 (1958).

[32] U. S. Patent 2,678,402 (1954).

[33] Harry, *Modern Cosmetocology*, 4th ed., p. 713.

[34] Keddie, Hexter, and Brown, *Archs. Derm.*, **74**, 504 (1956); *Drug Cosmet. Ind.* **79**, 114 (1956).

[35] Zentmayer, *Phytopathology*, **33**, 1121 (1943).

[35a] International Union against Cancer Symposium, Rome 1956.

[36] "Meteor," *Parfum. Kosmet.*, **34**, 15 (1953).

[37] Bechtold, Lawrence, and Owen, *Drug Cosmet. Ind.*, **78**, 403 (1956).

[38] L. J. Vinson et al., *J. Pharm. Sci.*, **50**, 827 (1961); Lemaire, Schramm, and Cahn, *ibid.*, **50**, 831 (1961); Lange and Mezikofski, *J. Soc. cosmet. Chem.*, **16**, 341 (1965); U. S. Patent 2,802,029 (1957).

[39] Lemon, Furia, Zussmann, *Soap, Perfum. Cosm.*, **33**, 609 (1960).

[40] Wilkinson, *Br. J. Derm.*, **74**, 295 (1962).

[41] See [19].

[42] *Z. ges. Hyg.*, **125**, 666 (1944).

[43] *Arch. sci.*, **7**, 497 (1954).

[44] *Z. Haut u. GeschlKrankh.*, **14**, 382 (1953).

[45] Yale, *J. Biol. Med.*, **23**, 277 (1950).

[46] *Am. Perfumer*, **61**, 361 (1953).

[47] Klarmann, *Ann. N.Y. Acad. Sci.*, **53**, 123 (1950).

[48] Domagk, *Dt. med. Wschr.*, **61**, 829 (1935); Valko and Du Bois, *J. Bact.*, **50**, 481 (1945).

[49] Seidenberg et al., *Schweiz. med. Wschr.*, **79**, 978 (1949).

[50] Rawling et al., *J. Am. pharm. Ass.*, **32**, 11 (1943).

[51] *Mfg. Chem.*, **22**, 143 (1951).

[52] Neu, *SÖFW*, **81**, 696 (1955).

[53] See [46].

[54] *Proc. scient. Sect. Toilet Goods Ass.* (June 1945).

[55] Freese and Andersen, *Am. Perfumer*, **71** (3), 37 (March 1956).

[56] *Schimmel Briefs*, **268** (1957); *Parfum. Kosmet.*, **38**, 654 (1957).

[57] Cantor, Most, and Shelanski, *J. Soc. cosmet. Chem.*, **7**, 419 (1956).

[58] *Soap sanit. Chem.*, **30**, 139 (1954); Ball, *Archs. Derm.*, **71**, 696 (1955); Tarnoff, *Am. Perfumer*, **77**, 35 (1962).

[59] *Drug Cosmet. Ind.*, **78**, 327 (1956).

[60] Miller and Elson, *J. Bact.*, **57**, 47 (1949); Vinson, *Soap sanit. Chem.*, **30**, 144 (1954); Baer and Rosenthal, *J. invest. Derm.*, **23**, 193 (1954).

[61] Meinhof, *Z. Haut u. GeschlKrankh.*, **33**, 124 (1962).

[62] *J. infect. Dis.*, **49**, 440 (1931).

[63] Clausen, *Medd. Norsk Farm. Selskap* **17**, 313 (1955).

[64] Baker, *Drug Cosmet. Ind.*, **80**, 458 (1957).

[65] *J. Am. med. Ass.*, **159**, 1736 (1955).

[66] *Hautarzt*, **8**, 518 (1957).

[67] Brune and Michell, *J. Am. pharm. Ass.*, Sci. Ed., **41**, 654 (1952); Varma et al., *ibid.*, **44**, 611 (1955); Plaxco and Husa, *ibid.*, **45**, 141 (1956).

[68] *Farmacentiske Tide.*, **64**, 208 217 (1954).

[69] *Am. Perfumer*, **77** (12), 32 (1962).

[70] *Ibid.*, **77** (1), 67 (1962).

[71] Babicka, paper read at the Czechoslovak Cosmetol. Soc. January 25, 1957, reported in *Parfum. Kosmet.*, **38**, 218 (1957); Nowak, *SÖFW*, **79**, 161 (1953); *Dragoco Rep.*, **5** (1962); Galloway, *Perfum. essent. Oil Rec.*, **43**, 82 (1952); Morelle, *Industrie Parfum.*, **12**, 91 (1957).

[72] *SÖFW*, **79**, 161 (1953).

[73] *Proc. scient. Sect., Toilet Goods Ass.*, **6**, 18 (1946).

[74] *Am. Perfumer*, **82** (12), 29 (December 1967).

[75] *SÖFW*, **83**, 153, 337, 459, 535, 580, 626 (1957).

[76] *J. Soc. cosmet. Chem.*, **8**, 30 (1957).

[77] Neidig and Burrell, *Drug Cosmet. Ind.*, **45**, 308 (1944).

[78] Krajkeman, *Perfum. essent. Oil Rec.*, **43** (June 1952).

[79] Mirimanoff and co-workers, *J. Pharm. Pharmac.*, 685 (1950); *Pharm. Acta Helv.*, **26**, 69, 284 (1951); **27**, 31 (1952); De Navarre and Bailey, *J. Soc. cosmet. Chem.*, **7**, 427 (1956) and later publications; Anderson, *Aust. J. Pharm.*, **37**, 8 (1956).

[80] Eisman, Cooper, and Jaconia, *J. Am. pharm. Ass.*, **46**, 144 (1957).

[81] De Navarre, *Am. Perfumer*, 37 (July 1957).

[82] Nowak, Die Konservierung nichtionischer Emulsionen, *Dragoco Rept.*, **5**, 12 (1962).

[83] *J. Am. pharm. Ass.*, Sci. Ed., **46**, 455 (1957).

[84] Puls, Lindgren, and Cosgrove, *J. Am. pharm. Ass.*, Sci. Ed., **44**, 85 (1955).

[85] *Am. Perfumer*, 29 (May 1956).

[86] U. S. Patent 2,773,834.

[87] *Schimmel Briefs*, **267** (1957).

[88] Lamanna and Malette, *Basic Bacteriology*, Williams & Wilkins, Baltimore, 1953, p. 609.

[89] Beam, Heman-Ackah and Thomas, *J. Soc. cosmet. Chem.*, **16**, 251 (1965).

[90] *Perfum. essent. Oil Rec.*, **43**, 82 (1952).

[91] *Drug Cosmet. Ind.* **38**, 37 (1936).

[92] *SÖFW*, **79**, 161 (1953).

[93] Rahn and Cohn, *Ind. Engng. Chem.*, **36**, 185 (1944).

[94] Garrett and Woods, *J. Am. pharm. Ass.*, Sci. Ed., **42**, 736 (1953).

[95] Dragoco Rept., 1962, No. 9.

[96] *Am. Perfumer*, **77** (1), 43 (1962).

# CHAPTER 4

# The Composition of Cosmetic Preparations

Cosmetic preparations may be classified according to their effect or purpose or, alternatively, to their physical/chemical composition. The second part of this book deals with the effect; the present chapter considers the basic physical/chemical types (anhydrous preparations, emulsions, aqueous/ alcoholic preparations, powders, and aerosols) and summarizes the most important raw materials for each as well as the principles of their formulation and production. General knowledge of the basic types and the part played by various raw materials will facilitate an appreciation of individual preparations and their composition because ultimately they can all be reduced to one of these categories.

## OILS AND ANHYDROUS CREAMS

The ingredients for these preparations may be subdivided as follows:

1. Mineral oils, petrolatums, mineral waxes.
2. Vegetable and animal oils and fats.
3. Oil and fat derivatives.
4. Vegetable and animal waxes and their derivatives.
5. Synthetic waxes.
6. Fatty alcohols and sterols.
7. Phospholipids and synthetic phosphoric acid esters.
8. Silicone oils and waxes.
9. Dispersed solids.
10. Antioxidants.
11. Preservatives.

### Mineral Oils, Petrolatum, and Mineral Waxes

Until the beginning of the century, cosmetics contained only vegetable or animal oils and fats. Good cosmetics could be produced with these materials

108

but they had one disadvantage: their stability was limited. They turned rancid after a certain time, showed signs of discoloration and unpleasant odors, and, if used nevertheless, caused skin irritations. Increased storage stability could be achieved by careful control of raw materials and cleanliness in preparation and packaging, but even at best preparations based on animal or vegetable fats lasted only 6–12 months.

When, at the turn of the century, paraffin hydrocarbons (mineral oil, petrolatum, paraffin wax, and ceresines) were introduced for use in cosmetics, they were hailed with considerable enthusiasm.

Fats that never turned rancid and were still odorless and tasteless even after years of storage had now been found. The increased stability of cosmetic preparations, originally regarded only as an advantage of mineral oils and fats, became even more important later on: this increase was the basic requirement for the development of cosmetics in the twenties.

Until then cosmetics had been a luxury for the "upper ten." Creams and skin oils were not in common use: if needed, a lady had them made up by her perfumer or pharmacist. Between 1920 and 1930, however, the use of cosmetic products increased enormously; they were no longer an upper class privilege; all women bought them. Sport creams, day creams, night creams, powder, even rouge and lipstick until then seen only on actresses and prostitutes, were used by everybody. Cosmetics went into mass production.

Under such conditions they had to meet a number of new requirements. A lapse of several months between production and sale had to be anticipated, as had the possible export of these perishables to countries with hot climates. Consequently cosmetic preparations were forced to meet the need for greater stability.

On the other hand, the mass market could hardly be conquered with products based on expensive refined oils. Low-priced raw materials were needed. Mineral oil and petrolatum met both requirements, stability and low cost, perfectly, and it is no exaggeration to say that the development of modern cosmetics depended on them. In view of their wide distribution, the medical profession sooner or later had to take notice of the increased use of cosmetic preparations. If millions of people (including those who are careless about personal hygiene) use certain preparations on their skins year after year, occasional undesirable effects are unavoidable, and must soon be brought to the physician's attention.

Initially the medical profession was highly critical of cosmetics. At best only "neutrality" was expected from their use as far as health was concerned; doctors knew all about negative results and certainly expected no therapeutic effects. As a matter of interest, it was the use of mineral oil in cosmetic preparations that provided a point of attack.

However, about 1930 this attitude began to change, and the collaboration that now exists between dermatologists and cosmetic chemists will hopefully become even closer. One question on which medicine and cosmetics have not yet fully agreed is the use of mineral oils.

For many years and even now, especially in Europe, objections have been raised from a medical point of view to the continued use of these raw materials.

We shall summarize the arguments against the use of paraffin hydrocarbons and then critically examine them one by one [1].

1. Paraffin hydrocarbons, as such, are harmful to the skin. Memmesheimer [2] describes the occurrence of a dermatitis and Schoch [3] tells of a cauliflowerlike growth that developed after extended use of a petrolatum-based brilliantine. Petrolatum has a strong positive reaction in the acanthosis test, which is supposed to point to its incompatability to the skin [4]. (The relation between chemical composition and effect in the acanthosis test is discussed by Schaaf [5].)

It has variously been assumed that mineral oils have a keratogenic effect on the hair-follicle epithel which leads to the formation of comedones and other symptoms of irritation [6].

2. Paraffin hydrocarbons are carcinogenic. The assertion, which goes back for many years, that petrolatum and paraffin oils are carcinogenic was confirmed by the specially created "Manchester Committee on Cancer" in 1926 after a thorough study of the problem.

3. Paraffin hydrocarbons form a water-impermeable layer on the skin which leads to entrapment of perspiration. Petrolatum, for example, has a water value of 8–15 and even this amount does not derive from the presence of emulsifiers but is based on the formation of pseudo-emulsions due to the viscosity of the petrolatum [7]. (Water value is defined as the maximum amount of water—in grams—that can be combined with 100 g of a water-insoluble substance to form a macroscopically uniform stable mixture.)

According to Rothman [8], petroleum inhibits the imperceptible sweat secretion by 40–60%, compared with 20–30% for zinc paste. If larger skin areas are covered with petrolatum, heat buildup might result. Hair-follicle and sweat-gland orifices would be obstructed. People with skin diseases cannot, for these reasons, tolerate paraffin hydrocarbons.

4. Paraffin hydrocarbons are alien to the body and therefore incapable of replacing skin fat. On the contrary, application and rubbing off may lead to a degreasing of the skin; important components of sebum dissolve in hydrocarbons and leave a physiologically ineffective alien coating on the skin.

5. Paraffin hydrocarbons do not penetrate the skin; they are not even absorbed by it. Many active substances are less well absorbed from a petrolatum base than from any other.

What attitude do cosmetic chemists adopt toward these arguments?

1. Every cosmetic chemist will seriously doubt the allegation that paraffin hydrocarbons are harmful; during the last 50 years millions have used brilliantines, hair oils, massaging oils, cold creams, cleansing creams, suntan oils, and many other cosmetic preparations that contain paraffin oil or petrolatum and damage has only rarely been caused. Even then the harm was due in most part to contaminations of the raw materials or components of the dye or fragrance. During World War II in particular inadequately purified paraffin hydrocarbons were used, as reported by Sidi in *Tolérance et intolérance aux produits cosmétiques* (Paris, 1955). The dermatoses caused by lubricating oils are also not due to saturated hydrocarbons but to impurities in the oils. The results of the acanthosis test cannot be accepted as evidence of the noxious effect of petrolatum on healthy human skin: the tests were made on animals, and it has been determined in many instances that results from animal tests cannot necessarily be applied to humans.

In any case, experience during the last decades has shown that there is little risk of harm to healthy skin if properly purified paraffin hydrocarbons are used; this risk is probably less than that incurred through rancidity of vegetable and animal oils and fats. In this connection the opinion of Sabetay [9] is of interest; that is, erythema caused by perfume occurs less often with products containing paraffin oil, petrolatum, or paraffin wax than with preparations in which hydrocarbons are lacking. According to this author, the mineral substances form a protective layer on the skin surface because of their inability to penetrate it, and the perfume oil remains in solution in this layer.

2. The report of the Manchester Committee in 1926 on the carcinogenic effect of mineral oils was not the last word in regard to this problem. After 1926 it continued to be studied by the Manchester Committee and independent physicians all over the world. (A bibliography is contained in Harry, *Cosmetic Materials*, London 1948, p. 235). These tests showed that saturated hydrocarbons (i.e., the main components of mineral oil) have no carcinogenic effect and that the symptoms are due rather to some aromatic constituents which occur in unpurified mineral oils in various amounts. Purified mineral oils, free from aromatic constituents, have no carcinogenic effect.

*Testing Methods for the Presence of Unsaturated or Aromatic Hydrocarbons in Petrolatum and Paraffin Oil:*

1. Thoroughly mix equal amounts of paraffin oil and concentrated sulfuric acid in a dry test tube and heat for 10 min in a water bath. The paraffin oil must not change its appearance; oils with a specific gravity above 0.880 may turn the acid yellow, lighter oils may brown it, but it must never be blackened. Petrolatum is tested by rubbing, say, 5 g with 5 ml of concentrated sulfuric acid in a porcelain bowl. After 30 minutes the mixture may be brown but never black.

2. Paraffin oils must show no fluorescence in UV light.

3. In its report for the year ending October 31, 1935, addendum to the 1932–1934 report, the Manchester Committee on cancer recommends the following quality stipulations for mineral oils used in the textile industry as spindle oils, which are also important in cosmetic preparations: the oils should have a specific refractivity of less than 0.5539 if the specific gravity (15.6°C/15.6°C, vacuo/vacuo) is above 0.895, or a specific refractivity below 0.5569 if the specific gravity is below 0.895. Specific refractivity is defined as $(n - 1)/d$, where $n$ is the refractory index for the $d$-line of sodium light and $d$ is the density in grams per milliliter at 20°C.

4. The presence of free acid in paraffin oil or petrolatum can easily be determined with litmus paper in a roughly 50/50 mixture with 95% ethyl alcohol.

The water impermeability of mineral oils and waxes has certainly been proved by many methods. If preparations containing petrolatum or mineral oils are applied to larger skin areas, heat congestions can therefore not be avoided. If a preparation contains a relatively high percentage of highly viscous or solid hydrocarbons and is not removed after use by washing, it may also cause an obstruction of the pores. Water permeability of paraffin hydrocarbons may be considerably increased by emulsifiers (as in all emulsified products), but there is the risk that only the emulsifier will be resorbed by the skin and not the hydrocarbon so that an impermeable layer will be left on the skin after all.

On the other hand, the water-repellent character of these substances makes them particularly suitable for preparations that are intended to protect the skin from contact with aqueous solutions and for other preparations that should resist being rinsed off with water (various protective products, suntan oils, etc.)

It is a fact that mineral oils are "alien" to the skin and cannot replace skin fat. Preparations intended to replace skin fat at least functionally will therefore not contain much mineral oil. Small quantities of skin-related fats are often added to cleansing creams and other preparations that contain a high percentage of paraffin hydrocarbons in order to avoid possible skin degreasing.

The argument that mineral oils have no effect on the lower skin layers is quite correct in itself: mineral oils and fats do not penetrate the skin at all. It should not be overlooked, however, that this effect is intended in only a very minor number of cosmetic preparations. Cleansing creams, massaging oils, powder bases, protective preparations, brilliantines, etc., do not require it, and the substances (hormones, vitamins, mercury, and sodium salt) that penetrate the skin more slowly or to a lesser degree from petroleum bases than from other bases are contained in only a few cosmetic preparations.

Summarizing, we may say that properly purified mineral oil, petrolatum, and paraffin waxes in cosmetic preparations cannot be regarded as damaging to the skin and that they are particularly suited to protective preparations because of their water resistance; they are not suitable for cosmetics intended to replace skin fat or to "nourish" the skin.

We need not dwell on the physical properties of mineral oils and petrolatum; these can be found in any reference book on cosmetics. Mineral oils and petrolatum are derived from crude petroleum. The mineral oils (paraffin oils with a specific gravity of 0.875 and higher; below this s.g. oils are called white oils; in practice, the terms paraffin and mineral oils are often used interchangeably; yellow mineral oils are not suitable for cosmetics) are high boiling and colorless and are marketed in different grades. The viscosity at 37.8°C may fluctuate between 15 and 100 cst. Petrolatum is an amorphous compound of higher saturated hydrocarbons which melts between 30 and 45°C over a wide temperature range. A yellow and a white grade are available; only white petrolatum is used in cosmetics.

After the preceding remarks regarding skin irritation and possible carcinogenic effects it is obvious that only completely purified material, absolutely free from unsaturated and aromatic compounds, may be used for skin and hair preparations.

Apart from genuine natural petrolatum, some artificial or synthetic petrolatums are used in cosmetics. "Unguentum paraffini" consists of a mixture of 15–25% ceresine with 75–85% viscous paraffin oil and sometimes hard paraffin wax. It never equals the viscosity and stringiness of genuine petrolatum.

A modern petrolatum replacement product consists of a 5% solution of high molecular polyethylene resins in high viscosity mineral oil [9]; it is a soft transparent jelly which compares favorably with genuine petrolatum because it shows no change in consistency between 5 and 38°C; it should not, however, be heated.

*Mineral waxes (paraffin, ceresine, ozokerite, and astrolatum)* also consist of high molecular saturated hydrocarbons. Consequently they are all insoluble in polar solvents, hydrophobic, and have little affinity with the skin but when properly purified have no toxic or allergenic properties. In view of the many contradictory data about the definition of mineral waxes found in reference books, we shall deal with this aspect here:

It is generally agreed that paraffin wax is derived from the higher petroleum fractions. This product is more or less translucent and has a crystalline structure that is occasionally visible. The melting point for hard paraffin waxes is between 50 and 60°C and sometimes as high as 75°C. Soft paraffin waxes, which are hardly ever used in cosmetics, melt around 40°C. Ozokerite is generally defined as a more or less purified grade of a natural mineral wax found in various parts of the world (Galicia, Russia, and the United States). Only white grades are used in cosmetics (semirefined grades are yellow or brown). The prime grade melts at 74–78°C, the secondary at 65–70°C. Contrary to paraffin wax, even thin layers of ozokerite are neither translucent nor crystalline but amorphous or microcrystalline in structure; ozokerite fails to crystallize and swells in solvents.

In the older chemical literature ceresine is usually described as a specially refined grade of ozokerite. This definition was also adopted by Janistyn [10] and Rothman [11], but Janistyn points out that ceresine is frequently adulterated with paraffin wax and that pure ceresine is hardly ever commercially available. De Navarre [12] describes ceresines as higher melting hydrocarbon waxes of petroleum origin. The situation is further complicated by the different nomenclature of the various national pharmacopoeiae. In Germany ceresine is described as *paraffinum solidum*, whereas in the United States, Great Britain, and France it appears as *paraffinum durum* and its derivation from crude oil is mentioned only occasionally.

In cosmetics ceresine is used for the same purposes as ozokerite because of its microcrystalline structure, its noncrystalline nature, and its oil retention. The more pronounced these characteristics are, the higher its value. Finally, particularly in American formulations, we find astrolatum (microcrystalline wax). The Toilet Goods Association describes it as "amorphous petroleum wax" [13] and defines it as a mixture of noncrystalline solid hydrocarbons derived from crude oil. According to Killingsworth (14) this product is made from petrolatum by removing the remaining oil content, and several grades are available, depending on the conditions of purification and production. According to the TGA [14], the cosmetic grade should be white or light yellow, odorless, and melt between 54 and 82°C. Like ozokerite, it fails to crystallize and has an even higher oil retention.

It follows that paraffin waxes can be divided into two groups:

1. *Macrocrystalline waxes* (*paraffin*). Used in oil mixtures, paraffin frequently provides the required thixotropic properties (a preparation is described as thixotropic if it is normally solid but liquefies under pressure). Their miscibility with liquid oils is limited, however, and they tend to crystallize.

2. *Microcrystalline waxes* (*ozokerite, ceresine, and astrolatum*). These waxes thicken oil mixtures without liquefying under pressure. They are often added to macrocrystalline waxes because they have a better miscibility with oils and also reduce the crystallization tendency of paraffin waxes.

### Vegetable and Animal Oils and Fats

These oils and fats are known to consist mostly of triglycerides of the higher saturated or unsaturated straight-chain fatty acids. Although they are also insoluble in water, they are not so decidedly nonpolar as paraffin hydrocarbons. Apart from long hydrocarbon chains, the molecules of these oils and fats also contain ester groups that impart certain hydrophilic properties to the molecules. In any case, these products do not show the same degree of inertness toward epidermal tissue as petrolatum and paraffin oil. They penetrate the hair follicle and possibly even the upper layers of the corneum with greater ease and are therefore "resorbed" by the skin. Compared with mineral oils, vegetable oils are more suitable for emollient and skin-nourishing cosmetics and less so for protective and water-repellent preparations. Especially beneficial effects are attributed to several vegetable and animal oils because of their content of vitamins, steroids, lecithin, and other agents (avocado oil, turtle oil, wheat-germ oil, and cod-liver oil). Excessive heating and oxidation must be avoided during the processing of these oils because they would then lose their special properties (see also Chapter 9).

## Oil and Fat Derivatives

**Hydrogenated Fats.** The main disadvantage of vegetable and animal oils and fats is their tendency to turn rancid. This is due primarily to their content of esters of unsaturated fatty acids. If the unsaturated fatty acid esters are modified by hydrogenation into saturated compounds, the stability of oils and fats is vastly increased. For this reason the many commercially available hydrogenated oils and fats have surpassed natural products in importance as raw materials. Any vitamins (A, D, F) present may, however, be destroyed in the hydrogenation process.

Apart from their greater stability, hydrogenated oils and fats are also harder and higher melting than natural oils and fats. Some hydrogenated vegetable oils have the consistency of lard and some are even harder.

In the United States hydrogenated vegetable oils are used extensively as edible fats. During production of these edible fats (e.g., Crisco) they undergo a special aeration process which results in a consistency that is neither hard nor tacky, but creamy soft, white, and light but not translucent. Such edible fats are excellent raw materials for cosmetics. If the special properties caused by aeration are to be retained, these products must not be heated beyond their melting point of 40–50°C.

Related to this group is perhydrosqualene (Cosbiol), a saturated hydrocarbon produced by hydrogenation of squalene which occurs in fish-liver oil (and in skin fat). Perhydrosqualene is a colorless, odorless, stable liquid and is used as a solvent for Vitamin A in hair oils, skin oils, and creams.

For some years synthetic triglycerides have been on the market. Similar to the hydrogenated oils, their greater stability is an advantage compared with natural oils, but they lack the natural nonsaponifiable component that may have a beneficial effect on the skin. A greater significance has been achieved by some esters of higher fatty acids with monohydric or dihydric alcohols.

The most important materials in this group at present are isopropyl myristinate, isopropyl palmitate (Deltol, Emcol IP), and isopropyl laurate (Emcol IL). These products are always esters of fatty acid mixtures which are designated according to the predominating fatty acid. These esters are more fluid than natural oils and have low surface tension. They form a thin layer on the skin which they can easily penetrate so that they leave no sticky or greasy feeling. They do not turn rancid and are a good solvent for mineral oils, vegetable and animal oils and fats, fat soluble vitamins, hormones, and other active substances. The main application for these products is in preparation with a high fat or oil content when a sticky-greasy feeling is to be avoided after application [15].

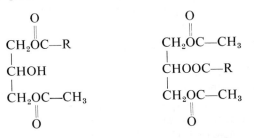

The socalled "Aceto fats" [16] resemble the products just described in their miscibility with mineral oil and vegetable and animal fats but leave no sticky-greasy feeling after application to the skin. Chemically, they are glycerol esters in which a hydroxyl group has been esterified with a higher molecular fatty acid, whereas one or both of the other hydroxyl groups have been acylated with acetic acid. The properties of these compounds depend on the basic fat and the degree of acylation. Two typical products of this group are Eastman Kodak's Myvacet 5-00 (from hydrogenated lard, predominantly monoacetate) and Myvacet 9-40 (from lard, mostly diacetate). In anhydrous preparations aceto fats reduce the tackiness of fat mixtures on the skin and increase the malleability of high viscosity fat or wax films; in this effect aceto fats are superior to materials such as isopropyl myristate.

### Vegetable and Animal Waxes and Their Derivatives

Vegetable and animal waxes are natural products that consist mainly of higher fatty acid esters of high molecular monohydric (occasionally dihydric) alcohols. Waxes also contain free fatty acids, alcohols, and higher hydrocarbons. Most waxes are hard solids, but liquid waxes (particularly spermaceti and sperm oil) are also occasionally used in cosmetics. Their higher content of free fatty acids and alcohols makes vegetable and particularly animal waxes more hydrophilic than oils and fats. The often reiterated statement that beeswax, spermaceti, and sperm oil are easily and quickly absorbed by the skin is also connected with this characteristic; fatty acids and alcohols probably have a higher wetting ability toward keratin than esters. This hypothesis is supported by the test results of Barail and Pescatore [17], who showed that cetyl palmitate (generally assumed to be the main constituent of spermaceti, although Wellendorf [18] suggests that the composition of spermaceti is more complex than usually believed) does not penetrate the skin. In the test cetyl palmitate was marked with radioisotope carbon ($C^{14}$). Solid vegetable and animal waxes also impart a firm consistency to fat mixtures.

Lanolin occupies a special place among animal waxes. It is produced from sheeps' wool. Of all natural raw materials it is closest to human skin and hair fat in its chemical composition and physiological properties. Lanolin contains about 50% unsaponifiable matter (mostly cholesterol and other sterols, cetyl alcohol and other fatty alcohols). The saponifiable part of lanolin, which consists of fatty acid esters of the sterols and fatty alcohols also contains free hydroxyl groups. Their occurrence is explained by the presence of partially saponified dihydric alcohols and of hydroxy acid esters [19]. Because of these free hydroxyl groups (free sterols and fatty alcohols, monoesters of dihydric alcohols, and hydroxy acid esters), lanolin has a hydrophilic character even if it contains almost no water-soluble components. Anhydrous lanolin (*adeps lanae anh.*) is capable of absorbing and binding 185% of its own weight of water. In an oil mixture lanolin acts as a W/O emulsifier. The affinity of lanolin with skin is at least partly explained by its high content of hydroxyl groups.

As we shall see in Chapter 8 in more detail, lanolin is a valuable ingredient in preparations that are designed to replace skin fat and to restore or maintain skin elasticity. It is neither toxic nor irritant and is well tolerated by the skin. Allergic reactions to lanolin are rare, but medical literature does report cases of lanolin hypersensitivity [20]. Sulzberger and collaborators found [21] that the allergenic factor is in the alcohol fraction and may be rendered ineffective by acetylation of the lanolin. In cosmetic processing, however, lanolin has certain disadvantages:

1. It has a rather strong odor, which is less pronounced in freshly refined lanolin but has a tendency to reappear after some time. Preparations containing considerable quantities of lanolin may also darken.

2. Lanolin is soluble in most organic solvents but can be blended in only small amounts with many cosmetic raw materials. It must also be used cautiously as a superfatting agent in soaps and shampoos because it may reduce the lathering capacity.

3. Lanolin leaves a viscous sticky film on the skin, a property sometimes noticeable even in products that contain only small amounts. Many lanolin

derivatives, available under a variety of trade names, have been developed with a view to overcoming one or more of these undesirable qualities [22]. The following different types can be distinguished:

(a) *Wool-fat alcohols* (also called wool wax) are produced by saponifying lanolin (or unpurified wool fat) and isolating the alcohol fraction. Obviously the hydrophilic properties of these preparations are even more pronounced than in lanolin itself. They also have a fainter odor and only little or no discoloration effect. Their films are not so tacky as those of lanolin. For all these reasons wool-fat alcohols are valuable cosmetic raw materials [23].

(b) *Wool-fat sterols.* Apart from sterols, wool-fat alcohols also contain higher fatty alcohols. If the latter are removed, the final products are wool-fat sterols. On a weight basis these sterols have an even stronger emulsifying effect than wool-fat alcohols. Whereas the alcohol fraction is still often yellow or brown, the sterols are almost or quite colorless. They are therefore preferred in some preparations.

(c) *Acetylated lanolin,* in which the majority of the free hydroxyl groups has been esterified with acetic acid, differs from lanolin in the following properties: it has no hydrophilic (emulsifying) properties but can be processed easily in O/W emulsions, and up to 10% is soluble in paraffin oil (lanolin itself is almost entirely insoluble) and can be combined more easily with oils and waxes than lanolin. Whereas lanolin often imparts a viscous sticky consistency to cosmetic preparations, the acetylated product has a waxlike consistency. Emulsions containing acetylated lanolin still remain soft at 0°C, whereas preparations containing lanolin may become stiff when cooled. The acetylated grade lacks the strong odor of lanolin; its odor is weak and not unpleasant. The likelihood of allergic reactions, already very slight in lanolin, is further reduced by acetylated lanolin.

(d) *Acetylated wool-fat alcohols.* According to Conrad and Motiuk [24], the product obtained by the acetylation of wool-fat alcohols is unsuitable for cosmetic purposes. One fraction isolated from this mixture has, however, proved very useful. The acetylated wool-fat alcohols are low viscosity oils which can readily be spread on the skin because of their low surface tension and can also penetrate it easily (probably mostly into the hair follicles). Esterification destroys the hydrophilic and emulsifying properties of wool-fat alcohols. The acetylated product is definitely hydrophobic but can easily be processed in O/W emulsions. In contrast to lanolin acetylated wool-fat alcohols are soluble in all proportions in mineral, castor, and vegetable oils as well as in 95% ethyl alcohol, isopropyl alcohol, silicone oil 555, isopropyl myristate and palmitate, and butyl stearate. Under the conditions prevailing in most cosmetics, no hydrolysis of these esters occurs.

(e) *Liquid lanolin* [25], a derivative produced by Croda Ltd., England, is described as a lanolin "extract" containing no solvents. It is similar to lanolin in its skin emollient and emulsifying properties but without its viscosity. It is solid below 20°C but melts above this temperature within a narrow range to a clear liquid. It can be combined with many materials with greater ease than lanolin itself and is miscible with mineral and vegetable oils, occasionally with clouding effects. Shaken with water in proportions of 40:60, 50:50, and 60:40, it yields soft smooth W/O emulsions that remain stable for at least six months.

(f) *Alcohol-soluble products* obtained by fractionating lanolin, for example, "Lanethyl" [26], are suitable additions to hair lotions and aerosol lacquer sprays.

(g) *Hydrophilic lanolin derivatives.* By condensing lanolin (or wool-fat alcohols) with polyoxyethylene compounds, the Atlas Chemical Co. and other manufacturers of cosmetic raw materials have developed hydrophilic lanolin derivatives some of which are water-dispersible and some even water-soluble.

(h) *Lanolin preparations.* One example, "Lanolin DAB 6" (German Pharmacopoeia), is prepared as follows: 139 g of *adeps lanae anh.* is melted in a water bath with 30 g of prime paraffin oil; at 45°C, 40 ml of distilled water is gradually stirred in.

## Synthetic Waxes

This apellation applies to many different substances which fundamentally have no more in common than their waxlike appearance and their miscibility with the standard ingredients of the oil phase. The following groups of synthetic waxes may be distinguished:

1. *Synthetic esters* are chemically related to natural waxes. Cetyl palmitate (artificial spermaceti) and cetiol are representatives of this group. Cetiol is a liquid mixture of esters of unsaturated fatty acids with alcohols of 12–18 C atoms. Its properties closely resemble those of sperm oil.

2. Products with only a few physical properties in common with natural waxes: Lanette wax, Tegin, and "Polywaxes" are occasionally grouped under this heading. We discuss them in greater detail later on.

## Fatty Alcohols and Sterols

Small amounts of fatty alcohols are often added to anhydrous creams with a high content of mineral oils and waxes. Cetyl and stearyl alcohols are most commonly used, but myristyl and lauryl alcohols are suitable also. The basic materials Lanette waxes K and D consist of pure myristyl alcohol and of a mixture of cetyl and stearyl alcohols respectively. We have already dealt with the significance of wool-fat alcohols (wool wax) and wool-fat sterols. Cholesterol in more or less purified form is also often used in cosmetic products, but wool-fat sterols, which also contain sterols other than cholesterol, are in many instances more economical because they are equally effective but cheaper than pure cholesterol.

From a cosmetic point of view, fatty alcohols and sterols have the following important properties:

1. They penetrate the skin easily and help to make it soft, smooth, and supple, thereby reducing the drying effect of mineral oils in cleansing creams and other products.

2. Similar to waxes, they impart a firm structure to fat mixtures.

3. They are neither toxic not irritating and do not turn rancid; they are light-resistant and stable in the presence of alkalies and acids.

4. They facilitate the blending of mineral oils and waxes with more polar raw materials.

5. They are surface-active and W/O emulsifiers. As such, they are frequently used in W/O creams. Added in small quantities to O/W emulsifiers, they have a stabilizing effect and act as auxiliary emulsifying agents. Also related to alcohols are the monofatty acid esters of polyhydric alcohols (e.g. diethylene glycol monolaurate or mono-oleate, polyethylene glycol stearate, etc.), although they contain ester and ether groups in addition to the hydroxyl group.

### Phospholipids and Synthetic Phosphoric Acid Esters

Phospholipids (particularly lecithin) occur in nature in nearly all cells and are also present, even if in very small amounts, in many vegetable and animal oils and fats. They increase the wetting properties of oil mixtures and thereby facilitate smooth spreading on the skin. "Nourishing" and emollient effects are also attributed to them.

Synthetic phosphoric acid esters have not yet found much use in cosmetics. Investigations by Winkler [27] and Schneider [28] indicate that they may well be suited to cosmetic and pharmaceutical applications. With water they form gels compatible with skin and are reported to promote the effect of incorporated active agents. Their water-absorbent capacity depends to a high degree on the pH.

A number of synthetic phosphoric acid esters is commercially available under the trade name of Hostaphates (Farbwerke Hoechst). Their properties are discussed by Eibel [29].

### Silicone Oils and Waxes

Silicone oils, which have been in commercial production only since the end of World War II, quickly developed to important cosmetic materials. Chemically they are organic/inorganic polymers that consist of long chains with alternating silicium and oxygen atoms and organic chains attached to the silicium atoms. A considerable number of different silicones have already been synthetized, and these products differ chemically and physically to such an extent from all other known compounds that they may be regarded

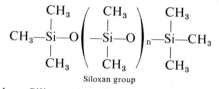

Siloxan group

as a class in themselves. Silicones are characterized by the following properties:

1. They are highly resistant against both saponification and oxidation and also against caustic chemicals. They are therefore stable in cosmetic preparations of every kind and moreover are suitable additives for industrial barrier creams.

2. They are strongly water-repellent, a particularly valuable characteristic in protective preparations. In spite of it, however, they are easily incorporated in cosmetic emulsions (i.e., combined with water!)

3. Silicones have a low surface tension and are therefore easily spread on skin and hair, and do not feel greasy. They easily penetrate the hair follicles and in this way transmit many active substances to the epidermal tissue.

4. Their viscosity is largely independent of temperature and hardly varies even with strong fluctuations. For this reason they are often used in theater, film, and TV cosmetics; standard cosmetics would melt under the strong lights.

5. Silicone oils show no toxic or irritant effect either on the skin or if taken orally or with intraperitoneal, intradermal, or subcutaneous injections. Contact with the conjunctiva of the eyes may result in temporary inflammations which disappear after 24 hours with no permanent damage. The complete innocuousness of silicones may be regarded as established after a thorough examination of these substances in laboratories and clinics all over the world. Silicone oils demonstrate strikingly that not much importance need be attached to the idea of cosmetics being "alien to skin", or "related to the body." No other raw materials are so alien to the human body as silicones and hardly any so harmless! A bibliography of the original literature is given by Leberl [30] and Ernst [31].

6. Heat conductivity is good and there is no congestion of heat as in petrolatums.

7. Silicones have a certain antioxidant effect which becomes noticeable with the addition of 1–3 % silicone oils in cream bases. Probably because of this effect silicones can act as stabilizers on certain chemically sensitive materials. Siebert [32] found that penicillin ointments on a silicone basis had

retained 50 % of their effectiveness after six months, whereas with other bases the penicillin had disappeared, in some after only seven weeks.

8. The foam-suppressing effect of silicones is advantageous in the preparation of larger batches of emulsions [33].

Silicone oils are produced by various manufacturers in a wide viscosity range from fluid oils to semisolid fats. The relationship between the viscosity and the number of siloxan units per macro molecule may be seen in Table 4-1 [34].

TABLE 4-1

| n | Viscosity cst/20°C |
| --- | --- |
| 50 | 60 |
| 110 | 140 |
| 280 | 680 |
| 400 | 1440 |

The solubility of silicones is generally that of nonpolar liquids. Next to the original and most commonly used grade (DC or MS 200), some manufacturers market a second grade, DC or MS 555 (Dow Corning Corp., Midland, Mich., and Midland Silicones Ltd., London) which has better compatibility with other cosmetic raw materials. These manufacturers supply the data in Table 4-2 for the miscibility of the two grades with the most important raw materials. Additional data on the subject are also given in the literature [30, 31]: miscible with cetyl alcohol, cocoa butter, lauric acid, polyethylene glycol 400-monostearate, and hydroxystearic acid sulfate; not readily miscible with potassium soaps, polyoxyethylene glycols, vegetable oils, cholesterol, ceresine, carnauba wax, and spermaceti. A certain confusion in the literature is due to the fact that no mention is made in some cases whether the data apply to grade 200 or 555.

More recent patents mention the suitability of another group of organic silicone oils in cosmetics, that is, Orthosilicates [35]. A typical grade in this group is tetracetylorthosilicate [$Si(OC_{16}H_{33})_4$].

Currie and Gergle [36] describe a new type of silicones that differs from the usual grades in that the end groups of the polysiloxan chains are not formed by alkyl groups but by ethers (or esters) of higher fatty alcohols. The formula of these substances therefore is

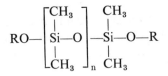

TABLE 4-2

| Substance | | DC⟩ 200 MS⟩ | DC⟩ 555 MS⟩ |
|---|---|---|---|
| Aliphatic hydrocarbons | All proportions | M | M |
| Aromatic hydrocarbons | All proportions | M | M |
| Bees wax | All proportions | I | M |
| Chlorinated hydrocarbons | All proportions | M | M |
| Diglycol stearate S | All proportions | I | M |
| Ethyl alcohol 95% | 50% silicone | I | M |
| Ethyl alcohol 95% | 90% silicone | I | I |
| Glycerol | All proportions | I | I |
| Glycerol monostearate | All proportions | I | I |
| Isopropyl alcohol 99% | 50% silicone | I | M |
| Isopropyl alcohol 99% | 90% silicone | M | M |
| Isopropyl alcohol 70% | All proportions | I | I |
| Lanolin | All proportions | I | I |
| Mineral oil | All proportions | I | M |
| Oleic acid | All proportions | I | M |
| Ozokerite | All proportions | I | M |
| Paraffin wax | 10% silicone | I | M |
| Paraffin wax | 50% silicone | I | I |
| Paraffin wax | 90% silicone | I | M |
| Propylene glycol | All proportions | I | I |
| Sesame seed oil | All proportions | I | M |
| Stearic acid | All proportions | I | M |
| Stearyl alcohol | All proportions | I | M |
| Petrolatum | All proportions | I | M |
| Water | All proportions | I | I |

M = miscible
I = immiscible

Until now the ethers were made with octyl, lauryl, stearyl, and behenyl ($C_{22}$) alcohols in two grades of each, one with a relatively high and one with a relatively low $n$-value (dimethylsiloxan content). Stearyl and behenyl ethers are waxlike substances that melt between 25 and 53°C; grades with shorter siloxan chains have higher melting points. These waxes spread easily on the skin, resemble paraffin wax in their water-repellent properties, and may be compared to silicone oils of the 555 grade as far as their compatibility with other cosmetic raw materials is concerned. With acids or alkali they can be split into silicone oils and fatty alcohols but they are stable under normal conditions of cosmetic application. They are reported to be similar to silicone oils in their other properties which are of interest in cosmetic preparations. Whether they have sufficient advantages compared with mineral waxes to warrant their considerably higher price seems doubtful at present.

### Dispersed Solids

A number of cosmetics also contain, in addition to the substances discussed so far, some finely dispersed solids. They are dispersed because they are insoluble in the fat vehicle. These are mostly inorganic substances whose use in cosmetic creams and oils may serve the following purposes:

1. Coloring of the preparation or the skin area on which it is applied. Zinc oxide and titanium dioxide, both white, have proved particularly suitable. (A "zinc oxide superfine" has been described [37] which is characterized by its brick-red color, very small particle size, high water-absorption capacity, and increased chemical reactivity.)

White coloring is used in cosmetics to give a semitransparent preparation a more attractive appearance (e.g., with some petrolatum creams), when the preparation is intended to cover skin blemishes (e.g., powder bases), or to make it immediately apparent to the user which skin areas have already been covered (e.g., nonfoaming shaving creams, depilatories). Stearates (e.g., zinc and magnesium stearate) are also used for this purpose, but they lack the covering capacity of zinc and titanium oxides. Many other insoluble pigments are used in preparations whose main purpose is a coloring effect (rouge, lipsticks, nail lacquers, etc.; see also Chapter 10).

2. To increase the protective effect, inert substances, such as zinc oxide, bentonite, kaolin, and talcum, are added to many protective preparations. These substances mechanically prevent the penetration of dust particles, allergenic matter, or certain liquids and also bar dirt from clogging the hair follicles.

Zinc oxide increases the action of light-protective preparations by reflecting part of the ultraviolet rays. Zinc oxide, titanium dioxide, and kaolin also play an important part in heat-protective preparations.

3. To obtain a cooling effect zinc oxide is most commonly used. Particularly in preparations with a high petroleum or paraffin oil content, which might lead to heat congestion, an addition of zinc oxide is very useful. According to Kleine-Nathrop [38], the heat conductivity of pastes is generally much better than that of ointments ("pastes are medicinal preparations with a doughlike consistency, which consist of a mixture of pulverized substances and fat. Ointments are soft, easily applicable pharmaceutical vehicles consisting mainly of fats and containing medicinal substances," [38a]).

4. To achieve an astringent effect, zinc oxide and zinc carbonate are the most commonly used materials. Zinc hydroxide, zinc phenol sulfate, and

other zinc salts are also used. The combination of cooling and astringent effects with a slight antiseptic action makes these substances particularly suitable for the treatment of burns (e.g., in antisunburn preparations).

5. In addition to zinc oxide and zinc carbonate, bentonite and certain grades of kaolin may be considered as drying and dehydrating agents. These substances are hygroscopic and therefore extract water from the underlying tissues if they are added to anhydrous preparations. It is possible that the dehydrating and astringent effects are basically the same. The use of kaolin in face packs is based on them.

6. Primarily the zinc salts mentioned under (4) but also zinc borate and boric acid are used as antiseptics.

7. As inert fillers to give semiliquid preparations a firmer consistency. In skin cleansers based on a detergent kaolin, bentonite, starch, and talcum are also used as inert fillers.

8. As emulsifying aids and dispersing agents, magnesium, calcium, and aluminum stearates may be used to stabilize W/O emulsions. Bentonite and special grades of kaolin are used as stabilizers for aqueous dispersions of chalk and zinc oxide and in O/W emulsions.

9. As scouring or polishing agents. In toothpastes calcium carbonate and various phosphates are mostly used for this purpose; in certain industrial skin cleansers, finely ground pumice or sand.

### Antioxidants

**Importance of Rancidity.** The phenomenon that vegetable and animal oils and fats as well as some waxes turn rancid and emit an unpleasant odor if they are exposed to air for any length of time is well known. In perfumed preparations and soaps the scent is soon overpowered by the odor of rancidity. Over and above this, rancid oils and fats (or cosmetic preparations that contain rancid ingredients) act as skin irritants. The revolutionary effect produced by the introduction of petrolatum and paraffin oil at a time when these products were not cheaper than vegetable and animal oils and fats proves better than long arguments that rancidity in cosmetic products really presents a serious problem.

**Causes of Rancidity.** Chemically, rancidity is the degradation of higher fatty acids by oxidation, generally produced by atmospheric oxygen. We cannot dwell here on all the chemical aspects of rancidity [39] and therefore we only summarize the aspects of the problem that have practical significance for the cosmetic chemist.

1. There are two types of rancidity: oxidative and "ketone." Ketone rancidity occurs with fatty acids that contain less than 14 carbon atoms and is the result of the action of certain molds (in particular, aspergillum and

penicillium) in the presence of moisture and nitrogenous substances. Ketone rancidity results in ketone formation (e.g., methyl nonyl ketone) which becomes noticeable by its odor and whose presence is easily demonstrated chemically. Since ketone rancidity is caused by fungi, it can be prevented by preservation of the cosmetic preparations.

2. "Oxidative rancidity" plays a much more important part in practice. It occurs mostly with unsaturated fatty acids and leads to splitting of the fatty-acid molecule at the point of the double linkage. The fragments are aldehydes which are responsible for the unpleasant odor and the skin irritation caused by rancid fats. Oxidative rancidity is an oxidation process caused by atmospheric oxygen and results primarily from contact of the fat (or oil) with air. Several factors may accelerate the onset of rancidity:

(a) The presence of heavy metal traces, for example, iron or copper; also Co, Mn, Sn, Ni, and, generally speaking, all metals that can assume different valences act as oxidation catalysts. The prevention of rancidity is a particularly important problem in soap production, and special measures are always adopted to eliminate the occurrence of heavy metal ions or molecules or to inactivate them in case they do occur.

(b) The effect of light; some wavelengths seem to be more effective than others. De Navarre [40] mentions tests that show that green or yellow cellophane and light brown glass afford good protection against rancidity.

(c) The presence of rancid fat. If a small amount of rancid fat is added to fresh fat, the whole lot will soon turn rancid.

(d) The presence of free fatty acids strongly promotes rancidity. It is not certain that fatty acids are more easily oxidized when they are free than when they are esterified or whether they have a catalytic effect on oxidation. In soap production free fatty acids must also be rigorously excluded. Care is always taken therefore to complete the saponification process of the neutral fats and to leave a certain, if small, excess of lye in the finished soap.

(e) The effect of factors that accelerate the formation of free fatty acids from neutral fats; that is, the presence of water which is responsible for hydrolysis of the glycerides; the presence of strong bases or acids which act catalytically on this hydrolysis; the presence of certain enzymes (from bacteria or fungi) which split the glycerides hydrolytically.

(f) Storage at elevated temperatures. The higher the temperature, the faster the chemical and enzymatic processes leading to rancidity.

**Prevention of Rancidity.** The methods that may be used to prevent rancidity logically follow from the previously listed causes of this phenomenon:

1. Contact of the product with air should be avoided as much as possible.

2. Traces of heavy metals in the product should be avoided. This can be done by using only vessels of stainless steel or aluminum with enamel or glass interiors in the production process.

3. The effect of light should be eliminated by packing the product in opaque (or colored) containers.

4. Fresh batches of fat should never be mixed with older batches. Storage vessels must be thoroughly cleaned before introducing fresh batches.

5. The hydrolysis of fats by bacteria and fungi can be avoided by preservation.

6. The fats should be stored in anhydrous condition.

7. Storage temperature should be as low as possible.

8. In practice the most important way of avoiding rancidity is by the use of antioxidants. These are substances which, added in small amounts to the fat mixture, will prevent the occurrence of rancidity or at least greatly retard its onset. To understand the effect of antioxidants it must be realized that oxidation of unsaturated fatty acids is a chain reaction. If a fatty-acid molecule is attacked by oxygen, not only is the molecule split oxidatively but in the course of this oxidation intermediary reaction products are formed which initiate the oxidation of another fatty-acid molecule. This second molecule will also be split into aldehydes and cause the oxidation of yet another fatty-acid molecule. Theoretically, the attack of atmospheric oxygen on a single fatty-acid molecule might well lead to the oxidation of all the unsaturated fatty acids present in a fat mixture. Antioxidants act by breaking the chains of the oxidation reactions. They react with the active intermediates which are formed in the oxidation process; they are themselves oxidized but do not activate a new fatty-acid molecule for oxidation. In this way the chain reaction is not continued.

The mechanism of this effect explains why only traces of an antioxidant are required to prevent oxidation of a fat mixture. In the purely theoretical case in which oxidation of all unsaturated fatty acids in a fat mixture would occur in one chain one molecule of an antioxidant would be sufficient to break the chain.

Not everything about this mechanism is understood; for example, why do excessive doses of antioxidants act as oxidation accelerators if they are added all at once (but not if they are added gradually)? Sfiras reports [41] that triethanolamine at 0.02% is a good antioxidant for certain aldehydes but acts as a pro-oxidant at 0.1% [42]. Antioxidants for cosmetic use should meet the following requirements:

(a) They must have no irritant or allergenic effect in the concentrations used.
(b) They must cause no discolorations or odors in the preparation.
(c) They must be sufficiently fat-soluble to develop their full effect.

**Antioxidants.** We list only a few of the many materials mentioned in technical and patent literature that meet these requirements [43]:

Nor-dihydroguaiaretic acid (NDGA) [44].
Ethyl gallate (Progallin A, Nipa 48) and propyl gallate (Progallin P, Nipa 49) [45].
Butylated hydroxyanisole (BHA) [46].
Butylated hydroxytoluene (BHT) [47].

According to Klim and Kummerow [48], substances in which one hydrogen of the methyl group in BHT has been replaced by alkoxy, alkylthio, or (preferably) alkyl amino groups, are more effective than BHT itself. The n-hexadecyl amine derivative is reported to be particularly effective.

Dihydroquercetine [49].
Diisoeugenol [50].
Amines (diphenylamine, triethanolamine, p-aminophenol).
Tocopherols (α-tocopherol, β-tocopherol, Vitamin E).
Dihydrochromans (chroman quinones).

The last two antioxidants occur in nature in many fats and oils and are responsible for the fact that these particular fats will only turn rancid after extended storage. During the refining process these natural antioxidants are often largely destroyed.

Reducing substances, such as ascorbic acid, sodium thiosulfate, or thiourea, may also act as oxidation inhibitors either by themselves or, better still, in conjunction with one of the above mentioned antioxidants. It is advisable to add antioxidants to the oils and fats as soon as possible after refining. Only if it cannot be done in any other way should the antioxidant be added to the cosmetic in the course of preparation.

The optimum dose of antioxidants depends on the kind of fat and is generally much higher for animal fats than for vegetable oils. With lard the optimum dose of tocopherol amounts to 0.05 % and for soybean oil to 0.001 % [51]. Generally, additions between 0.01 and 0.03 % are sufficient.

The effect of antioxidants may be increased two- or threefold by adding a synergist; citric, tartaric, phosphoric, and some amino acids (particularly methionine), maleic, and ethylene diamine tetraacetic acids act synergistically and are added in equal quantities to the antioxidants. Substances that absorb ultraviolet rays (e.g., hydroxybenzophenon) may also help to prevent oxidation [52]. A particularly good effect is often achieved by using several antioxidants in combination with synergists. The following are recommended mixtures:

| Di-*tert*-Butyl *p*-cresol | 10% | *tert* Butyl hydroxyanisole | |
|---|---|---|---|
| *tert* Butyl hydroxyanisole | | (BHA) | 20% |
| (BHA) | 10% | Propyl gallate | 6% |
| Dodecyl gallate | 6% | Citric acid | 4% |
| Citric acid | 4% | Propylene glycol | 70% [54] |
| Hexylene glycol | 70% [53] | | |

Some important cosmetic raw materials have an antioxidant effect that is much less pronounced than that of the typical antioxidants themselves and can develop only in higher concentrations but is nevertheless interesting in practice. According to Vogt [55], additions of 1–3% silicone oil have an antioxidant effect. Lecithin acts in a similar way even at concentrations of 0.05–0.1% [56]. Some ingredients of perfumes as well act as antioxidants in their regular concentrations. De Navarre [57] lists the raw materials of perfumes with an antioxidant action and others that accelerate oxidation of fat mixtures. Benzoic and guayac resin in concentrations of 2–4% also act as antioxidants in fat mixtures.

**Experimental Determination of Rancidity.** There are two methods to determine rancidity in a fat mixture: organoleptic detection and chemical determination. Organoleptic detection is much easier and is the method used by the consumer.

Chemical methods have the advantage of being objective and reproducible as well as more sensitive, occasionally even too much so. Oils and fats with a high peroxide or aldehyde number may still be acceptable to smell and taste. Positive readings are sometimes caused by impurities not derived from the oxidation of fatty acids. The most reliable method for determining rancidity (and the effectiveness of antioxidants) is the combined use of several chemical tests and olfactory and taste impressions.

The chemical tests are divided into two groups: the determination of aldehydes and the determination of peroxides; aldehydes as well as peroxides are developed in the course of fatty acid oxidation by atmospheric oxygen.

1. Determination of aldehydes. (a) In its simplest form the Kreis test (1902) is conducted as follows: 1 ml of the oil or molten fat is shaken for one minute with 1 ml of concentrated hydrochloric acid; to this is added 1 ml of a 0.1% ether solution of phloroglucin and shaking is resumed for another minute. A pink to red coloration of the acid layer (at the bottom) is a sign of rancidity and the intensity of the color shows how far it has progressed. The red color is caused by the presence of epiphydrin aldehyde. A modification of the Kreis test has been described by Jones [58].

(b) Lea [59] has described a method that determines even traces of aldehydes in a rancid fat by simple titration with sodium sulfite.

(c) Schiff's aldehyde test may also be used to determine rancidity in oils and fats.

(d) The benzidine test according to Wode [60] is based on the formation of condensation products by benzidine and aldehydes; the absorption of the compounds is measured in the ultraviolet spectrum at 350 or 420–435 m$\mu$. Pokorny [61] describes a modified method used to analyze cosmetic creams.

2. Determination of peroxides [62]. (a) The iodometric method according to Wheeler is quick and easy; 3–10 g of the fat or oil are dissolved in a mixture consisting of 30 ml of glacial acetic acid and 20 ml of pure chloroform to which is added 1 ml of a saturated aqueous potassium iodide solution. Exactly one minute after the addition of the potassium iodide 100 ml of water are added. The freed iodine is then titrated with a standard solution of sodium thiosulfate, with an addition of starch as an indicator. Strong shaking is required to remove the last traces of iodine from the chloroform layer. The peroxide content is calculated according to the following equation:

$$\text{peroxide content (in millimoles per kilo)} = \frac{TN\,500}{W}.$$

$T =$ ml of thiosulfate solution, $N =$ normality of this solution, and $W =$ weight of the oil/fat in grams.

(b) A colorimetric method [63] is based on the decolorization of methylene blue by peroxides. About 2 ml of a 0.025 % alcoholic solution of this indicator are added to 20 ml of the test oil (or molten fat). The paling of the blue color gives a measure of the rancidity.

(c) Lips, Chapman, and McFarlane [64] describe a method based on titration with potassium ferrocyanide. This method is reported to be easy to carry out and very sensitive. The results obtained depend on the presence or absence of atmospheric oxygen during the test but are reproducible, provided the procedure is strictly adhered to.

### Preservatives

Apart from the additives that prevent oxidation of fats, all cosmetic preparations require the addition of substances that will protect them from the effect of bacteria and fungi. These substances were discussed in detail in Chapter 3.

### COMPOSITION

A number of possible combinations of the raw materials listed in the preceding paragraphs and the difficulties that might occur are now discussed.

Formulations that illustrate the principles covered will be found in the second part of this book.

## Thixotropic Creams

Cleansing and massaging creams are often required to be thixotropic; that is, they should be gels while they are in the container but should liquefy immediately on being applied to the skin. In anhydrous creams this behavior can be achieved by combining paraffin wax and mineral oil. If the cream is poured into jars before cooling, the paraffin wax crystallizes in a three-dimensional net structure which imparts firmness to the preparation but collapses as soon as pressure is applied. In practice the combination of paraffin wax and mineral oil is not very satisfactory because the oil is not bound in the paraffin net and starts bleeding out after a short time. In order to prevent bleeding, petroleum jelly or one of the microcrystalline waxes (ceresine, ozokerite, astrolatum, or possibly beeswax) is added. This yields very good thixotropic preparations. Spermaceti and cetyl palmitate resemble paraffin wax in their effect and may also be used in thixotropic preparations. Petrolatum as such behaves similarly because it is firm at room temperature but melts at body temperature (i.e., in contact with skin), but it melts much more slowly than a genuine thixotropic preparation.

The tendency of liquid components of a preparation to bleed out is increased with their increasing fluidity. The very fluid mineral and silicone oils, synthetic oils such as isopropylmyristinate, cetiol, and sperm oil particularly tend to bleed out; creams containing a high proportion of these materials must therefore be formulated with an adequate quantity of binders (apart from petrolatum and micro waxes, cetyl alcohol and Lanette O are also useful) to avoid bleeding.

## Nongreasy Products

Cosmeticians are often called on to formulate anhydrous preparations that will not leave a sticky-greasy feeling on the skin.

It is difficult to pinpoint the reasons why some anhydrous oils, creams, and W/O emulsions leave this sticky feeling. Experience shows, however, that this sensation is usually related to a film on the skin which is fairly thick, or has high viscosity, or a high surface tension. Viscous paraffin oils, petrolatum, many vegetable and animal oils and fats as well as lanolin are known to cause this feeling. This sensation does not occur, however, if substances with low surface tension that penetrate into wrinkles and hair follicles are used; substances with low viscosity that permit them to be spread in a thin layer (low-viscosity petrolatum and silicone oil, isopropyl myristate, acetylated lanolin derivatives, aceto fats, and cetiol); or dry waxlike substances that have a good affinity with the skin (cetyl alcohol, lanette wax, spermaceti etc.).

Whether a cosmetic preparation will cause a greasy feeling depends on the ratio of its greasy and nongreasy constituents. The greasy effect may often be reduced by replacing some greasy ingredients with nongreasy ones.

## Protective Preparations

Here it is matter of finding the correct proportion of substances with high affinity to skin keratin and substances that remain on the skin surface. A protective preparation is effective only if at least part of it does not penetrate the skin but remains on the surface; however, it must at least adhere to the skin, for otherwise it would be rubbed off too easily. The adherence of the film may be increased by increasing the viscosity; this again causes the greasy feeling which should be avoided in protective preparations. Finally, the film must often be water-repellent and water-impermeable; yet a completely impermeable film will lead to heat congestion and the loosening of the film from the inside by the accumulation of perspiration. The problem with its many contradictory requirements can be solved only by some kind of compromise.

## Pastes

Pastes are dispersions of more or less finely distributed solids. As we noted in Chapter 2 particles in such systems show a tendency to lump together, with the result that larger particles accumulate at the top or bottom of the preparation. Small additions of lecithin, phosphoric acid esters, and alkylolamides facilitate the preparation of such pastes because they facilitate wetting of the solids by the fats.

## Preparation

Generally the method of preparation is very simple. Waxes and other solids are melted and the oils are stirred in. All components, solid and liquid, are often heated together in one container and stirred until the mass is homogeneous. Care must be taken not to heat it longer or to a higher temperature than is required for the fusion of the raw materials because all chemical changes in the basic materials are considerably accelerated at higher temperatures. Oils that are rich in vitamins (if they are being used because of their vitamin content) and vitamin concentrates should be heated as little as possible. The two most important fat-soluble vitamins are A and $D_2$. Vitamin A is oxidized by atmospheric oxygen and an increased temperature will accelerate oxidation. Vitamin $D_2$ is not stable at higher temperatures.

If antioxidants have not been added to the basic materials before processing, they are dissolved in the oil or oil mixture or alternatively in the finished product while it is still hot and liquid.

In the production of pastes the solid pulverized ingredients are added at the end when the preparation is still liquid. Stirring must be continued until the mass has thickened, since otherwise the solids do not remain well dispersed.

## WATER-IN-OIL EMULSIONS

## RAW MATERIALS

### The Raw Materials of the Oil Phase

The raw materials for anhydrous preparations discussed in the first section of this chapter are used in these products as well.

### The Raw Materials of the Aqueous Phase

Here, too, we can be very brief. With few exceptions, additions to the aqueous phase of W/O emulsions serve no purpose. No moisture-binding substances (glycerol, or sorbitol) are needed to prevent the drying of the cream because the water is protected from evaporation by the surrounding oil phase. Nor do such additions to W/O creams have an emollient effect on the skin; they are insoluble in the fat film and therefore have little contact with the skin. At best, they improve the spreadability of the emulsions.

Substances that increase the viscosity of the aqueous phase have no particular effect on the viscosity of W/O creams, which is determined by the viscosity of the oil phase and the quantity and dispersion of the water droplets in it but not by their viscosity. Water-soluble active substances usually have a weaker effect in W/O emulsions (and should therefore not be incorporated in them) than in O/W emulsions. Polano [65] established, for example, that water-soluble antilight agents are effective only in O/W emulsions.

Water-soluble emulsifying agents or bases and basic salts, which form emulsifiers with the acids contained in the oil phase, are occasionally important components of W/O creams. By reducing the surface tension between both phases they facilitate the breaking of the aqueous phase into fine droplets. They may also at times increase the stability of the emulsions. Their use often results in creams of the dual emulsion type.

### Emulsifying Agents

Most of the typical W/O emulsifying agents have already been mentioned in a different context. They are fat-soluble substances such as lanolin, wool-fat alcohols or sterols, beeswax, cetyl alcohol and other fatty alcohols, certain fatty-acid esters of polyhydric alcohols (e.g., sorbitan sesquioleate) and magnesium, calcium, or aluminum salts of the higher fatty acids. Their use as W/O emulsifying agents is now discussed in detail.

**Lanolin, Wool-Fat Alcohols and Sterols, and Fatty Alcohols.**   The hydrophilic character of these substances is due to their free hydroxyl group. (As previously mentioned, lanolin can absorb almost twice its own weight in water, whereas acetylated lanolin, in which the hydroxyl groups are esterified, is definitely hydrophobic and does not absorb water.) It is amazing, and at the same time of great importance to cosmetic practice, that mixtures of small amounts of these emulsifiers with fats and oils with little or no hydrophilic properties will have an even greater water-absorbing capacity than the emulsifying agents alone; 3–10 % solutions of these substances in petrolatum, paraffin oil, hydrogenated peanut oil, etc., often absorb a multiple of their total weight in water in the form of a W/O emulsion.

In Europe a number of blends based on this principle are commercially available. They are called "absorption bases." In addition to lanolin, wool-fat alcohols or sterols, and cetyl alcohol, commercial absorption bases may also contain cholesterol or monofatty acid esters of polyhydric alcohols (sorbitan sesquioleate, Spans, Cremophor FM, etc.) as emulsifiers and beeswax, sterol esters, spermaceti, or lecithin as stabilizers. Janistyn [66] and Rothemann [67] give good descriptions of the preparation of absorption bases and a listing of commercial products. The advantage of using absorption bases in cosmetic formulations lies in their well-balanced composition which often simplifies formulation and processing. In most cases the manufacturers of absorption bases also provide suggestions for their use in a number of cosmetic preparations. The advantage of starting from the basic raw materials instead of absorption bases lies in better knowledge of their composition so that the formulator who uses them is less dependent on one supplier.

**Beeswax.**   Beeswax as such is rarely used as an emulsifying agent, although it has certain emulsifying properties due to its content of free high-molecular fatty acids and fatty alcohols. These properties are utilized in the traditional cold creams; formulations of these preparations go back to the Middle Ages and can still be found in the pharmacopoeiae of various countries.

In addition to many original formulations, Renaud [68] lists prescriptions for cold creams from 20 different pharmacopoeiae.

*Ceratum Galeni* (French Codex)

| | | |
|---|---|---|
| Cera alba (bleached beeswax) | 12.0 | Wax and oil are melted together |
| Almond oil | 50.0 | and rosewater is added under |
| Rose water | 37.5 | intensive stirring. |

*Genuine Cold Cream* (German Pharmacopoeia)

| | | |
|---|---|---|
| Cera alba (bleached beeswax) | 7.0 g | The waxes are melted, almond |
| Spermaceti | 8.0 g | oil is stirred in, and stirring is |
| Almond oil | 60.0 g | continued until cool; then water |
| Water | 25.0 g | and finally attar of roses are |
| Attar of roses | 2 drops | added under intensive stirring. |

These formulations are based on a recipe by Galen in the second century, of which even he may not have been the inventor: "Melt carefully in a porcelain bowl one part refined beeswax together with 3–4 parts olive oil into which rose leaves have been ground. After the mixture is cool, as much water as can be held by the mass is stirred in."

Emulsions made in this way have no great stability. As soon as the cream melts after application to the skin the water separates. The evaporation of the water on the skin causes the cooling effect that gave the preparation its name.

Prescriptions such as the two preceding are unfortunately useless in modern cosmetic practice because their stability, particularly in fluctuating temperatures, is much too low. On opening a new jar the consumer would probably find a preparation that would show large drops or even a whole layer of water on the surface.

The stability of beeswax emulsions may be increased if small quantities of borax are added during processing. This reacts with the fatty acids in beeswax leading to formation of sodium salts.

It is often stated in the literature that cerotic acid ($C_{26}$), melissic acid ($C_{30}$), and the corresponding alcohols (ceryl and melissyl alcohols) occur in beeswax. The substances so described are not really chemically defined compounds but rather mixtures of homologous high-molecular fatty acids and alcohols.

The over-all equation for the beeswax/borax reaction is

$$2RCOOH + Na_2B_4O_7 + 5H_2O \rightarrow 2RCOONa + 4H_3BO_3.$$

The acid content of beeswax is expressed as the "acid number" in pharmaceutical and cosmetic literature. This number shows how many milligrams of potassium hydroxide are required to neutralize the acids contained in 1 g of beeswax. Normally the acid number for good beeswax lies between 17 and 24. A beeswax with an acid number of 20 requires 20 mg of potassium hydroxide or 68 mg of borax ($Na_2B_4O_7 \cdot 10 H_2O$) per gram to be completely neutralized. The proportion of borax to beeswax here would be about 1:15. Most cold cream formulations approximate this proportion. The change from a free fatty acid (in the traditional prescriptions) to a fatty-acid salt (in the borax formulations) means changing from an emulsifying agent with a low HLB value to one with a much higher HLB value (see Chapter 2), that is, from a W/O emulsifier to an O/W emulsifier. Actually the beeswax/borax cold creams are no longer pure W/O emulsions but belong to the dual type, which is discussed in more detail in the following section.

In addition to the fatty acids and their salts, the fatty alcohols contained in beeswax also play an important part in the emulsifying properties of this wax. Pickthall [69] found that cold creams made with beeswax whose hydroxyl groups had been blocked by acetylation showed a coarser dispersion of the aqueous phase and less stability than creams made with untreated beeswax. It follows in practice that apart from the acid number the alcohol content (acetyl value) of the wax must also be taken into consideration as an indication of its emulsifying capacity.

**Fatty Acid Esters of Polyhydric Alcohols.**   In this group sorbitan sesquioleate (Arlacel 83, Atlas Chemical Co.) has proved particularly effective. The manufacturer reports that a 10% solution of Arlacel 83 in petrolatum can bind 16.3 times its weight in water as a W/O emulsion. W/O emulsions prepared with this emulsifier are more stable in fluctuating temperatures than lanolin or beeswax emulsions. Other fatty-acid esters (e.g., the "Spans" of Atlas Chemical Co. and the monofatty acid esters of glycol, glycerol, or polyethylene glycols) are hardly, if ever, used as W/O emulsifiers, but they act as auxiliary emulsifying agents in O/W emulsions.

**Zinc, Magnesium, Calcium, or Aluminum Salts of Higher Fatty Acids.**   The stabilizing effect of these salts is due in part to surface activity and in part to the swelling property of these substances in the oil phase which increases its viscosity. They are never used alone but always in conjunction with other W/O emulsifying agents.

### Preservatives

It is advisable to use preservatives for both the aqueous and oil phase of all cosmetic preparations (see Chapter 3). Antioxidants should be added to the oil phase.

### General Remarks

Most of the remarks regarding anhydrous products may also be applied here. A suitable composition of the oil phase will impart to products of this type protective, conditioning, emollient, or cleansing effects. Compared with anhydrous preparations, W/O emulsions have certain advantages: the evaporation of the water may cause a pleasant cooling sensation on the skin; because of their water content, these preparations are often more economical in preparation and use; in cleansing preparations the aqueous phase may play a certain part in removing water-soluble impurities. A remark by Harry [70] is of interest in this connection: according to him, anhydrous cleansing creams are also able to remove water-soluble impurities because they are dissolved by the perspiration on the skin which is enclosed or emulsified by the fatty cream and then removed with it.

Water-in-oil emulsions are more attractive in consistency and appearance (smoother, less greasy, lighter in color) than most anhydrous preparations. They are easier to perfume because they present no solubility problems.

The great disadvantage of W/O emulsions compared with anhydrous preparations is their relatively low stability. Anhydrous preparations also sometimes become hard on cooling or soften or even liquefy in high temperatures, but they always return to their normal consistency as soon as the temperature returns to normal. With W/O emulsions there is always a risk that they will separate after too much cooling or too much heat, and at room temperature the preparation will then show two distinct layers that are all too noticeable to visual inspection. W/O emulsions in which a high water-absorption capacity of the fatty base is not exhausted by the water in the emulsion exhibit relatively good stability.

As we saw in Chapter 2, the mutual electrostatic repulsion of the droplets in the dispersed phase, which is important in the stabilization of O/W emulsions, plays no part in W/O emulsions. Here the important factors are the stability of the interfacial film and the viscosity of the external (oil) phase. Münzel evaluates these factors in a fundamental study of the stability of W/O emulsions [71]. His microscopic examinations show that the interfacial film in these emulsions is usually hard and tough and belongs to the "solid" type. The drops of the internal phase are shaped irregularly. (O/W emulsions have an elastic film of the "liquid" type and the droplets are always spherical.) It frequently happens that in W/O emulsions the combination of two surfactants will lead to a stronger interfacial film than the use of any one of them alone. Since the stabilizing effect of emulsifiers and pairs of emulsifiers depends largely on the composition of the oil phase, Münzel could not establish generally valid rules. It would be interesting to examine the possibility of using the HLB system to obtain some clarification on this point.

Among the emulsifying agents tested beeswax was the most effective in stabilizing water-in-mineral-oil emulsions, and beeswax and magnesium stearate were the best emulsifiers for water-in-peanut-oil emulsions. It is remarkable that in these instances the emulsifying agent did not reduce the interfacial tension between the phases but even slightly increased it. The interfacial tension is therefore not an important factor in the stability of these emulsions. Münzel observes that beeswax as well as magnesium stearate are oil-soluble only to a limited extent and assumes that their stabilizing effect is related to their capacity of thickening the oil phase by colloidal swelling.

The dependence of the emulsion stability on the viscosity of the oil phase was noticeable in all tests made. Microcrystalline waxes and petrolatums had a better stabilizing effect than macrocrystalline waxes, such as paraffin wax. This dependence is also the reason for the sensitivity of W/O emulsions to temperature changes. The separation of emulsions at low temperatures may probably be explained by the fracturing of the interfacial film by the aqueous phase.

### Preparation

Generally the components of the oil phase are melted together, with the temperature being kept as low as possible. The water, containing whatever water-soluble ingredients are used, is heated to 2–5°C above the temperature of the melt and stirred into the oil phase. Since the viscosity is so important to the stability of the emulsion, which tends to separate as long as the oil phase is liquid, stirring must be continued until the mass is cool enough for the oil phase to have thickened. In some cases the water is even stirred into the cold or almost cold fat mass (see Galen's prescription for cold cream). According to a private communication by H. H. Daute, emulsification of W/O emulsions based on wool fat or wool-fat alcohols can be effected only by cold processing. These emulsions may be more finely dispersed in roller mills. Emulsification of a similar preparation with sorbitan sesquioleate, cetyl alcohol, or saponified beeswax succeeds only if fat and water are heated for mixing. In these instances a finer dispersion can be obtained only with homogenizers.

If a small amount of surfactant is added to the aqueous phase to reduce the interfacial tension between oil and water, this helps the dispersion of the aqueous phase and may increase the stability of the emulsion. Such an addition, however, may often result in a dual rather than a pure W/O emulsion.

Subsequent homogenization usually increases the stability considerably. We shall not dwell here on the technology of emulsification. This problem is thoroughly discussed by Becher [72].

In pastes on a W/O basis the finely ground solids are usually added at the end. Occasionally they are added to the phase that would provide a better wetting agent before emulsification.

## DUAL EMULSIONS

Cosmetic literature divides emulsified preparations into two main groups: W/O and O/W emulsions. Emulsions based on absorption bases are typical representatives of the first, stearate creams representative of the second type. A number of tests are known to determine whether an emulsion belongs to the W/O or O/W type. Nevertheless, there are a number of emulsified preparations for which agreement has not been reached regarding the type of emulsion. The beeswax/borax creams are a good example. Janistyn, Harry, and De Navarre usually describe them as O/W emulsions but add that the type of emulsion depends on the ratio of the phases and on the emulsifiers used; Keithler and Rothemann describe these creams throughout as W/O emulsions.

In our opinion beeswax/borax emulsions and many others containing both O/W and W/O emulsifiers in which the oil phase amounts to 50–75% of the system are neither pure water-in-oil nor pure oil-in-water emulsions but "dual" types. It is difficult to picture in these emulsions how the available hydrophilic and lipophilic constituents are dispersed in the system. There might be an O/W dispersion in one part and a W/O dispersion in another, that is, a mixture of both types. However, the situation is probably even more complicated and the so-called double emulsions may also play a part here (W/O/W or O/W/O).

It has been known for a long time that the transition from W/O to O/W emulsions is not clearly defined. Parsons and Wilson [73], for instance, have carried out a series of tests in which the oil phase was mineral oil, the aqueous phase, pure water, and a mixture of sodium and magnesium oleates was used as the emulsifier. They found that stable W/O emulsions were obtained only if the emulsifying mixture contained 91% + of magnesium oleate and stable O/W emulsions resulted only if the mixture contained 50% or more sodium oleate. In the intermediary range dual emulsions were formed. In a similar series of experiments with a mixture of potassium and magnesium palmitates as emulsifier, van der Minne [74] found the critical emulsifier composition to be 18% and 79% potassium palmitate, respectively; mixtures with more than 18% and less than 79% potassium palmitate resulted in dual emulsions. Some authors have also recognized that such dual emulsions may occur in cosmetic and pharmaceutical practice [75]. Generally, however, the high incidence of this type of emulsion in cosmetics has not yet been fully appreciated.

What practical conclusions can be drawn from the fact that an emulsion belongs to the dual type? Unfortunately there is no answer: no research has yet been carried out on the basic aspects of this emulsion type. We have no clear picture of its physical structure, so that we are not in a position to make logical deductions regarding the factors that affect the stability of these emulsions as we were able to do for O/W and W/O emulsions. This would appear to be a fruitful field for further research.

The only conclusion we can draw today is the following: if an emulsion belongs to the dual type, it is an error to assume that it is either a W/O or a O/W emulsion. It may well be that steps taken to ensure the stabilization of such an emulsion will have the opposite result. An awareness of the dual character of the emulsion will lead to the special caution required.

## Comparison with W/O and O/W Emulsions

1. Compared with W/O emulsions, dual emulsions are usually more stable. It is known that the addition of borax to the old-style cold creams increased their stability and, after all, this was the reason why this added ingredient was universally accepted. This increase in stability in cold creams has a certain inherent disadvantage: the cooling effect due to the evaporation of the water has largely been lost in modern formulations.

It may well be that the addition of a water-soluble O/W emulsifier, which reduces the tendency of the water droplets to coalesce, is important to better stability. Nevertheless, the viscosity of the oil phase is also an essential factor in these emulsions.

2. Dual emulsions differ from pure O/W emulsions primarily because of their higher content of W/O emulsifiers. Since these substances have many emollient and smoothing properties, dual emulsions seem to be the type most indicated for emollient creams.

Although some O/W emulsions have a very high oil content, generally speaking the oil content of dual emulsions is higher. Preparations whose effectiveness is due in particular to the oil phase (barrier, cleansing, or hair creams) can therefore be presented in a more "concentrated" form as dual emulsions than as O/W emulsions.

## Preparation

Dual emulsions are made usually in the same way as W/O emulsions but other methods are occasionally recommended. It is interesting to note that with this type of emulsion the processing decisively affects the quality of the preparation. The following remarks are made about beeswax/borax creams [76]:

1. If the water is stirred into the melted oil phase at 70°C, a semisolid cream is obtained which easily melts on application.

2. If the water, heated to 55°C, is stirred into the melted oil phase and the mixture heated first to 90°C before cooling starts, a semisolid cream is obtained which has a high gloss and melts slowly.

3. If both phases are melted together at 55°C without any subsequent heating, a somewhat granular soft cream results, which melts easily. Keithler gives the following formulation for a "lubricating cream":

| | |
|---|---|
| Beeswax | 14 |
| Cetyl alcohol | 2 |
| Stearyl alcohol | 2 |
| Mineral oil | 54 |
| Lecithin | 2 |
| Borax | 1 |
| Water | 25 |

The temperature of both phases should be between 60 and 70°C for mixing but as near to 60°C as possible. Two methods of preparation may be followed:

(a) All ingredients of the oil phase are heated together and the aqueous borax solution is stirred in.

(b) The solids of the oil phase are melted together; the mineral oil is heated in another vessel, the borax/water solution in a third. When all three constituents have reached 65°C, a small part of the aqueous phase is added to the melted waxes; the remainder of the water and the mineral oil are added simultaneously under intensive stirring in such a way that the addition of both is finished roughly at the same time. Both methods are reported to result in good emulsification, but the second yields a smoother product with better gloss.

## OIL-IN-WATER EMULSIONS

### The Raw Materials for the Oil Phase

**Oils and Fats.** The materials used in anhydrous preparations are also suitable here.

**Waxes.** Waxes play a less important part in O/W creams than in anhydrous or W/O preparations. One of their functions in any preparation is the thickening of the oil phase which tends to stabilize the emulsion. Since the stability of O/W emulsions does not depend on the viscosity of the oil phase, waxes are correspondingly less important. Only lanolin and its derivatives play a major part as skin smoothing agents.

**Fatty Alcohols.** Fatty alcohols are also of importance in O/W emulsions. Cetyl alcohol is a valuable emollient. Lanette Wax N (a mixture of cetyl and stearyl alcohols, with small additions of sodium cetyl sulfate and sodium stearyl sulfate which makes the mixture self-emulsifying) is used in European formulations as the basis of many O/W emulsions and of many pharmaceutical ointment bases as well. In this system fatty alcohols act as auxiliary emulsifying agents and thereby contribute to the stabilization of the emulsion. Generally speaking, the emulsifier component in O/W emulsions may be reduced, the higher the fatty alcohol content of the oil phase.

**Monoesters of Polyhydric Alcohols.** The most important representative of this group is glycerol monostearate. There are, however, many other related esters that have assumed importance in the cosmetic industry: glycol monostearate, diethylene glycol monostearate, polyethylene glycol monostearate, sorbitan monostearate ("Span 60"), and the corresponding monoesters of other fatty acids. More recent representatives of this type are the monofatty acid esters of saccharose (cane sugar).

The commercial grades of these substances are not chemically pure but are mixtures of mono- and di- (occasionally even tri-) esters which also contain free acids and free alcohols (glycerol, glycol, etc.). Moreover the fatty acid is usually not uniform but a technical product in which the name merely indicates the predominating acid in the mixture.

So-called self-emulsifying grades of glycerol monostearate (and similar fatty acid monoesters) contain small additions of an emulsifier, usually the sodium salts of the fatty acid used—in this case sodium stearate. If such a self-emulsifying product is mixed with water, a very stable O/W emulsion results.

**Fatty Acids.**    These are much more important in O/W than in W/O emulsions. Stearic acid is the most important material in this group. Here as well the addition of small amounts of a O/W emulsifier results in a self-emulsifying grade: the traditional "vanishing cream," which exists in many variations, is fundamentally nothing more than a stearic acid-in-water emulsion with an alkali stearate acting as emulsifier. Such products are prepared in practice by adding a little alkali to the aqueous phase which reacts with stearic acid and forms an emulsifier. In contrast to the alcohols, fatty acids have no emollient effect on the skin; stearate creams have a definitely "dry" effect.

**Preservatives and Antioxidants.**    Microbiological decomposition is much more pronounced in O/W than in W/O emulsions. Suitable preservation is absolutely essential and must be particularly effective if the emulsions contain any vegetable mucins, biological complexes, or vitamins (particularly of the B group). Products containing vegetable oils require antioxidants.

### The Raw Materials of the Aqueous Phase

**Water.**    Distilled water is preferred in cosmetics because the substances dissolved in normal tap water may cause difficulties in certain circumstances: electrolytes may reduce the stability of many emulsions, and calcium and magnesium salts may act as W/O emulsifiers in the system and thus also reduce the stability. Traces of iron cause coloration in phenols (which might be present as preservatives or disinfectants), and probably in triethanolamine, and promote rancidity of vegetable and animal oils.

Organic impurities (in particular those containing nitrogen or sulfur) may lead to unpleasant odors. The presence of magnesium, copper, zinc, and manganese promotes the growth of microorganisms. Calcium salts increase the risk of bacteria penetrating the skin. Mellon [77] and Jones and Lorenz [78] found that the penetration of bacteria from the aqueous into the oil phase is facilitated by the presence of calcium salts. Microorganisms then enter hair follicles and sebum glands and may cause infections. This also explains the frequency of staphylococcus infections if calcium compounds are used in the treatment of wounds. Precipitates of calcium fatty-acid salts which accumulate on the skin may also protect bacteria from the action of disinfectants, soap, or other microorganisms. In calcium soaps bacteria are capable of reproducing for two weeks or longer.

For all of these reasons it is advisable to use only distilled water or water that has been desalted by an ion exchange process [79] in cosmetic preparations. It is also important to use freshly treated water; it is astonishing how many microorganisms can be found in distilled water that has been kept in storage for several months.

**Humectants.** Almost all cosmetic O/W emulsions and some W/O emulsions contain one or more hygroscopic substances in the aqueous phase. This addition may serve several purposes [80].

1. Preventation of at least retardation of "shrinkage" of the cream by water evaporation.

2. Smoothing of the skin surface and prevention or curing of a rough or broken condition of the horny layer.

3. Ease of application of the cream and prevention of the "roll effect."

The main water-binding substances in cosmetics are glycerol, propylene glycol, and sorbitol. Polyethylene glycols, with molecular weights of 200–600, polypropylene glycols, and diethylene glycol monoethylether as well as honey [81] are also used but less frequently. Sodium lactate has been recommended as a moisturizer [82].

The three purposes of these substances are now discussed in detail:

1. *Prevention of shrinkage.* The effect of moisture-binding substances has been fully discussed in an article by Griffin, Behrens, and Cross [83]. These authors point out that two properties must be differentiated in humectants: the equilibrium hygroscopicity which determines how much water can be held by a definite amount of the substance when a balance has been established between the solution and the atmosphere (the amount of bound water also depends on the moisture content of the atmosphere); and the dynamic hygroscopicity that indicates the speed at which the substance or its solution attracts moisture from the atmosphere or releases water before equilibrium has been established. In older publications these two properties are rarely differentiated. Since a high equilibrium hygroscopic capacity is not always linked to a strong dynamic hygroscopocity, conflicting data have often been published. In cosmetics it is not the equilibrium but the dynamic hygroscopicity that is important and this should be as low as possible, however much of a paradox this may appear. In practice even a relatively high content of hygroscopic substances is usually not sufficient to protect the emulsions

from evaporation of the aqueous phase or a major part of it. Griffin et al. [83] found that even with high atmospheric humidity O/W emulsions must contain at least three parts of humectants (glycerol, etc.) for each part of water in order to prevent evaporation altogether. This is obviously quite impossible from a dermatological point of view. Even if the hygroscopic substances cannot completely prevent evaporation, they can considerably retard it. They can reduce evaporation so that it is of no practical significance during the time the jar of cream is in use, even if it is left open for many hours. The most effective substance will be the one that in solution is the slowest to attract or release water: the substance with the lowest dynamic hygroscopicity. Griffin and co-workers made a series of experiments in which they compared the effectiveness of glycerol, propylene glycol, and sorbitol. Velon made similar tests but only compared glycerol with propylene glycol [84]. Creams containing various humectants (and control batches without such additions) were exposed for periods of 5 minutes to 48 hours to an atmosphere with a definite degree of humidity and the evaporation was then measured for these periods. The tests were made at 30, 50, and 70% of relative humidity, with concentrations of the hygroscopic agents between 0 and 20%. Three types of emulsion were examined: two stearic acid-in-water-emulsions, one with potassium stearate as the emulsifying agent, the other with nonionic emulsifiers, and a W/O emulsion. The following results are of interest:

When the O/W creams without humectants were left open for 48 hours, they lost water amounting to 10–20% of their total weight. The W/O creams did not suffer any appreciable loss in weight.

In the O/W creams with potassium stearate as emulsifier the three tested humectants showed widely differing effects that also depended on atmospheric humidity. At 70% relative humidity additions of less than 10% glycerol (based on the total) were ineffective because they did not reduce the loss in water after 48 hours. Propylene glycol was effective only in concentrations above 5%. Sorbitol reduced evaporation in every concentration, even at 2%. At a lower atmospheric humidity glycerol is more effective than propylene glycol. In every instance sorbitol proved to be the only substance that acted as an effective protection at concentrations of 5% and less. In some instances it was most interesting to note that small additions of glycerol and propylene glycol not only failed to reduce the speed of evaporation but actually increased it. This may be due to a crust formation of stearate creams in the course of drying out which inhibits further evaporation. Small additions of glycerol and propylene glycol apparently prevent this crust from forming. In O/W creams with nonionic emulsifiers all three substances showed a retarding effect on evaporation in all concentrations, provided the relative air humidity was 50 to 70%. Crust formation plays a less important part here.

It is reported that the hygroscopicity of low-molecular polyethylene glycols lies at 90% (polyglycol 200) and 50% (polyglycol 600), respectively, compared with the value for glycerol [85]. These data probably refer to the equilibrium and not to the dynamic hygroscopocity. With the higher molecular polyethylene glycols hygroscopicity is much lower; they are therefore not used as humectants.

Ossipow [86] recommends sodium lactate in combination with lactic acid as a buffering agent as well as a highly effective humectant. Another advantage of this system is its weakly acid pH. Lactic acid as such is widely used for acidifying cosmetics. It has certain bactericidal properties. Its calcium salt is water-soluble and is used in medicine as a calcium source. Sodium lactate is a hygroscopic compound that crystallizes only with difficulty. It is commercially available as a viscous, aqueous solution with a sodium lactate concentration of 70–80%. The salt is compatible with almost all cosmetic ingredients. The only important incompatibility occurs in the salting out of soaps from aqueous solutions. The above mentioned mixtures are suitable for antiperspirants, hand, face, and shaving creams, and hair lacquers.

2. *The smoothing of the skin surface.* Traditionally, glycerol is one of the main active constituents (sometimes the only one) of hand creams that are intended to prevent roughening and chapping of the hands. As we shall see in more detail in Chapter 8, skin roughness is due to loss of water from the uppermost layers of the corneum. A thin glycerol film on the skin surface is effective because of its moisture-retaining capacity. In this instance the binding capacity (equilibrium hygroscopicity) rather than the moisture attraction (dynamic hygroscopicity) is probably operative because equilibrium with the environment is quickly established in a thin film. Tests by Powers and Fox [87] are interesting in this connection. No tests have been carried out on the relative effectiveness of the available substances. Most experience has been gathered in connection with glycerol. It is completely nontoxic and nonirritating when used in aqueous solutions at concentrations not above 30%.

It has repeatedly been pointed out in the literature that glycerol acts as an irritant in combination with stearate soaps and that such combinations should therefore not be used in facial preparations. Actually many available stearate creams also contain glycerol; the combination of glycerol and soaps also occurs in many toilet and shaving soaps. We cannot therefore take these allegations very seriously. Among the other substances that may be used for this purpose sorbitol, propylene glycol, and the polyethylene and polypropylene glycols also appear to be nontoxic and nonirritating. Ethylene glycol may be absorbed by the skin and oxidized to the noxious oxalic acid in the body. For the same reason the use of diethylene glycol is also not recommended. Diethylene glycol monoethylether (Carbitol) is harmless in this connection, but its use leads to the appearance of beads of perspiration on the skin [88].

3. *The ease of application of creams.* It is a widely known phenomenon that stearate creams with a high content of stearic acid and other O/W creams in which the oil phase contains solids or waxes tend to dry out on application so that in extreme cases the cream rolls off the skin in small flakes. Generally this property of creams is undesirable; it is used only in some massaging creams. An addition of glycerol, sorbitol, etc., to the aqueous phase reduces this tendency to roll off. Sorbitol in particular (and its derivatives such as sorbitol sesquioleate) imparts a velvety consistency to the film during spreading. Propylene glycol also results in a soft film; glycerol is stickier. According to De Navarre [89], glycerol may adversely affect the stability of W/O emulsions, whereas propylene glycol and sorbitol have an unfavorable effect on some O/W emulsions that causes them to stiffen after a short time. Cessna, Ohlmann, and Roehm [90] have made similar observations. According to Griffin, Behrens, and Cross [83], these substances will effect the stability or formation of emulsions only if they were not particularly stable or easy to prepare because of improperly selected raw materials.

The incompatibility of emulsions containing borax with glycerol, which has occasionally been reported, is probably due to complex formation of borax and glycerol—the complex has an acid reaction. According to Tschakert and Gathen [91], a borax solution had a pH 6.5 after the addition of glycerol: sorbitol resulted in a pH 4 and should therefore be even more unfavorable than glycerol in beeswax/borax cold creams. "Polyglycol 200" did not form a complex with borax; the pH of this solution was 8.5.

**Substances which Increase the Viscosity of the Aqueous Phase.** The viscosity of an emulsion depends on the following factors: the viscosity of the external phase, the concentration and dispersion of the internal phase (the higher the concentration and the finer the dispersion, the higher the viscosity in general), and the characteristics and concentration of the emulsifier system.

As far as the last factor is concerned, it is known, for instance, that stearate creams with triethanolamine stearate are much softer and smoother than stearate creams with sodium stearate. The reason for this phenomenon is not quite clear. Generally the viscosity of an emulsion increases with the emulsifier concentration [92].

The viscosity of the internal phase is almost of no importance. Many O/W emulsions may be thickened by the addition of cetyl alcohol, but this is due to the effect of cetyl alcohol as an auxiliary emulsifying agent and not to the thickening of the oil phase. Paraffin wax or petrolatum, which cause a similar stiffening without being surfactants, do not thicken O/W emulsions. Since the concentration of the internal phase is also one of the factors determining the viscosity of emulsions, those with a low proportion of the dispersed phase (hand lotions, certain hand creams, cream shampoos, etc.) will be fluid. Thickening agents are used partly in order to give a thicker consistency to preparations with low viscosity; for example, a dilute O/W emulsion. The preparation can then be spread more smoothly and in a thicker layer on the skin so that it will not run off.

The thickening agents also have another effect: they stabilize cosmetic emulsions. As we have already seen in Chapter 2, one of the factors affecting the stability of an emulsion is the viscosity of the external phase. Just by thickening the aqueous phase thickening agents act as stabilizers in O/W emulsions. However, the situation is more complicated: the thickening agents form colloidal suspensions in water, and in the case of emulsions there is a pronounced tendency to form a colloidal protective sheath around each dispersed droplet which leads to further stabilization. In some instances (methyl cellulose, sodium alginate, and gum arabic) the protective colloidal effect is so strong that the thickening agents by themselves may act as emulsifiers. Chun, Joslin, and Martin [93] have even determined the HLB values of thickening agents. Other substances in this group act only as stabilizers.

Actually, some of the materials listed here as thickening agents have been grouped together with emulsifying agents in other technical publications; for example, Janistyn [94] lists all these substances as emulsifiers of the O/W type. As far as their chemical structure is concerned, thickening agents differ from the products we have described so far as emulsifying agents by the absence of the contrast between polar and nonpolar groups which characterizes genuine emulsifying agents but is not present in those with a colloidal action. Nearly all cosmetic emulsions contain one or more emulsifiers of the polar/nonpolar type; only a few contain a substance that acts as a protective colloid, and this is never used by itself but always in combination with an emulsifying agent of the other kind. In cosmetic practice, therefore, it seems more realistic to us to continue to describe as emulsifying agents only the polar/nonpolar substances and to classify the colloidal materials as thickening agents or, at best, stabilizers. Of the many materials that belong to this group we list only the most important [95]:

1. *Vegetable mucins.* Gum tragacanth, gum karaya, gum arabic (gum acacia), quince mucilage, marsh mallow, etc., form mucilages with water that are more or less stable and nonirritating and therefore suitable for cosmetics. (Figley [96] did observe allergic reactions to gum karaya.) It would be impossible here to list fully the individual characteristics of the different mucins. De Navarre [97] gives many valuable suggestions for their use.

2. *Alginates* [98]. The most commonly used thickening agent of this group is sodium alginate which is commercially available under a number of different

trade names. It is considerably more economical than the various gums and resins, and alginate solutions and gels are less sticky than those based on tragacanth and similar gums. Additions of calcium salts (e.g., calcium citrate or gluconate), particularly at pH 4–5, thicken alginate solutions even more. Sodium alginate and its solutions are completely harmless and nonirritating; they are therefore valuable cosmetic raw materials [99].

The carrageenates also belong to this group of thickening agents [100]. Agar-agar, an important thickening agent in the food industry, is hardly ever used in cosmetics.

3. *Cellulose derivatives and similar compounds* [101]. The following have gained particular importance in modern cosmetics: methylcellulose and the sodium salt of methylcellulose carboxylic acid, called CMC, or carboxymethylcellulose. Compared with vegetable gums and resins, CMC has certain advantages: its physical and chemical properties are the same from batch to batch; solutions and gels can be made in cold water; the solutions are not susceptible to fermentation and provide only a poor culture medium for bacteria and fungi.

Methylcellulose as well as sodium carboxymethylcellulose have a neutral reaction and their use is physiologically unobjectionable.

Methylcellulose is available in various grades that differ in molecular weight and the viscosity of their solutions. Low-viscosity grades yield gels at 10% concentrations; high-viscosity grades at 7–8%. In or near the neutral range the viscosity does not depend on the pH. In a strongly acid or strongly alkaline environment the fluctuation of the viscosity is partly due to the degradation of the polymeric chains.

Strong or continued heating of methylcellulose solutions leads to an irreversible reduction of viscosity [102].

Methylcellulose has a surfactant effect. Its solutions have a lower surface tension than water and they foam. Methylcellulose and CMC are used as stabilizers and even by themselves as emulsifying agents for O/W emulsions of animal and vegetable oils and fats, mineral oils and waxes, and essential oils. Such emulsions are reasonably stable after being passed through a high-pressure homogenizer. These emulsions have no practical importance in cosmetics; however, the stabilizing effect that cellulose derivatives exercise on emulsions is important in many instances. It must be borne in mind in the preservation of preparations containing methylcellulose that this substance is able to inactivate *p*-hydroxybenzoic acid esters and probably the other phenolic preservatives [103].

Sodium carboxymethylcellulose is much less surface-active than methylcellulose but nevertheless has a good stabilizing effect on emulsions and a high dispersing capacity for suspended solids. It is used frequently as a skin-protective agent in detergents. Although methylcellulose solutions coagulate when tanning agents, carbonates, phosphates, or silicates are added, CMC mucins are considerably more stable and only sensitive toward polyvalent metal ions (Fe, Al, Cr, Cu, etc.). Davies and Rowson showed that CMC mucins are sensitive to light but methylcellulose is not [104].

Chemically, the three groups of thickening agents we have discussed so far are closely related: they are all derivatives of polysaccharides. In addition, representatives of various other classes of material are also used as thickening agents.

4. *Proteins and degradation products.* Among these products gelatin in particular is used occasionally, often with vegetable gums (e.g., gum tragacanth). The viscosity of gelatin solutions depends on temperature and pH.

5. *Inorganic gels.* Various inorganic gels have the property of swelling in water and of forming viscous solutions or gels. Important representatives of this group are colloidal aluminum silicates: bentonite and "Veegum" (Vanderbilt Co.), which are differentiated by their crystal structure. Certain grades absorb up to 15 times their own volume of water. Additions of small amounts of magnesium oxide or other basic oxides increase the water affinity of bentonite even further, and in weakly alkaline solutions (also in the presence of soap) bentonite and Veegum form smooth stable gels with thixotropic properties. According to Ewing, Polite, and Shackleford [105] a 2% suspension of bentonite has a pH of 9–10. Concentrations of 1–3% impart a smooth consistency to the aqueous phase of emulsions (particularly of weakly alkaline preparations) and also act as suspending agents in insoluble solids. Bentonite and Veegum appear to be completely harmless on the skin; bentonite gels have even been used as dermatological unguent bases with good effect on damaged skin.

A light flocculent and incredibly finely dispersed grade of silicic acid (particle size 4–20 m$\mu$), which also acts as a thickening agent, is commercially available under the trade name Cab-o-Sil. As opposed to bentonite suspensions, those of Cab-o-Sil are slightly acid (a 10% suspension has a pH of 4–5).

Inorganic thickening agents have certain advantages when used in cosmetic preparations: ointments and creams are made particularly smooth and nonsticky; these preparations have a good temperature stability and the basic materials as well as their suspensions are completely immune to microorganisms. Inorganic thickening agents are also remarkable because of their ability to swell both in water and in mineral oil, and other nonpolar solvents (see Table 4.3).

6. *Synthetic polymeric substances.* Polyvinyl alcohol, polyvinylpyrrolidone, polyacrylates, and other similar substances yield highly viscous solutions in water; at higher concentrations they form gels. The solutions have a neutral reaction and are completely nonirritating to the skin. They dry to flexible

TABLE 4-3 PROPERTIES OF SOME THICKENING AGENTS

| Thickening Agent | pH | Stable at pH | T | M | Thickened by | Thinned by | Precip. by | Properties of the Solution | Remarks |
|---|---|---|---|---|---|---|---|---|---|
| Agar agar | | 4–8.5 | + | − | Little alkali | Acid, strg alkali | | Emollient | Rarely used |
| Bentonite | $b$ | | + | + | MgO a.o. basic oxides | | | | Good suspension effect; swells also in fatty vehicles |
| Carbopol 934 | $a$ | 6–10 | + | + | Little alkali | All salts, many preservatives | | Smooth, transparent, highly viscous | Dries to very thin film; light sensitive |
| Gelatin Grade I | IEP 8.0 | abt. 3 | | | | Tragacanth, gum arabic | Tannin, acids | Largely dependent on the pH; at optimum pH very smooth and stiff | Good protective colloidal effect |
| Gelatin Grade II | IEP 4.7 | abt. 8 | + | − | Tragacanth, etc. | | | | |
| Gum arabic | $a$ | | | | | | Lead salts | Thin, tacky, emollient | Stronger emulsifying than thickening effect |
| Gum karaya | $a$ | | − | − | Borax $K_2CO_3$ | | | Viscous, stringy | For a few days after preparation mucilage thickens, then gradually thins |
| Carrageenates | $b$ | 4–10 | + | − | $K^+$, $Ca^{2+}$ $Mg^{2+}$, $NH^+$ | | | Smooth, emollient | Surface-active |
| Methylcellulose | $n$ | 3–10 | ± | + | | | Tanning agents, $CO_3^{2-}$, $PO_4^{3-}$ | Smooth; viscosity independent of pH | |

| Thickening agent | | pH | T | M | Compatible with | Soluble in / incompatible | Precipitated by | Consistency | Remarks |
|---|---|---|---|---|---|---|---|---|---|
| Sodium alginate | n | 4–8.5 | ± | + | Glycerol, $Ca^{2+}$ little acid | Alcohol, alkali, Na salts | Salts, acids | Smooth, highly viscous | Odorless, colorless, tasteless |
| Na carboxy. methylcellulose | n | | + | + | | | $Al^{3+}$ $Pb^{2+}$, etc. | | Not surface-active but good dispersing agent; light sensitive |
| Polyvinyl alcohol | n | abt. 7 | | + | Borates, Si compounds, alcohols | Acids | High salt concentrations | Smooth; viscosity depends on degree of polymerization | Good emulsifying and dispersing effect; dries to a tough film |
| | | | | − | | Alkali | | Smooth, stringy | |
| Quince seed | a | | | − | Little KOH | Acid | | Highly viscous, stringy | Expensive |
| Tragacanth | | | | − | Little borax | Gum arabic | | stringy | |

*Notes.* Column "pH" refers to the reaction of an aqueous suspension of the thickening agent. "IEP" stands for "isoelectric point." Column "Stable at pH", indicates the pH range within which the thickening agent may be used without any difficulties.
Column "T" indicates whether the mucilage is stable in strong temperature fluctuations; + signifies a stable, − an unstable mucilage. Column "M" indicates whether the mucilage is susceptible to mold and bacterial attack. Mucilages and gels of thickening agents designated − must be preserved.

thin films which are particularly useful in protective preparations. The film of polyvinylpyrrolidone is hygroscopic.

High-molecular ethylene oxide polymers have recently appeared on the market: "Polyox" resins [106], at 1% solutions in water, are reported to yield highly viscous slippery mucins. They show no tendency to biological decomposition, no irritant or sensitizing effect on the skin, and a low toxicity in animal tests. They are compatible with detergents, high concentrations of electrolytes, and numerous organic solvents and will probably find many applications in cosmetics.

The thickening agent "Carbopol 934" [107] also belongs to this group. It is described as a "polycarboxymethylene" and yields acid mucins in water whose viscosity can be strongly increased by neutralization with the usual alkalies (sodium hydroxide, triethanolamine, etc.). The neutralized mucins are transparent and colorless, have a good slip effect, and are harmless to the skin. In the pH range between 6 and 10 their viscosity is almost constant and remains unchanged even with temperature fluctuations. The viscosity of a 1% Carbopol 934 dispersion corresponds to that of 4% gum tragacanth or 2.5% high-viscosity CMC. Carbopol 934 is therefore particularly suitable for aqueous preparations with a high viscosity which leave only a small residue after the water has evaporated. A certain film is always left, of course; this film is especially elastic if triethanolamine is used for neutralization instead of potassium hydroxide. The application range for Carbopols is much restricted, however, by their sensitivity to salts; even small amounts of soluble salts considerably reduce the viscosity of the mucins. This also applies to various preservatives [108]. Carbopol gels are light sensitive [109]. If Carbopol 934 is neutralized with a mixture of a water-soluble base and an oil-soluble amine, it can act as an O/W emulsifying agent [110].

**Water-Soluble Film Formers.**    The higher molecular polyethylene glycols leave films on the skin that have a consistency similar to those formed by stearic acid; the polyethylene glycols are also water-soluble. Although they may be used in O/W creams to impart a nongreasy hydrophilic character to the film on the skin, they are used mostly in nonfatty preparations.

### Emulsifying Agents

Chapter 2 may have created the impression that there is an infinite variety of substances that may be used as cosmetic emulsifiers. Although many materials might indeed be useful, the range for practical cosmetics is at present rather restricted. In 95% of all cosmetic O/W emulsions the emulsifying agent is an alkali metal soap or a triethanolamine soap, the sodium or triethanolamine salt of a sulfated fatty alcohol, or one of the nonionic polyoxyethylene derivatives. The presence of one of these emulsifying agents is not always apparent from the formulation. It must be borne in mind that emulsifiers are marketed under different trade names, that Lanette Wax N contains sodium salts of fatty-alcohol sulfates as emulsifying agents, that the self-emulsifying grades of glycerol monostearate contain sodium soaps of fatty-alcohol sulfates, and so on. In addition to the pure O/W emulsifying agents, surfactants with a low HLB value in many instances also act as auxiliary emulsifiers: fatty alcohols, lanolin or lanolin fractions, fatty acids, and mono-fatty-acid esters of polyhydric alcohols (e.g., glyceryl monostearate, sorbitan sesquioleate). All of these substances considerably increase the stability of oil-in-water emulsions. The thickening agents discussed in the preceding paragraphs are often used as stabilizers.

**Anionic Emulsifying Agents.** The best way of appreciating the specific properties of this class of emulsifying agent is to consider the three types of O/W emulsions based on them: stearate creams, emulsions based on fatty alcohol sulfates and the creams based on glycerol monostearate.

*Stearate Creams.* These creams are O/W emulsions in which stearic acid is the main constituent of the oil phase and in which the emulsifying agent is an alkali stearate formed by the reaction of an alkali dissolved in the aqueous phase with part of the stearic acid. The formula and method of preparation for these creams may be very simple; for example [111],

| | |
|---|---|
| Triple pressed stearic acid | 15 |
| Glycerol 28°Bé | 10 |
| Sodium hydroxide | 0.7 |
| Perfume | 0.8 |
| Distilled water | 73.5 |

The stearic acid is melted and heated to 85°C. The sodium hydroxide is dissolved in another vessel in the water/glycerol solution. The stearic acid is slowly stirred into the aqueous solution (this method is also often reversed). Stirring is continued until the mass has cooled to about 30°C; the perfume is added at 40°C.

As Harry points out [112], even such an elementary emulsion is chemically not a simple system: first of all even the triple-pressed stearic acid is not chemically pure but contains oleic and palmitic acids, and, second, the partial neutralization of fatty acids does not only yield fatty acid and "neutral salts" (e.g., sodium stearate) but also "acid salts," that is, different complexes of salt and acid.

Nevertheless, we have a good idea of the properties of stearate creams which also coincides with practical experience if we assume at the same time that stearic acid represents the oil phase and the auxiliary emulsifying agent, that sodium stearate is the emulsifying agent, and that the aqueous phase is formed by glycerol in water.

The oil phase is stearic acid: the cream is therefore nongreasy and does not smooth the skin. The creams deposit no oily film on the skin; hence most vanishing creams are stearate. When the water has evaporated, the stearic acid precipitates on the skin in finest crystals. The result is a matting effect (very often day creams are based on stearic acid) and a characteristic feeling that may be described as a reduction in smoothness of the skin. (The micro-crystalline stearic acid acts on the skin in a way similar to sand on a slippery road.) The majority of powder bases therefore are also stearate creams. The main emulsifying agent is sodium stearate, a soap. Stearate creams are there-fore sensitive to all substances that reduce the effectiveness of soaps: acids, calcium salts, magnesium salts, heavy metal ions, and any high-ion con-centrations. Many publications maintain that stearate creams have an alkaline reaction because of their soap content. Often this does not apply: Harry et al. [113] have demonstrated that stearate creams usually have a pH between 6.0 and 6.9. The occasionally observed irritating effect of these creams is probably due to the precipitation of calcium soaps, which occurs if the face is washed with hard water, when some remnants of the cream are still present.

Emulsions of this type may be varied by substituting other fatty acids and/or other alkaline substances. Palmitic acid acts in a way similar to stearic acid; oleic or ricinoleic acid results in softer creams. Other acids are rarely used, and stearic acid remains the most commonly used basic material. As Schmidt-La Baume and Lietz [114] observed, the salts of myristic acid, for example, have at least equally good emulsifying properties as stearates but the latter are more suitable for creams because of their more pronounced colloidal qualities which stabilize the emulsion as protective colloids.

The selection of alkali will strongly affect the properties of the cream. The most common bases are sodium or potassium hydroxide and triethanolamine. As shown in Table 4.4, the HLB values of sodium, potassium, or triethanol-amine soaps of the same fatty acids differ widely.

In practice, this means that sodium oleate yields a relatively hard triethanol-amine, a soft cream; potassium oleate lies in between these two. The desired

TABLE 4-4   HLB VALUES OF SOME
OLEATES [115]

| Substance | HLB Value |
| --- | --- |
| Potassium oleate | 20 |
| Sodium oleate | 18 |
| Triethanolamine oleate | 12 |

consistency is often achieved by using two alkalies together. With triethanol-amine there is a risk of the cream's darkening, but a special grade of tri-ethanolamine is available which does not show this effect. It is prepared by adding 1–2% of sulfurous acid (or $SO_2$) to the amine [116]. Darkening can also be prevented if, instead of triethanolamine, triisopropanolamine is used. In any case, it is always advisable to heat these amines as little as possible. Usually the amines are added only to the preheated aqueous phase just before it is stirred into the oil phase. There are some references to sensitivity caused by triethanolamine soaps in dermatological literature [117]. Very probably they are occasioned by impurities; triethanolamine is generally considered the mildest of the three alkalies used. Laufer [118] gives an extensive report on the use of triethanolamine in cosmetics.

Several other amines are also being recommended in the more recent literature for use in stearate creams; for example, "Aminoglycol" [2-amino-2-methyl-propandiol-(1,3)], which is reported to yield creams of a consistency similar to those based on sodium hydroxide.

In older formulations ammonia or sodium carbonate are often suggested, but these substances cannot be recommended; the unavoidable hydrolysis of ammonium salts imparts an unpleasant odor to the creams and the emulsions are not stable. If sodium carbonate is used, the strong carbon dioxide develop-ment causes heavy frothing which is particularly bothersome in bulk pro-duction. Borax, which plays such an important part as an alkali in cold creams, is hardly used at all in stearate creams. One of the reasons is its incompatibility with glycerol, a constituent of most stearate creams; glycerol (also sorbitol but not propylene glycol or polyoxyethylene glycols) forms acid complexes with borax. Stearic acid is particularly suitable for day creams, powder bases, etc. This type of cream is also used for other purposes, when nongreasy bases are required: protective creams, antisun creams, nonfoaming shaving creams, even nourishing creams. Stearate creams have the following advantages:

1. They are made easily and at low cost.
2. They remain stable over a wide range of temperatures.
3. The oil phase does not easily turn rancid.
4. The emulsifying system is strong: in addition to the emulsifying agent (sodium stearate), an auxiliary emulsifying agent (stearic acid) is also present. (In emulsions of this type the emulsifying agent is formed only during prep-aration by reaction of the water/alkali solution with the fatty acid. It is generally assumed that such emulsifiers *in statu nascendi* form particularly stable emulsions. To my knowledge this assumption has never been critically examined, but it is quite possible that the local heat engendered by the reaction alkali/fatty acid has a favorable effect on the developing interfacial

film.) There is an excess of emulsifier over and above the quantity required to form a monomolecular layer around the dispersed droplets. This excess accumulates around the droplets in the aqueous phase and acts as a protective colloid. An addition of moisture retaining substances, for example, glycerol, is important, since otherwise the creams have a tendency to dry out.

5. These creams are very attractive; they are pure white and may be produced in different degrees of hardness by selecting the appropriate alkali. If a high-grade stearate is used, they will have a weak odor that can be covered by almost any perfume. Suitable formulation will result in creams in which the stearic acid does not crystallize in microscopically small crystals but more slowly in larger flakes, and this often imparts a pearly sheen to the creams [119].

These advantages have led to the wide use of stearate creams in cosmetics, but these creams also have certain disadvantages:

1. Because of their soap content, persons with very sensitive skins do not tolerate them well.
2. Stearic acid has no smoothing or nourishing effect.

As already mentioned, the emulsifying agents of these creams are generally sensitive to acids, polyvalent metal ions, and higher salt concentrations.

*Fatty Alcohol Sulfate-Based Creams.* Here the oil phase is usually a mixture of stearyl and cetyl alcohols, substances that are outstanding in their smoothing and emollient effects. This type is therefore particularly suitable as a base for emollient creams. Additions of cetiol increase the nourishing properties and enhance the action in depth of fat-soluble active ingredients. In central Europe creams of this type are often made with Lanette Wax N, a mixture of stearyl and cetyl alcohols that contains sodium cetyl and sodium stearyl sulfate as an emulsifier. An excellent summary of the various applications of Lanette creams is given by Schmidt-La Baume-Lietz [120]. In contrast to fatty-acid soaps, fatty-alcohol sulfates are not acid-sensitive and form water-soluble calcium and magnesium soaps. For this reason nearly all cosmetic and dermatological active ingredients may be incorporated into fatty-alcohol creams, which represents an advantage over stearate creams. Fatty alcohols are effective as auxiliary emulsifiers, and Lanette creams therefore retain excellent stability over a wide temperature range. Other points of comparison between stearate and fatty-alcohol sulfate creams are the following:

1. Like stearate creams, Lanette creams are also easily prepared but not at the same low cost. As in stearate creams, the water content, hence the consistency of the emulsions, may be varied as required from liquid to firm and stiff preparations.

2. Lanette creams, particularly if they also contain cetiol, show less tendency to dry out than stearate creams; 10% glycerol is quite sufficient to prevent drying out entirely [121].

3. The appearance of Lanette creams is also highly satisfactory: they are pure white and almost odorless; generally they are slightly softer than stearate creams. Schmidt-La Baume-Lietz give two formulations for Lanette creams which may be regarded as fundamental:

| | | |
|---|---|---|
| Lanette N | 24 | 15 |
| Cetiol | 6 | |
| Glycerol (or Karion/Merck or 1.2.4-butantriol pure/BASF) | 10 | 10 |
| Water | 60 | 75 |

The fats are heated together to 70°C; the water (in which glycerol has been dissolved) is heated to the same temperature and stirred into the oil phase.

*Creams Based on Glycerol Monostearate.* The so-called "glycerol monostearate" and all related products are not chemically uniform. Apart from the compound after which it is named, it also contains varying amounts of glycerol di- and tristearate, glycerol, and small quantities of free stearic acid; moreover the corresponding compounds of oleic and palmitic acids, as far as they occur in commercial stearic acid, are also present. It is obvious therefore that glycerol monostearate will vary according to the supplier; it is marketed under different trade names. Lower [122] discusses composition and properties of the various grades of glycerol monostearate in detail.

Three types are available:

1. Self-emulsifying products, in which a small addition of soap, usually sodium stearate, acts as the emulsifying agent.

2. Acid-resistant self-emulsifying products in which sodium lauryl sulfate often acts as the emulsifying agent.

3. Products without emulsifiers (i.e., not self-emulsifying). In many respects the properties of preparations based on glycerol monostearate lie between those of stearate and Lanette creams. Their smoothing effect is much better than that of stearate but not so strongly developed as that of Lanette creams. They leave a less oily film than the latter; neither have they the matting or friction-increasing effect of stearic creams.

The emulsions are possibly even easier to prepare than the other types: if desired, all raw materials may be heated in one container until the solids melt; the mixture is then stirred until cool. In this way, one part of the self-emulsifying glycerol monostearate yields an attractive white cream with 10 parts of water or a liquid emulsion with 30 parts of water. Just as in the two other types of cream, the oil phase here also acts as an auxiliary emulsifying agent. The creams are white and show a neutral to weakly alkaline reaction according to the emulsifier used; they have a very faint odor that is easily covered by any perfume.

One of the attractive properties of these creams is the possibility of re-reheating them to melting temperature to correct any faults that might have become apparent after emulsification was originally completed (too fluid, too stiff, too hard, too soft, too greasy, and too dry) by adding suitable agents. They are again stirred until cool. Fatty-alcohol sulfate emulsions may also frequently be corrected in this way.

Obviously, glycerol monostearate emulsions with soaps as emulsifying agents are sensitive to the same additives as stearate creams. Even the "acid-resistant" grades with acid-resistant emulsifying agents (such as sapamine salts) do not remain stable at higher concentrations of strong acids or alkalies because hydrolysis of the glyceryl esters may then occur.

The pure basic stearate, Lanette, and glycerol monostearate creams have hardly any significance in cosmetic practice today. There are two reasons nevertheless for discussing them in such detail: first, to exemplify how the properties of an emulsion result from its components, and, second, even if these types occur only rarely in pure form they provide the basis for many different preparations.

Suitable additions to oil or aqueous phase will modify basic stearate creams to protective creams or foamless shaving creams. Occasionally such preparations deviate so much from the basic type that the oil phase hardly contains any free fatty acids and only alkali soap is present as an emulsifying agent. Obviously such preparations will show only those properties of fundamental stearate creams that are a function of the emulsifying agent. Contrary to pure stearate creams, these preparations will probably have an alkaline reaction because the alkalinity of the emulsifying agent will not have been neutralized by an excess of fatty acid.

Lanette and glycerol monostearate creams and their variations have also found many uses and occur in many formulations in cosmetics. Mixed types that contain glycerol monostearate and stearic acid and alkali also occur frequently.

**Nonionic Emulsifying Agents.**    In addition to alkali soaps and the sodium and triethanolamine fatty-alcohol sulfates, various nonionic substances play an important part as O/W emulsifying agents in modern cosmetics. One example of their application is discussed in detail by Sfiras [123]. The most commonly used products of this type are probably the Tweens of Atlas Chemical Co. and in Germany the Cremophores of BASF, which are mono-fatty-acid esters of polyethylene glycol. Tweens are mostly used with small amounts of "Spans" as auxiliary emulsifying agents. With Cremophores

O, A, AP, and EL, an addition of Cremophor FM as an auxiliary emulsifying agent has occasionally proved advantageous.

Although these emulsifying agents are more expensive than alkali soaps, their use in cosmetics is becoming increasingly widespread. Their most important property is probably their mild effect on the body [124]; they cause irritations even more rarely than anionic emulsifiers, are less toxic if taken orally, and irritate the conjunctiva of the eye even less (see Table 2.2). They have even been credited with an emollient effect, which is not surprising because they are monofatty-acid esters of polyhydric alcohols (or their derivatives), that is, substances related to glyceryl monostearate. Nonionic emulsifying agents have another advantage: there is a whole range of similar products that differ only in their HLB values. Fine nuances may be achieved by mixing a number of these products because careful experimentation will identify the most effective emulsifying agent (or pair of emulsifiers) for the particular purpose. The HLB system is an important tool in this selection.

Generally, nonionic emulsifying agents are insensitive to acids, alkalies, and salts of every kind. Hydrolysis of the ester linkage leading to inactivation of the emulsifying agent occurs only in very strongly acid or alkaline solutions. For such solutions fatty-alcohol polyoxyethylene ethers are recommended for they contain no ester linkage and are therefore also resistant to hydrolysis.

The only important group of products that is incompatible with polyoxyethylene compounds (including all nonionic emulsifying agents mentioned except "Spans") are phenols and tannic acids with which complexes are formed. This reduces the stability of emulsions with high phenol content (about 5%) [125] and phenolic disinfectants [126] and preservatives [127] may be inactivated if nonionic emulsifiers are used at the same time.

Mono fatty-acid esters of saccharose belong to a more recent class of nonionic emulsifying agents. They are prepared from fatty acids and cane sugar and may eventually be considerably cheaper than the older emulsifying agents of this category [128].

### Insoluble Solids

The incorporation of such substances in O/W emulsions is not unusual. We have already summarized the substances available and the purposes for which they are used. A preparation will usually have paste consistency if it contains about 20–30% solids. Higher solid concentrations result in a cake or crumbling consistency.

**Formulation.** The stability of O/W emulsions is principally determined by the following factors:

1. *The characteristics of the emulsifying agents used.* When using anionic emulsifiers, it is particularly important to avoid substances that might

destroy or diminish their effectiveness. With nonionic emulsifiers a correct selection is important.

2. *Concentration of emulsifying agents.*   It can generally be accepted that emulsion stability will increase with the emulsifier concentration; there are nevertheless some arguments against high concentrations:

(a) Of all regular cream constituents, anionic emulsifying agents are most likely to cause skin irritations.

(b) Nonionic emulsifying agents are comparatively expensive.

(c) With an increasing emulsifier concentration, emulsions become harder and stiffer.

In practice it is best to work with both emulsifying and auxiliary emulsifying agents and to add protective colloids to fluid preparations. The quantity of emulsifier to be used depends on the required stability.

3. *Fine dispersion of the oil phase.*   With O/W emulsions, as with the W/O type, the stability improves with an increasingly fine dispersion of the internal phase. Creaming is all the more likely (hence homogenization is more necessary) the thinner the emulsion. Here it should be borne in mind that the finer the dispersion of the oil phase, the more emulsifier required; a fine dispersion means extensive interfaces. If an emulsion with a low emulsifier content is dispersed to very fine droplets, the effect achieved will be only temporary. As long as the interface is so large that it is not completely covered by an emulsifier film, the small droplets will coalesce until the interface has shrunk to an extent at which the emulsifying agent is able to cover it completely.

4. *Viscosity of the aqueous phase.*   As we have seen already, O/W emulsions and, in particular, fluid emulsions with low oil concentration are stabilized by increasing the viscosity of the aqueous phase.

**Preparation.**   Properties of completed O/W emulsions depend less on the method of preparation than do the properties of W/O or dual emulsions. In general oil and aqueous phases are heated separately to 70°C. (Occasionally temperatures up to 90°C are recommended but lower temperatures are usually preferable because the basic materials are less affected.) The phases are then mixed. Many formulations require the oil phase to be added to the aqueous phase: this method often yields very good results, but the dispersion is even better if the aqueous phase is stirred into the oil phase, which results in an unstable W/O emulsion that inverts to an O/W emulsion after further stirring (probably via the stage of a dual emulsion). The dispersion of the oil phase is made even finer by homogenizing the emulsion. It is not necessary to stir O/W creams until they are cool; in most cases stirring may be discontinued at approximately 50°C. The stability of the emulsion depends less on the viscosity of the external phase, and this in turn not so much on the temperature. With stearate creams it is occasionally even undesirable to continue agitation below 45°C because in these circumstances consistency and appearance of the emulsion is conditioned by the crystal form of the precipitating stearic acid. Brisk stirring at low temperatures while the acid is in the process of crystallizing out may prevent the formation of relatively large crystals; this may make the cream thin and prevent the development of a pearly sheen.

Solids are stirred into the completed emulsion or added to the phase with the better wetting effect on them. It should be realized that in pastes the solids may absorb water from the aqueous phase, which would make the paste harden further after preparation. This may be prevented (a) by introducing the solids into the emulsion when it is very hot (in some instances this speeds up the water absorption by the solids); (b) by soaking the solids before preparing the emulsion in part of the aqueous phase; (c) by passing the completed cream through a colloid mill. The water absorption by the solids is then accelerated by close contact. Similar results may be obtained by long and thorough mixing of the cream after the addition of the solids.

## COSMETIC PREPARATIONS WITHOUT OIL

Although today's public thinks first of creams and fat-containing preparations in connection with "cosmetics," products without oil, based on water or alcohol, do play an important part. Such preparations are usually liquid: hair, mouth, and face lotions, extracts, toilet waters, sun-screen, and astringent lotions, body deodorants, pre- and after-shave lotions, etc. Sometimes they are jellies (e.g., for the hands) or pastes (toothpastes). Solid preparations free of fat are marketed as cologne sticks, deodorant sticks, and so on.

Preparations without fat are pleasant to use because only active substances remain on the skin or hair after a quick evaporation of the solvents. They are easy and cheap to prepare and often are stable indefinitely. In many cases they represent the most economical form of applying active substances. As with previously described preparations, we cover the most important raw materials in connection with their function in individual products but leave a discussion of specific active ingredients to Part II.

## RAW MATERIALS

### Water and Low Molecular Alcohols

Nothing much need be said about water: it is of all cosmetic raw materials, the most compatible and completely nontoxic. It is therefore irreplaceable when it is a question of diluting other substances which might have an irritating effect in high concentrations (ethyl alcohol, glycerol, etc.) It is also cheap.

Since the introduction of nonionic solubilizers (see below), it has become possible to formulate preparations with lower alcohol and higher water concentrations than before.

**Ethyl Alcohol.**  Probably the most important function of alcohol in cosmetics is that of solvent: it dissolves perfume oils, organic agents of disinfectants and sunscreen lotions, oily substances occasionally contained in hair lotions, and pigments in hair dyes. It also acts as a disinfectant (most active at 65% concentration) and an astringent. It has a cooling effect on the skin because of its quick evaporation and facilitates the application of aqueous solutions to skin and hair by reducing surface tension.

Although ethyl alcohol may penetrate the skin, no harmful effects need be feared, since it evaporates very quickly after application. As a raw material ethyl alcohol is nontoxic and normally nonirritating. In high concentrations alcohol used regularly leads to a hardening of the horny layer and to irritations; it causes coagulation of skin proteins. Alcohol solutions above about 50%, dissolve the major part of the skin fat. If such solutions are removed immediately after application, they have a degreasing effect that might in certain circumstances be harmful. This effect, however, does not occur if the alcohol is left on the skin until it has evaporated, which is usually the case. Since 95% alcohol (fine spirits) is comparatively expensive as a raw material, attempts have been made to replace it with other products of a similar effect. Denatured ethyl alcohol (industrial methylated spirits) has been in use for a long time. Only those grades may be used, of course, in which the substances added in the denaturing process are dermatologically harmless. In recent years, n-propyl and isopropyl alcohols have been widely used especially in Europe as replacements for costly spirits. Rothemann [129] gives a good summary of their properties compared with ethyl alcohol. They (in particular isopropyl alcohol) are superior solvents compared with ethyl alcohol and can therefore be used in lower concentrations. Their disinfectant effect is also stronger than that of ethyl alcohol; according to Rothemann [129], 50% isopropyl alcohol and 30% n-propyl alcohol correspond to 70% ethyl alcohol in effectiveness. Propyl alcohols reduce the surface tension of aqueous solutions in the same way as ethyl alcohol. Cooling and astringent effects are less pronounced with propyl alcohols. Similar to glycerol, undiluted n-propyl alcohol leaves a warm sensation on the skin. These substances have no iritating action on the skin, and although their toxicity (particularly that of n-propyl alcohol) is higher than of ethyl alcohol, no objection can be raised on this account against their use in cosmetics. The one great disadvantage of these substances is their odor. Pure ethyl alcohol has a very faint and not unpleasant odor and develops all perfumes dissolved in it extremely well; but propyl alcohols have an unpleasant odor of their own. Isopropyl alcohol has a pungent smell which turns sweetish; *n*-propyl alcohol smells sweetly stale. These solvents certainly do not bring out a fine perfume to advantage; on the contrary, it is difficult for the perfumer to create fragrances to cover their odor.

## Emollients

The same products discussed in the section on humectants in connection with O/W emulsions are also widely used in preparations that are free from fat. Here their main function is their emollient effect. One of the oldest cosmetic preparations is a hand lotion consisting of 50% glycerol (far too high a concentration according to present opinion!) in rose water. The same substances also act as solubilizers for products with slight water solubility. Carbitol (diethylene glycol monoethylether) and the polyethylene glycols (also high-molecular solids which have no moisture-retaining or emollient action) are used for this purpose.

## Thickening Agents

The most important materials in this category were discussed in the section on O/W emulsions. Perhaps the description of "thickening agents" is not quite correct. These products not only increase the viscosity of aqueous solutions, facilitate slow pouring, and prevent them from running off the skin, but also impart a peculiar soft and smooth consistency and easy applicability which cannot be obtained even with emulsions. Vegetable mucins such as gum tragacanth or sodium alginate are suitable in this connection, since they also impart an often desired stringy consistency to the preparation. An interesting type of thickening agent is described in French Patent No. 1,068,586 [130]. These thickening agents are reported to be especially suitable for hair dyes and permanent wave lotions because they remain stable with both ammonium thioglycolate and hydrogen peroxide and are prepared by allowing the acid (not the salt!) of anionic surfactants to react with a quaternary ammonium compound. The examples cited are the waxlike compounds of stearic acid and sapamin, oleic acid and sapamin (liquid) and of stearic acid with the distearyl amide of dihydroxy-diethylene triamine. According to this patent, 0.5–5% of these substances result in stable creamlike jellies. Water/alcohol mixtures are also reported to be thickened by adding these products. The thickening agents mentioned above are used to impart to products without fat a thick-to-jellylike consistency. It is also possible to thicken alcohol/water mixtures to a hard waxlike mass suitable for cologne sticks, deodorant sticks, and similar preparations. This is usually done with sodium stearate.

## Film-Forming Substances

Basic materials that are water-soluble, yet deposit on the skin a film similar to that left by stearic acid or glycerol monostearate, have recently become available: polyethylene glycols. They are represented by the general formula

$$HO—CH_2—(CH_2—O—CH_2)_n—CH_2—OH.$$

Products of various chain lengths are commercially available; the molecular weight of the shortest chain grade is around 200, the longest available polymer around 9000. The consistency of these polymers ranges from liquids (at the low molecular weight end) through lardlike and soft waxy textures to the hard waxy consistency of the highest molecular weight members in the series.

Polyethylene glycols are easily soluble even in hard water (see Table 4-5). They are unsaponifiable, do not turn rancid, and are chemically stable because they contain only hydroxyl groups and ether linkages. They are soluble in standard organic solvents and are compatible with film formers such as nitrocellulose, polyvinylpyrrolidone, casein, and shellac, which makes them suitable as ingredients for hair lacquers and certain protective agents.

TABLE 4-5   PROPERTIES OF POLYETHYLENE GLYCOLS [131]

| Average Molecular Weight | Average Melting Point (°C) | Water Solubility (grams/100 g of water at 20°) | Hygroscopicity* (glycerol = 100) |
|---|---|---|---|
| 200 | — | Complete | 90 |
| 240 | — | Complete | — |
| 300 | 8 | Complete | 70 |
| 400 | 9 | Complete | 60 |
| 500 | 11 | Complete | 53 |
| 600 | 16 | Complete | 50 |
| 700 | 19 | Complete | — |
| 800 | 24 | 90 | — |
| 900 | 30 | 80 | — |
| 1000 | 36 | 70 | — |
| 1200 | 37 | 67 | — |
| 1600 | 40 | 65 | — |
| 4000 | 52 | 62 | — |
| 4500 | 55 | 60 | — |
| 6000 | 60 | 50 | — |

* This probably refers to static hygroscopicity.

They have only a limited solubility in the standard fats, oils, and waxes used in cosmetics. Liquid polyethylene glycols are hygroscopic but less so than glycerol; wherever hydroscopicity need not be too strong they may therefore replace it.

The high molecular waxlike compounds of this group are suitable dispersing agents for water-insoluble pigments in hair dyes. The toxicity of short-chain polyethylene glycols is higher than that of the high-molecular compounds; the $LD_{50}$ (the amount of substance per kilo of body weight that kills 50% of the test animals within 24 hours) for polyethylene glycol 200, the shortest chain substance of this group, is 38.3 ml/kilo for mice [132]. No irritations on normal skin or sound mucous membrane were observed after short-term application, nor could any irritating effect be noticed after intracutaneous, subcutaneous, or intravenous applications.

Polyethylene glycols are incompatible with phenolic compounds because of the formation of complexes. Polyethylene glycol derivatives, in which one of the hydroxyl groups has been esterified with higher fatty acids ($C_{12}$—$C_{18}$), have surface-active properties and are used as nonionic emulsifying agents and dispersing agents. The same applies to monoethers of polyethylene glycol with fatty alcohols and derivatives of sorbitol.

### Suspended Solids

Finely dispersed solids are used in fat-free cosmetic preparations as abrasives (calcium carbonate and calcium phosphates in toothpastes), for their light reflecting properties (zinc oxide in some sunscreen lotions), for their dehydrating and astringent effect (kaolin in face masks), their cooling effect (zinc carbonate or zinc oxide in sunburn lotions), or for their mechanical barrier action (zinc or magnesium stearates in hand jellies).

### Solubilizers

The difference between a solvent and a solubilizer is the uniform distribution of a solvent throughout the solution, whereas a solubilizer through its colloidal-chemical properties remains firmly linked to the solute. Hence the required amount of a solvent depends on the total quantity of the solution (two liters of 50% alcohol contain twice as much alcohol as one liter), but for a solubilizer the required quantity depends on the amount of insoluble substance to be dispersed (a 1% aqueous perfume requires twice as much solubilizer as one containing $\frac{1}{2}$% perfume oil). Surfactants with solubilizing effect permit the incorporation of perfume oils and other water-insoluble substances without clouding even in preparations with low or no alcohol content. The nonionic "Tween 20" (Atlas Chemical Co.) is used for this purpose; 2–5 times the amount of perfume oil is the required addition for Tween 20 to achieve a clear dispersion in water.

## The Preparation of Fat-Free Cosmetic Products on an Alcohol or Water Basis.

Generally the preparation of fat-free products causes no difficulties. If the formulation contains alcohol as well as water, the water-soluble substances are dissolved in the water, the water-insoluble ones in the alcohol, and the two phases are stirred together at room temperature. The mixture is then stored for some time to allow the perfume to "mature"; it depends on the quality of the perfume and the water-content of the solution whether this maturing process takes days or months: the more water, the more quickly maturation is complete. Before bottling the mixture is cooled to 0–5°C and filtered through magnesium carbonate or some other filter material.

Thickening agents are incorporated by first allowing them to swell in a portion of the water until a mucilage has formed, which is then mixed with the other ingredients. In some instances (e.g., with CMC) complete swelling occurs overnight (with brisk stirring, even after a few hours); in others the mucilage reaches the required viscosity only after a few days (e.g., with gum karaya).

When water-insoluble substances, such as perfume oils, are to be solubilized to achieve a clear dispersion, they are first mixed with the solubilizer and then combined with the aqueous solution. Finely dispersed solids are usually mixed into the completed preparation.

## POWDERS

All preparations discussed so far in this chapter are applied to the skin in a liquid layer. Powders differ fundamentally from these preparations in their physical characteristics and their most important cosmetic properties are determined exactly by these characteristics. The minute particle size causes a large surface per unit weight which again results in strong light dispersion and therefore visual covering of the skin underneath.

The surface of powdered skin exposed to air is much larger than that of unpowdered skin which leads to a cooling effect if the powder has good heat conductivity. Finally, because of the fine particle size and light weight, powder adheres to the skin by the stickiness of the fat film and by the skin relief and neither gravity nor rubbing will easily remove it.

## RAW MATERIALS

Since the properties of powder are determined by its physical characteristics, all finely dispersed solids may be considered suitable raw materials for powder, provided they meet the following requirements:

1. They must not be hard and their crystals must not have sharp edges or points that might damage the skin.
2. Their solubility in water and in fat mixtures (skin fat!) must be slight.
3. They must not be irritating or toxic, and chemically neutral.

The most important raw materials for powders include representatives of many different classes of material: silicates (talcum, kaolin, Cab-o-Sil), carbonates (calcium carbonate, magnesium carbonate), metal oxides (zinc oxide, titanium dioxide), metal salts of organic acids (zinc and magnesium stearates, magnesium undecanate, aluminum stearate), polysaccharides (starch, ultraamylopectine, dextrans), protein degradation products ("Labilin," "powdered silk"), plant spores (lyopodium), and synthetic organic polymers. As in all cosmetic products, the raw materials of powder must be selected according to their purpose. In the following section we discuss the most important raw materials according to their applications.

## Materials which impart Softness and Slip

These materials are, in particular, talcum, aluminum hydrosilicate, and the zinc and magnesium soaps of higher fatty acids.

Talcum is the most commonly used powder base. It is distinguished by its great softness and slip and is almost neutral if adequately purified. Many baby and body powders consist exclusively or largely of talcum.

Since talcum penetration of wounds may cause talcum granulomae, its use has been discouraged, even in cosmetics. Meyer [133] showed that these inflammations are caused by a slow splitting off and dissolution of silicic acid in colloidal form and that this does not occur only with talcum but with all silicates and most of all with silicic acid itself. The damage is caused only under certain conditions, and, generally speaking, talcum may be regarded as a harmless raw material. If talcum is not considered sufficiently safe, aluminum hydrosilicate may be used instead which, according to Meyer [133] has far less tendency than talcum to split off silicic acid.

It is important to use properly purified and disinfected grades of talcum which have no coarse or hard admixtures.

These admixtures can be recognized microscopically or they may be isolated [134] by thoroughly stirring 5 g of talcum into 100 ml of water and allowing the suspension to settle for one minute, pouring off the cloudy water and repeating this procedure about 10 times; finally the residue of coarse admixtures left in the vessel is dried and weighed. Talcum should contain only small amounts of alkaline substances (such as calcium carbonate): according to Rothemann not more than 0.3%, according to Auch not more than 6.6% [135]; they are determined after boiling the talcum with water and titrating with acid. The density of talcum is not constant and depends on purity and origin. It may simply be determined by measuring the volume of, say, 100 g of talcum in a measuring cylinder. The color of a talcum grade is determined simply by observation against a light or dark background; wetting of the samples with turpentine is reported to be helpful. Talcum must be free of spores of pathogenic substances (e.g., tetanus: in New Zealand in 1946 five deaths were caused by tetanus spores found in baby powders based on talcum). All basic materials from mineral sources carry the risk of such spores. Sterilization can be achieved by heating the product for several hours to 150–160°C.

Softness and slip of talcum are examined by rubbing, and here experience is the only guide.

*Aluminum Hydrosilicate.* According to Meyer (133), this is a valuable basic material for powder if it has been treated with acid, washed in water, dried, finely ground, and rubbed. It is an extremely fine powder which, like talcum, feels smooth and fatty if it is rubbed between the fingers and clings to the skin surface. It has a certain cooling effect and absorbs fatty secretions and small amounts of water (up to 3 % of its own weight, whereas talcum does not absorb any water). It is completely nontoxic, even if taken orally, and is tolerated by skin and mucous membrane without any symptoms of irritation.

Of the metal soaps, zinc and magnesium stearates and zinc and magnesium undecanate are used. The undecanates in particular are soft and have excellent slip but are relatively expensive. Stearates are used extensively. Objections have been raised to zinc stearate because of its toxicity, but properly purified grades are harmless to the skin. Magnesium stearate has similar qualities and is nontoxic and nonirritating. These metal salts are especially distinguished by their excellent adhesion to the skin (see below).

## Materials which impart Adhesion

These materials are primarily the metal soaps just mentioned: zinc and magnesium stearates and undecanates (lithium stearate is also recommended [136]. They improve adhesion not only to the skin surface but also to the powder puff, which facilitates taking powder from its container.

Fissan colloid (a fluorosilicic acid colloid of Deutsche Milchwerke/Zwingenberg) and powdered silk [137] are also reported to have excellent adhesion. Adhesion of powders is sometimes improved by adding 1–2 % petrolatum, cetyl alcohol, lanolin, or similar fats.

## Materials which impart Covering Power

The ability to cover small skin imperfections, enlarged pores, etc., is requisite, particularly in face powders. The best covering agents are titanium dioxide [138] and zinc oxide, but kaolin, zinc and magnesium stearates, and starch are also being used for this purpose. Titanium dioxide has by far the best covering power and, on an equal weight basis, is one and one half to two times as effective as zinc oxide. Apart from the chemical characteristics of a material, covering power also depends on other factors.

Generally, the covering power per unit weight is stronger, the finer the powder. According to Grady [139], the optimal particle size for zinc oxide is 0.25 $\mu$. Below this the covering power diminishes considerably.

The medium in which the powder is dispersed is also of considerable importance. Generally, the covering power of powders is better if they are surrounded by air (or on dry skin) than in a moist environment (or perspiring skin), and it is weakest in a greasy environment (petrolatum, greasy skin). According to Grady, the covering power of zinc oxide in a moist environment is 37% of that of dry powder and in petrolatum, 21%. The covering power of titanium dioxide does not decrease so much as that of zinc oxide from dry, to moist, to greasy environments, but that of other raw materials decreases even more. Zinc oxide and titanium dioxide are nontoxic and may be regarded as dermatologically harmless. It has been reported that constant use of zinc oxide causes increased cornification of the skin, but there is no clinical evidence. Both metal oxides have a certain cooling effect because of their good heat conductivity [140].

Zinc oxide also has a pronounced protective effect against ultraviolet rays which cause erythema, whereas titanium dioxide is much less effective in this respect [141].

An ultrafine grade of zinc oxide is available [142] with an average particle size of 0.02 $\mu$. This "hyperfine" grade is characterized by its brick-red color, strong dynamic hygroscopicity, and increased chemical reactivity.

### Materials which impart Absorbency

For different reasons good absorbent properties in aqueous and fatty liquids are required for baby powders, dusting powders (after bath), deodorant foot powders, and healing powders. Face powders as well should have a certain absorbency to prevent smudging of make-up by perspiration. The following raw materials show good absorbency:

Colloidal kaolin [143] is a fine, soft, white powder, chemically resembling aluminum hydrosilicate but produced in a different manner. It is nontoxic and nonirritating, has a good absorbent capacity for aqueous and fatty substances, and good covering power. It is therefore a valuable raw material for powders, some of which contain up to 50%. Its relatively slight slip is a disadvantage, and if used by itself, it is somewhat dry.

Bentonite is chemically related to kaolin, but it differs strongly in its crystal structure. It has extraordinary swelling power and is able to absorb up to 15 times its own weight in water. It is only rarely used in cosmetic powders, but it is an excellent thickening and dispersing agent in emulsions and gels.

Calcium carbonate has good absorbent powers for water and fatty substances and is fine, white, and soft. Some special grades are available which absorb only fats but no moisture and therefore have no drying effect. Although this material is used extensively in England and the United States, German authors (e.g., Rothemann and Janistyn) have advised against it because small amounts of calcium carbonate dissolve in skin moisture and thus cause an alkaline reaction. The presence of calcium salts on the skin is also undesirable if the face is washed with soap after powder has been used or if creams containing fats are present with the calcium salts.

Magnesium carbonate is less alkaline than the calcium salt. It has good covering power and adhesion and is light and fluffy. If it is used with other powder ingredients, it renders the mixture lighter and looser. It has good absorbency for moisture and fats. This property is utilized frequently in the addition of perfume oils to powders: the oils are mixed with magnesium carbonate which is then added to the other ingredients.

Starch (rice, wheat, corn, potato, etc.) is being used much less in powders than formerly, when rice starch was one of of the most important raw materials. It has good moisture absorbency and good adhesion, a neutral reaction, and is completely nontoxic. The unsuitability of rice starch because it becomes sticky in a moist environment (therefore on the skin) and obstructs the orifices of the hair follicles [144] is denied by Harry [145, 146]. It is a fact, however, that starch is an ideal culture medium for bacteria and other pathogenic germs, and for this reason Rothemann warns of its use in baby, body, wound, or foot powders. On the other hand, the risk of bacterial impurities may be reduced by adding suitable disinfectants; sometimes even the perfume oils used have this preservative effect.

Powder based on starch has the unique property of achieving a peach-bloom effect on the face by adhering to the lanugo hairs and accentuating them. Only in face powders has rice starch a well-earned place.

Ultra amylopectine (sodium amyl pectine glycolate) may be used in small amounts in absorbent powders because of its excellent moisture absorbency. Silicic acid as well may be used in powders in different forms: all are characterized by their strong water absorbency. Kieselgur (diatomaceous earth) consists of hollow particles that swell when they absorb moisture and may thus enlarge the pores; it should be used only in foot powders in which a particularly strong absorbency is required. Cab-o-Sil [147] is extremely light and fluffy.

Fissan colloid is a silicic acid colloid which also contains degradation products of milk proteins. It is also very light and has good moisture-absorbent properties. A powder that is based on this colloid has frequently been used in Europe as a wound powder. According to Meyer [148], colloidal silicic acid should not be used in powders that might come in contact with damaged skin areas because here the risk of talcum granuloma is considerably greater than with talcum itself. "Orbacid," a raw material made from ground formaldehyde urea resin (Organa Schaumchemie, Frankenthal, Pfalz) is also reported to be particularly absorbent of moisture and oil [149]. This powder is acid (pH 4.5), stable, completely nonirritating and has a very fine structure and great adhesion.

### Preparation of Powders

The preparation of powders is simple in principle (if not always in execution) because it is only a matter of mixing dry, finely dispersed ingredients. Perfume oils are either incorporated in an absorbent powder component or stirred in solution into the mixture during the mixing process. Pigments are added in a similar way if they are not mixed in as dry powders. With fat additives there is also a choice of adding them pure or spraying in a solution.

## AEROSOL PREPARATIONS

Aerosols are among the newest types of cosmetic preparation. In the few decades of its development the spray can has proved to be a versatile vehicle. Cosmetics are only part of its applicability, but even in this single sector it gained great importance. All the products we have discussed so far—oil preparations, emulsions, aqueous and alcoholic products, powders, and also shaving creams and shampoos—have been produced as aerosols. We could have discussed aerosol creams under creams, aerosol powders in the section on powders, and so on, but it seems more useful to deal with aerosol preparations separately because they have important properties in common that differentiate them from other products.

### History

The idea of expelling a substance from a container by encasing it with a gas under pressure is not new in itself (Helbing and Pertsch took out U. S. Patent 628,463 in 1899 for a self-spraying product), but it was only practically developed during World War II. American forces in the Pacific met an ever-present adversary, always troublesome, and at times as dangerous as the actual enemy: insects. Many insecticides had been developed around 1940, but the problem lay in their application. It has been found that they gain in effectiveness the more finely dispersed they are in the atmosphere. How could such an atomization best be achieved?

The "insecticide bomb," a solution of an active agent with an inert gas as propellant, packed under pressure in a metal cylinder, was the practical solution to the problem and at the same time the first modern aerosol product. During the war Allied forces used about 50 million of these insecticide bombs.

The propellant in these products was dichlorofluoromethane (Freon 12, E. I. Du Pont de Nemours), and the internal pressure at 20°C was almost 6 atm (hence the description "bomb"). To avoid explosions heavy cast-iron containers had to be used.

The aerosol principle became commercially practicable when other propellants were found that enabled the preparation to be packaged under lower pressure, in lighter, handier, and cheaper containers. It took about eight years before aerosol products could be packaged in light metal, even glass containers, without risk. In these years aerosol products increased enormously; the push button can became very popular and all possible and impossible preparations, from lubricating oils to pharmaceutical preparations, from shaving cream to Christmas tree snow, were brought out in aerosols. Aerosol cans were also tried in cosmetics for almost all existing products, and in some instances aerosol preparations gained a permanent place next to the more traditional forms.

### Advantages and Disadvantages

What are the advantages from the cosmetic chemist's point of view that have made aerosol products so popular in such a short time?

Aerosol cans facilitate fast and uniform application of different products (oils, alcoholic solutions, and powders) to skin and hair. Preparations that are effective as foams (shaving soaps and shampoos) can be dispensed in this form directly from the can.

Up to the last drop the contents of the can are completely sealed off from the environment so that the influence of atmospheric oxygen and moisture, microorganisms and spores from the air, and the evaporation of water and solvents are completely excluded. Against these advantages, we have the following disadvantages:

Apart from the usual problems inherent in preparing cosmetics, which are similar for both traditional and aerosol presentation, additional problems occur: the possible decomposition of the propellant; the effect of degradation products on the cosmetic perfume, or container; emulsification of the propellant in the preparation, obstruction of the valves, and so on. The solution to these problems and the preparation of a stable product is always tricky and requires the work of experienced specialists.

Another disadvantage of aerosol products is that fundamentally they are rarely economical. The container must be strong because higher demands are made on it than on traditional packs. Aerosols also require rather complicated valves and contain a propellant which has no cosmetic effect in itself and literally disappears without trace during use.

It is quite correct that, considering the value of the contents, the cost of the containers, valves, and propellant is only a small part of the total; nevertheless, it is an additional cost and is quite sizable in most cosmetic products. It is theoretically feasible that aerosol packing could make use of inexpensive basic materials that might not have been utilized because of their sensitivity to air or moisture; that cheaper products might be made in this manner; or than an active substance would develop greater effectiveness if it were atomized and would actually be more economical. However, at present aerosol preparations are generally more expensive than the same preparations in traditional packages.

## PRINCIPLES OF ACTION

### Two-Phase Aerosols

The aerosol package contains two phases (see Figure 5). The liquid phase $L$ consists of a solution of the propellant in the active ingredients. The gaseous phase $G$ consists mostly of the vapor of the propellant. The gaseous phase exerts pressure on the container and the liquid phase; the magnitude of the pressure depends on the character of the propellant and its concentration in the preparation (i.e., the proportion of the propellant to the active ingredients). The basic condition for the practical application of the aerosol principle is the fact that pressure does not depend on the amount of propellant present in the container and therefore remains constant until the liquid phase has been almost exhausted. This pressure is always higher than the external pressure (1 atm). When the opening of the valve $V$ establishes the connection with the external air, the liquid phase is pressed out through the tube $T$ and the valve.

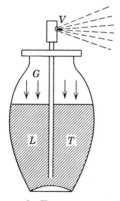

FIGURE 5   TWO-PHASE AEROSOL.

The liquid phase immediately leaves the valve, the propellant dissolved in it evaporates, and the resultant quasi-explosion of the liquid phase leads to atomizing of the active ingredients in very fine droplets. With some space aerosols (e.g., insecticides) vaporization may be so fine that the droplets remain in suspension for two hours. Cosmetic products which are not dispersed in rooms but on skin and hair do not require the same fine dispersion. The degree of atomization depends on several factors:

1. The vapor pressure of the propellant at the existing room temperature; the higher the vapor pressure, the greater the "explosion" and atomization.

2. The proportion of the propellant to the active ingredients in the liquid phase: the higher the propellant component, the finer the atomization.

3. The solubility of the propellant in the active ingredients: the less soluble the propellant, the quicker it evaporates and the finer the atomization. (This principle is utilized in "ultra-low pressure aerosols.")

The spraying pattern (whether the liquid is sprayed in a wide angle over the room or in a narrow far-reaching jet) depends on the construction of the valve. To understand fully the action of two-phase aerosols, we must also consider what happens inside the container during spraying. Since part of the liquid phase is being forced out of the container, its volume inside the container decreases and the gaseous phase must therefore expand to a larger volume. This would lead to a decrease in pressure if it were not immediately equalized by the evaporation of part of the propellant contained in the liquid phase. As soon as the level of the liquid falls, part of the propellant in the liquid phase evaporates so that the vapor pressure remains almost constant until the liquid phase is exhausted. It does not remain absolutely constant (because the proportion of the propellant to the active ingredients changes slightly during the use of the container), but this has no practical significance.

From a technical point of view the two-phase system is the best because it offers less chance of complications and difficulties than the three-phase system. It is therefore used in almost all cases in which a liquid is to be dispensed and in which the active ingredients can be formulated to permit the propellant to be dissolved in them.

### Three-Phase Aerosols

Here, the propellant is not soluble in the active ingredients so that there are two liquid phases in addition to the gaseous phase, hence the classification "three-phase aerosols."

**Nonemulsified Type (Figure 6).** The liquid phase settles in two layers; according to the specific weights of the phases, the liquid propellant will be above or below the active ingredient solution.

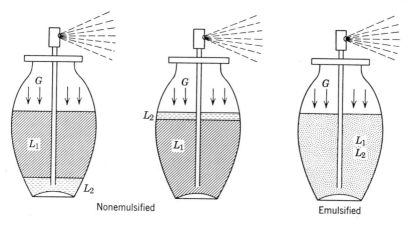

Nonemulsified

Emulsified

FIGURE 6 THREE-PHASE AEROSOLS.

Contrary to the situation with two-phase aerosols, the vapor pressure here is always that of the propellant at the prevailing temperature and not dependent on the proportion of propellant to active ingredient solution.

When the valve is opened, the pressure of the gaseous phase forces the active ingredients through the tube and valve to the outside. Since the solution of active ingredients does not in this instance contain any dissolved propellant, there is no further vaporization in the air. Spraying can be achieved only by the appropriate construction of the valve, and it is never so fine as in good two-phase aerosols.

As in two-phase aerosols, the vapor pressure inside the container is kept constant by the evaporation of liquid propellant when part of the liquid phase is forced out of the container. If the propellant is heavier than the solution of active ingredients and lies below it, there is no direct contact between liquid and gaseous propellant: they are separated by a liquid layer. The evaporation of the liquid propellant may therefore be retarded considerably and then occur suddenly. The result is an uneven, jerky spray pattern. This tendency of three-phase aerosols may be reduced by adding a few boiling stones to the liquid propellant.

This type of three-phase aerosol has the advantage of requiring only relatively small amounts of propellant because the latter is not being used up. Actually, it is not a "genuine" aerosol because the propellant acts only by forcing the liquid out of the container and does not contribute toward the spraying effect. During development of a liquid aerosol product the question arises occasionally whether it should be presented as a two-phase or three-phase system. In Table 4-6 Hans [150] lists some considerations for and against three-phase systems which should be taken into account.

TABLE 4-6   THE THREE-PHASE SYSTEM

| Pro | Con |
| --- | --- |
| Spraying of aqueous solution is possible | Activating pressure not necessarily constant |
| Little propellant, much active ingredient, hence very economical | Risk of loss of propellant if sprayed under conditions in which the tube dips into the propellant phase; the container then becomes unusable |
| Excellent surface wetting without room spraying, hence no loss of ingredients in space, no undesirable inhalation of vapors | Restricted possibility of influencing the spray pattern |

When developing a three-phase system, the matter of patents must be borne in mind. Chemway Corporation is an important patent holder.

Herzka [151] describes an interesting modification of the three-phase system in which the solution of active ingredients is contained in a flexible bag and is therefore not in contact with the propellant.

**Foam Emulsion, O/W Type.**   The most commonly used emulsified three-phase aerosols are foam products. Here the liquid phase is a propellant-in-concentrate emulsion. The vapor phase above it consists of gaseous propellant; the pressure always equals the vapor pressure of the propellant at the prevailing temperature. When the valve is opened, the liquid phase is forced out of the container. The propellant, as the internal phase of the emulsion, evaporates suddenly and is replaced by air. The result is an emulsion of air-in-concentrate or foam. With foam aerosols the liquid phase does not immediately escape from the container as it leaves the valve; it remains enclosed in a small tube; this prevents the liquid phase from "exploding" and flying in all directions when the propellant evaporates. The active ingredients are captured in the tube during evaporation of the propellant and ejected as finished lather. According to the composition of the concentrate, the foam may be dry and stiff, or moist and elastic, or (if the vapor pressure is too low or the concentrate unsuitably formulated) it may be a slack viscous mass. All factors must be controlled in order to achieve a first-class foam aerosol [192]. The speed of foam formation depends on the evaporation rate of the propellants used. Very low boiling propellants (e.g., dichlorodifluoromethane) result in instant foam formation; if part of the propellant has a higher boiling range, foam builds up more slowly and may even continue to develop on the hand of the user. The most important foam aerosol is shaving cream, but foaming aerosol shampoos and hand creams have also been produced.

Although most aerosol foams are required to be stable, formulations have recently been developed [152] in which the foam breaks immediately on leaving the valve and almost disappears into the skin.

**Foam Emulsion, W/O Type.** Here the propellant is dissolved in the external (oil) phase and hardly any foam formation occurs on evaporation of the propellant; there is only a moist, slack, and unstable foam. Root [153] describes a method that will yield an ample stable foam for this type as well: first the can is filled with a concentrate (W/O emulsion). The can is sealed and a propellant-in-water emulsion is added under pressure. The result is really a W/O—O/W mixed emulsion or a O/W/O dual emulsion.

**Spray Emulsions, W/O Type [154].** Here an aqueous solution of the active ingredients is the internal phase, the propellant, often dissolved in a solvent, the external. On spraying, the propellant evaporates, and the aqueous internal phase remains, mainly or exclusively, in fine drops. The character of the spray depends on the amounts of water and emulsifying agents used, the quality of the propellant, and the absence or presence of propellant solvents. Root [155] suggests how fine, medium, and coarse sprays can be obtained, and a systematic study of the behavior of surfactants with propellants has been made by Kanig and Desai [156].

**Spray Emulsions, O/W Type [157].** The development of this type became practicable only when spraying heads that are able to atomize liquids mechanically were introduced. These products are propellant-in-water emulsions. The propellant level may be kept very low (3–5%), and these products are therefore inexpensive. The internal pressure is low; hence they are safe. A disadvantage is the difficulty of preparing stable emulsions, and shaking before use is always required. Because of the external aqueous phase these products are likely to corrode, and some foam formation during spraying is almost unavoidable.

### Aerosols with Inorganic Propellants

The aerosol systems discussed above all have the common property that the propellant partly liquefies under pressure in the container and that the liquid propellant is blended with the other ingredients to form a homogeneous solution or at least an emulsion with them (only the unemulsified three-phase aerosols are an exception). This is actually the basis for the action of aerosols.

Aerosols with inorganic propellants, which neither liquefy nor dissolve in the concentrate nor form an emulsion with it, are therefore based on a fundamentally different system.

The principle of their action is actually simpler than that of the previously described aerosols: here the propellant mechanically forces the concentrate from the container. In practice this system produced so many difficulties that it was not marketed in the United States until 1957, 10 years after the triumphant entry of the "classical" aerosols. (This is not absolutely correct: "whipped cream aerosols" with carbon dioxide as a propellant already existed but they were specialized products designed for large restaurants and bakeries and were much too heavy and cumbersome for household use.)

At present the most important inorganic propellants are nitrogen and carbon dioxide. Argon and laughing gas ($N_2O$) have also been suggested but so far have not been found acceptable.

**Nitrogen [158].**     We have found that in "classic" aerosols the gas pressure inside the container remains constant because the liquid propellant evaporates as soon as the level of the liquid drops, the gas volume increases, and the pressure temporarily decreases. There is no liquid, hence no evaporating propellant in nitrogen aerosols; therefore the gas pressure must drop while the container is in use.

This is the root of most of the difficulties in the production of nitrogen aerosols. It is very difficult to adjust the contents in such a way that the concentrate will be forced out of the valve at the same rate at the beginning, when the pressure is high, as at the end, when it has dropped considerably. It is hardly possible to prepare them in such a way that they can be used until they are exhausted, and if any propellant is allowed to escape from the valve part of the contents will be left in the container.

These aerosols must be filled under an initially rather high internal pressure, and the container is always only partly filled. If, for example, it were filled to 90% of its capacity, the pressure would have to be 10 times as high at the beginning as at the end when the container is almost empty, which is impracticable. In practice the containers are filled to 60% of capacity, and gas is added up to an internal pressure of about 100 psi; this means that when the container is almost empty the pressure amounts to about 40 psi, or 25 psi excess pressure. This high internal pressure is less "dangerous" in nitrogen aerosols than in aerosols with halogenated and nonhalogenated hydrocarbons as propellants because with nitrogen the internal pressure rises less rapidly with increasing temperature. If it is 100 psi at 21°C (70°F), it will be only 123 psi at 55°C (130°F). Nevertheless, nitrogen aerosols should be packed in metal containers (preferably seamless); plastic and glass are dangerous. Widely differing preparations are suitable for nitrogen aerosols: viscous or nonviscous products and even creams and pastes. These preparations are not, as in other aerosol systems, dispensed as fine droplets or foam but in their normal form: liquid, syrup, or paste. In many products (creams, toothpastes, medicines, etc.) this is an advantage. In others (and in particular the most important aerosol products—insecticides, hair lacquer, and shaving creams) the spray or foam is the most important factor, so that it would be pointless to use nitrogen.

The advantages of nitrogen aerosols compared with others is the low price of the propellant, the absence of risk of corrosion, and (particularly interesting for pharmaceutical products) the possibility of sterilizing filled and sealed containers in autoclaves.

Compared with traditional packaging (bottles, tubes, jars), nitrogen aerosols have the following advantages: the contents have absolutely no contact with the outside, and the influence of atmospheric oxygen or the entry of microorganisms is completely excluded after filling. The contents are conveniently removed from the container by pushing a button. The manufacturer can determine the speed of dispensing by selecting the valve and dip tube; a metered valve can dispense the contents in measured portions. Furthermore, the container remains fully intact until the contents are exhausted (it need not be pinched and rolled like collapsible tubes) and the printed instructions remain legible to the very end. This is certainly an advantage for the manufacturer, possibly less so for the user.

Until now nitrogen aerosols have not earned any major share of the cosmetic market. They probably will do so only if there is some major development in this category.

**Carbon Dioxide Aerosols.**   Carbon dioxide as a propellant is recommended in particular for pharmaceutical and food aerosols. It differs from nitrogen mainly in that it is water-soluble and can be solidified and transported in solid form. Standard carbon dioxide snow is not suitable for aerosols, but a "carbon dioxide ice," developed by Professor L. W. Haas [159], is reported to be quite acceptable for this purpose.

### Powder Aerosols

Powder aerosols contain three phases: a gaseous phase (i.e., the propellant vapor) a liquid phase (i.e., liquid propellant that often incorporates suspending agents and other additives), and a solid phase (i.e., the powder). The powder is suspended in the propellant: when the valve is opened, this suspension is ejected from the container. The propellant evaporates and the powder reaches the skin in a dry state (if other liquids and suspension agents are present, it will be moist).

Practical suggestions for formulating these products are given by Kanig and Cohn [160].

### RAW MATERIALS

### Propellants [161]

Theoretically any substance that is gaseous at room temperature but liquefies under pressure at this temperature can be used as propellant. In practice, however, a good propellant must meet quite a few additional requirements:

1. It must be nontoxic and nonirritating to the skin. The physiological properties of propellants are discussed by Kuebler [162]. Although the major part of the propellant has evaporated by the time the active ingredient reaches the skin, some traces may be left in solution and could affect the skin.

2. It must not react with the active ingredients, the other raw materials of the preparation, or solvents and must not chemically affect containers or valves.

3. It should be soluble in the standard cosmetic solvents; two-phase aerosols require the propellant to be soluble to a certain extent in the solution of active ingredients.

4. It should be almost entirely odorless, noninflammable and, finally, as inexpensive as possible.

No known propellant meets all of these requirements completely.

**Halogenated Hydrocarbons.** As previously mentioned, the first practical aerosol used dichlorodifluoromethane ($CCl_2F_2$) as a propellant. This has remained the most commonly used propellant. It is neither toxic nor irritating and is chemically inert to all important cosmetic raw materials. In the presence of water there is a slight tendency to split off hydrogen chloride; nevertheless, small amounts may be incorporated in aqueous products without problem.

The chemical designations for these propellants are complicated and somewhat confusing; we are therefore using the simpler trade names in the text. We have chosen the Freon series because they were the first commercially available propellants and are still in very wide use, not because they are superior to other similar products.

*Dichlorodifluoromethane* (Freon 12) is miscible in all proportions with mineral oil, aliphatic and aromatic hydrocarbons, anhydrous ethyl, isopropyl or *n*-propyl alcohols, and most organic solvents. Its miscibility with glycerol and propylene glycol is restricted. Producers of propellants give further details about the solubility range and physical-chemical properties of their materials.

Freon 12 is completely noninflammable and even reduces the flammability of other raw materials so that alcoholic aerosols, for example, become inflammable only at alcohol concentrations above 25%. Unfortunately it is not inexpensive. Although dichlorodifluoromethane meets many of the requirements of a good propellant, it has one disadvantage: its vapor pressure at 70°F is 88 psi. The vapor pressure strongly increases with rising temperatures and amounts to 216 psi at 130°F. For this reason aerosol products with dichlorodifluoromethane as the only propellant must be packed in heavy cast-iron containers. This did not particularly matter for the insecticide bomb of the Allied forces but it would be cumbersome and unattractive for cosmetic products.

New propellants that would combine the desirable properties of dichloro-difluoromethane with a lower vapor pressure were sought and several materials were developed. The most important in cosmetics are dichloro-tetrafluoroethane (Freon 114) and trichloromonofluoromethane (Freon 11).

*Dichlorotetrafluoroethane* (Freon 114) has a vapor pressure of about 29 psi at 70°F (about 15 psi excess pressure), which means that this propellant may be used in light metal and even glass containers which are safe up to 73 and 50 psi, respectively. Another important advantage of Freon 114 is its chemical inertness, which is even more pronounced than that of Freon 12. Dichloro-tetrafluoroethane may be used safely in any aqueous aerosol preparations with risk of splitting off hydrogen chloride. The disadvantages of this material, apart from its price, which is high even in comparison to Freon 12, is its limited miscibility with polar substances.

It is more or less miscible with mineral oil, aromatic, and aliphatic hydro-carbons, and pure alcohols, and these products are therefore often used as solvents with Freon 114.

*Trichloromonofluoromethane* (Freon 11) has an even lower vapor pressure than Freon 114. Its boiling point is at 75°F; at room temperature its vapor pressure is less than 14.7 psi. This material cannot be used by itself as a propellant but it plays an important part as a diluent for Freon 12 to reduce the pressure inside the container. Freon 11 is far less expensive than Freon 114 and also has a much better solvent action for many materials. Its disadvantage is that it easily splits off hydrogen chloride and thus forms hydrochloric acid when it comes in contact with water inside the container. According to Bergwein [163], the hydrolysis value in one year at 50°C is 28.0 g/l for Freon 11, 9.5 g/l for Freon 12, and 3.0 g/l for Freon 114.

Hydrochloric acid may affect a metal container, the metal parts of valves, the perfume, and certain active ingredients. Even very small amounts of hydrochloric acid may have serious effects. When working with Freon 11, anhydrous raw materials should be used, or, if this is not practicable, con-tainers, valves, and perfumes that are not affected by small amounts of hydrochloric acid should be selected. If the active ingredients in aqueous preparations are not hydrochloric-acid resistant, Freon 11 cannot be used. The generation of hydrochloric acid is probably the reason why patch tests have shown that Freon 11 is irritating to the skin after a year's storage.* Aerosol products made with Freon 11 which had been stored for a year and more are reported to have occasionally caused skin irritations. Great caution

---

* Personal communication from Ing. J. Bossina.

is required therefore if Freon 11 is to be used in cosmetic preparations. Small additions of nitromethane help to stabilize Freon 11 in the presence of water. The commercial propellant 11 S contains such an addition [164]. Hoffman [165] questions the usefulness of such nitromethane additions, however. Apart from the three propellants mentioned, a few other fluorinated hydrocarbons are also used, but they are less important in cosmetics. The most important properties as well as the trade names used in various countries are summarized in Table 4-7. A few years ago, E. I. Du Pont de Nemours added Freon C 318, boiling point $-6°C$, to its range; the vapor pressure at $21°C$ is 2.3. It is specifically recommended for food aerosols.

*Freon 21*, and to a slightly lesser extent *Genetron 100*, *Freon 22*, and *113*, has a relatively good solvent action for substances containing oxygen. Du Pont classifies its propellants according to increasing solvent effect: Freon 114, 12, 22, 113, 11, 21.

*Genetron 101* is especially recommended by the manufacturers for use in cosmetic preparations. It is reported to develop perfumes fully and to be stable in the presence of water.

*Methylene chloride* and *vinyl chloride* have also been used as propellants or propellant diluents. In the presence of water they split off hydrochloric acid but less so than Freon 11. Their flammability may be considerably reduced by small additions of Freon. The narcotic effect of these substances may become noticeable if aerosol preparations incorporating them are sprayed in closed rooms; even Freon 12 vapor, when concentrated, has this effect. Particular caution is recommended in connection with vinyl chloride because it tends to polymerize in the presence of ingredients that have an acid reaction or are capable of splitting off acids, in which case a resin would form and the contents would become unusable.

**Hydrocarbons [166].** In addition to the halogenated hydrocarbons, unsubstituted hydrocarbons, in particular *n*-butane, are sometimes used as propellants; *n*-butane is neither toxic nor irritating to the skin; it cannot split off hydrochloric acid in any circumstances and may be combined at will with the halogenated hydrocarbons. It is much less expensive than they are but has one disadvantage: it is highly inflammable. Some countries therefore have prohibited its use as a propellant. There must be some warning about not using this aerosol near an open flame. Admixtures of Freon will reduce the inflammability. If *n*-butane is used, it should be almost pure. Sulfurous impurities cause unpleasant odors; unsaturated hydrocarbons might react with some product ingredients or, in the presence of hydrogen chloride, initiate the formation of tars that would clog the valve. A mixture of saturated hydrocarbons would have a rather wide boiling range. During the use of the container something like a fractionated distillation of the propellants would

TABLE 4-7 PROPELLANTS

| | | | | | Trade Names | | | | | | |
|---|---|---|---|---|---|---|---|---|---|---|---|
| Chemical Name | Formula | Molecular Weight | Boiling Point, C° (14.7 psi) | Vapor Pressure (psi at 70°F) | Hoechst German | Du Pont United States | Penn Salt United States | General Chemical United States | I.C.I. Great Britain | Electro-chimie d'Ugine France | Montecatini Italy |
| Trichloromonofluoromethane | $CCl_3F$ | 137.4 | +23.8 | 12 | Frigen 11 | Freon 11 | Isotron 11 | Genetron 11 | Arcton 9 | Electro CF 11 | Algofrene 1 |
| Dichlorodifluoromethane | $CCl_2F_2$ | 120.9 | −29.8 | 85 | Frigen 12 | Freon 12 | | Genetron 12 | Arcton 6 | Electro CF 12 | Algofrene 2 |
| Dichloromonofluoromethane | $CHCl_2F$ | 102.9 | +8.9 | 23.5 | Frigen 21 | Freon 21 | | | | | |
| Monochlorodifluoromethane | $CHClF_2$ | 86.5 | −40.8 | 138 | Frigen 22 | Freon 22 | | Genetron 141 | | Electro CF 22 | Algofrene 5 |
| Trichlorotrifluoroethane | $C_2Cl_3F_3$ | 187.4 | +47.5 | 6 | Frigen 113 | Freon 113 | | Genetron 226 | | Electro Forane 233 | |
| Dichlorotetrafluoroethane | $(CClF_2)_2$ | 170.9 | +3.5 | 27 | Frigen 114 | Freon 114 | | | | | Algofrene 6 |
| Difluoroethane | $(CH_2F)_2$ | 66.0 | −25 | 73 | | | | | | | |
| Monochlorodifluoroethane | $CHClF-CH_2F$ | 100.5 | −9.5 | 44 | | | | | Arcton 33 | Electro Forane 242 | |
| Methylene chloride | $CH_2Cl_2$ | 84.9 | +40 | | | | | | | | |
| Vinyl chloride | $CH_2{:}CHCl$ | 62.5 | −12 | 35 | | | | Genetron 320 | | | |
| n-propane | $C_3H_8$ | 44.1 | −42.2 | 131 | | | | Genetron 100 | | | |
| n-butane | $C_4H_{10}$ | 58.1 | −0.6 | 35 | | | | Genetron 101 | | | |

183

occur; the highest boiling substances would accumulate inside the container and vapor pressure would drop accordingly, which is, of course, undesirable. *Isobutane* and *n-propane* have also occasionally been used as propellants.

**Inorganic Propellants.** *Nitrogen* is sometimes used in cosmetic and pharmaceutical preparations and *carbon dioxide*, in food aerosols. Both are inexpensive, nontoxic, chemically inert, and noninflammable. They differ fundamentally from the other substances inasmuch as they never liquefy inside the container and are almost insoluble in all standard products. Argon and laughing gas ($N_2O$) are also mentioned as propellants in the literature but are hardly ever used in practice.

**Propellant Mixtures.** In many instances the use of a single propellant does not achieve the desired end effect in an aerosol preparation. The vapor pressure in Freon 12 alone is too high; in Freon 11, too low, and Freon 114 is often too expensive. Generally, therefore, a mixture of propellants will be used. It is always important, of course, to know the vapor pressure of the mixture used; how this may be calculated for a mixture is demonstrated in the following with a 60:40 mixture of Freon 114 and Freon 12.

100 g of this mixture contains 60 g of Freon 114 and 40 g of Freon 12, or

$$\frac{60}{170.5} = 0.3511 \text{ moles Freon 114}$$

and

$$\frac{40}{120.9} = 0.3308 \text{ moles Freon 12.}$$

The mole fraction of Freon 114 in the mixture is therefore

$$\frac{0.3511}{0.3511 + 0.3308} = 0.5149$$

and of Freon 12,

$$\frac{0.3308}{0.3511 + 0.3308} = 0.4851.$$

The partial pressure of Freon 114 vapor at 70°F is then $0.5149 \times 28 = 14.4$ psi; the partial pressure of Freon 12 vapor is $0.4851 \times 86 = 41.7$ psi. If it is assumed that the total vapor pressure of the mixture equals the sum of the partial pressures, the total vapor pressure of this mixture will be $14.4 + 41.7 = 56.1$ psi. This assumption is, however, justified only for gas mixtures that are "perfect" in the chemical-physical sense and does not altogether apply to most propellant mixtures. The vapor pressure of a 60/40 Freon 114/12 mixture, experimentally determined, is about 54 psi. Generally the actual vapor pressure deviates less than 10% from the calculated value.

The propellant mixture described above is often used in practice. Another widely used mixture is 50/50 Freon 11/12 with a vapor pressure of 50 psi at 70°F. "Propellant A" widely used in the United States, consists of a mixture of Freon 11 and 12 with isobutane. Details of various propellant mixtures may be obtained from the suppliers of propellants.

## Active Ingredients

In an aerosol powder the active ingredient is the powder; in an aerosol shampoo it is the aqueous detergent solution; in an aerosol lotion, the perfume oil, and so on. The composition of these ingredients of course resembles that of traditional preparations, but it is not true that any good shaving cream, any good perfume, or any good powder may be packed in aerosol containers without further change. Often drastic alterations in formulation are required for aerosols. The main problem is usually the solubility of the active ingredients in the propellant. With powder aerosols complete insolubility is required; in two-phase aerosols, on the other hand, complete solution even at low temperatures is necessary.

Mucins used as thickening agents in emulsions and resinoids in perfume compositions tend to flocculate after the propellant has been added. Solids with limited solubility, which occur in suntan lotions or perfume compositions, may crystallize out on strong cooling caused by the addition of the propellant (at least during cold filling) and not redissolve. In some cases such precipitations may clog the valve; in glass containers they are unattractive. In all instances crystallized substances lose their effectiveness.

## Solvents

The problem of solubility is often eliminated by the addition of a solvent in which both the propellant and the concentrate are soluble. Ethyl and propyl alcohols are widely used solvents in cosmetics. The solvent effects of glycol ethers on several propellants are listed in Table 4-8. In any case, the solution of active ingredients must be cold-filtered before it is introduced into the

TABLE 4-8   QUANTITY OF PROPELLANT (IN GRAMS) SOLUBLE IN 100 GRAMS OF SOLVENT AT 90°F UNDER THE PRESSURE INDICATED

| Composition | Freon 11 (6.17 psi) | Freon 12 (52 psi) | Freon 22 (84 psi) | Freon 14 (15.2 psi) |
|---|---|---|---|---|
| Diethylene glycol diethyl ether | 49.5 | | 112.7 | 30.0 |
| Tetraethylene glycol diethyl ether | 21.6 | 25.8 | | 12.0 |
| Tetraethylene glycol dimethyl ether | 30.2 | 21.5 | 109 | |
| Diethylene glycol monoacetate monoethyl ether | 33.8 | | 114.3 | 15.5 |

aerosol container. If the cold-filling process is used, precooling should be effected to below the boiling point of the propellant.

When there are no solubility problems because the active ingredients are soluble in the liquid propellants, the solvents used are mostly paraffin oils, odorless petroleum fractions, or methylene or ethylene chloride. "Chlorethene," 1,1,1-trichloroethane, is also recommended [167]. Organic propellants are miscible with these solvents in all proportions.

### Emulsifying Agents

The preparation of emulsified three-phase aerosols gives rise to the problem of emulsifying a liquid propellant in an aqueous vehicle or an aqueous solution in a liquid propellant (with or without additional water-insoluble solvents). These emulsification problems have been fully discussed by Root [168]. This author states that triethanolamine soaps and alkylolamides are good emulsifiers when it is desired to emulsify halogenated hydrocarbons (such as Freons) in an aqueous product, such as shaving creams. For the emulsification of hydrocarbons in aqueous products sulfated fatty-acid amides and the "Spans" and "Tweens" of the Atlas Chemical Co. have also proved useful.

Nonionic emulsifying agents are recommended for water-in-propellant emulsions: "Emcol 14" (Emulsol Chemical Division, Chicago, described as "fatty-acid polyglycerideester"), "Span 20" (sorbitan monolaurate), and "Polyethylene glycol-400-ditriricinoleate" (Glyco Products, New York).

### CONTAINERS

The aerosol industry quickly overcame the initial stage when only heavy and expensive iron containers could be used because of high internal pressure. Today, cosmetic manufacturers have a wide choice of many types of handy, attractive, and less expensive packages.

### Glass Bottles

The most attractive container for liquid cosmetic products, including aerosols, is and always will be the glass bottle. In glass bottles the contents are given full visual value, the level of the liquid is easily observed at all times, and any number of attractive shapes are available. The required pressure resistance restricts the design of glass bottles to a considerable extent, but many variations are still possible. Glass bottles also have the great advantage of being corrosion-resistant to all raw materials used in cosmetic products. Their disadvantage is their breakability: a bottle will break either when the internal pressure is too high or after a strong mechanical shock. With good construction, adequate wall thickness, and not too much contents (United States law prescribes a maximum of 80 ml for glass aerosols), glass bottles are perfectly safe under normal conditions of use up to a pressure of 25 psi. Even at low pressure there is always the risk that the bottle will break if it is dropped or explode if it is left standing in too high a temperature, in which case glass splinters could be blasted off with great force up to 30 ft [169].

To eliminate this risk many glass bottles today are coated with a tough elastic polyvinylchloride film that would hold the splinters in case of breakage. This synthetic sheath may be made colorless and transparent, but it can also be clouded or pigmented, and the selection of the plastic coating offers further possibilities for the presentation of the product.

### Metal Containers [170]

In spite of the esthetic superiority of glass, metal cans remain the most important containers for aerosol cosmetics. At present all three-phase aerosols (shaving cream, shampoos, powder, etc.) and all preparations that require pressure above 35 psi (air deodorants, hair lacquers, etc.) are packed in metal containers.

Drawn, seamless cans play a particularly important part. These cans are manufactured by drawing the cylindrical body with head and orifice collar (the bottom part) in one piece; the bottom (curved inward) or the head is then rolled on.

Welded or soldered tin containers are less expensive than the seamless ones; the cylindrical bodies are made from tinplate with a vertical seam; head and bottom are rolled on. These forms have the disadvantage of showing a certain weakness at the seams. Technical aspects of aerosol containers of steel or tinplate are discussed in detail by Johnson [171].

The body and head of aluminum cans [172] are always drawn in one piece; sometimes the bottom is also included so that the whole container consists of one piece, and sometimes a piece of tinplate, rolled on, serves as the bottom. Aluminum cans may be made in various shapes; they are light in weight and comparatively inexpensive. Attractive lipstick-sized aluminum cans with a metered valve are also available as handbag perfume dispensers [173]. Even more than tin containers, aluminum cans are likely to corrode. Corrosion in metal containers may be actuated by various substances; for example, metal salts and alcohols. In most instances this is due to hydrolysis of the propellant in the presence of water. Freon 11 may cause considerable damage in this connection. Aluminum containers, in particular, tend to corrode in the presence of ethyl or isopropyl alcohol. It is interesting to note that with aluminum ethyl and isopropyl alcohols free of water cause much stronger corrosion than alcohols containing small amounts of water (even as little as 1%) [174].

In order to prevent corrosion, metal containers are usually provided with internal protective lacquers with good adhesion to the metal, insoluble in the contents, and generally inert to chemical reactions. This lacquer must form an unbroken coating, free of bubbles, particularly in products containing surfactants, since otherwise corrosion would begin in the gaps and spread underneath the lacquer.

All metal aerosol containers are supplied with the standardized valve orifice of 1 in. diameter with a collar into which all regular valves may be inserted. All have been designed to be safe up to 60 psi.

### Plastic Containers [175]

Various synthetic resins may be used for aerosol containers; the most common is probably "Zytel" nylon (Du Pont). The containers are break- and corrosionproof but presently very expensive. Technical difficulties limit the possibility of varying shapes.

### Valves [176]

Different types of valve are used for cosmetic aerosols. In some designs the contents on their way out come in contact only with plastic parts; in others, with rubber or metal. Spraying angle, speed, and the degree of atomization depend on the construction of the valve.

Metered valves spray only small predetermined amounts in a single actuation.

### Protective Caps

Finally, caps that cover the can when it is not in use, protect the valve and provide the finishing touch to the package.

## FORMULATION OF AEROSOL PRODUCTS

The main requirements to be met by an aerosol product are the following:

1. *Effectiveness.* The preparation must be effective; that is, it must fulfill its cosmetic purpose. This effectiveness depends primarily on the composition of the active ingredients.

2. *Stability.* The aerosol must be stable. Active ingredients, perfume, propellant, container, and valve must be selected to avoid completely all symptoms of insolubility and after longer storage nearly all chemical reactions between components. In many instances this is the requirement that presents the most difficult problems.

One of the main difficulties with aerosol products is the risk of corrosion of the inner wall of the container. Occasionally constituents of the concentrate react with the container (e.g., alcohol with aluminum, particularly when anhydrous alcohols are used; corrosion may be considerably reduced by small additions of water [177]). Mostly, however, corrosion is caused by hydrochloric acid formed by hydrolysis of the propellants. Whenever there is a risk of hydrochloric acid formation, metal containers are commonly coated inside with one or more layers of an acid-resistant lacquer. In many cases this precaution is effective, but it often fails in preparations that contain surfactants (e.g., aerosol shampoos). This is due to the difficulty of achieving a completely impermeable protective layer. Almost invariably it will contain fine bubbles and cracks which normally have no adverse effect. In the presence of surfactants, however, which always have a certain wetting effect, the contents penetrate even the finest openings and cause corrosion of the metal wall which then spreads underneath the lacquer. Various protective lacquers for aerosols are discussed by Morris [178]. Oxygen in the container may promote corrosion and should be avoided as far as possible [179].

Another precaution against corrosion is the addition of substances that would react with any liberated hydrochloric acid and inactivate it. Organic nitrites and aluminum palmitate have been suggested as possible additives; triethanolamine has also been successfully used; Hopf [180] recommends the "epoxidized oils" produced by Boake Roberts Ltd., London. These materials may, of course, be used only when they are compatible with the active ingredient.

3. *Safety.*    Aerosol containers and their contents must be harmless.

PRESSURE. With preparations under pressure there is a risk of the container not tolerating the internal pressure, particularly if it is raised by heat, and exploding. It is essential therefore to use containers that are strong enough for these products. In many countries minimum requirements for aerosol containers are prescribed by law.

FIRE [181]. Another risk is fire. The aerosol process atomizes inflammable organic substances in the air. The large surface covered by the sprayed material and the fast evaporation of volatile organic matter considerably increase the risk compared with that offered by products in conventional packing. A product is "flammable" if the spray on being directed onto an open flame from a distance of about 20 in. burns back in the direction of the valve over a distance of more than about 1 in. (this is the so-called "torch effect"). If the flame shows more intensive burning and the spray also burns behind the flame but does not backfire, the product is classified as "combustible." Generally, only aerosol products that contain large amounts of organic solvents (e.g., more than 25% ethyl alcohol) or a flammable propellant (propane, butane, vinyl chloride) are flammable. Fluorinated hydrocarbons are not flammable and even reduce the flammability of other aerosol constituents. Nonflammable aerosol products may be formulated with flammable organic solvents if sufficient quantities of Freons or other similar propellants are added. Nonflammable aerosols may also be prepared by mixing propane, butane, or vinyl chloride with nonflammable propellants. The flammability of the finished product should in any case be determined by the torch test (spraying into an open flame). The law in various countries requires nonflammability of aerosol products, but the danger from flammable products should not be exaggerated; as soon as pressure on the valve is released, burning stops [182]. Fulton and Yeomans describe a device to test the flammability of aerosols [183].

OTHER RISKS. Further risks with aerosol products lie in halogenated hydrocarbons used as propellants which may form the highly poisonous gas phosgene ($COCl_2$) if they come in contact with flames or hot surfaces or which may cause spasms of the respiratory muscles with resulting asphyxiation if inhaled in high concentration. Butane and propane, which are heavier than air and also used as propellants, may accumulate on the ground and combine to an explosive mixture [184]. These risks cannot be avoided but consumers must be warned.

4. *Costs of Production.* These costs should be as low as possible. More than with other products, the scale of production is a contributive factor to cost. In the United States, where aerosol products are mass produced, the cost per unit is considerably below that in other parts of the world, where production is still on a much smaller scale.

The cost is also influenced by formulation. Without cheapening the product by cutting the cost of the active ingredients, the adjustment of the propellant mixture is still an effective tool for controlling the price. The last important requirement must not be forgotten in this connection.

5. *Spraying Pattern.* The product must be easily sprayed. Cosmetic products do not require the same fine dispersion as room insecticides, for instance, whose droplets remain suspended in the atmosphere for several hours. On the other hand, a thick wet spray is undesirable for liquid products, and a foam aerosol should not produce a slack semiliquid lather.

TWO-PHASE AEROSOLS. As already mentioned, a fine spray of two-phase aerosols is promoted by the following factors: a high proportion of propellant in the finished product, high vapor pressure of the propellant or propellant mixture, and not too high a solubility of the propellant in the solution of active ingredients.

A practical example will best demonstrate how control over these factors will achieve a satisfactory spray pattern. Assume an aerosol perfume with the following composition: 2% perfume oil, 53% ethyl alcohol 95%, 45% Freon 114. On spraying, this preparation is dispensed in a thick wet jet, which may be improved in three different ways:

(a) By increasing the propellant component. 2% perfume, 45% ethyl alcohol 95%, and 53% Freon 114 results in a better spray pattern. This method has the disadvantage of increasing the cost of the product because Freon 114 is not cheap. Furthermore, the internal pressure is increased which is admissible with glass aerosols only to a limited degree and never desirable.

(b) Spraying may also be improved by replacing part of Freon 114 by Freon 12; a mixture of 2% perfume oil, 53% ethyl alcohol 95%, 35% Freon 114, and 10% Freon 12 will again yield a good spraying pattern; and the cost of the product is not increased but lowered. However, vapor pressure is again increased, and Freon 12 is not quite so stable in the presence of water as Freon 114; in the case of hydrolysis of the propellant, the perfume would be affected.

(c) Finally, the solubility of the propellant in the concentrate may be reduced by diluting the alcohol used with water; for example, 2% perfume, 53% ethyl alcohol 92%, and 45% Freon 114 may again have good spraying properties. This direction might be pursued even further by taking, say, 2% perfume oil, 74% alcohol 80%, and 24% Freon 114. A satisfactorily spraying product could thus be obtained with low vapor pressure, and low propellant content (meaning low price). Products of this type are classified as "ultralow pressure" aerosols. As long as Freon 114 is used exclusively there is no risk of propellant hydrolysis and separation of hydrochloric acid. Working with diluted alcohol and Freon 114 is an excellent solution of the problem and is applied whenever possible in two-phase aerosols. It must be borne in mind that "ultralow pressure" systems are covered by certain patents held by Chemway Corp.

The alcohol obviously cannot be diluted indefinitely. Many active ingredients, and among them perfume oils, have only a limited solubility in dilute alcohol and strong dilution increases the risk of flocculation. Moreover, if the solubility of the propellant in the concentrate is too small, spraying is no longer satisfactory. Mina [185] demonstrates in Table 4-9 how the required proportion of propellant depends on the alcohol concentration.

THREE-PHASE AEROSOLS.   The last-mentioned method cannot be used with three-phase aerosols to improve the spraying pattern. Here the only way is to adjust the propellant mixture to achieve a higher vapor pressure. To increase the proportion of propellant beyond a definite point is useless: there must be sufficient propellant to last until the content is used up. To add more is pointless; vapor pressure would not be increased.

TABLE 4-9

| Alcohol Concentration (vol. %) | Proportion of Freon 114 soluble in Alcohol (vol. %) | Proportion of Freon 114 Required for Good Spraying Effect (vol. %) |
|---|---|---|
| Ethyl alcohol | | |
| 85 | 17 | 16.5 |
| 88* | 24 | 23.2 |
| 90 | 32 | 30.6 |
| 93 | 50 | 35·6 |
| 100 | unlimited | 64 |
| Isopropyl alcohol | | |
| 75 | 23 | 22.2 |
| 80* | 31 | 29.5 |
| 85 | 50 | 36.0 |

* These are regarded as the optical concentrations. If the alcohol is still further diluted and the propellant concentration lowered, the spray characteristics are impaired.

POWDER AEROSOLS.    It is particularly difficult to achieve a good spraying pattern for powder aerosols. The difficulties are twofold: powder particles may become entrapped in or at the valve, and either clog it or force a leak. They may also coalesce at the bottom of the container.

The concentration of solids in powder aerosols rarely exceeds 10%. With such concentrations it is still possible to disperse the solid particles in the propellant and to prevent their coalescence (see below). During use the powder dispersion is forced through the narrow channels of the valve with the risk that the powder particles may coalesce, form a cake, and clog the valve. If this cake does not form in the valve but at its base, spraying continues, but in the end the valve is no longer able to return to its closed state and leaks will occur. To prevent this effect a valve appropriate for the particle size of the powder must be selected, and the powder itself must have a particle size as uniform as possible. Larger size particles, even in small amounts, often lead to difficulties. It also becomes clear in this connection why the solids must be insoluble in the propellant or propellant mixture. If there is any solubility, the result is a tendency for the particles to grow; small particles dissolve, the dissolved substance precipitates to larger particles, and they continue to grow. Even more important than the size is the shape of the powder particles: almost spherical particles show less tendency to become entrapped than elongated needleshaped ones.

The tendency of powder to form lumps on the bottom of the container may be counteracted by selecting a propellant mixture with a specific gravity as close as possible to that of the powder. Substances with a dispersing effect on powder may also be incorporated. Di Giacomo [186] recommends iso-propyl myristate for this purpose. Sometimes small metal or glass beads are placed in the aerosol containers which mechanically break up cakes that have formed on the bottom.

## Preparation [187]

All usual propellants are either gaseous or at least near their boiling point at room temperature. Since they should be introduced into the aerosol container in more or less definite quantities in liquid state, it seems obvious to liquefy them before filling. This can be achieved in two ways: either by cooling the propellants below their boiling points or by compression at room temperature. Corresponding to these two methods, are two filling techniques: cold filling and pressure filling. In cold filling the propellant, which is taken from the storage cylinder in the gaseous state, is liquefied by cooling. It is then added through a metering device to the precooled concentrate in the aerosol container, the valve is inserted and the container sealed. This filling method is easily carried out in the laboratory with simple apparatus and has also proved satisfactory in bulk production. Careful operating is essential to avoid condensation of atmospheric moisture inside the container or at its rim, since water in the aerosol system, particularly with Freon 11 as a propellant, gives rise to complications. Losses of propellant can also only be avoided by careful working. This technique is not applicable to products which cannot tolerate strong cooling (aerosol creams, etc.).

Pressure filling is more generally applicable. The propellant is already compressed and liquid in the storage cylinder, and pressure of this cylinder may be utilized for filling. The propellant is then passed into the aerosol container, already provided with a valve, through a pressure-resistant gas-impermeable filling system containing some measuring or metering device. This method requires simpler and less expensive equipment than the cold-fill system but is not so rapid. With pressure filling metering is less accurate and less easily adjusted than with cold filling. The higher requirements on valves is another disadvantage of pressure filling because the propellant is forced from outside into the container through the valves. A number of valve types therefore cannot be considered for this filling method, for there is always some risk of damage. Most modern plants use both methods side-by-side because what may be suitable for one product may not be for another. For both methods preliminary cleaning of the propellant is recommended to remove all possible rust particles. After sealing, the containers are dipped into a water bath of about 120°F in order to uncover leaks and weak spots.

Honisch [188] describes still another filling method that might be regarded as halfway between cold and pressure filling. There is a risk, in particular with pressure filling, that air will become trapped in the filled container. This may be air that has been present in the container from the beginning, or introduced during filling into the propellant or concentrate.

The following example shows that the internal pressure is considerably increased by entrapped air [189]: a typical aerosol insecticide (15% concentrate, 85% Freon 11:12, 50:50) was pressure-filled into a container from which air had not been previously removed until it was filled to 70% capacity. The internal pressure measured at 70°F was 22 psi higher than in an identical preparation without air. If half the air present in the container were removed before filling, pressure would be about 9 psi too high. With other propellants conditions are similar. Enclosed air may be removed after filling by reversing the container and releasing the air mixed with some propellant by brief pressure on the valve. This method is easily carried out with two-phase aerosols but it encounters difficulties with foam aerosols. However, the working pressure with foam aerosols is so low that enclosed air hardly interferes at all. Air may also be removed before filling by flushing the containers with small amounts of propellants, which is easy because they are heavier than air, and is the method most commonly used, or by evacuating the containers. If air is introduced with the propellant or concentrate, it obviously remains enclosed.

# TESTING OF AEROSOL PRODUCTS

Bergwein [190] gives an excellent summary of the methods used to test newly developed or finished products. We have already mentioned the torch test for flammability or combustibility and the impermeability test by dipping the sealed containers into a warm-water bath. Other important tests are the following:

## Spraying Tests

**Spraying Pattern.** Here the spraying behavior is observed primarily to determine whether the preparation has the correct degree of atomization, whether a three-phase aerosol sprays jerkily, an aerosol foam has the required consistency, or a powder causes clogging or leaking of the valve. Root describes various methods to get a more exact picture of the spraying pattern [191].

**Spraying Speed.** This is measured by spraying with a fully opened valve for a definite number of seconds, weighing the container before and after, and calculating the loss in weight per second. Spraying speed should be as high with an almost empty container as with one newly filled.

## Storage Tests

The only reliable method of determining whether an aerosol product changes in the course of storage over many months is actually to keep it for that period and to observe the changes. Since in practice it is often desirable to bring out a newly developed product quickly, attempts have repeatedly been made to circumvent these lengthy methods and to accelerate testing. No reliable method has yet been found. In some cases storage at increased temperatures accelerates the processes inside the container so that possible modifications become apparent after weeks instead of months. This does not always occur; cases have been known in which these processes occurred more speedily at room temperature than in an incubator. It has become common usage therefore to test for storage stability simultaneously at room temperature and in incubators (at about 130°F) [184]. Observation time should be 1–2 months for incubators and six months for room temperature. During this period, the following are tested:

**Loss in Weight.**   According to Bergwein, this should not exceed 2.5 g/yr.

**Corrosion.**   After the usual observation time, the test products are emptied from the containers at room temperature and the internal wall of the container examined. Tests with metal disks sawn out of the walls of the containers are unreliable because they present the possibility of corrosion at the edges of the disks which do not exist in sound containers.

**Shelf Life.**   In storage tests the stability of the active ingredients and the perfume must be tested. Depending on the product, the stability of the active ingredients may be determined by chemical analysis or tests of effectiveness. In many instances minor changes are not easily discerned. It is easier to check the stability of the perfume by olfactory tests. The perfuming of aerosol preparations has developed into a specialized branch of the fragrance industry because of the particular requirements that must be met by perfume compositions for aerosol products regarding their solubility and their stability to chemical reactions also because perfumes develop differently in a fine spray instead of in conventional packing. Hydrochloric acid, which might have developed through hydrolysis of the propellant, not only causes corrosion in metal containers it is also the most dangerous adversary of perfume compositions and certain active ingredients. Additives that prevent corrosion (organic nitrites, aluminum palmitate and triethanolamine) also act as protective agents for perfumes and active ingredients.

# REFERENCES

[1] Czetsch-Lindenwald and Schmidt-La Baume, *Salben, Puder, Externa*, Springer-Verlag, Berlin/Goettingen/Heidelberg, 3rd ed., 1950.

[2] *Dermat. Wschr.*, **40** (1937).

[3] *Mschr. Krebs-Bek.*, **11**, 31 (1943).

[4] Vonkennel, *Parfum. Kosmet.*, **37**, 249 (1956).

[5] Schaaf, *Dermatologica* (Basel), **123**, 362 (1961).

[6] Rajka and Viucze, *Berufsdermatosen*, **V**, 164 (1955).

[7] Meyer, *Dissn. Bern*, 1936.

[8] *Arch. Derm.*, **131**, 549 (1932); Weitzel, Fretzdorff, and Heller, Hoppe-Seyler's *Z. physiol. Chemie*, **301**, 26 (1955); Kleine-Nathrop, *Hautarzt*, **8**, 421 (1957).

[9] Trade Marks: "Jelene 50W" and "Plastibase," *Schimmel Briefs*, **254** (May 1956); Mutimer, Riffin, Hill, and Cyr, *J. Am. pharm. Ass.*, **45**, 101 (1956).

[10] *Riechstoffe, Seifen, Kosmetika*, Bd. I, Hüthig Verlag, Heidelberg, 1950, p. 306.

[11] Rothemann, *Das grosse Rezeptbuch der Haut-und Körperpflegemittel*, 3rd ed., Hüthig Verlag, Heidelberg, 1962, p. 312.

[12] De Navarre, *The Chemistry and Manufacture of Cosmetics*, 2nd ed., Van Nostrand, Princeton, New Jersey, 1962, p. 359.

[13] Board of Standards Specification No. 8.

[14] *Am. Perfumer*, 33 (January 1944).

[15] Bergwein, Seifen-Öle-Fette-Wachse, **82**, 469 (1956); Nowak, *SÖFW*, **83**, 9 (1957).

[16] Newman, *J. Soc. cosmet. Chem.*, **8**, 44 (1957); Sisley, *Kosmetik Parf-Drogen*, No. 5/6, 62é (1957); Janistyn, *Parfum. Kosmet.*, **37**, 406 (1956); McDonough and Edman, *Drug Cosmet. Ind.*, **78**, 171 (1955).

[17] *J. Soc. cosmet. Chem.*, **5**, 277 (1951).

[18] Wellendorf, *Nature* (London), **198**, 1086 (1963).

[19] Conrad and Motiuk, *Am. Perfumer* (April 1956); Dietrich, *Industrie Parfum.*, **12**, 177 (1957).

[20] Harry, *Cosmetic Materials*, London, 1948, p. 168.

[21] *J. invest. Derm.*, **15**, 453 (1950); **20**, 33 (1953).

[22] Conrad, *Am. Perfumer*, **71** (6), 70 (1950); De Navarre, *op. cit.* II, 200 ff; Barnett, *Drug Cosmet. Ind.*, **80**, 744 (1957); **83**, 192 (1958); Colbert, *op. cit.*, **82**, 221 (1958); Herzka, *Aerosol Rept.*, **2**, 119, 150 (1963).

[23] Stejskal and Vyhnanek, *Parfum. Kosmet.*, **38**, 566 (1957).

[24] *Am. Perfumer*, **71** (4), 35 (April 1956).

[25] Lower, *Perfum. essent. Oil Rec.*, **47**, 403 (1956).

[26] *Perfum. essent. Oil Rec.*, **47**, 179 (1956).

[27] Winkler, *Dissn. Tübingen*, in Profand, *Kosmetic-Parf.-Drogen* 3, 93 (1956).

[28] *Hautarzt*, **4**, 560 (1953); **5**, 29 (1954).

[29] *Parfum. Kosmet.*, **38**, 686 (1957).

[30] *Kosmetik-Parf.-Drogen*, 45 (May–June 1954).

[31] *SÖFW*, **82,** 543 (1956).

[32] *Pharm. Zentralhalle*, **94,** 166 (1955).

[33] Gergle, Gregory, and Todd, *Drug Cosmet. Ind.*, **82,** 36 (1958).

[34] *Angew. Chem.*, **66,** 41 (1954).

[35] German Patent DAS 1 018194, Wella A.G.

[36] *J. Soc. cosmet. Chem.*, **7,** No. 3, 6 (May 1956).

[37] Conn et al., *J. Am. pharm. Ass.*, Sci. Ed., **45,** 311 (1956); Drug *Cosmet. Ind.*, **79,** 101 (1956).

[38] *Arch. Derm. Syph. Vienna*, **193,** 503 (1951); **195,** 310 (1953).

[38a] Volk and Winter, *Lexikon der kosmetischen Praxis*, Springer-Verlag, Vienna 1956, p. 472.

[39] Thorvik, *Riechst. Aromen*, **8,** 49 (1950) et seq.; Ostendorf, J. *Soc. cosmet. Chem.*, **16,** 203 (1965).

[40] De Navarre, *op. cit.*, **I,** 301.

[41] J. Sfiras, *Recherches*, No. 4, 9 (August 1954).

[42] Heimann and Petzold, *Fette Seifen*, 1957, p. 330.

[43] Schneider, *Riechst. Aromen* **8,** 15 (1950); Janecke and Senft, *Arch. Pharm.*, **290,** 178, 200, 472 (1957).

[44] *Oil Soap*, **21,** 33, 160 (1944); *J. Am. Oil Chem. Soc.*, **28,** 477 (1951).

[45] *SÖFW*, **80,** 542 (1954); *Oil Soap*, **19,** 144 (1942); **22,** 81 (1945).

[46] *J. Am. Oil Chem. Soc.*, **26,** 449 (1949).

[47] *Schimmel Briefs*, **269,** (1957); *Parfum. Kosmet.*, **38,** 654 (1957).

[48] Klim and Kumerow, *J. Am. Oil Chem. Soc.*, **39,** 150 (1963).

[49] *J. Am. Oil Chem. Soc.*, 433 (October 1951).

[50] *Oléagineux*, 726 (1949); **86,** 478 (1950).

[51] Petzold, Jubilee Convention DGF Hamburg, October 1956.

[52] Rosenwald, *Am. Perfumer*, **78,** (10), 41 (1963).

[53] A. Ruys, *Parfum. Kosmet.*, **38,** 149 (1957).

[54] *Schimmel Briefs*, **269** (1957).

[55] *Pharm. Zentralhalle*, **94,** 166 (1955).

[56] Royce, *Soap* (September 1931) 25; Evans, *Ind. Engng. Chem.*, 329 (March 1935).

[57] De Navarre, *op. cit.*, **I,** 301.

[58] *J. Am. Oil Chem. Soc.*, **27,** 128 (1944).

[59] *Ind. Engng. Chem.*, Anal. Ed., **4,** 209 (1932).

[60] Holm, Ekbom, and Wode, *J. Am. Oil Chem. Soc.*, **34,** 606 (1957).

[61] Pokorny, *Parfum. Kosmet.*, **46,** 33 (1965).

[62] Finholt and Hopp, *Riechst. Aromen*, **8,** 15 (1958).

[63] *Oil Soap*, **12,** 187 (1935).

[64] *Oil Soap*, **20,** 240 (1943).

[65] *Dermatologica*, **91,** 297 (1945).

[66] Janistyn, *op. cit.*, **I,** 3.

[67] Rothemann, *op. cit.*, 113.

[68] R. Renaud, *Parfums Cosmét. Savons*, **13**, 21 (1958).

[69] *J. Cosm. Chem.*, **6**, 263 (1955).

[70] Harry, *Modern Cosmetocology*, 4th ed., Leonard Hill, London, 1955, p. 126.

[71] *Pharm. Acta. Helv.*, **21**, 123, 145, 204, 286 (1946); **22**, 12, 86, 247 (1947); Benson, Griffin, and Truax, *J. Soc. cosmet. Chem.*, **13**, 437 (1962).

[72] Becher, *Emulsions*, Reinhold, New York, 1957; Janistyn, *op. cit.*, II; Klempson-Jones, *Am. Perfumer*, **71** (6), 88 (1958).

[73] *J. Ind. Engng. Chem.*, **13**, 1116 (1921).

[74] Van der Minne, *Diss. Utrecht*, 1928, p. 94.

[75] Schmidt-La Baume-Lietz, *Die Emulsionen in der Hauttherapie*, 2nd ed., Stuttgart 1951, p. 22.

[76] *Soap, Perf., Cosm.*, **11**, 625 (1938).

[77] *J. Bact.*, **15**, 13 (1928).

[78] *J. invest. Derm.*, **4**, 69 (1941).

[79] Kunzmann, *SÖFW*, **85**, 227 (1957).

[80] Bryce and Sugden, *Pharm. J.*, 311 (November 1959).

[81] Trutey, *Industrie Parfum.*, **11**, 295 (1956).

[82] Osipow, *Drug Cosmet. Ind.*, **88**, 438 (1961).

[83] *J. Soc. cosmet. Chem.*, **3**, 5 (March 1952).

[84] Velon, *SÖFW*, **81**, 89 115 (1955).

[85] Tschakert and von zur Gathen, *SÖFW*, **11**, 403 (1951).

[86] Osipow, *Drug Cosmet. Ind.*, **88**, 4 (1961); *Kosm-Parf-Drogens R.*, **7/8** (1961).

[87] Powers and Fox, *Drug Cosmet., Ind.*, **82**, 32 (1958).

[88] De Navarre, *op. cit.*, 1st ed., 245.

[89] *Proc. scient. Sect.* Toilet Goods Ass., **4**, 22 (1945).

[90] *Ibid.*, 6, 20 (1946).

[91] Tschakert and von zur Gathen, *SÖFW*, **77**, 483 (1951).

[92] Sfiras, *Recherches*, **5**, 38 (June 1955).

[93] Chun, Joslin, and Martin, *Drug Cosmet. Ind.*, **82**, 161 (1958).

[94] Janistyn, *op. cit.*, II, 51.

[95] Chong, *J. Soc. cosmet. Chem.*, **14**, 123 (1963).

[96] Figley, *J. Am. med. Ass.*, **123**, 747 (1940).

[97] De Navarre, *op. cit./*II, 2nd ed., 151 et seq.; Cook and Peterson, *Drug Cosmet. Ind.*, **82**, 446 (1958).

[98] Schofield, *Soap, Perfum., Cosmet.*, **37**, 59 (1964).

[99] Sfiras, *Recherches*, 68 (June 1956).

[100] Sommer, *Parfum. Kosmet.*, **39**, 204 (1958).

[101] Klema, *SÖFW*, **82**, 549 (1956); Batdorf and Francis, *J. Soc. cosmet. Chem.*, **14**, 117 (1963).

[102] Davies and Rowson, *J. Pharm. Pharmac.*, **9**, 672 (1957).

[103] Tillman and Kuramoto, *J. Am. pharm. Ass.*, Sci. Ed., **46**, 211 (1957).

[104] *J. Pharm. Pharmac.*, **9**, 672 (1957); 10, 30 (1958).

[105] Ewing, Polite, and Shackelford, *J. Am. pharm. Ass.*, Sci. Ed., 129 (May 1945).

[106] Osipow and Berger, *Drug Cosmet. Ind.*, **82,** 166 (1958).

[107] *Schimmel Briefs*, **257,** (August 1957); Dittmar, *Drug Cosmet. Ind.*, **81,** 446 (1957); Secard, *Drug Cosmet. Ind.*, **89,** 718, 763, 804 (1961).

[108] Schwarz and Levy, *Drug Stand.*, **25,** 154 (1957).

[109] Schwarz and Levy, *J. Am. pharm. Ass.*, Sci. Ed., **47,** 442 (1958).

[110] Kalish, *Drug Cosmet. Ind.*, **81,** 98 (1957).

[111] Janistyn, *op. cit.*, II, 323.

[112] Harry, *op. cit.*, 156.

[113] *Ibid.*, 155.

[114] Schmidt-La Baume-Lietz, *op. cit.*, 34.

[115] Griffin, *J. Soc. cosmet. Chem.*, **1,** 311 (1949).

[116] Wolff, *Fette Seifen*, 142 (1952).

[117] Curtis and Netherton, *Archs. Derm. Syph.*, **41,** 729 (1940); Mumford, *Brit. J. Derm.*, **50,** 540 (1938); Ray and Blanc, *Archs. Derm.*, **42,** 285 (1941).

[118] Lauffer, *Am. Perfumer*, **71** (6), 55 (1958).

[119] *Parfum. Kosmet.*, **39,** 801 (1958).

[120] Schmidt-La Baume-Lietz, *op. cit.*, 37–39.

[121] *Ibid.*, 41.

[122] Lower, *Riv. ital. Essence, Profumi*, **45,** 240, 289 (1963), in *Parfum. Kosmet.*, **45,** 320 (1964).

[123] Sfiras, *Recherches*, **5,** 38 (June 1955).

[124] Ullman, *Mitt. dent. pharm. Ges.*, **27,** 1 (1957).

[125] Anderson, *Australasian J. Pharm.*, **37,** 8 (1951).

[126] Bouchardy and Mirimanoff, *Pharm. Acta Helv.*, **26,** 69 (1951).

[127] De Navarre, *Am. Perfumer*, 31 (May 1956).

[128] Osipow, *J. Soc. cosmet. Chem.*, **7,** 249 (1956); Nobile, Svampa, and Rovesti, *Parfums, Cosmet., Savons*, **6,** 495 (1963).

[129] Rothemann, *op. cit.*, 109 et seq.

[130] *Schimmel Briefs*, **253,** (1956).

[131] *Chemische Courant*, **55,** 632 (1956).

[132] Loeser and Stuermer, *Fette Seifen*, **54,** 87 (1952).

[133] *Parfum. Kosmet.*, **37,** 409 (1956); **37,** 470 (1956).

[134] Rothemann, *op. cit.*, 620.

[135] Auch, *Am. Perfumer*, **28,** 45 (1933).

[136] *Riechst. Aromen*, **1,** 275 (1957).

[137] *Parfumerie Moderne* 1947, No. 4, p. 29.

[138] Brews and Fisk, *Am. Perfumer*, **79** (10), 89 (1964).

[139] *J. Soc. cosmet. Chem.*, 17 (July 1947).

[140] Kleine-Nathrop, *Riechs.-Parf.-Seifen*, 5 (April 1956).

[141] Luckiesh, Taylor, Cole, and Sollman, *J. Am. med. Ass.*, **130,** 1 (1946).

[142] Conn et al., *J. Am. pharm. Ass.*, Sci. Ed., **45,** 311 (1956).

[143] Conley and Torok, *Am. Perfumer*, **79** (10), 57 (1964).

[144] McDonough, *Drug Cosmet. Ind.*, 110 (1937).

[145],[146] Harry, *op. cit.*, 189; Czetsch-Lindenwald, El Khawas, and Tawashi, *J. Soc. cosmet., Chem.*, **16**, 251 (1965).

[147] Rothemann, *Parfum. Kosmet.*, **38**, 691 (1957); Leideritz, *ibid.*, **32**, 9 (1951).

[148] See (133).

[149] Czetsch-Lindenwald and Schmidt-La Baume, *Die äusseren Heilmittel* 1950–1955, p. 109; Czetsch-Lindenwald, *Pharm. Ind.*, **18**, 4 (1956).

[150] *Parfum. Kosmet.*, **38**, 46 (1957).

[151] *Perfum. essent. Oil Rec.*, **48**, 176 (1957); British Patent 740 735.

[152] *Aerosol Age*, **5** (5), 50 (1960).

[153] *Am. Perfumer*, **71** (6), 63 (1958).

[154] *Techn. Memorandum No.* 21, E. I. du Pont de Nemours; Pickthall, *Am. Perfumer*, **70** (7), 23 (1957); Root, *Am. Perfumer*, **71** (6), 63 (1958).

[155] Kanig and Desai, *J. Soc. cosmet. Chem.*, **15**, 549 (1964).

[156] *Am. Perfumer*, **71** (6), 63 (1958).

[157] Root, *Drug Cosmet. Ind.*, **79**, 473 (1956); *Am. Perfumer*, **71** (6), 63 (1958).

[158] J. Kalish, *Drug Cosmet. Ind.*, **81**, 441 (1957); Mina, *ibid.*, **82**, 321 (1958); *Parfum. Kosmet.*, **39**, 205 (1958).

[159] *Parfum. Kosmet.*, **39**, 205 (1958).

[160] Kanig and Cohn, *Proc. scient. Sect.* Toilet Goods Ass., No. 37, 19 (1962).

[161] Lessenich, *Parfum. Kosmet.*, **38**, 42 (1957).

[162] Kuebler, *J. Soc. cosmet., Chem.*, **14**, 341 (1963).

[163] *Parfum. Kosmet.*, **37**, 71 (1956).

[164] Saunders, *Soap Chem. Spec.*, **36**, (7), 95 (1960); *Aerosol Rept.*, **2**, 178 (1962).

[165] Hoffman, *Aerosol Rept.*, **2**, 17, 182 (1962).

[166] Helfer, *Aerosol Age*, **7** (12), 34 (1962).

[167] Barker, *Soap chem. Spec.* (February 1957).

[168] *Am. Perfumer*, **71** (6), 63 (1958).

[169] Pickthall, *Soap, Perfum. Cosm.*, **30**, 171 (1957).

[170] Genzsch, *Parfum. Kosmet.*, **38**, 659 (1957).

[171] Johnson, *Aerosol Age*, **7** (6), **20** (7), **29** (8), **39** (9), **39** (1962).

[172] *Parfum. Kosmet.*, **39**, 209 (1958); Appleton, *Aerosol Age*, **7** (12), 83 (1962).

[173] *Parfum. Kosmet.*, **39**, 212 (1958); *Am. Perfumer*, **71** (6), 93 (1958).

[174] "Freon" Bull., No. 2, 115; Minford, *J. Soc. cosmet. Chem.*, **15**, 311 (1964).

[175] *Parfums, Cosmét., Savons*, 54 (March 1956); Ryan, *Drug Cosmet. Ind.*, **80**, 615 (1957); *Parfum. Kosmet.*, **38**, 50 (1957).

[176] *Parfums, Cosmét., Savons*, 60 (March 1956); *Parfum. Kosmet.*, **38**, 532 (1957).

[177] "Freon" Bull. No. 2., 115.

[178] Morris, *J. Soc. cosmet. Chem.*, **13**, 2 (1962).

[179] Lychalk and Webster, *Aerosol Age*, **8** (3), 28 (1963).

[180] Pickthall, *Am. Perfumer*, **71** (2), 62 (1958); *Aerosol Rept.*, **2**, 103 (1963).

[181] Kempe, *Aerosol Rept.*, **2,** 1 (1963).

[182] Roth and Ferrati, *Mitt. Gebiete Lebensmittelunters. Hyg.* (Bern), **52,** 433 (1961) in *Parfum. Kosmet.*, **45,** 166 (1964).

[183] Fulton and Yeomans, *Soap Chem. Spec.*, **39** (3), 136 (1963).

[184] Foresman, *Parfum. Kosmet.*, **39,** 45 (1958).

[185] *Drug Cosmet. Ind.*, **78,** 45, 192 (1956).

[186] *Drug Cosmet. Ind.*, **79,** 328 (1956).

[187] Honisch, *Parfum. Kosmet.*, **38,** 140 (1957); Hass, *ibid.*, **38,** 46 (1957); **39,** 45, 112, 393 (1958).

[188] *Parfum. Kosmet.*, **39,** 804 (1958).

[189] "Freon" Bull. No. 1, 35.

[190] *Parfum. Kosmet.*, **37,** 81 (1956).

[191] *Drug Cosmet. Ind.*, **78,** 178 (1956).

[192] Saunders, *Soap Chem. Spec.*, **39** (9), 63 (1963).

# PART II

# CHAPTER 5

# Cleansing Preparations

Keeping the body clean is surely the first and most primitive demand on personal hygiene and, therefore, one of the main purposes of cosmetics.

The healthy body participates in the cleansing process just as it does in protecting itself against external disturbances. Surface impurities, even if they have penetrated the corneal layer to some small degree, are removed by the skin in the constant sloughing off of the uppermost horny cells. Impurities migrate to the surface with the corneal cells and are rubbed off by the normal activities of the body. The skin's bacterial resident flora also assists in the degradation and removal of organic impurities (cellular degradation products, excretory remnants, etc.). Cleansing of the hair is effected by continuous self-renewal: old hair is shed and replaced by newly grown clean hair. In the oral cavity saliva has a certain cleansing effect on the teeth, and the bacterial flora assists in the decomposition of food remnants.

The natural process cannot be regarded as adequate from the cosmetic point of view; modern man demands a higher degree of cleanliness. Physiological self-cleaning becomes even more inadequate in view of the many unnatural influences and impurities (among which cosmetics occupy an important place) to which the body of modern civilized man is exposed, whereas his teeth suffer from an unnaturally sophisticated diet. Since oldest times man has therefore used washing to help nature. The purposes of washing are the following:

Removal of visible soil from skin, hair, and nails.

Removal of dried perspiration or remnants of cosmetic preparations that make the skin and hair sticky.

The action of bacteria on perspiration or skin fat components (particularly in the arm pits and between the toes), excretory remnants (in the anal and urogenital regions), and food remnants (between the teeth) may cause the formation of substances that are either malodorous or have an adverse effect on the surrounding tissue. We probably consider the smells of substances such as butyric, valeric, and capric acids, amines, and sulfur compounds as unpleasant because we associate them with the decomposition of organic matter, that is putrefaction and uncleanliness. Washing removes the substrates and the end products of these undesirable reactions and frequently also inactivates or removes part of the bacterial flora (here the effects of washing and disinfectants overlap).

Apart from fulfilling these requirements as completely as possible, the washing process must not affect the underlying tissue unduly. This requirement also applies to the washing of textiles, glass, and lacquered surfaces but is particularly important when the surface to be cleaned is living tissue. Research on new cosmetic cleansing agents therefore centers on problems different from detergent research in general. It is not so much a matter of finding agents that are more effective in removing dirt but those that are as mild as possible.

The characteristics and physiology of skin, hair, and nails as well as the types of soil encountered on each differ in many respects; the cleansing of these different parts of the body is discussed separately in the following.

## CLEANSING OF THE SKIN

Fundamentally, we may differentiate between various methods of cleansing the skin:

1. Cleansing with water.
2. Cleansing with oil.
3. Cleansing with solids that adsorb impurities.
4. Mechanical cleansing (scraping or rubbing).

According to these four methods, cosmetic skin cleansers may be divided into four groups.

In modern cosmetics the fourth and most primitive method corresponds to "peeling." Since it does not wholly belong to cosmetic practice but rather to dermatology or plastic surgery, it is not discussed in this context.

### Water-Based Skin Cleansers

The simplest and still most commonly used cleanser is water. It is liquid and therefore easily brought into contact with any part of the body. It softens the corneal layer. Mechanical rubbing, brushing, or scouring then loosens the dirt along with the uppermost horny cells which are subsequently rinsed off with water. Water is cheap, nontoxic, and completely harmless to normal skin. As a modern cosmetic, however, it has certain shortcomings:

Pure water does not have a good wetting effect on the skin. This becomes apparent on leaving the bath: the remaining water collects in drops. (The water-repellent nature of the skin is primarily due to keratin, not to sebum, which contains hydrophilic constituents and is able to bind water in the form of a W/O emulsion.) Washing with pure water therefore necessitates a comparatively long period of contact and thorough mechanical distribution (rubbing) to bring the whole skin surface into contact with it. Pure water penetrates skin folds and follicle orifices, the very areas in which dirt particles lodge, only with difficulty.

Although skin fat is water-permeable, penetration of the lipid layer by water still takes some time; the fat is certainly not immediately soluble in water. Particles of dirt and bacteria embedded in skin fat are therefore not completely removed by water alone.

Bacteria and most types of dirt are not water-soluble and must therefore be flushed off the skin with large amounts of water. If only a limited quantity is used, part of the dirt is redeposited on the skin. The final result of washing then is only redistribution, not removal of the dirt.

To counteract these failings, various substances are added to water. One type of simple skin cleanser, the so-called face lotions, is prepared by adding alcohol.

**Face Lotions.**    Basically, face lotions consist of dilute (20–40%) alcohol; the main active ingredient is water. The addition of alcohol results in

(a) reduced surface and interfacial tension with the skin and consequently better wetting;

(b) a pleasant refreshing sensation caused by the rapid evaporation of the alcohol;

(c) a mild degreasing effect (according to Neis [1], 33–35% alcohol has a slower but almost the same degreasing effect as 70–90% alcohol);

(d) better solubility of the perfume used;

(e) slightly increased solubility for fatty soil and

(f) a slight astringent and disinfectant effect.

The two last-named effects are only weakly developed because of the low alcohol concentrations (higher concentrations would be degreasing and possibly irritating).

Ethyl alcohol may be replaced with isopropyl alcohol that can be used in lower concentrations. Solvent and disinfectant effects of isopropyl alcohol are superior to those of ethyl alcohol, but it is less refreshing and perfumes do not develop their fragrance in it so well.

Face lotions are used to remove water-soluble impurities (e.g., dried perspiration) and for freshening up; they are often applied after oil-based cleansers.

Occasionally astringents are added to face lotions: small amounts of a salt such as alum (potassium aluminum sulfate), zinc phenol sulfate, or a vegetable product such as witch hazel. It should be borne in mind that the astringent effect of vegetable extracts is due to their tannic acid content. Distillation products such as witch hazel are less effective because the tannic acid remains in the distillation residue. In cleansing lotions the astringent constituents must be kept low because the astringent effect (closing of the pores) counteracts the cleansing effect. Additions of glycerol, glycols, or sorbitol have a smoothing effect; small additions of borax increase the cleansing action but make the lotion weakly alkaline. Antiseptic agents are added occasionally (boric acid, benzoic acid, or *p*-hydroxy benzoic acid esters) but only very small doses are permissible to avoid irritation.

Very small amounts of perfume are sufficient for face lotions because it has a high fragrance yield in diluted alcohols (particularly in ethyl alcohol). Most perfumes are not immediately soluble in alcohols diluted to this extent; a clear solution can be prepared according to two methods:

1. *With magnesium carbonate.* A small quantity of alcohol is set aside when the lotion is being prepared so that the first solution is somewhat too dilute. The perfume oil mixed with an equal quantity (in weight) of magnesium carbonate is then stirred into this solution. The mixture is left for 24 hours, stirred occasionally, and then filtered. Finally the remaining alcohol is added. Probably the effectiveness of magnesium carbonate is due here to a considerable increase in the contact area of the perfumed oil/water. In any case, this method facilitates adequate scenting even with very weak alcohol solutions. Addition of the last alcohol portion after filtering protects against subsequent clouding of the preparation which might otherwise occur, particularly at low temperatures.

2. *With solubilizing agents.* The perfume is mixed with the solubilizing agent, and then stirred into the completed face lotion. Formerly, Turkey red oil was used; presently, mostly "Tween 20" (Atlas Chemical Co.). Depending on the characteristics of the perfume oil, 2–5 pt/wt Tween 20 are used per part perfume oil. Even solutions without alcohol may be perfumed in this way without clouding, but a certain frothing of the product is unavoidable.

Face lotions are often colored to avoid similarity with water.

It may occur that initially clear preparations become cloudy or precipitate after some time. It is therefore advisable to allow the preparation to mature for about two weeks after preparation and to filter shortly before bottling. Clouding and precipitation can be still further inhibited by refrigerating the preparation before bottling for about 24 hours to 0–10°C and subsequent cold filtering.

|                       | 1    | 2    | 3  | 4    |
|-----------------------|------|------|----|------|
| Water                 | 58.9 | 57.9 | 61 | 53.6 |
| Ethyl alcohol 96%     | 28.4 | 32.0 | 34 |      |
| Isopropyl alcohol     |      |      |    | 36.4 |
| Glycerol              |      | 6.5  | 2  | 1.5  |
| Propylene glycol      | 6.7  |      |    |      |
| Hamamelis water       |      |      |    | 5    |
| Normolactol           |      |      |    | 0.5  |
| Boric acid            | 2.0  | 2.0  |    |      |
| Sodium alum           |      | 1.0  |    |      |
| Zinc phenolsulfonate  | 1.1  |      |    |      |
| Benzoic acid          | 2.1  |      |    |      |
| Menthol               | 0.1  | 0.2  |    |      |
| Perfume               | 0.7  | 0.4  |    |      |
| Orange-blossom water  |      |      | 3  |      |
| Rose water            |      |      |    | 2    |

REMARKS.  1 and 2, Keithler, *The Formulation of Cosmetics and Cosmetic Specialties*, pp. 318 and 321. Dissolve the solids in the mixture of propylene glycol (or glycerol) and water. Stir in the solution of menthol and perfume oil in alcohol. Filter after a maturing period of about two weeks. (Menthol has a cooling effect on the skin. The perfume concentration seems too high.)

3 and 4. Janistyn, *Riechstoffe, Seifen, Kosmetika*, II, Hüthig Verlag, Heidelberg, 1950, 185/186. Normolactol is a buffered (pH 3.7) aqueous lactic acid solution with 13–15% sodium lactate.

**Surfactants.**  Although an addition of alcohol improves the cleansing effect of water in some respects, face lotions are far from being perfect skin cleansers; their soil dissolving and suspending properties are too slight.

Better and stronger cleansers can be obtained by adding surfactants to the water. In Chapter 2 we fully discussed how small additions of surface-active substances improve the cleansing properties of water. These substances act by facilitating the wetting of the skin and preventing dirt particles from redepositing on it by emulsifying, solubilizing, and dispersing them.

Because of the efficiency of many of these substances, the removal of normal dirt from the skin is no longer a problem. The question that has been studied almost exclusively in recent years is how skin cleansers can be manufactured from interface-active substances that will have no undesirable side effects on the skin.

**Materials.**  We consider first the most important surfactants used in skin cleansing preparations and then discuss the preparations briefly.

SOAPS.    Soap in this context means a mixture of sodium salts of stearic, palmitic, and oleic acids containing smaller components of myristic and lauric acids. Of all the skin-cleansing agents used today soap is by far the oldest. For centuries it was the only known detergent. Although it has been superseded by synthetic detergents for technical and textile washing, it still plays a major part in skin care.

Soap owes its position mainly to the following properties:

It has an excellent cleansing effect, particularly in soft water, and compared with other surfactants is fairly harmless to the skin.

Soap is manufactured from universally occurring, normally easily obtainable raw materials and is inexpensive. It can be manufactured in handy solid cakes in a simple process. These cakes represent by far the most popular version of skin-cleansing agents due perhaps to the century-old monopoly of soap for this purpose.

In the past few decades, attempts have been made to find new surfactants for skin cleansing. This search for other materials was prompted by the ineffectiveness of soap in hard water and because, although the majority of users tolerate it, some showed symptoms of incompatibility. Historically the introduction of soapless detergents for body care was occasioned by the scarcity of fats during World Wars I and II in Europe; they retained their position for the other reasons mentioned above, even when the fats required for soap production again became available. The loss of soap effectiveness in hard water is due to its chemical composition: a mixture of salts of weak acids whose calcium and magnesium salts are insoluble; this has been fully discussed in Chapter 2.

The intolerance for soap experienced by some users is due to soap solutions affecting the skin in various ways. The effect of soap and other detergent solutions on the skin has been discussed in detail by Carrié [2], Ruf [3], Jacobi [4], Stüpel and Szakall [5], and Götte [6]. We summarize the results regarding soap solutions:

1. *Alkalization.*  Fatty acids are weak acids, and hydrolysis of the soaps occurs in aqueous solutions, according to the equation

$$RCOO^- + Na^+ + H_2O \rightleftharpoons RCOOH + Na^+ + OH^-.$$

Free hydroxide ($OH^-$) ions are therefore always present in an aqueous soap solution and give it an alkaline reaction; the pH of the solutions is generally between 9.5 and 10.8. Normal skin has a pH of about 5. Washing with soap solutions will always result in a temporary increase of the skin pH. The pH value of the uppermost skin layers rises even after washing with pure water because certain water-soluble substances that contribute to the acid reaction are dissolved; but here the pH can never rise beyond 7. Washing with soap solutions may cause a temporary inversion to the alkaline range which does not, however, occur normally. Szakall's studies on living skin showed that the increase of the pH on normal skin ceases within a few minutes if washing is followed by thorough rinsing; natural acidifying occurs after 5–10 minutes and the original pH is re-established within 30 minutes [7]. It is still uncertain whether this buffering action is caused by inorganic salts (Szakall), phospholipids (Schneider), the skin protein itself (Wohnlich), or a combination of these factors.

Alkalization will cause damage only if it lasts too long, if rinsing is insufficient and soap remains in the skin folds, or if washing is very frequent (dentists, physicians, and laundry personnel). With some persons the natural buffering effect of the skin is strongly reduced [8], and after the skin reaction has been shifted into the alkaline range the original pH is re-established only after several hours. Such persons have a low tolerance for soap.

The question arises, however, whether this low tolerance is due to continuous alkalization or is caused by anomalies in the skin protein. If the latter applies, the disturbance in the buffering property would be merely a symptom of the anomalies and not the cause of the lesions.

Although it is often stated in professional publications that soap damages the skin because of its alkaline reaction, it has never been proved that a change in the skin pH, even if it is actually of longer duration, has an adverse effect; nor have any reasons for such an adverse effect been given. Degradation of skin keratin is not to be expected at a pH hardly higher than 7. Perhaps the swelling of the keratin or the increased activity of certain skin bacteria at pH 7 in comparison to pH 5 play some part. In any case, the results of Edwards and Emery [9] are interesting: they found that no lesions were caused on patch tests that for 4 hours expose skin areas to pH 8.8–10.9.

2. *Swelling.* As we have seen, the absorbent capacity of any protein for water is lowest at the isoelectric point of the protein. The swelling effect of an aqueous solution on protein will be all the stronger, the further removed its pH is from the isoelectric point of the protein. Even pure water (pH 7) is able to make keratin swell (isoelectrical point about pH 5); the swelling action of soap solutions (pH about 10) is considerably stronger. Swelling in itself is not harmful, but it softens the corneal layer and facilitates the diffusion of foreign matter from outside.

Götte [10], using bovine skin, observed a change in the effect of a soap solution on skin at the "critical concentration" (at which micell formation starts): Below this concentration the different layers of the epidermis swell at the same rate, whereas swelling above the critical concentration is differentiated: the basal layer swells more strongly than the upper layers. Götte also determined the critical concentration for several synthetic detergents and believes that a correlation exists between the irritating effect of various detergents and their critical concentrations. The fact that he used animal skin *in vitro* throws some doubt on the validity of his findings for human skin.

3. *Degreasing.* One of the purposes of detergent solutions in cosmetics is the removal of dirt embedded in skin fat and the loss of at least part of the skin fat in this process is unavoidable. Even washing with pure water removes certain hydrophilic constituents of the skin fat, and the fat content of the epidermis drops to 75.8% of its original value (Szakall, *loc. cit.*). Washing with soapy water also removes part of the water-insoluble components, and the fat content of the epidermis drops to 64.4% of the original. Most of the other detergents have an even stronger degreasing action than soap. We discuss the undesirable results of epidermal degreasing in Chapter 8.

4. *Adsorption of soap to skin keratin.* Jäger [11] points to the risk of surfactants, forming a thin film on the horny cells when they are brought into contact with the skin. This would prevent the adsorption or absorption of externally applied fatty substances and would lead to brittle and broken skin. It seems somewhat improbable to us that rough skin should be caused by a fat deficiency of the corneal cells, but, even so, a film of alien molecules may very well have an adverse effect on the skin keratin.

Keratin is a protein characterized by its comparatively high sulfur content. The sulfur occurs in the amino acids cysteine [$HS-CH_2-CH(NH_2)-COOH$] and cystine [$-S-CH_2-CH(NH_2)-COOH]_2$. Normally there are hardly any free mercapto (SH) groups in keratin. This may be due to sulfur occurring in the form of cystine which does not contain free mercapto groups; or perhaps the long protein chain of the keratin is folded in such a way that any free mercapto groups are "buried" inside the molecule and not able to react.

According to Anson [12], anionic detergents react with keratin in such a way that they make the mercapto groups titratable, that is, chemically active. According to the way the composition of the keratin is visualized, this may be regarded as a shift in the balance cysteine $\rightleftharpoons$ cystine [i.e., a shift in the oxidation-reduction balance (redox potential) of the skin] or as a degradation of the keratin chains, with the originally "hidden" mercapto groups emerging at the surface of the molecule [13]. Van Scott and Lyon [14] suggested measuring the skin compatibility of detergents by titrating the liberated mercapto groups: the fewer the mercapto groups, the better the skin compatibility. This method must still be evaluated in practice.

Ramsey and Jones [15] found that skin fat showed an abnormally high oleic acid content 3 hours after washing with sodium oleate. Hopf and Burmeister [16] demonstrate in tests with detergents containing radioactive sodium that considerable quantities of detergent remained on the skin even after rinsing. It remains arguable, however, whether such a fatty acid film deposited on the skin after washing with soap is harmful or, as believed by

Peukert [17], beneficial. Fatty-alcohol sulfates and sulfonated alkyls certainly have a less favorable effect than soap because they are more strongly adsorbed by keratin [18].

5. *Irritating action by acid molecules or ions.* It has been known for a long time that coconut-oil soap is much more irritating than, for example, tallow soap; this is a matter of primary irritation, not of allergic reactions. Kröper [19] pointed out that the irritating effect of soaps runs parallel to their dialyzation capacity through a semipermeable cellophane membrane. According to Emery and Edwards [20], $C_{12}$ soaps have the strongest irritating effect; $C_{14}$ soaps are still quite strong, but the soaps of higher and lower fatty acids are much less irritating. Oleic acid is more irritating than stearic acid [21]. These results, however, were based on patch tests and may be, as Czetsch-Lindenwald and Schmidt-La Baume [22] point out, quite misleading, particularly in the evaluation of detergents.

The fact that soap based on coconut oil with its relatively high sodium laurate ($C_{12}$) content is more strongly irritating than soap based on tallow, which consists mostly of sodium stearate, has been known for a long time. This is especially interesting because sodium stearate is more strongly hydrolyzed in aqueous solution and therefore has a stronger alkaline effect than sodium laurate. The acid group thus plays a larger part in causing the reaction than the degree of alkalization.

6. *Precipitation of calcium soaps.* Calcium and magnesium salts of the higher fatty acids are insoluble in water. The use of soap in hard water therefore leads to the formation of gelatinous precipitates on the skin. These may cause skin lesions even quite mechanically by blocking the follicle mouths and encapsulating any foreign matter present. Moreover, according to Jones and Lorenz [23], bacteria in calcium soap precipitates are protected from disinfectants and retain their germinative capacity for at least two weeks. Jones and Lorenz also found that the presence of calcium salts facilitates the entry of bacteria into the oil phase of water/oil mixtures (which include all cosmetic emulsions). With the oil phase, bacteria may cause inflammation by penetrating into the follicles and sebaceous glands. This kind of mechanism might explain the skin lesions occurring in women who use cosmetic face creams and wash before or after with soap and hard water. According to Kowalczyk [24], skin lesions would also be caused by soap inter-reacting with calcium and magnesium ions in the epidermis. Ruf [25] quite rightly states that calcium occurs in the lower lying connective tissue and that contact of soap with this layer is most unlikely. In the upper epidermis potassium is the predominant ion.

PROTEIN FATTY ACID CONDENSATION PRODUCTS. These materials are prepared by condensing fatty-acid chlorides and protein degradation products and should be regarded as modified soaps into which a polypeptide chain has been inserted between the alkyl chain and the polar end group. They are commercially available under the trade names "Maypons" and "Hostapons"; for example,

$$C_{17}H_{33}\text{---}(\underset{\overset{\|}{O}}{C}\text{---}\underset{\overset{|}{H}}{N}\text{---}\underset{\overset{|}{R}}{CH}\text{---})_x COONa.$$

The hydrophilic part of the molecule is strengthened by the accumulated amide groups so that not only the sodium salts but calcium and magnesium salts as well become water-soluble in every proportion, hence protein/fatty-acid condensation products show good efficiency in hard water. The wetting effect of these products is slight, but their emulsifying and dispersing (soil suspension) capacity is good.

Aqueous solutions have a neutral or weakly alkaline reaction and the skin is therefore not alkalized. The swelling effect is much weaker than with soap solutions. There is no irritating action of the acid component of the molecule; protein/fatty-acid condensation products in combination with less compatible detergents even develop a good protective colloidal effect and reduce irritating properties.

According to Szakall, the degreasing effect is stronger than that of soap. After washing with a cleanser based on protein/fatty-acid condensates the fat content of the epidermis dropped to an average of 57.2% of the original value.

Such cleansers have been successfully used on a broad basis and are also tolerated by patients with soap sensitivity [26/27].

FATTY ACID CONDENSATION PRODUCTS.   Although these compounds are prepared from fatty acids or their chlorides, their properties differ considerably from soaps. The carboxyl group is blocked and a sulfonic acid group is the end group. One example is Igepon T formed from oleic acid chloride and the amino sulfonic acid taurine:

$$CH_3(CH_2)_7CH\text{=}CH(CH_2)_7\text{---}\underset{\overset{\|}{O}}{C}\text{---}\underset{\overset{|}{CH_3}}{N}\text{---}CH_2CH_2SO_3Na.$$

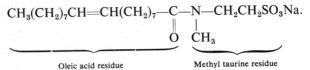

Oleic acid residue              Methyl taurine residue

These products have good wetting and detergent effects and are characterized by their excellent dispersing property. As salts of strong acids whose calcium and magnesium salts are also water-soluble, their detergent action is good even in an acid environment or in hard water.

Aqueous solutions of fatty-acid condensates react neutrally: an inversion of the skin reaction into the alkaline range need therefore not be feared. Instead of the swelling effect, Igepons may cause dehydration of the epidermis (Szakall) that may possibly even lead to skin cracks if they are not completely rinsed off. Degreasing is much stronger than with soap: according to Szakall, washing with Praecutan, a skin cleanser based on Igepon T, only preserves 48% on an average of skin surface fat, whereas washing with soap leaves an average of 64.4%. However, Praecutan has proved satisfactory for soap-sensitive skin.

SULFONATED OILS (TURKEY RED OILS) [28]. When castor oil is treated with concentrated sulfuric acid, the result, apart from the hydrolysis of the triglycerides, is an esterification between the sulfuric acid and hydroxyl groups of the ricinoleic acid and produces

$$CH_3 \cdot (CH_2)_5 \cdot CH \cdot CH_2 \cdot CH{=}CH \cdot (CH_2)_7 \cdot COOH.$$
$$|$$
$$O \cdot SO_2 \cdot OH$$

After removing the glycerol and the free sulfuric acid the product is carefully neutralized with soda lye or soda, and Turkey red oil, an oil with surfactant properties, is formed. A similar product may be obtained by treating the free castor-oil fatty acids with sulfuric acid.

In cosmetic publications these products are usually referred to as "sulfonated" oils. Chemically, this description is not correct. "Sulfonated" compounds contain one sulfur atom directly linked to carbon; for example,

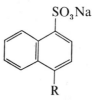

a sulfonated naphthaline derivative. If, on the other hand, the sulfur-atom is not linked directly but by an oxygen atom to carbon, it is an organic sulfate (monoalkyl ester of sulfuric acid); for example,

$$CH_3(CH_3)_{12}OSO_3Na \text{ (sodium myristyl sulfate)},$$

which is produced by sulfating myristic alcohol.

Since castor oil consists of only about 82% glycerides of ricinoleic acid and the remaining components cannot be sulfated, Turkey red oil always contains some sulfonated constituents as well. Sulfation is often not completed so that some free ricinoleic acid is retained.

Similar products may be prepared from oils with a high unsaturated fatty acid content; for example, linseed oil or olive oil. Here the sulfuric acid adds across the double bond. The grades of Turkey red oil will differ in accordance with the basic fat and the degree of sulfatization. The different types are marketed in grades that are differentiated according to their water content.

Turkey red oils have good wetting and dispersing properties, moderate emulsifying and very weak foaming effects, and are moderate to good cleansing agents. Turkey red oils have been used in skin cleansers for soap-sensitive patients with good results [29]. Sodiumoxystearylsulfate, which is used as a "skin-protecting" component in a German skin cleanser, "Praecutan," is closely related to Turkey red oils [30].

OTHER ANIONIC SURFACTANTS. A great number of anionic substances with a detergent effect are known today (see Chapter 2), many of which may be considered for skin cleansing.

Some types used widely for applications other than skin cleansing include sulfated fatty alcohols, alkyl sulfonates, alkyl aryl sulfonates, and the sodium salts of glycerylmonosulfate monofatty-acid esters. Space does not permit a discussion of the effect of individual materials in detail, but we have grouped them together and describe their general characteristics.

In all instances these materials are the salts of stong acids whose calcium and magnesium salts are water-soluble. There is therefore no precipitation even in hard water and most of these substances are effective in hard water or a salt-rich environment. This property constitutes their main advantage in comparison with soaps. Alkalization cannot occur when these products are used, since their aqueous solutions have a neutral reaction. The skin pH can rise to a maximum of 7 only. The critical concentration (according to Götte) is much lower than for soaps; in normal use these substances have a dehydrating rather than a swelling effect on the corneal layer.

The degreasing of the skin is an important problem in the cosmetic use of these products because it is more drastic and affects lower lying layers than does the use of soap [31]. According to Neuhaus [32], the fat regeneration capacity is inhibited to a larger extent by washing with synthetic detergents than with soap. Although degreasing in itself is not dangerous, it exposes skin to the risk of secondary irritations.

Adsorption of detergent molecules by the skin protein is much stronger according to Stüpel [33] in organic sulfates and particularly sulfonates than in soap. With these detergents, the major portion can be rinsed off more readily than soap, but the residue has stronger adhesion. Possible consequences of such adsorption have already been described.

Irritation by anions has been observed in synthetic detergents as well as in soap. Again, compounds whose alkyl residue contains 12 to 14 carbon atoms have the strongest irritating effect. According to patch tests by Emery and Edwards [34], sodium alkyl sulfates are far less irritating than the corresponding sodium or potassium soaps. Willmsmann [35] suggested using the inhibition of saccharase activity as a measure for the physiological compatibility of anionic surfactants.

CATIONIC, AMPHOTERIC AND NONIONIC SURFACTANTS. Cationic surfactants a recompletely unsuitable as skin cleansers. They are strongly adsorbed from aqueous solutions by the skin protein (except from acid solutions with a pH below 5) and thereby lose their effectiveness in the cleansing process.

Theoretically, nonionic detergents should be suitable for skin cleansing because they are mild. Until recently, however, the nonionics could not compete with soap because of their much higher price, but it would not surprise us if these substances gained more significance in the future.

Amphoteric detergents have been used in shampoos but not in skin cleansers because of their high price.

It can be seen from this summary that during the last 20 years the advantages and disadvantages of soap and synthetic detergents have been widely studied and a number of soapless skin cleansers have been developed.

Practitioners and the public seem to agree, however, that none of the soapless washing agents that have been marketed so far is so generally satisfactory as soap. Whether this is inherent in the basic materials themselves or is due to our insufficient experience with these substances only the future will tell.

### Skin Cleansers Based on Surfactants

We subdivide these preparations into skin cleansers for normal use and for heavily soiled skin.

**Skin Cleansers for Normal Use.** Milled toilet soap has for many years been the most important cleansing agent for the skin. The production of toilet soap that meets the highest requirements in appearance, consistency, foaming capacity, and stability is an art and a science in itself, and we cannot possibly discuss it fully here.

To provide a basis for comparison with other preparations we merely give the normal composition of a toilet soap:

| | |
|---|---|
| Fatty acids (as sodium salt) | 78–80% |
| Glycerol | 0–1% |
| Common salt | 0.2–0.5% |
| Free alkali | 0.03–0.05% |
| Rosin | 0–2% |
| Superfatting agents | 0–2% |
| Antioxidants, chelating agents, whitening, pigments | q.s. |
| Perfume | 0.5–3% |
| Water | ad 100 |

Toilet soap retains the disadvantages of its active ingredients, the fatty-acid salts: loss of effectiveness in hard or salt-rich water and the fact that some persons cannot tolerate it (particularly on the face).

Skin irritations caused by perfumed soap must be discussed separately. The observations made in this connection at the Institute for Constitutional Research in Berlin with dermatological patients and later with persons with apparently normal skin are interesting [36a]. In a majority of cases in which patch tests with perfumed soap caused irritation both the perfume by itself and unperfumed soap were tolerated without irritation. This was not a matter of cross sensitization but of primary irritation. Perhaps skin resistance was weakened by the soap or the surface activity of the soap permitted the perfume to penetrate into deeper skin layers.

There are two ways to prepare a skin cleanser with the effectiveness of soap but without its undesirable properties: the performance of the soap may be improved by suitable additives or it may be replaced altogether by other surfactants with better characteristics. Skin cleansers for normal use have usually represented the first approach. The second possibility, the development of soapless skin cleansers, has also been thoroughly studied in recent years. First we discuss "improved soaps" and then soapless preparations.

**Improved Soaps.**   As a result of the recognition of the significance of the physiological acid mantle of the skin by Marchionini et al. [36b], the alkaline reaction of soap solutions was held responsible for observed skin lesions. It is difficult to change this alkaline reaction itself because it is not caused by a surplus of lye in the soap but by the structure of the soap molecule or ion and is based on the reaction of the ion with water:

$$R—COO^- + H_2O \rightleftharpoons R—COOH + OH^-.$$

It is impossible to neutralize the hydroxide ion by adding small amounts of a strong acid because acid reduces the ionization of the soap (and its effectiveness) according to the formula

$$RCOO^- + H^+ \rightleftharpoons RCOOH.$$

If an excess of free fatty acid is added instead of a strong acid, the washing effectiveness of the soap is less strongly reduced but the tendency to rancidity is promoted.

Some authors have seen in the addition of neutral fats the possibility of eliminating the alkalinity of soap solutions but this idea is not practicable either. It is reported of "Dove," a product based on a detergent/soap mixture, that it has a neutral reaction even though it contains soap [37]. Szakall observed that milled soaps cause a stronger alkalization of the skin than the poured household soaps.

As already discussed, the swelling action of soap solutions is closely related to alkalinity. Since the swelling effects of soaps and sulfonated fatty alcohols differ, soap/detergent mixtures tend to cause less skin swelling.

Superfatting agents are often added to reduce the degreasing effect of soap. These are lanolin, lanolin derivatives, fatty alcohols, fatty acid monoglycerides, fatty acid alkylolamides, and lecithin. Theoretically, superfatting agents may act in two ways: either by replacing fat removed in the washing process or by reducing in one way or another the degreasing effect of soap.

The first effect would apply only to superfatting agents with a pronounced skin affinity because soap generally removes lipid matter from the skin. Lanolin is said to act in this way [38].

As a rule, however, the effectiveness of superfatting agents is probably based on lessening the degreasing effect of the soap solution. The studies by Schneider and Schädel [39] and Carrie and Neuhaus [40] point in this direction. However, it would be surprising if an addition of fat did not reduce the cleansing effect along with the degreasing effect; this actually occurs according to Greither and Ehlers [41] and McCords [42]. Various authors have expressed doubts about the beneficial effect of superfatting agents on the skin (e.g., Greither and Ehlers [41]). A clarification of this question seems important.

From a technical point of view, small additions of superfatting agents have a beneficial effect on soap because they make the lather firmer and the bubbles finer; cakes feel smoother and their tendency to crack when dry is reduced.

According to Stüpel [43], additions of carboxymethylcellulose (CMC), polyacrylic condensates, and protein/fatty acid condensation products also act as skin protectors. Weber [44] also mentions neutralized Rohagit (a polymerized high-molecule organic acid; after neutralization, particularly with triethanolamine, its aqueous solution is water-white and viscous). Janistyn [45] refers to proteins (e.g., milk protein) in this connection. Here, as well, the reason for the effectiveness of these protective agents is not quite clear; a protective colloidal effect is assumed in which the additive forms a film around the individual soap micells and thus moderates the action of the soap. This need not reduce the cleansing properties of the soap which may even be improved, since the protective colloids also promote emulsification and dispersion of the dirt particles (and possibly precipitated calcium soap particles).

Moreover, small additions of these substances have a good effect on the gloss and smoothness of the soap cake and the quality of the foam, which is made soft and creamy. For this reason the abovementioned products, in particular CMC, are often incorporated into present-day soaps.

The tendency of soap molecules and ions to be adsorbed on the skin keratin may be inhibited by adding substances with an even stronger affinity to the skin without affecting it adversely. Tanning agents have been proposed for this purpose (e.g., the "Dermolanes," developed and patented by Jäger [46]). There is no certainty, however, that the fatty-acid and soap molecules adsorbed on the corneal cells will have an adverse effect and that the addition of tanning agents is indeed an improvement.

Finally, the precipitation of calcium soaps must be borne in mind. Products with a protective colloidal action are suitable here because they are able to hold calcium soaps in suspension and prevent them from precipitating on the skin. Unfortunately, it is technically impossible to add sufficient protective colloids to prevent altogether the precipitation of calcium soaps in very hard water.

Many substances are able to form water-soluble complexes (so-called "chelates") with polyvalent metal ions [47] and in this way take them out of circulation; the most important are polyphosphates (Dulgon, Calgon, etc.) and ethylene diamine tetra acetic acid, which is commercially available under various trade names in the form of its sodium salt. Although these substances are useful in soap production by binding copper and iron traces in the soap mass and thus reducing the tendency toward rancidity and spot formation, their concentration in the soap is not sufficient to bind the calcium ions in hard water and prevent the precipitation of calcium soaps.

The best method of preventing calcium soap precipitation in hard water is an addition of surfactants with good dispersing effect (such as Igepon T) whose own calcium salts must of course be water-soluble. A correctly balanced combination of soap and surfactants will then result in an increase of the detergent and foaming action of soap, also in soft water. These are the combined "soap-detergent" preparations that have been on the market in a number of countries for some years.

According to U.S. Patent 2 749 313 (Colgate-Palmolive Co.) [48], "Vel-Beauty-Bar" contains at least 50% anhydrous soap and 10–45% of a mixture of glycerylmonosulfate-monofatty-acid esters and higher fatty-acid amides of $n$-methylaminomethanesulfonate (Sarcoside). The proportion of the two detergents lies between 1:4 and 4:1. The moisture content is 5–15%. The patent gives the following typical formulation:

| | |
|---|---|
| Sodium salt of an amide of a higher fatty acid with aminomethane sulfate | 8.0 |
| Sodium salt of a monosulfate of a mono fatty-acid glyceride | 10.0 |
| Sodium dodecylbenzene sulfonate | 15.0 |
| Sodium soap chips (10% moisture) | 63.4 |
| Guanidine carbonate | 2.0 |
| Titanium dioxide | 0.4 |
| Preservative | 0.2 |
| Perfume | 1.0 |
| | 100.0 |

Swanson [49] reports that "Dove" (Lever Brothers) was tolerated by 85% of 200 patients, the majority of whom could not tolerate soap. Such preparations have come to play an important part side by side with traditional soaps. However, a prediction made in the mid-fifties that solid detergents will in time replace 65–75% of toilet soap [50] today appears to be greatly overstated.

**Soapless Skin Cleansers in Solid Form [51].** Although soaps with a moisture content of 20–40% can be made into handy solid cakes without further additives, synthetic detergents are not quite so easily processed into solids with the required properties. The main problem in the manufacture of solid skin cleansers on a detergent basis is not to achieve sufficient cleansing action and foam effect but to produce a solid cake with a certain gloss and smooth feel, neither too hard or becoming brittle in dry storage, nor too soft in a moist atmosphere and too water-soluble. It might, of course, soon appear old-fashioned to try to imitate soap in all its properties with solid detergents just as the young automobile industry rejected the trend of imitating the appearance of horse-drawn carriages. At present the problem is still important and is mainly solved by selecting good fillers and binders.

The binding agents have the purpose of imparting the desired consistency to the cake and preventing the cake from dissolving too rapidly because of the high water solubility of many detergents. High-grade detergents are usually more expensive than soaps but are effective at lower concentrations; "extending" detergents with binding agents is therefore also important for reasons of cost.

The following materials have been mentioned as suitable binding agents for solid detergents; many of these binders are patented.

1. *Insoluble inorganic compounds* (e.g., barium sulfate, talcum powder, or ground Sorel cement) [52]. Additions of these substances should not exceed 25%, in some cases 10%, lest both the consistency and foaming capacity of the detergent cake be affected.

2. *Finely dispersed solids able to swell in water* (e.g., bentonite, kaolin, diatomaceous earth, or starch). These solids may constitute a considerable proportion in weight of the detergent cakes.

3. *Substances that form highly viscous solutions in water* (e.g., cellulose ether, possibly dissolved in glycerol, and polyvinyl acetate [53]).

4. *Organic salts* (e.g., zinc stearate, zinc undecanate [54], aluminum stearate, which is reported to have a skin protective effect; calcium and magnesium salts of alkyl sulfonic acids are also mentioned). These salts should be used only in small quantities because large amounts have an adverse effect on the foaming capacity of the detergent.

5. *Waxlike organic compounds* (e.g., paraffin wax, stearic acid, carnauba wax, cetyl and stearyl alcohols, glyceryl monostearate, and lecithin). According to Snell [55], fatty alcohols as such should not be added to solid detergents because they affect the consistency; they may, however, be used in the form of solid complexes with urea; in aqueous solutions such complexes are soon degraded and fatty alcohol and urea (both substances beneficial to the skin) are liberated. Several of the other substances also have a beneficial effect on the skin and, added in small quantities, may improve the foam quality. Lanolin and neutral fats are not recommended because they tend to reduce foam formation, even in small amounts.

Best results are obtained with combinations of binding agents of various types; the selection will, of course, depend on the other ingredients of the formulation.

Apart from binding agents, "builders" are occasionally added to the detergent: these substances have no cleansing effect on their own but increase that of the detergent in combination with it. Since builders are of particular interest in cleansing agents for badly soiled skin, they are discussed in a later section.

Finally, skin-protecting additives are important in cosmetic detergents. The same substances mentioned in connection with soaps may be used. Materials that prevent the adsorption of the active ingredient by the skin keratin (tanning agents, dermolanes) are more important here than in soaps, but the problem of calcium-soap precipitation does not arise. A few simple formulations follow. None is completely satisfactory but all show the type of formulations used.

|  | 6 | 7 | 8 | 8a |
|---|---|---|---|---|
| Sodium lauryl (or ceytl) sulfate | 17 | | | |
| Alkyl aryl sulfonate | | 48.5 | 15 | 20 |
| Talcum | | 16.0 | | |
| Bentonite | 22 | | 10 | 76 |
| Starch | 28 | 16.0 | 10 | |
| Methylcellulose | 1.5 | | | |
| Ester gum | | | 1 | |
| Paraffin wax, refined | 6 | | | |
| Beeswax | 2 | | | |
| Carnauba wax | 4 | | | |
| Stearic acid | | | 20 | |
| Triethanolamine | 1 | | | |
| Sodium carbonate | | | 5 | |
| Sodium silicate | | | 5 | |
| Casein (soluble) | 13.5 | | | |
| Soy lecithin | | 19.5 | | |
| Lanolin | | | | 3 |
| Water | 5 | | 30 | |
| Perfume | | | 1 | |

REMARKS

6. Waddans, *Soap, Perfum., Cosm.*, **23**, 1019 (1950).

7. Keenan, *Soap sanit. Chem.*, **27**, 27 (1951). The alkyl aryl sulfonate is "Ultrawet K" (Atlantic Refinery). The added lecithin reduces tackiness, starch hardens the product, and talcum prevents softening during storage.

8. Blumenthal, *Mfg. Chem.*, **19**, 153 (1948). Stearic acid, ester gum, and paraffin wax are melted together and the other ingredients mixed in. The mixture is cooled in molds to

tablets. Other detergents may be used instead of alkyl aryl sulfonate and, instead of bentonite, either kaolin or talcum may be used.

8a. Schwartz, in Harry, *Modern Cosmetocology*, 4th ed. p. 639. Alkyl aryl sulfonates (Nacconol NRSF, Santomerse D), fatty-acid condensates (Igepons), or sulfated fatty alcohols (Duponol) may be used as detergents.

**Detergent-Based Skin-Cleansing Jellies.** These products are marketed as "dry hand cleansers." They may be used without water and are therefore suitable for travel; they are usually packed in tubes. Washing is done by rubbing the preparation over the hands and removing it with a cloth or paper towel.

| | 9 | 10 | 11 | 12 |
|---|---|---|---|---|
| Igepal CA 630 | 5 | | | |
| Tween 80 | | 6.25 | | |
| Tween 85 | | | | 5 |
| Arlacel C | | 1.25 | | |
| Ultrawet | | | 8 | |
| Vinyl methyl ether-maleic anhydride polymer | 0.4 | | | |
| Sodium carboxymethylcellulose | | 2.50 | 6 | |
| Lanolin | | | 5 | |
| Glycerol | 5 | | | |
| Polyethylene glycol, mol. wt. 1500 | 5 | | | |
| Dioxane | | | 20 | |
| Kerosene, odorless | | | | 65 |
| Water | 90 | 89 | 32 | 15 |
| Preservative | 0.01 | 1 | | |

REMARKS

9. U.S. Patent 2 702 277 (General Anilin and Film Co.), in *Schimmel Briefs*, 251, February 1956. 8-hydroxyquinoline, prescribed as a preservative, is mixed with the Igepal and the melted polyethylene glycol. The mixture is then stirred into the aqueous PVM-MA polymer solution which has previously been adjusted to pH 7 with potash lye.

Igepal CA 630 is a polyoxyethylene ether of isooctyl phenol. Possible alternatives are Igepal CA 430, the corresponding derivative of isononylphenol, Tween 80, or Renex 20, a polyoxyethylene derivative of a mixture of fatty and resinic acids. The potassium salt of the vinyl methyl ether-maleic acid anhydride copolymer acts as a thickening agent and imparts to the preparation the feeling of "slip" which is so popular with soap solutions. Instead of this, sodium carboxymethylcellulose may be used. The polyethylene glycol acts as a plasticizer.

Since the preparation has a weak odor, 0.3–0.4% perfume is sufficient.

10. Lesser, *Drug Cosmet. Ind.*, 326 (1953). Add the other ingredients to the CMC mucilage (the preservative concentration seems unnecessarily high).

11. Readers Questions, *Drug. Cosm. Ind.*, **75**, 250 (1954). Mix the ingredients by stirring at high speed in the following order: CMC, water, polyethylene glycol, Ultrawet (an alkyl aryl sulfonate), sodium pyrophosphate, lanolin, glycerol, and dioxane (an organic solvent miscible with water).

12. Lesser, *Drug and Cosmet. Ind.*, 326 (1953).

Skin cleansing jellies occur in two grades: as a 5% aqueous detergent solution (approx.) brought to the required consistency with a thickening agent or as the emulsion of an organic solvent. The solvent removes tar, lacquer, etc.; the surfactant acts at the same time as an emulsifying agent for the solvent and a cleansing agent for the skin. In any case, the detergent must have a very mild effect on the skin, since it can never be so thoroughly removed from the skin as by rinsing with water. Here, nonionic detergents are most commonly used.

**Preparations for Cleansing Heavily Soiled Skin.** Preparations of this type are intended for industrial workers, mechanics, painters, and other groups whose hands are exposed to heavy soil in the course of their activities. In view of the steadily growing popularity of "do it yourself" projects, heavy-duty cleansers are also finding increasing use in the home. The emphasis on these products lies in strong detergent action and low price. Since they are intended only for the hands, the requirements for skin compatibility are not excessive, but even so they must not act as irritants.

These preparations are divided into soap-based and soapless types, but we prefer a physical classification for the following discussion.

**Solid Preparations.** Solid soaps with an addition of mechanically active fillers are important here. The fillers most commonly used are fine scouring powder, powdered pumice, finely ground quartz, feldspar, and barite. Before being added to the soap mass, these substances are frequently steeped in a methylcellulose or CMC mucilage which facilitates their incorporation. Paste preparations are frequently based on soft soap (potassium soaps of the higher fatty acids). Pure soft soap is still being used as a hand cleansing agent. Hand-washing pastes with a detergent base often contain fatty-alcohol sulfate pastes (abt. 35% activity) as the surface-active ingredient. Detergent pastes may be higher priced than soaps but are active in lower concentrations. According to Franz [56], the following additives may be used for both soap and soap preparations:

Methylcellulose, carboxymethylcellulose, polyacrylates, and other substances with a protective colloidal effect act as skin protective agents, facilitate the dispersion of mechanically active solid fillers, and are important as thickening agents in detergent pastes. Usually they are added in amounts up to 2%.

*Mechanically Active Fillers.* The same materials may be used here as mentioned in connection with solid soaps. Franz also lists bentonite, Veegum, diatomaceous earth, and Aerosil (Cab-O-Sil), but they have a far higher swelling capacity than the preceding ones, and although they have a thickening and lubricating effect they do not act as abrasives.

Organic solvents which may be water-soluble (alcohol, dioxane, acetone) or water-insoluble (mineral oil, hexaline, methylhexaline, tetralin, trichloros and perchloroethylene). The water-insoluble solvents in particular are useful in removing paint, varnish, tar, and lubricants. Protective agents, such as lanolin and fatty alcohols are sometimes used in small amounts.

Most hand-washing pastes contain water, but some anhydrous preparations do exist. Liquid hand cleansers usually consist of aqueous soap solutions, possibly with an addition of organic solvents.

Hand-cleaning powders [57] usually contain about 5% of an active ingredient, which may be a soap powder or a detergent, such as sulfated fatty alcohol, a fatty-acid condensate, or alkylaryl sulfonate.

Larger quantities of inorganic salts added to these surfactants serve to increase the effectiveness of the surfactants and are designated "builders." Polyphosphates, in particular sodium tetrapolyphosphate and sodium tetra-tripolyphosphate [58], act as water softeners by binding calcium and magnesium ions in water-soluble complexes. They promote the foaming effect of soaps and detergents, contribute to the soil-suspending capacity, and moreover are reported to act as protective agents. Potassium metaphosphate, insoluble in water, is soluble in salt solutions, forming colloidal solutions. It thickens the washing liquid and gives it softness. Sodium pyrophosphate is not easily soluble and its solutions are strongly alkaline but it has the advantage of not being hygroscopic.

Metasilicates are also used in hand-cleansing powders. They resemble polyphosphates in their effect, buffer the alkalinity of the washing liquid, and contribute to the dirt-suspension capacity in their emulsifying effect.

Alkaline salts (phosphates, carbonates) lower the price of the preparation, but if used in high concentrations they reduce the skin compatibility. Neutral salts such as sodium sulfate are primarily extenders. Cellulose ethers (e.g., methylcellulose) act as skin protectors and promote the cleansing effect.

In his articles, Franz [59] describes many formulations for hand cleansers; a few follow:

13. Hand-cleansing paste based on soap. Dilute 29 g of soy fatty acid with 50 g of trichloroethylene and saponify with slightly less than the theoretically required quantity of potassium hydroxide. The finished paste is made by diluting with water.

14. Aqueous hand-cleansing paste based on detergents.

| | |
|---|---|
| 30 parts | fatty alcohol sulfate paste (e.g., Texapon CS) are mixed with |
| 30 parts | water and |
| 12 parts | methylhexaline and then mixed with |
| 28 parts | water |
| 100 parts | |

Thirty-two parts of this mass are mixed with 68 parts of filler; this hand-cleansing paste contains 10% active ingredients. It may be diluted further with both water and fillers to 3% active ingredients.

15. Anhydrous hand-cleansing paste based on detergents (thixotropic). According to

Franz, preparations of this type contain 70–88% of a fatty alcohol sulfate paste (Sulfopon OK, Texapon Extract A), 5–10% methylhexalin, and 2–25% trichloroethylene. Aerosil (or Cab-o-Sil) is reported to be a suitable binding agent.

16. Liquid hand cleansers.

| | | |
|---|---|---|
| Sodium oleate | 34 | |
| Potassium oleate | | 36 |
| Ethyl Alcohol | 13 | 17 |
| Tri- or perchloroethylene | 17 | 14 |
| Water | 36 | 33 |

Clear yellow solutions are obtained from these formulations which remain clear and stable when diluted with 1–60 parts of water.

17. Hand-cleansing powder.

| | |
|---|---|
| Sodium fatty alcohol sulfate (converted to 100% activity) | 5 |
| Trisodium phosphate | 10 |
| Disodium phosphate | 5 |
| Potassium metaphosphate | 5 |
| Soda | 35 |
| Sodium metasilicate | 40 |

| | |
|---|---|
| Sodium fatty alcohol sulfate (100% active) | 4 |
| Sodium polyphosphate | 10 |
| Sodium metasilicate | 70 |
| Tetrasodium silicate | 10 |
| Potassium carbonate | 3 |
| Methylcellulose | 3 |

## Oil-Based Skin Cleansers

All the preparations we have discussed so far in this chapter have one thing in common in spite of their considerable differences: the main active ingredient is water. Before discussing oil-based preparations, we compare water and oil in their capacity as cleansing agents and list their specific advantages and disadvantages.

The advantages of oils may be summarized as follows:

They are more effective then water in removing oil-soluble, water-insoluble grime, and are therefore most appropriate whenever the matter to be removed is mainly oil-soluble (e.g., make up). Every woman can easily test the higher effectiveness of oil-based preparations by first washing her face with soap and water and subsequently using a cleansing cream. Considerable amounts of make up will be removed by the latter which were left behind by the soap and water treatment.

When oils are used, there is less risk of the skin becoming brittle and cracked. At first glance, this might appear to be obvious, since oils have a greasing effect and preserve the skin from drying out. Actually, matters are not quite so simple; oil-based cleansing preparations dissolve the skin fat which is then removed with the cleanser. The thin film of cleanser deposited on the skin does not suffice to replace the skin fat. It contains considerable amounts of petrolatum or mineral oil and its physical and chemical properties differ strongly from skin fat. In this connection it is quite justifiable to refer to the "degreasing" effect of cleansing creams. On the other hand, it is a fact that the removal of oil-soluble constituents of skin fat is not a cause of the development of rough skin. The most important factors here are the removal of water-soluble constituents and the enlargement of the skin surface by partial removal of the smooth fatty layer. It is obvious that in view of these factors washing with water, particularly with surfactants, is more harmful than cleaning with oil-based preparations.

As we have already shown, water by itself is not a perfect cleansing agent. All surfactants that might be added to increase the cleansing action have some kind of undesirable side effect. Many oil-based preparations also contain surfactants but they have more affinity with the skin than those used in combination with water.

The advantages oils have as skin cleansers in comparison with water are offset by several important disadvantages:

All purified oils, even mineral oil, are quite expensive compared with water and are therefore used in much smaller quantities than water. Rinsing with pure oil, which would be important in removing the last remnants of grime, is usually omitted.

The water left behind after washing can nearly always be completely removed with an absorbent towel. Any remaining moisture in excess of that normally present on skin dissppears soon by evaporation. Because of its high viscosity, any oil remaining after cleansing with creams can be only partially removed with even strongly absorbent paper tissues or cotton. The remnants do not evaporate and are not resorbed by the skin. If the cream has been prepared with high-grade raw materials, this oily residue is not harmful; nevertheless, the skin surface after oil cleansing is further removed from its normal state than after washing with water.

Water-soluble dirt particles are not as easily removed by oil cleansers as by water-based preparations; however, certain substances may be added to oils that enable them to remove this type of grime as well.

**Liquefying Cleansing Creams.** These preparations are simple mixtures of oils and waxes. The least complicated but very effective and compatible representative of cleansing oils is pure olive oil.

Creams without water must be thixotropic; that is, they liquefy under pressure (on application to the skin). The preparation of thixotropic fat mixtures has already been discussed in Chapter 4.

The viscosity of cleansing preparations should not be too high at skin temperature so that there will be as little friction as possible during application and removal. On the other hand, the preparations must not be too fluid, so that impurities will be entrapped.

The lower the viscosity, the better the removal of the preparation after use. A certain amount of fat, however, is always left as a thin film on the skin and in the follicle mouths. Additives such as lanolin, cetyl alcohol, or other W/O emulsifying agents increase the water permeability of this film and the skin affinity of the preparation. Colloidal solutions of lanolin in vegetable or mineral oils, isopropyl palmitate, oleyl alcohol, butyl glycol ethers, or mixtures of these solvents are well suited to skin cleansing. Such preparations are discussed by Heald [60].

Cleansing preparations without water might be expected to be completely ineffective in removing water-soluble soil. Surprisingly, though, tests by Harry show [61] that this is not true. Harry applied an O/W cream with fluorescein in its aqueous phase, which is a water-soluble, mineral-oil-insoluble compound. After 30 minutes part of the treated skin area was cleaned with an anhydrous fat cream, another part simply wiped with a face tissue. Radiation with ultraviolet rays (which make fluorescein fluorescent) showed that the fluorescein had been removed by the cream but was still present on the skin area that had only been wiped. Harry explained this as the result of the constant presence on the skin of some skin fat and moisture. The skin fat which has hydrophilic components is absorbed by the creams, thus enabling it to absorb the water (as W/O emulsion or in micells), with the fluorescein dissolved in it.

| | 18 | 19 | 20 | 21 | 22 | 23 | 24 |
|---|---|---|---|---|---|---|---|
| Mineral oil | 15 | 60 | 62 | 25 | 40 | 30 | 55.5 |
| Isopropyl palmitate | | | | 25 | | | |
| Cetiol V | | | | | | | 24 |
| Petrolatum | 85 | 25 | 15 | 30 | 41.5 | 20 | 30 |
| Prime paraffin wax | | | | | 20 | 18 | |
| Ceresine | | 15 | 18 | | 12 | | |
| Soft ozokerite | | | | | | | 12 |
| Beeswax | | | | | | | 2.5 |
| Spermaceti | | | | 5 | | | |
| Cetyl alcohol | | | | | | 8 | |
| Stearic acid | | | | | 6 | | |

REMARKS

18, 19, 20. De Navarre, *The Chemistry and Manufacture of Cosmetics*, Van Nostrand, Princeton, New Jersey, p. 270–271. The author prescribes a low-viscosity mineral oil, petrolatum with a melting point of 49–54°C, and Ceresine M. P. 64°C. Melt the ceresine, stir in the petrolatum and then the mineral oil. Add perfume at 45°C and fill into jars preheated to 37–40°C. The jars should be filled first to three-quarter capacity and the balance added only when the first portion is almost cold. This procedure avoids funnel formation in the cream surface.

21. *The Use of Isopropyl Myristate in Cosmetics*, A Boake Roberts & Co., London. Melt the ingredients at 65°C, stirring vigorously. Continue stirring the mixture until cool.

22. Keithler, *The Formulation of Cosmetics and Cosmetic Specialties*, p. 48. Perfume 0.5%.

23, 24. Rothemann, *Das grosse Rezeptbuch der Haut- und Körperpflegemittel* 3rd ed. HüthigVerlag, Heidelberg, 1962, p. 523. Melt all ingredients together; after cooling to 50°C add 0.2–0.3% perfume oil and pour into jars while warm.

**Skin-Cleansing Emulsions of the W/O Type.** In many respects these preparations can be compared with anhydrous creams. The water content results in a somewhat smoother consistency and possibly increases the effectiveness of the preparation in removing water-soluble grime. It also has a clouding effect and improves the appearance of otherwise glassy-looking fat creams. (Small additions of titanium dioxide also have a whitening effect on such preparations.) If the creams contain only small quantities of emulsifying agents and separation occurs on application to the skin, evaporation of the water will also cause a pleasantly cooling sensation.

Emulsified preparations usually contain larger amounts of hydrophilic (lanolin, cetyl alcohol, etc.) than anhydrous substances. This reduces the degreasing effect because through these hydrophilic substances the film deposited on the skin after cleansing is made to resemble skin fat to a much larger extent than pure petrolatum or mineral oil. An excess of these materials inhibits the cleansing effect, however: they adhere to the skin surface and entrap impurities.

| | 25 | 26 | 27 | 28 | 29 |
|---|---|---|---|---|---|
| Mineral oil | 45.5 | 60 | 68 | 20.0 | 48 |
| Petrolatum | 24.0 | 2 | | 31.0 | |
| Paraffin wax | | | | 7.0 | |
| Ceresine | | 1 | | | |
| Beeswax | 18.0 | 8 | | | 6 |
| Spermaceti | | | | | 6 |
| Lanolin | 3.0 | 10 | 6 | 3.0 | 1 |
| Cetyl alcohol | | 4 | 2 | | |
| Glyceryl monostearate self-emulsifying | | | 8 | | |
| Arlacel 83 | | | | 4.0 | |
| Turkey red oil, prime grade | | 5 | | | |
| Triethanolamine lauryl sulfate | | | 1 | | |
| Magnesium sulfate | | | | 0.2 | |
| Water | 8.85 | 10 | 15 | 32.3 | 38 |
| Sorbitol syrup 70% | | | | 2.5 | |

REMARKS

25. Keithler, *The Formulation of Cosmetics and Cosmetic Specialties*, p. 48; 0.5% perfume oil and 0.15% preservative should also be added.

26. Janistyn, *Riechstoffe, Seifen, Kosmetika*, II, 345. Emulsification is at 80°C and stirring is continued until cool. (A reduction of the cleansing effect may be expected because of the high lanolin content, and the addition of cetyl alcohol.)

27. Keithler, *The Formulation of Cosmetics and Cosmetic Specialties*, p. 48. Stir the aqueous solution of triethanolamine lauryl sulfate at 65–70°C into the melt of the other ingredients (65–70°C) and continue stirring until cool.

28. "Drug and Cosmetic Formulation," Atlas Chemical Co. Arlacel 83 is sorbitan sesquioleate. Astrolatum may be used instead of paraffin wax. Stir the aqueous solution of sorbitol syrup and magnesium sulfate (70–75°C) slowly into the melt of the other ingredients (70–75°C). Perfume and homogenize at 55–60°C and pour.

29. Harry, *Modern Cosmetocology*, 4th ed., p. 116. Melt the fats and waxes and allow the clear melt to cool to 45–50°C. Slowly stir in the water (45–50°C) and continue stirring until 25–30°C. Perfume is added at 40°C.

**Cleansing Emulsions, Dual-Emulsion Type (Cold Creams).** Among cleansing emulsions cold creams occupy an important place. Expertly made from high-grade raw materials, they combine good cleansing action (because of their high fat content) with smooth consistency, easy spreadability, and snow white color.

The "heart" of all modern cold creams is the beeswax/borax emulsifier system that we have already discussed in Chapter 4. Cold creams are used not only for cleansing but as moisturizing creams, protective creams, and sunscreen creams (with the addition of ultraviolet screens). It is quite usual to apply the same product for various purposes: as a cleansing cream, it is spread on thickly and removed immediately with an absorbent tissue or cotton pad; as a moisturizing cream, it is massaged into the skin in small quantities and left on the skin overnight. Books and articles reflect this custom: cold creams are fully discussed without mentioning their end use.

It seems uneconomical to manufacture or buy a cream without knowledge of its intended end use. Cold creams with a high mineral oil content have no great value as night creams (probably this is the reason for the common prejudice against mineral oils in cosmetics); on the other hand, it is pointless to use an expensive cream containing valuable vegetable oils and vitamin concentrations as a cleansing cream if a lower priced product with a high mineral-oil content meets the purpose as well if not better.

As we mentioned in Chapter 4, we do not yet know very much about beeswax/borax cream systems (and all dual emulsions). Since it is not quite clear how the various components are distributed within the system, it is hard to tell how certain modifications of a formula (proportions or procedure) might affect the quality of the end product.

The formulations listed below illustrate how the consistency of creams of this type depends, often in unpredictable ways, on the method of preparation. From the innumerable cold-cream formulations published, we have selected a few that appear to us to be especially well suited as cleansing creams.

| | 30 | 31 | 32 | 33 | 34 |
|---|---|---|---|---|---|
| Paraffin oil | 50 | 55 | 50 | 45 | 25 |
| Isopropyl myristate | | | | | 20 |
| Petrolatum | | | | | 10 |
| Ozokerite | | | | 8 | |
| Paraffin wax | | | | 4 | |
| Spermaceti | | 8 | | | |
| Lanolin | | | 1 | 2 | 2 |
| Beeswax | 16 | 8 | 20 | 10 | 12 |
| Borax | 1 | 0.5 | 0.7 | 0.7 | 1 |
| Water | 33 | 28.5 | 27.8 | 30.3 | 25 |

REMARKS

30, 31. De Navarre, *The Chemistry and Manufacture of Cosmetics*, p. 214 and 215. The aqueous borax solution (70–74°C) is stirred quickly into the clear fat and wax melt (68–72°C); slow constant stirring is continued until cool; perfume (abt. 0.5%) is added at 45–50°C; pouring follows. At 45°C the cream may also be passed through a colloid mill which results in a soft cream. In another method of preparation the cream is stirred until cool, and left overnight; it is stirred again on the following day and put through a colloid mill. The jars are filled cold.

The first formulation represents a cold cream in its simplest form; in the second the beeswax/borax constituent is much smaller. This product more closely resembles the classic cold cream without borax. It has a stronger cooling effect but is less stable than the cream made according to formula 30. Spermaceti is used to stiffen the cream, which, because of the low beeswax content, would otherwise be too soft.

32, 33. Keithler, *The Formulation of Cosmetics and Cosmetic Specialties*, pp. 41 and 40. The waxes (beeswax, lanolin, petrolatum, etc.) are melted together and heated to 65°C. Stirring quickly, a small amount of aqueous borax solution (65°C) is added first; mineral oil (65°C) and the balance of the borax solution (65°C) are then added simultaneously or alternately under vigorous stirring; the last portions of both liquids should be added more or less simultaneously.

It is also possible to melt together all components of the oil phase and to stir in the borax solution, but the creams are less stable and have less luster.

In spite of the high beeswax content, the beeswax/borax system in 32 is weaker than in 30 because there is less borax. The lanolin (a W/O emulsifying agent) promotes the stability of the product, however. This cream resembles the pure W/O creams closer than products 30 and 31.

In 33 the emulsifier system is the same as in 32, but the "free" beeswax is replaced by mineral waxes. The lanolin content is higher here, and the W/O character is accordingly more pronounced. Additions of lanolin make cold creams softer; therefore Formula 32 provides for mineral oil with light viscosity, Formula 33 with medium viscosity.

Formula 32 prescribes 0.15% preservative and 0.5% perfume. Formula 33 also contains 0.002% butyl-*p*-hydroxybenzoate.

34. *The Use of Isopropylmyristate in Cosmetics*, A. Boake Roberts & Co., London. The aqueous borax solution (70°C), which also contains preservatives, is stirred into the fat melt; pour warm.

A number of modern cold creams have been measured for their electrical conductivity which was found to be higher than that of the familiar W/O emulsions. This might lead to the conclusion that they are O/W type creams [62]. It is a familiar and often demonstrated fact that the viscosity of an emulsion depends on that of its external phase but is hardly affected by the viscosity of its internal phase. Consequently, if a cold cream belongs to the O/W type, additions of paraffin wax or spermaceti which only alter the viscosity of the internal phase should have no or only little effect on the viscosity of the cream. Everybody who has ever worked with these creams knows that this does not correspond with the facts.

We may be tempted to say "if it is not an O/W cream, it must be a W/O cream." We have another rule that has been confirmed by many emulsions—that the viscosity of an emulsion increases with the concentration of its internal phase. Accordingly, a W/O cream ought to thicken if, all other proportions remaining equal, the water content is raised from, say, 15 to 25%. With cold creams, the opposite usually occurs and the assumption that we are dealing with a W/O system would also lead to faulty predictions.

We are obviously faced with mixed systems, and because our theoretical knowledge is inadequate here empirical observations and practical tips assume special importance. We quote some observations of De Navarre [63].

Cold cream becomes harder and more lustrous, the more oil it contains; with more water, it becomes softer. If more than 60% mineral oil is present, it tends to bleed. Vegetable oils occasionally make the creams granular. A smooth consistency is achieved in such instances by reducing the wax component or adding lanolin or an absorption base. The wax content of a cold cream should be between 10 and 20%. A high beeswax content makes the cream ductile and salvelike. Spermaceti, ceresine, and paraffin wax impart gloss. Lanolin makes the cream softer; this effect may be compensated by adding spermaceti or mineral waxes. An excess of high melting waxes may cause the water to bleed out during cooling.

Borax and the products that may develop in the cream from borax have a limited solubility in water. Hard granules may therefore form in creams with a high borax content. Here an addition of glycerol helps to prevent crystallization of borax and its hydrolysis products. [It should not be overlooked, however, that borax and glycerol form a strongly acid complex. Author's note.] Insufficient borax may cause instability of the emulsion.

Controlling the temperature during preparation is also important. Overheating of fats and waxes may lead to discolorations of the cream, which may also be caused by impurities in the raw materials or an unsuitable perfume. If the aqueous phase being stirred into the fat melt is too cold, granular creams may result. If the cream is too warm when the jars are filled (about 50°C), the stability will be affected. If warm cream is poured into cold jars, it may happen that water will separate within a short period.

Homogenizing the completed cream (either at 40°C or at room temperature) makes it softer and more stable.

Often, perfuming cold creams is not easy because beeswax, lanolin, and various other vegetable oils used have a rather strong natural odor themselves. Experience has shown that the "rose" type is particularly suited to mask this fatty kind of odor. The perfume oil selected must, of course, not have an irritating effect. Dosage should be as low as possible, just enough to mask the unpleasant odor of the cream mass or to modify it to a pleasant one.

**Skin-Cleansing Emulsions, O/W Type.** Liquid emulsions are commercially available under a number of labels, such as "face milk", and "beauty milk," whose end purpose is, as with cold creams, not always quite clear. These emulsions are used as powder bases and also as cleansing preparations.

Here, as well, efficacy in both applications is not really possible for one and the same product. In a powder base the oil phase should consist of stearic acid and possibly glyceryl monostearate; mineral oil and isopropyl palmitate, on the other hand, are indicated for cleansing creams. Occasionally beauty milks are also used as moisturizing preparations; this application would again require different compositions.

Emulsions with a high water content represent something of an intermediate stage between oil-based and water-based skin cleansers. They are used for the same purpose as the fat-rich cleansing creams, that is, for makeup removal. Although they are considerably less effective, they enjoy a certain popularity, possibly because they seem "cleaner," that is, less fatty.

| | 35 | 36 | 37 | 38 |
|---|---|---|---|---|
| Paraffin oil | 10 | 5 | 40 | 35 |
| Petrolatum | | | | 10 |
| Isopropyl myristate | | 20 | | |
| Peanut oil | | 7 | | |
| Cetyl alcohol | 0.5 | | | |
| Stearyl alcohol | | 1 | | |
| Stearic acid | 3 | 3 | | 8 |
| Diglycol laurate | | | 14 | |
| Triethanolamine lauryl sulfate | | 2 | | |
| Triethanolamine | | | | 3 |
| Amino glycol | 1.8 | | | |
| Water | 84.7 | 62 | 46 | 39 |
| Glycerol | | | | 5 |

35. Harry, *Modern Cosmetocology*, 4th ed., p. 132. Stir the aqueous solution of triethanolamine and preservative (70°C) slowly into the molten oil phase (70°C); continue stirring until 25°C. Perfume at 40–45°C. If required, this emulsion may be homogenized.

36. Keithler, *The Formulation of Cosmetics and Cosmetic Specialties*, p. 88. Add the aqueous solution of triethanolamine lauryl sulfate (85°C) to the fat melt (85°C), stirring vigorously. Continue agitation until cold, perfume, stir again, and fill.

37. Harry, *op. cit.*, p. 132. This emulsion may be prepared at room temperature. Mix diglycol laurate and water containing a preservative with fast stirring. Add mineral oil under continued rapid agitation. The product may subsequently be perfumed or, alternatively, the perfume may be added to the mineral oil and incorporated with it.

38. Harry, *op. cit.*, p. 130. The solution of glycerol, amino glycol [2-amino-2-methyl-propandiol-(1,3)], and preservative in water (75°C) is carefully stirred into the fat melt (75°C). Continue agitation until cold but avoid stirring in air. Perfume at 45–50°C. (This formula results in a stiff cream. Products of this type have not become as popular as the liquid "milks.")

Beauty milk is often tinted a faint pink. An eosine solution or a 1–2% solution of erythrosine are suitable for this purpose.

The emulsifying agent in these products is usually an amine soap; for example, triethanolamine stearate (amine soaps yield soft emulsions) or a nonionic emulsifying agent. Generally speaking, these products are better, the less complicated their composition. Neither vitamins nor other active biological ingredients are indicated here. Glycerol and mucins may be added in small amounts; larger quantities lead to stickiness. Lanolin and cetyl alcohol in small amounts are beneficial; larger additions reduce the cleansing action of the cream.

## Solid Cleansing, Soil Adsorbing Preparations

Preparations whose cleansing effect is based on the adsorption of soil to solid crumbs are divided into two groups: those that are applied in solid form and creams in which crumbs develop only after evaporation of the solvent or the external emulsion phase.

Such preparations frequently have an excellent cleansing effect, and as long as they do not contain strong alkalies or abrasives or have a high disinfectant content their effect on the skin is mild. They are therefore suitable for persons who cannot tolerate soap. However, allergies against specific preparations of this type occur rather frequently.

Most of these preparations also contain colloidal materials (cellulose or protein derivatives), and apart from soil adsorption the cleansing is based on the capacity of the colloids to hold dirt particles in suspension.

Preparations in solid form are still used to a considerable extent in Europe, especially in central Europe. The basic raw material is almond meal, that is, the dried and pulverized filter cake of pressed almonds, which, in view of its high price, is usually extended or replaced by filter cake of peach and apricot kernels. Other materials used are powdered orrisroot, starch, talcum, and some mild abrasives. In Germany these preparations are commercially available as *Mandelkleie* [64].

**Rolling Creams.** The active ingredient, that is, the substance that "crumbles" on the skin after the evaporation of the preparation, is usually a cellulose ether and occasionally starch or fully refined paraffin wax. These preparations often contain alcohol as well as water because it promotes the drying of substances in colloidal solution and the rolling effect. Glycerol, lanolin, and disinfectants are also used in rolling creams. If hand cleansing preparations are intended to remove heavy oily soils, water-insoluble organic solvents are also added occasionally.

|  | 40 | 41 | 42 |
|---|---|---|---|
| Carboxymethylcellulose | 14 | | |
| Methylcellulose | | 10 | 14.3 |
| Water | 54 | 52 | 74 |
| Alcohol | 30 | 10 | 5.5 |
| Trichloroethylene (or methylene chloride) | | 25 | |
| Glycerol (or replacement) | 2 | 3 | 5.5 |
| Lanolin | | | 0.3 |

REMARKS

40 and 41. Franz, SÖFW, **82**, 58 (1956).

42. Lesser, *Drug Cosmet. Ind.* 326 (1953). The addition of 0.1% menthol (to achieve a cooling effect) and 0.3% preservative is recommended.

43.  Cornstarch              14.3
       Distilled water         66.9
       Boric acid               2.8
       Paraffin oil             2.7
       Ammonium stearate        8.5
       Prostearin               1.0
       Glycerol                 3.3
       Perfume (lavender/rosemary).   0.5

Janistyn, *Riechstoffe, Seifen, Kosmetika*, II, 357. The glycerol is mixed into the transparent starch mucilage and subsequently stirred together with the paraffin oil/stearate melt at

90°C. (Prostearin is a self-emulsifying propylene glycol monostearate with soap as an emulsifying agent.) Stir until cold.

| | |
|---|---|
| 44.   Paraffin wax (abt. 55°C MP) | 22.5 |
| Span 40 (sorbitan monopalmitate) | 1.5 |
| Tween 40 (polyoxyethylene sorbitan monopalmitate) | 1 |
| Distilled water | 75 |
| | 100 |

Janistyn, *op. cit.*, p. 390. The paraffin wax is melted with the emulsifying agents and emulsified at 55°C with the water which has been heated to 60°C. Perfume is added and stirring continued until cold. The initial portions of water must be added slowly and in very small amounts.


# CLEANSING OF THE HAIR AND SCALP


Although skin-cleansing preparations may be grouped into several fundamentally different types (water-based, oil-based, and dirt-absorbent), only one type of product has prevailed in hair preparations: water-based products containing a surfactant. (Even so-called oil shampoos must be regarded as water-based preparations because the dirt is actually emulsified and dispersed in water and then rinsed off with water [65].) The main reason is probably because such preparations are removed from the hair with water, whereas oil-based or rolling creams can be removed only mechanically, by wiping with cotton or tissue. Such mechanical removal naturally is not practical.

The main purpose of shampoos is, of course, the washing of the hair: removal of fat, dust, and loose corneal cells. Quite apart from this purpose, however, all shampoos must meet a number of additional requirements to be competitive. After shampooing the hair should be left soft, lustrous, fragrant, and manageable. Also, the hands should never become rough and chapped from using these preparations.

In hard and soft, warm and cool water the shampoo should almost immediately form abundant foam, and this lather should not be affected too much by the presence of a certain amount of soil and fat. Actually, foam formation is not related to the cleansing effect. Nevertheless the public demands a richly lathering shampoo. It is ironic that chemists should try so hard to develop shampoos with good foaming characteristics in the full knowledge that they are only satisfying the public's whim. A good shampoo should be completely and easily removed from the hair by rinsing with water. If it comes in contact with the eyes, it must cause no more than temporary irritation, but no lasting damage. Nor should it irritate the scalp. Lesions of the scalp hardly ever occur because of the high resistance [66] of this skin area, but the risk of damage to the eye conjunctiva is considerable. If a little well diluted shampoo gets into the eyes, it is usually quite harmless, but undiluted or nearly undiluted shampoo is a different matter.

Draize and Kelly [67] established several years ago that some of the shampoos then available on the American market not only caused temporary irritations but lasting clouding of the cornea. Cationic surfactants are the most dangerous raw materials in this connection; according to Draize and Kelly, even 0.5–1% concentrations can cause damage to the conjunctiva of albino rabbits that is still noticeable after seven days. In the same tests the maximum concentration of sodium lauryl sulfate which did not result in lasting damage to the conjunctiva after seven days was found to be 20%, whereas the nonionic Spans and Tween caused no damage after seven days even in 100% concentration. Other nonionic and anionic detergents, however, showed a caustic effect in lower concentrations. Martin, Draize, and Kelley [68] found that some surfactants had a localized anaesthetic effect on the eye conjunctiva which suppressed the natural defense mechanism and thus promoted lesions. Nonylphenoxypolyoxyethylene ethanol has a strong anesthesizing effect in 1.25% concentration, and other polyoxyethylene condensates of alkyl aryl compounds as well as some fatty-acid/amine condensates have a similar effect.

Eye damage caused by detergent solutions were studied by several authors [69]. The quantitative results of the different investigators do not completely coincide but certain general conclusions nevertheless may be drawn:

1. Cationic substances are by far the most dangerous.
2. The irritating effect of Spans, Tweens, and some other nonionic detergents is very slight.
3. Anionic surfactants, including soaps, fall between these two extremes.
4. It is impossible to predict irritating action on the conjunctiva on the basis of other properties such as wetting effect or pH.
5. Mixtures of surfactants may be more strongly irritant than might be expected from the irritation potential of the individual components.

It is advisable therefore to test every new shampoo before it is marketed for its irritating effect on animals.

Powers investigated the properties that are most important to consumer selection of shampoos [70]. In 16 leading American shampoos Powers tested soil-suspension capacity, foaming effect (volume and stability) in soft, hard, and seawater, foaming effect in the presence of perspiration, hair cream, and (synthetic) hair fat, formation or absence of precipitation in hard water, and the average cost of each shampoo. He tried to establish a relation between the properties of the shampoos and their share of the market. Powers found that it was not possible to link market success with any one of the properties investigated. A leading shampoo, for instance, had an excellent cleansing effect in every kind of water, whereas another, which also sold in considerable quantities in spite of its comparatively high price, had a very low cleansing effect in soft water and hardly any in hard. How little the market success of a shampoo depends on its measurable properties may be illustrated by the following example: one shampoo that had come out rather badly in comparison with others in a consumer test was again compared with competitive products at a later date; the formulation was unchanged but the fragrance was altered. In the second test this shampoo was rated best: the better perfume had influenced the testers to such an extent that better cleansing and foaming effect were also attributed to the shampoo.

Apart from the perfume, advertising, and packaging, consistency and appearance also determine the reaction of the buying public to a considerable extent. This definitely does not mean that the manufacturers of shampoos should ignore the cleansing and conditioning properties of their products because the public cannot evaluate them anyhow. In the long run only high-quality products will prevail in the market.

As with skin cleansers, we first discuss the most important raw materials individually and later the different types of preparations based on them. Table 5-1 summarizes the most important properties of various detergents which are common in present cosmetic practice. Not everything can be expressed in a table, and we therefore discuss it more fully in the notes that follow.

NOTES

We do not claim that this table is complete. We have listed only a small part of the detergents commercially available, and in many cases we could not find data in the literature regarding the properties of several of the substances included. The reader may be able to fill in certain details himself. We have omitted any quantitative details about most of the properties because they have been measured in different laboratories under different conditions and the figures available are therefore not comparable. We have given only numerical values in the columns for pH and toxicity. The pH value refers to an aqueous solution of the detergent, with the concentration appearing in parentheses. Figures under Toxicity are the $LD_{50}$ values for rats, that is, the dose (in gram per kilogram weight of each rat) that kills 50% of the test animals after one administration. The higher the $LD_{50}$, the lower the toxicity of the substance.

The other columns are to be understood as follows:

WE = wetting effect.
DE = detergent effect.
FE = foaming effect.
WS = water solubility.

TABLE 5-1  SUMMARY OF DETERGENTS

| Chemical Type | WE | DE | FE | WS | SI | EI | Toxicity | pH(%) | MC |
|---|---|---|---|---|---|---|---|---|---|
| *Anionic* | | | | | | | | | |
| Sodium tallow soap | C | B* | B* | D* | − | | | 9.1–9.7(0.25) | − |
| Potassium coconut soap | C | | A* | B* | + | + | 10+ | 9.4(2.5) | |
| Potassium stearate | C | B* | C* | D* | + | | | | |
| Triethanolamine oleate | C | B* | B* | C | + | | | 8.8(2.5) | |
| Sodium lauryl sarcoside | | B | A | | | | | 7.5–8.5(10) | |
| Sodium lauryl sulfate | C | B | A | B | + | + | 1.5 | | ++ |
| Triethanolamine lauryl sulfate | A–B | | A | | + | + | 2.7 | 7.1(10) | |
| Sodium sec. fatty alcohol sulfates | C | B | D | | | | 1.3 | | |
| Sodium fatty acid monoglyceride sulfate | D | A | A | A | | | | | |
| Sodium polyoxyethylene lauryl sulfate | B | B | B* | B | | | | 7.5–8(10) | ++ |
| Turkey red oil | D | C | D | B | | | 25+ | | − |
| Sodium lauryl isoethionate | | A | D | D | | | | | |
| Sodium oleyl taurate | B | A | C | C | | | 6.6 | | ++ |
| Sodium isopropylnaphthyl sulfonate | A–B | D | C | C | | | 7.1 | | ++ |
| Sodium dioctylsulfosuccinate | AA | D | C | D | + | + | 1.8 | 5(1) | ++ |
| Sodium alkyl aryl sulfonate | A–B | | A | | − | | | | ++ |
| Triethanolamine alkyl aryl sulfonate | A | A | A | | | + | | 7.1(10) | |

TABLE 5-1 (*continued*)

| Chemical Type | WE | DE | FE | WS | SI | EI | Toxicity | pH(%) | MC |
|---|---|---|---|---|---|---|---|---|---|
| *Cationic* | | | | | | | | | |
| Alkyl (C$_9$—C$_{15}$) cetyl trimethylammonium chloride | B | D | (A) | | + | +++ | | 7.3(10) | |
| Alkyl (C$_{10}$—C$_{14}$) dimethyl benzyl ammonium chloride | C | D | C | | + | +++ | 0.3–0.4 | 7.3(10) | |
| *p*-diisobutyl phenoxyethoxyethyl dimethyl benzyl ammonium chloride | C | D | (A) | | + | +++ | | 7(10) | |
| N-soy-N-ethyl oleyl amide acetate | D | D | (B) | | + | +++ | | 7.1(10) | |
| N-soy-N-ethyl morpholiniumethosulfate | D | D | (B) | | + | +++ | | 7.1(10) | |
| Cetylpyridinium chloride | D | D | (A) | | + | +++ | | 4.8(10) | |
| Diethylaminoethyl-oleyl amide acetate | B | C | (B) | | + | +++ | | 6(10) | |
| *Amphoteric* | | | | | | | | | |
| Lauryl imidazolin | D | B | A | | – | + | 3.2 | 9.3(20) | |
| Triethanolamine-lauryl-β-aminopropionate | | | A | B | – | + | | 8.2–8.4 | |
| "Solubilized" sodium lauryl-β-aminopropionate | | | B | A | – | + | | | |
| *Nonionic (71)* | | | | | | | | | |
| Sorbitan monolaurate | D | | D | | – | – | | | |
| Polyoxyethylene sorbitan monolaurate | D | | B | | – | – | 25$^+$ | 6.8(10) | ++ |
| Polyoxyethylene lauryl ether | C–D | | B | | – | – | | 6.0(10) | |
| Polyoxyethylene-2-butyloctanol | AA | | A | | – | + | | 4.4(10) | |
| Alkyl phenol polyglycol ether | A | A | C | A | | ++* | ca. 2 | 7(10) | |
| Fatty acid (C$_{10}$—C$_{12}$) monodiethanolamide | C* | B* | B* | C | | +* | ca. 3 | 9.3(1) | ++ |

The degree of effectiveness is indicated with capital letters; AA for "excellent," D for "moderate." An asterisk after a letter (e.g., B*) indicates that the respective degree of effectiveness refers to solutions in distilled water and that the effect in hard water is much poorer. In measuring the foaming effect, both the "immediate" foam level and that after a few minutes have been taken into consideration. Whenever the degree of effectiveness reflects one measurement only, it appears in parentheses.

SI = skin irritation.

EI = eye irritation, designated as follows:

+ + + indicates that the maximum concentration of the substance causing no permanent damage to the eye conjunctiva amounts to 1 % or less.

+ + indicates that the maximum concentration tolerated is 1–5 %.

+ indicates that the maximum concentration tolerated is 5–20 %.

− indicates that even 100 % of the substance does not cause any permanent damage to the conjunctiva.

* indicates that the substances have an anesthetizing effect on the conjunctiva and therefore promote damage [72].

MC = metal corrosion through aqueous solutions of the detergent. + + stands for strong corrosion, + indicates moderate corrosion, and − the absence of corrosion.

## Active Ingredients

The perfect active ingredient in a shampoo should have the following properties: it should be easily soluble even in hard water and not form precipitates. It should have a good cleansing effect in every kind of water without being too degreasing. This means that its emulsifying effect (soil-suspension capacity) should be strong and its wetting effect less pronounced.

On being adsorbed to the hair shaft, the perfect active ingredient should make it supple and not brittle or unmanageable. The peculiarly brittle feel of hair after the use of a shampoo with fatty alcohol sulfates or, more strongly yet, with alkyl aryl or alkyl naphthyl sulfonates is due to a degreasing of the hair shaft and subsequent adsorption of the surfactant, according to Zussman [73]. Possibly an electrostatic charge of the hair also plays a part. The brittle feel disappears by using hair cream or rinsing with highly diluted solutions of cationic substances. This brittleness does not seem to occur when surfactants are used in whose molecules the hydrophilic portion is not too small but extends over several groups of atoms (e.g., fatty acid condensation products, polyethylene oxide compounds).

The perfect active ingredient for shampoos must obviously not have an irritating effect on the scalp and no corrosive effect on the eye conjunctiva. A good discussion of testing methods for eye conjunctiva damages in shampoos is given by Gaunt and Harper [74].

It should develop its full effectiveness in neutral weakly alkaline solutions.

Since the shampoo should not only be effective but also have sales appeal, some additional requirements must be met.

The perfect active ingredient should quickly develop in any water a smooth, rich, stable, soaplike foam. Foaming action should be maintained even in the presence of small amounts of fat, lanolin, and soil. It must have no unpleasant odor and, finally, should not be too expensive.

Not one of the known cleansing surfactants meets all these requirements. Nevertheless, good shampoos can be made from many detergents by using certain additives.

**Anionic Detergents.** In soft water soaps have an adequate detergent action and good foam formation. They do not degrease hair and scalp too strongly and leave the hair smooth and manageable. They are inexpensive and less dangerous to the eyes than most synthetic detergents. The drawbacks are the alkalinity of their solutions and their calcium sensitivity. Foaming and cleansing effects are considerably reduced if soap is used in hard water. Moreover, the precipitated calcium soaps adhere to the hair shaft and make it look gray and dull. The precipitation of calcium soaps may be prevented partly or completely by adding surfactants with a good dispersing effect (Igepon T, alkylolamides) which represents an important improvement.

Chemically related to soaps are "Medialanes" or "Sarcosides," amides of fatty acids with the α-amino acid sarcosin [75]. For use in shampoos the sodium salt of the lauryl derivatives is most suitable. It is commercially available in the United States as a 30% solution under the trade name "Sarcosyl NL."

$$C_{11}H_{23}CO{-}N{-}CH_2COONa$$
$$|$$
$$CH_3$$

Sarcosyl NL

In aqueous solution the sodium salt has a weakly alkaline reaction and yields a thin foam which may be stiffened by adding an organic acid; the optimum pH is about 5.5. This, then, is a mixture of sodium salt and the free acid of Sarcosyl NL. In hard water Sarcosyl NL has good detergent action up to a calcium content of about 0.025%. If the water is very hard, a nonionic dispersion agent should be added to maintain the foaming capacity and to prevent the precipitation of calcium soaps.

Sarcosides have a strong affinity for hair keratin and make the hair smooth and supple.

The fatty acid-protein condensation products such as Maypons differ from Sarcosides by a "multiplication" of the amide group in the interior of the molecule. They are frequently used in shampoos because they combine a good detergent and foaming action with a mild effect on hair and scalp. Fatty acid condensation products such as the Igepons may also be used—both those with an ester group inside the molecule (type Igepon A) and those with an amide group (type Igepon T).

$$C_{11}H_{23}COOCH_2CH_2SO_3Na$$

Sodium lauryl isoethionate
(type Igepon A)

$$C_{17}H_{33}CO—N—CH_2CH_2SO_3Na$$
$$CH_3$$

Sodium oleyl methyl aminoethyl
sulfonate (type Igepon T)

Cleansing and foaming effect are very good, particularly for Igepon T; this has better stability than Igepon A against acids, alkalines, and calcium ions. Igepon T is the best dispersing agent for calcium soaps we know; even small additions to soaps or soap solutions prevent the precipitation of calcium soaps in hard water.

The monofatty acid esters of glycerol monosulfate (Artic Syntex A and T) should also be regarded as fatty acid condensation products; they share with the other raw materials of this group a mild effect on hair and scalp. The sodium salt, the basis of one of the leading American shampoos, has an excellent detergent and foaming effect and good calcium stability but only within a narrow pH range (pH 5–8).

The most commonly used synthetic detergents for shampoos are probably alkyl sulfate salts, particularly sodium and triethanolamine lauryl sulfates. They are inexpensive and economical, have a strong detergent action, and foam well even in hard water. Their good water solubility results in quick action on the hair and facilitates rinsing.

Sodium lauryl sulfate is the least expensive and most frequently used substance of this group. Aqueous solutions of triethanolamine sulfate cloud at lower temperatures than those of the sodium salt; for this reason "tri" salt is often preferred. Solutions of triethanolamine salt are rather thin, but this disadvantage may be compensated by adding thickening agents. The ammonium salt is less alkaline in solutions than sodium and tri salts and is occasionally used for this reason. The magnesium salt which is also only weakly alkaline and has a lower cloud point (i.e., the temperature at which the shampoo starts clouding) has hardly been used at all up to now.

The most important disadvantages of the alkyl sulfates are their rather strong degreasing effect and their tendency to adsorb to the hair shaft which makes the hair feel dry and resistant. These effects, however, can be reduced by suitable additives.

Recently salts of alkyl polyether sulfates have also been recommended as basic materials for shampoos, such as "Sipon ES" (American Alcolac Corp.) [76].

$$C_{12}H_{25}O(CH_2CH_2O)_nSO_3Na$$
Sipon ES

These salts are characterized by good water solubility (hence a low cloud point of the solutions), excellent acid, alkali, and calcium resistance, and good foaming effect and have a mildly alkaline reaction in aqueous solution (pH 7.5–8). According to Powers [159] the detergent action is mild, although the wetting effect is reportedly stronger than that of sodium lauryl sulfate.

During the first postwar years "Teepol" (Shell) was frequently used as a basic material for shampoos. Here the active ingredient is a mixture of sodium salts of higher secondary alcohols. Although the detergent action of this product is very good, even in hard water (and even if the foaming effect is slight), Teepol is presently hardly used at all because of its unpleasant odor. Chemically, the "Tergitols" (Carbide and Carbon Chemical Co.) belong to the same type but they are purer and less odorous.

Tschakert [77] reports on the use of sodium and triethanolamine alkyl aryl sulfonates in shampoos. The detergent and foaming effect of these inexpensive and economical raw materials is good. They are also effective in hard water, but it may happen, if the washing liquid is too highly diluted (during rinsing), that calcium salts will precipitate or at least adsorb on the hair shaft, which makes the hair sticky and dull. An addition of calcium soap-dispersing agents (usually nonionic surfactants) may overcome this draw-back. The most important weakness of the alkyl aryl sulfonates as shampoo bases is (as in lauryl sulfates) their degreasing effect on the hair and the ad-sorption of the detergent molecules to the hair shaft, which makes it brittle and difficult to manage. A fat-replacing agent would have to be adsorbed even faster and more strongly than the sulfonate in order to compensate for this effect.

The sulfosuccinates (e.g., Aerosol OT, sodium dioctylsulfosuccinate) are characterized by their excellent wetting effect and for this reason have a strongly degreasing action. Their detergent effect is moderate. They are therefore not particularly suitable as basic materials for shampoos but may be considered as additives.

Turkey red oils cleanse effectively and have a mild effect on skin and hair but a very low foaming effect. For this reason the so-called "oil shampoos" based on Turkey red oils never achieved great popularity. The most important Turkey red oils are sulfonated castor oil and sulfonated olive oil. The former is viscous and sticky; the latter is thin. Usually they are used together.

**Cationic Detergents.** Among these materials, only sapamines may be considered detergents. They are salts of diethylaminoethyl oleyl or stearyl amides with weak acids, such as acetic, phosphoric, citric and, lactic:

$$C_{17}H_{35}CONHCH_2CH_2\overset{+}{N}(C_2H_5)_5CH_3COO^-.$$

(Stearyl) Sapamine acetate

In aqueous solution these salts have a weakly acidic reaction. An addition of alkali inactivates the solutions, just as an addition of acid inactivates soap solutions. Solutions of the sapamine salts are absolutely calcium resistant and yield an abundance of large-bubbled but not very stable foam. Their wetting effect is better but their detergent action not quite so good as that of soap. Quaternary ammonium salts are unsuitable for shampoos because they are strongly adsorbed by the hair (except from strongly acid solutions) and in this way removed from the aqueous solutions in which they should develop their detergent activity. They are used occasionally in small quantities because of their disinfectant action but never in shampoos based on anionic surfactants because these would inactivate them.

**Amphoteric Detergents.**   To a certain degree these cleansing agents combine the detergent action of the anionics with the disinfectant effect of the cationics. To a considerable extent they meet the requirements of a "perfect" basic material for shampoos and should find wider use in the future, although they are higher priced than most of the anionic surfactants. Salts of N-alkyl $\beta$-aminopropionic acids are marketed under the trade name ("Deriphats" (General Mills) [78]. Particularly suitable for shampoos is the triethanolamine salt of N-laurylaminopropionic acid which is commercially available as a 50% aqueous solution "Deriphat XD-150 B",

$$C_{12}H_{25}NHCH_2CH_2COO^-\overset{+}{H}N(CH_2CH_2OH)_3.$$

In shampoos it can be combined with a great variety of anionic, cationic, and nonionic substances. The cleansing action is excellent, the disinfectant effect rather weak. The foam, even in hard water, is rich and smooth, and after shampooing the hair is soft and manageable. "Deriphat XD-150 B" also has a favorable effect if it is added in small quantities (about 10%) to other detergents, in particular, to anionics: it stabilizes the foam and counteracts the dryness of the hair.

The corresponding sodium salt ("Deriphat XD-150 A") is not so easily combined with the various anionic shampoo bases. The antiseptic action is less pronounced than that of the "tri" salt. In solution Deriphat XD-150A has a strong alkaline reaction and must be adjusted before use to a pH 6.5– 9.5 (at which it is most effective) by adding an acid.

The same applies to "Deriphat XD-160," a solubilized Deriphat XD-150 A. This product is characterized by an extremely high water solubility and is also able to solubilize insoluble phenols and quaternary ammonium salts. It can be combined even more easily than other Deriphats with various anionic detergents and has a mild effect on skin and eyes. For this reason it is particularly suitable for use in baby shampoos. The foam volume is slightly less than that of other "Deriphats."

"Miranols," another group of amphoteric detergents [79], are imidaz-
inium derivatives. The most suitable for shampoos is "Miranol SM
concentrate."

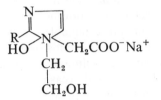

In Miranol SM concentrate R = isocapryl.

$$-CH(CH_2)_5CH_3$$
$$\mid$$
$$CH_3$$

Miranol SM concentrate has an excellent foaming effect which is also
maintained in the presence of soil and fats. It has a mild effect on skin and
hair (which is attributed to its slight wetting action) and on the eye conjunctiva; it also has a weakly disinfectant effect which can be strengthened by
adding quaternary ammonium salt.

It is of interest that amphoteric shampoo bases have no corrosive effect on
metal when used in aerosol or other metal containers. Even small additions
of a Deriphat reduces the metal corrosion of lauryl sulfate shampoos.

**Nonionic Detergents.** In shampoos these detergents are hardly ever used
alone because of their slight foaming action and comparatively high price,
but some of them play an important part as additives for shampoos based on
anionic surfactants.

The most important representatives of this class are fatty acid alkylolamine condensation products [80] such as lauric acid diethanolamine condensate. This material cannot be described with an unambiguous chemical
name or formula because it is a mixture of four or five different substances
[81], the most important of which is the amide $C_{11}H_{23}CONH(C_2H_5OH)_2$.

According to Kritchevsky and Sanders [82], these products have the
following effects:

They promote immediate foam formation, also with fatty hair.

They increase foam stability.

They increase the viscosity of the shampoo and give it a smoother, more
soaplike consistency.

They can prevent the stickiness of the hair caused by adsorption of detergent calcium salts on the hair shaft. A similar effect is also attributed to
alkyl- (octyl or nonyl)phenol polyoxyethylene ethers and other polyoxyethylene condensates.

They can remove or prevent the brittleness of the hair caused by an alkyl sulfate or alkyl aryl sulfonate shampoo.

These condensation products are marketed in different grades and with different properties [83]. Among the technical (i.e., not highly purified) grades the most important are capric or lauric acid diethanolamine condensates.

### Preparations

At present shampoos are available in four different forms: clear liquid preparations, creams, gels, or dry powder. We discuss these four types separately.

**Clear Liquid Shampoos.** These products consist in principle of aqueous solutions of detergents, whose surfactant concentration varies between 10 and 30%. Apart from the general requirements that must be met by all shampoos, two more are added here.

The preparation must have a suitable consistency. If it is too thin, it can too easily run from the scalp to the face (eyes!) and down the neck. If it is too thick, it will pour too slowly from the bottle and will not mix easily with water on the hair; thus it will lose its full effectiveness. The preparation must remain clear under normal storage conditions. Its cloud point should therefore be below 5°C.

To impart the desired properties to a liquid shampoo several additives are frequently used. These may be divided into the following groups, according to their effect:

*Calcium-salt dispersing agents.* The purpose of these products is the prevention of calcium soap precipitation and the dullness or tackiness of the hair caused by it. This action results in increased foaming. Calcium salt dispersing agents are particularly important in soap shampoos, but they are also used with alkyl aryl sulfonates, and sarcosides. Among them are Igepon T, alylolamine fatty-acid condensation products, polyoxyethylene alkyl phenols, and other nonionic ethylene oxide condensation products.

*Sequestrants.* These substances also prevent the precipitation of calcium soaps and are therefore particularly important in soap shampoos. Whereas the effectiveness of the dispersing agents is based on their surface activity, sequestrants have a purely chemical effect: they bind calcium and other polyvalent metal ions to a stable water-soluble complex and in this way prevent the formation of insoluble calcium salts.

Even small additions (about 1%) of sequestrants clarify all clouds caused by calcium-rich water in soap shampoos and also prevent flocculation which may occur in bottles by leaching calcium salts from the glass. They also counteract darkening or rancidity of the shampoo by binding any present traces of copper and iron. Larger quantities of sequestrants may act as water softeners and thereby improve the foaming of the shampoo. There are both organic and inorganic sequestrants. Important among the inorganic are polyphosphates; among the organic, the salts of ethylene diamine tetra acetic acid [84].

*Solvents.*  As we have seen in Chapter 2, it is inherent in the character of detergents that they cannot be easily soluble in water; the water-insoluble part of the molecule must be strong enough to drive the molecule to the interface of the solution. In the preparation of a reasonably concentrated shampoo it is occasionally necessary to approach the limit of solubility, above which the solution becomes cloudy. However, a shampoo that was absolutely clear during preparation may cloud after extended storage or when exposed to low temperatures. Solvents are added to prevent this cloudiness; those most frequently used are alcohols (ethyl, *n*-propyl, or isopropyl alcohols), glycols (1,2-propylene glycol, 1,3-butylene glycol, polyglycols), and glycerol. Solvents often increase the foaming action of the shampoo but lower the viscosity.

*Thickening agents.*  In addition to the substances generally used to thicken aqueous solutions (alginates, polyvinyl alcohol, methylcellulose, and colloidal silicates), several other types are also suitable: inorganic salts (ammonium chloride is the most effective and most commonly used, although it develops a slight ammonia odor which has to be masked with perfume), polyethylene glycol esters (e.g., polyethylene glycol 400 distearate), and nonionic surfactants (most commonly used are the alkylolamine fatty-acid condensation products). The required consistency may also be achieved with a mixture of surfactants as a shampoo base. Sulfated castor oil, for example, increases the viscosity of a shampoo based on sulfated olive oil, and a triethanolamine alkyl aryl sulfonate-based shampoo may be thickened by adding the corresponding ammonium salt.

*Hair and skin conditioning agents.*  As previously mentioned, some detergents have a strongly defatting effect on the hair. This, as such, is undesirable; if, in addition, the surfactant tends to be adsorbed on the hair, it may lead to a peculiar brittleness and the hair will become unmanageable.

The skin of the hands may also be degreased during shampooing. Several substances have been used successfully as conditioning or fat-restoring additives.

Lanolin and lanolin derivatives [85], cetyl and oleyl alcohol have a good effect but must be used sparingly; concentrations above 2% usually affect the foaming action of the shampoo. Lanolin often has a pronounced thinning effect on the consistency of the shampoo.

Lecithin as well must be added only in small amounts. Egg yolk and dried egg, which are ingredients of egg shampoos, also contain lecithin, cholesterol, and proteins which act as hair conditioners through their protective colloidal effect.

Certain mild surfactants used as additives are supposed to mitigate the effect of strong detergents, and alkylolamine fatty-acid condensation products are often used for this purpose. The dry feel of the hair, attributed to an electro-static charge of each strand, is also counteracted by N-alkyl-$\beta$-amino-propionates ("Deriphats"). A number of theories have been advanced about the mechanism involved in the effectiveness of hair conditioners. It may be that these substances are adsorbed more quickly on the hair than alkyl sulfates or alkyl aryl sulfonates and in this way prevent their adsorption: they occupy the hair first. It is also possible that the conditioning substances do not become effective at the beginning of the washing process because they are emulsified by detergents which are present in high concentration. Only when the washing liquid is strongly diluted, that is, during rinsing, are the conditioners adsorbed on the hair; this causes the conditioning effect. According to a third theory, hair conditioners act by enveloping the detergent micells (protective colloid effect) to mitigate their action.

It appears to us that different substances act differently. Alkylolamine fatty acid condensation products may well be effective according to the first hypothesis; lanolin and its derivatives may act as fat-restoring agents (second hypothesis), and proteins may be effective as protective colloids.

*Finishing agents.* Many of the conditioning agents also improve the gloss of the hair after washing; defatted hair has no luster. Sequestrants and calcium soap dispersants also prevent the hair from becoming dull after certain shampoos have been applied. The gloss-increasing effect of substituted 4-methyl coumarins is based on a different principle. These substances are described as "fluorescent hair brighteners" [86]. They have the capacity of converting invisible ultraviolet rays into visible white light and of reflecting it as such to impart a luminous brightness to the surface (the hair, in this instance). Especially suitable for shampoos are 4-methyl-7-diethylamino-coumarin and 4-methyl-5,7-dihydrocoumarin; they are incorporated in amounts between 0.2 and 1%. In a weakly acid solution (pH 4.5–6) these compounds are substantive to the hair and are therefore useful only in shampoos that develop their full effect in this pH range. They usually give a clear solution in the common shampoo formulations but occasionally a solvent is required (e.g., alcohol).

*Foam builders.* In soap shampoos sequestrants improve the foam by inhibiting the formation of calcium soaps which suppress foam development. In shampoos based on sulfated fatty alcohols an addition of 1–2% free alcohols (e.g., cetyl alcohol) reduces the foam volume but makes it denser and more stable. Small portions of alkylolamine fatty acid condensation products are often added to anionic detergents to achieve quick development of smooth and dense foam. The amphoteric "Deriphats" are reported to have the same effect.

*Preservatives.* According to Bryce and Smart [87], commercially available shampoos often contain great quantities of gram-negative germs. Phenyl mercury salts and formaldehyde are occasionally used, although the stability of both is inadequate. Bryce and Smart recommend the use of 2-bromo-2-nitropropane-1,3-diol.

In the following we group liquid shampoos into soap shampoos, shampoos based on fatty alcohol sulfates, and shampoos based on other detergents.

SOAP SHAMPOOS. The usual liquid soap shampoos are aqueous solutions potassium soaps of coconut oil and other vegetable oils. Coconut oil soaps of are easily soluble and develop ample foam which is connected with the high lauric acid content of the oil. Coconut oil may be wholly or partly replaced by palm oil which has also a high lauric acid content but contains less caprylic and capric acids. The addition of olive oil (consisting mostly of trioleine) yields a fine textured more stable lather and mitigates the skin irritant action of coconut oil soaps.

There are three ways to prepare soap shampoos:

1. The completed basic soap may be dissolved in water.
2. Free fatty acids may be neutralized with alkali.
3. The soap may be prepared by saponifying neutral fats.

The first method is simple but uneconomical and is used only by small plants. In the last decades the trend has been to change from the traditional third method to the second because it offers a number of advantages.

In the use of natural oils and fats the composition of these raw materials imposes certain restraints on the fatty acid composition of the shampoo; the use of free fatty acids, however, permits the mixture of the desirable fatty acids in any proportion and the omission of the undesirable. High-grade distilled lauric acid, for example, is preferable to coconut oil fatty acid because lauric acid causes fewer skin irritations.

It also leaves a wider choice as far as alkali is concerned because there is no need to heat over a long period and, instead of potassium lye, tri- or mono-ethanolamine may be used. In particular, if triethanolamine is used, soaps will have a less strong alkaline reaction. (The pH of a 2.5% potassium/coconut soap solution is 9.5; of the corresponding "tri" soap, 8.5). The foam volume may be less than that of potassium soap solutions, but the foam is more stable.

The method of preparation is simpler for free fatty acids than for neutral fats. Production of a good liquid soap by total saponification of neutral fats is an art which requires much experience and cannot be learned from a textbook.

We give no details regarding the preparation of the following suggested formulations; they can be found in any text or reference book on soap production [88].

| | 45 | 46 | 47 | 48 | 49 |
|---|---|---|---|---|---|
| Coconut-oil fatty acids | 4 | 4 | 6.5 | | |
| Coconut oil | | | | 21 | 15 |
| Oleic acid | 5 | 5.5 | 4.9 | | |
| Olive oil | | | . | 3 | 5 |
| Castor oil | | | | | 5 |
| Potassium hydroxide 85% | | | | 4.1 | |
| Potassium hydroxide 38° Bé (36%) | | | | | 12 |
| Sodium hydroxide 95% | | | | 1.9 | |
| Triethanolamine | 5.4 | 5.8 | 3.31 | | |
| Monoethanolamine | | | 1.47 | | |
| Potassium carbonate | | | | | 0.5 |
| Polyoxyethylene alkyl phenol | | | 2.42 | | |
| Tetrasodium pyrophosphate | | 1.2 | | | |
| Disodium ethylene diaminetetra acetate | | | | 0.5 | |
| Tetrasodium ethylene diaminetetra acetate | 0.4 | | | | |
| Alcohol | | | | 15 | |
| Propylene glycol | 5 | 5.2 | 6.4 | | |
| Glycerol | | | | | 3.5 |
| Water | 80 | 78.3 | 75.0 | 54 | 56 |

REMARKS

45, 46. Keithler, *The Formulation of Cosmetics and Cosmetic Specialties*, pp. 189 and 190. Heat fatty acids, triethanolamine, and propylene glycol under constant agitation to 65°C until the mixture is homogeneous. Stir in sequestrant and water and avoid introducing air.

47. *Schimmel Briefs*, **248** (November 1955). The fatty acids are mixed and stirred into the propylene glycol. The amines are added and stirring is continued until the solution is clear; polyglycol ether is added subsequently (Tergitol NPX), and the mixture is diluted with the requisite amount of water. This formulation contains a slight excess of amines which is supposed to keep the solution clear and to facilitate rinsing. The pH of this preparation is about 8.

48. Keithler, *op. cit.*, p. 190. This is an example of cold total saponification. Dissolve the alkali in water to make a 50% solution. Melt the fatty acids and let them cool to slightly above room temperature and add the alkali solution in a thin jet, under constant stirring.

Add the alcohol in which the perfume has been dissolved and continue stirring until the mixture is perfectly clear. The remaining water is to be stirred in next day. Allow the product to mature for two weeks, cool for two days to about 5°C, filter, and fill.

49. Rothemann, *Das grosse Rezeptbuch der Haut- und Körperpflegemittel*, 3rd ed., p. 500. We are reproducing Rothemann's hints and working methods in abridged form:

The potash lye (60°C) is added to the fat melt (60°C) in a thin jet and under constant agitation. The heat is removed and stirring is continued for some time. The kettle which should have heat insulation is covered and sheathed and the mixture is left; at this state it generates heat [the reaction heat of saponification]. When, after some time, dark clear soap liquor has developed, it is adjusted to the required pH. If any unsaponified fat is left [the reaction is not alkaline with phenolphthalein], more lye must be added. If the reaction is too strongly alkaline, more fat is added and saponification is continued or neutralization is effected with Turkey red oil, boric acid, or benzoic acid until a phenolphthalein strip turns faint pink. The remaining water and potash (in aqueous solution) are then stirred into the completed soap. Glycerol (or alcohol) is added only when the mixture is almost cold. The liquid soap is stored for at least a week at a temperature as low as possible. The perfume is added and the soap filtered and filled.

*Perfuming of Soap Shampoos* [89]. Oleates have a strong soap odor and require a masking perfume that must also be stable in an alkaline environment. Amine soaps tend to darken; it is advisable to select a perfume that does not promote this darkening effect.

## SHAMPOOS BASED ON FATTY ALCOHOL SULFATES

| | 50 | 51 | 52 | 53 | 54 | 55 |
|---|---|---|---|---|---|---|
| Sodium lauryl sulfate | 46 | 40 | 37.5 | | | |
| Triethanolamine lauryl sulfate | | | | 30 | 49 | |
| Sodium cetyl sulfate | | | | | | |
| Sodium oleyl sulfate | | | | | | 46 |
| Castor oil sulfonic acid | | | | | | 10 |
| Triethanolamine oleate 50% | | | | | 9.8 | |
| Ethylene glycol monostearate | | 1.5 | | | | |
| Alkylolamine fatty acid condensation product | | | | 10 | | |
| Coconut oil fatty acid monoethanolamide | | 5 | | | | |
| Ammonium chloride | 5 | | | | | |
| Polyethylene glycol 400 distearate | | | 6.2 | | | |
| Octylene glycol | | | | | 2.0 | |
| Lanolin | | 1 | | | | |
| Oleyl alcohol | | | | | 1.0 | |
| Acetic acid | | | 1.8 | | | |
| Lactic acid | | | | | | 1 |
| Water | 49 | 52 | 56.3 | 58.2 | 38.2 | 79 |

REMARKS

These formulations are incomplete because the concentrations of sodium and triethanol-amine lauryl sulfates are not accurately stated. These materials are commercially available in different grades and under different brand names and their content of active substances fluctuates between 25 and 60% in the usual paste products. These formulations are of interest primarily because of the additives they contain.

50. Keithler, *The Formulation of Cosmetics and Cosmetic Specialties*, p. 184.

51. Powers, *Drug Cosmet. Ind.*, **79,** 694 (1956). This formulation is based on a grade of sodium lauryl sulfate with 28% active substance. An addition of glycolic acid adjusts the product to a pH of 7.4.

52. Keithler, *op. cit.*, p. 185.

53. Zussmann, in Harry, *Modern Cosmetocology*, 4th ed., p. 427.

54. Harry, *op. cit.*, p. 426. The brand of "tri" lauryl sulfate used is "Sipon LT/6" (American Alcolac Corp.). The 50% triethanolamine oleate is prepared by mixing 32.7% oleic acid, 17.4% triethanolamine, and 49.9% distilled water.

55. Rothemann *Das grosse Rezeptbuch der Haut- und Körperpflegemittel*, 3rd ed., p. 507. Perfume: 0.5%.

## SHAMPOOS BASED ON VARIOUS DETERGENTS

|  | 56 | 57 | 58 | 59 | 60 | 61 | 62 |
|---|---|---|---|---|---|---|---|
| Fatty acid–protein condensation products | 30 | 20 | | | | | |
| Triethanolamine lauryl sulfate | 20 | | | | | | |
| Glyceryl monolaurate monosulfate | | 20 | | | | | |
| Sodium alkyl benzene sulfonate (60%) | | | 33 | | | | |
| Sodium lauryl sarcoside (30% active) | | | | 66 | | | |
| Sodium dioctyl sulfosuccinate (20%) | | | | | 80 | | |
| Sapamine citrate | | | | | | 20 | |
| Sulfated castor oil 90% | | | | | | | 60 |
| Sulfated olive oil 80% | | | | | | | 25 |
| Glyceryl monolaurate | | | 2 | | | | |
| Coconut oil fatty acid monoethanolamide | | | | 3 | | | |
| Sequestren No. 3 | | | | 0.5 | | | |
| Sodium alginate solution (3%) | 5 | | | | | | |
| Glycerol | 3 | 5 | | | | 2 | |
| 2-amino-2-methylpropanol-1 | | | | | | | 1 |
| Mineral oil | | | | | 5 | | 4 |
| Cetyl alcohol | | | | | 5 | | |
| Lecithin | | | | | 1 | | |
| Citric acid | | | | | | 0.5 | |
| Water | 42 | 55 | 65 | 30.5 | 9 | 77.5 | 10 |

REMARKS

56, 57. Janistyn, *Riechstoffe, Seifen, Kosmetika*, II, p. 129. The fatty acid-protein condensation product used is Maypon A (40% active material) or Maypon Special (increased foam effect).

58. Harry, *Modern Cosmetocology*, 4th ed., p. 428.

59. *Schimmel Briefs*, **260** (November 1956). Sequestren No. 3 is an ethylene diamide tetra acetic acid derivative.

60. "Manoxol" Techn. Bulletin, in Harry, *op. cit.*, p. 427.

61. Janistyn, *op. cit.*, II, p. 128.

62. Keithler, *The Formulation of Cosmetics and Cosmetic Specialties*, p. 204. An oil shampoo.

**Cream Shampoos.** It is considered a serious esthetic fault if liquid shampoos begin to cloud after prolonged storage or strong cooling. The cosmetic chemist is somewhat restricted in his formulations by the requirement that the product remain clear under normal circumstances. Certain detergents may be added only in limited concentrations; for example, many grades of fatty alcohol sulfates with a high sodium sulfate content (which crystallizes at low temperatures). Clouding can hardly be avoided when the addition of fats is more than 5%.

These difficulties have been solved in the most ingenious way by making a virtue out of necessity and artificially increasing the cloud. The result was a new product: cream shampoo.

Apart from permitting a freer selection of raw materials, cream shampoos have another advantage: new consistencies can be achieved. The viscosity of clear liquid shampoos ranges from a thin waterlike fluid to a viscous syrup, whereas liquid and solid cream shampoos can be adjusted so that they neither run off nor are too viscous but can be easily and quickly mixed with water.

On the other hand, the preparation of cream shampoos is technically more difficult than that of liquid shampoos. It is possible to achieve a nice creamy consistency with these products, but it is not quite so easy to stabilize it for longer storage and normal temperature fluctuations. Patterson [90] gives a good survey of the technical difficulties and the measures leading to stable consistency. Cream shampoos in general are more expensive to produce and therefore higher priced than liquid preparations.

In addition to the basic materials we have already discussed in connection with liquid shampoos (all of which may be used for cream shampoos as well; only solvents are not so important), cream shampoos also contain one or more opacifying agents. Probably the most commonly used is sodium stearate; this is hardly ever added as such but develops during the preparation process from stearic acid and sodium lye. In correct procedure sodium stearate crystallizes in shampoos as a net of fine needles which solidifies the preparation. To achieve the desired consistency it is essential to control the temperature very strictly during the cooling period, during filling, and the first days of storage. If the preparation cools too quickly after filling, the sodium stearate may crystallize into crystals that are too small and the result will be a thin and glossy paste. If the product is stored at too high a temperature, slow crystallization may result in a soft, flocculent product.

Sodium stearate may be replaced by zinc or magnesium stearates, which are added as such to the shampoo mass. Sodium cetyl sulfate also crystallizes and has an effect similar to that of sodium stearate; it also improves the cleansing action of the shampoo.

| | 63 | 64 | 65 | 66 | 67 | 68 |
|---|---|---|---|---|---|---|
| Sodium lauryl sulfate | 50 | | | | | |
| Sodium fatty alcohol sulfate paste (3%) | | 45 | 30 | | | 60 |
| Triethanolamine lauryl sulfate (50%) | | | | | 40 | |
| Ammonium lauryl sulfate | | | | 49 | | |
| Protein fatty acid condensation product (25%) | | | | | 10 | |
| Glyceryl monolaurate | | 2 | | | | |
| Ethylene glycol monostearate | | | | 1.4 | | |
| Glyceryl monostearate | | | | | | 2 |
| Propylene glycol | | | | 2 | | |
| Alcohol 95% | | | | | 5 | |
| Polyvinyl alcohol (10%) | | 6 | 20.5 | | | |
| Methylcellulose (3%) | | | 9 | | | |
| Polyethylene glycol 400 distearate | | | | 2.6 | | |
| Veegum, dry | | | | | | 1.5 |
| Cetyl alcohol | | 2 | | | | |
| Lanolin | 1 | 1 | 0.5 | | | |
| Lanolin, acetylated | | | | | | 2 |
| Amerchol L-101 | | | | | | 4 |
| Atlas G-1441 | | | | | 1 | |
| Egg yolk | | | | | 10 | |
| Magnesium stearate | | 2 | 1 | | | |
| Stearic acid | 5 | | | | | 8 |
| Sodium hydroxide | 0.75 | | | | | 0.5 |
| Potassium hydroxide | | | | | | 0.5 |
| Triethanolamine | | | | | | 1.5 |
| Water | 43.25 | 42 | 38 | 49 | 34 | 20 |
| | 100 | 100 | 99 | 104 | 100 | 100 |

REMARKS

63. Harry, *Modern Cosmetocology*, 4th ed., p. 340. The sodium lauryl sulfate is "Sipon LS" (American Alcolac Corp.). A solid cream shampoo.

64. *Am. Perfumer*, June 1956. Mix the fatty-alcohol sulfate paste with the magnesium stearate. Add polyvinyl alcohol solution and water, heat the mixture to 77°C, and stir it into the melt of lanolin, cetyl alcohol, and glyceryl monolaurate (77°C). This product is also solid.

65. Pantaleoni, Shanks, and Valentine, *Proc. scient. Sect. Toilets Goods Ass.*, 9 (December 1949). Working method as in (64). (This product is liquid and differs from the preceding in its lower detergent and greater water content.)

66. Keithler, *The Formulation of Cosmetics and Cosmetic Specialties*, p. 198.

67. Rothemann, *Das grosse Rezeptbuch der Haut- und Körperpflegemittel*, 3rd ed., p. 493.

The original formulation prescribes "Texapon Extract T" for the triethanolamine lauryl sulfate 50%. This may be replaced by Texapon Extract A (ammonium lauryl sulfate 33–35%). The protein-fatty acid condensation product in Rothemann's formulation is Maypon 4 BC (potassium or triethanolamine salt, 25%). Atlas G-1441 is a polyoxyethylene sorbitol lanolin derivative. The original formulation also provides for 0.25% of a preservative, Nigapin M, 0.5% perfume oil, and egg yolk coloring ad lib. (example of an egg shampoo).

68. Conrad and Motiuk, *Am. Perfumer* 35 (April 1956). The acetylated lanolin may also be replaced by liquid acetylated lanolin alcohols. Both, as well as Amerchol, are products of American Cholesterol Products Inc. "Veegum" (R. T. Vanderbilt Co.) is a colloidal magnesium aluminum silicate.

(Whereas natural lanolin above 2% would inhibit the foaming effect of the shampoo, purified lanolin derivatives may be used in larger quantities).

**Gel Shampoos.** If the content of thickening agents in liquid or cream shampoos is strongly increased, the result is a transparent jellylike product (91).

According to Dijkstra [92], a good base for this type of preparation consists of equal parts of triethanolamine lauryl sulfate and triethanolamine myristinate. Harry (93) gives the following formulation based on a mixture of soap and alkyl sulfate:

| 69. Triethanolamine lauryl sulfate | 20 |
|---|---|
| Sodium lauryl sulfate | 10 |
| Coconut fatty acids | 15 |
| Triethanolamine (tech.) | 10 |
| Sequestering agent | 1 |
| Water | 44 |
| Perfume and color | q.s. |

**Dry Shampoos.** Dry shampoos represent the least expensive kind of hair-cleansing preparation: 5 g of a detergent powder are sufficient for one application, and low cost packs are also practicable. Moreover, it is easy to package in single-application portions which is definitely an advantage. (Liquid-clear and liquid-cream shampoos are also available in single-application packs; although this method of packaging is comparatively expensive, it is rather popular, especially in Europe.) On the other hand, it is a disadvantage of dry shampoos that hair-conditioning agents can be added only in rather limited quantities. Apart from the active detergent, these shampoos usually also contain some inorganic salts; since these salts have a weakly alkaline reaction in solution (bicarbonate of soda, borax), they increase the cleansing power to a certain extent. Their main function, however, is the psychological effect on the buyer: they increase the volume of the powder. If the user found only a teaspoonful of powder in a shampoo pack, she might feel cheated.

Dry shampoos occasionally contain powdered sequestering agents, cellulose ether, or egg powder (these act as hair conditioners). It is important that all ingredients be easily soluble but not hygroscopic.

Here are a few formulations from various publications:

|  | 70 | 71 | 72 | 73 | 74 |
|---|---|---|---|---|---|
| Prime basic soap, powdered | 60 | 60 | 50 | 30 | |
| Coconut soap, prime, powdered | | 10 | 25 | | |
| Sodium lauryl sulfate, powdered | | | 5 | 40 | 40 |
| Igepon T | 10 | | | | |
| Tetrasodium pyrophosphate | | | | 10 | 6 |
| Trilon A | 10 | | | | |
| Whole egg powder | | 5 | | | |
| Borax, powdered | 5 | 10 | 5 | | |
| Sodium carbonate, powdered | 15 | 15 | 15 | 20 | 54 |

REMARKS

70. Janistyn, *Riechstoffe, Seifen, Kosmetika*, II, p. 121. Trilon A is a sequestering agent, $N(CH_2COONa)_3$.

71. Rothemann, *Das grosse Rezeptbuch der Haut- und Körperpflege*, 3rd ed., p. 509. The formulation also requires 0.5% perfume oil. A particularly mild product for sensitive hair.

72. Rothemann, *op. cit.*, 509. The basic soap should contain a maximum of 0.05% free alkali. 0.5% perfume oil is also prescribed. This is a product for heavily soiled hair. It is suggested to provide a twin pack of hair conditioner for an acidifying rinse.

73, 74. Harry, *Modern Cosmetology*, 4th ed., pp. 426 and 425. Harry recommends a light voluminous grade of sodium lauryl sulfate; for example, Empicol LZ (Marchon Products, Inc.).

**Special Shampoos.** So far we have discussed products in this section whose purpose is the cleansing of the hair, leaving it lustrous, smooth, and manageable. Shampoos with special properties are also commercially available. The most important are disinfectant shampoos against dandruff and scalp infections. These preparations once contained tar products or simple phenols, such as *p*-cresol; today the same modern disinfectants used in soaps are frequently incorporated. Since dandruff is not entirely a problem of infection, it can only rarely be cured by disinfectant shampoos. Nevertheless, there is always a certain market for disinfectant shampoos, probably because by disinfecting hair and scalp they also prevent infections of the facial skin, particularly the forehead.

Cream shampoos containing colloidal sulfur have also achieved widespread acceptance as antidandruff shampoos. Shampoos containing selenium sulfide (see Chapter 9) can be obtained only by medical prescription because of the toxicity of this material, which is frequently not tolerated on the skin. Color rinses are discussed in Chapter 10.

**Rinses.** The purpose of these preparations is not to cleanse, but we discuss them here because their use is closely related to shampooing. Their purpose is the elimination of the undesirable side effects of shampoos, the most common being the dulling effect or tackiness caused by precipitating calcium salts, in particular after using soap shampoos, and brittleness resulting from the use of alkyl aryl sulfonates or fatty alcohol sulfates.

1. *Rinses to impart luster to dull "grayed" hair.* If the calcium salts of the higher fatty acids were completely insoluble in water, it would not be possible to release them from the hair with rinsing preparations. Actually, however, they do dissolve a little and then dissociate according to the equation

$$[CH_3(CH_2)_nCOO]_2Ca \rightleftharpoons 2CH_3(OH_2)_nCOO^- + Ca^{2+}.$$

This is a reversible reaction. The chemical law applicable here permits a complete dissolution of calcium salts by chemically binding the liberated calcium ion ($Ca^{2+}$). If precipitated calcium salts are to be entirely removed, this can be achieved with solutions of sequestrants; that is, substances that form water-soluble complexes with earth alkali and heavy metal ions. The effectiveness of the rinsing preparation increases with the stability of the $Ca^{2+}$/sequestrant complex; that is, the more powerfully calcium is bound by the sequestrants. Table 5-2 shows the dissociation constants of the calcium complexes of various sequestering agents as a measure of the stability of the complexes (the higher the value of log K, the more stable the complex); 1–2% solutions of the products at the top of the list are efficient rinses. These preparations should first be rubbed into the hair undiluted and then rinsed off. It is important that they be allowed sufficient time to act on the hair (several

TABLE 5-2   STABILITY OF CALCIUM COMPLEXES OF VARIOUS SEQUESTERING AGENTS [94]

|  | Log $K$ |
|---|---|
| N-benzylethylene diamine triacetic acid | 10.59 |
| Amino triacetic acid | 6.41 |
| Ethylene diamine N-benzyl-triacetic acid | 6.20 |
| 2-carboxyethyl amino acetic acid | 5.04 |
| Citric acid | 3.2 |
| Malic acid | 2.06 or 2.66* |
| Tartaric acid | 1.8 or 2.8* |
| Lactic acid | 0.9 or 1.4* |
| Acetic acid† | 0.53 or 0.62* |

* Different methods of determination have resulted in differing values.
† With acetic acid the complex formation with calcium is only of theoretical interest.

minutes) because calcium salts with little solubility dissolve only slowly under their influence.

Diluted acetic acid is also sometimes recommended for hair rinses. Since it does not form stable complexes with $C^{2+}$ ions, this acid is not able to remove precipitated calcium salts from the hair. The dull appearance of the hair after washing may also be due to the swelling of keratin in alkaline solutions. Any acid rinse would then improve the appearance of the hair by its action. The hair may also lose its gloss because of the degreasing effect of washing. In this case sequestering agents would not help, but the hair should be treated with brilliantine or conditioning cream.

Rinses based on sequestering agents are helpful before cold-wave setting and coloring because they not only bind calcium ions but also other heavy metal ions that interfere with these processes.

2. *Rinses to make the hair smooth and manageable.*   As we have seen, the brittleness shown by the hair after shampooing with certain detergents is due to the adsorption of detergent molecules or ions by the hair shaft. It has been found that cationic substances will neutralize this effect.

We may imagine the manner in which these cationic substances act; the surfaces of the hair cells have weakly positive and negative centers that result from the distribution of the carboxyl, carbonyl, and amino groups in the keratin molecule (see Chapter 1). If an anionic shampoo is used, the anions accumulate at the free positive centers of the keratin cells (after the fat layer has been removed). In keratin negative centers normally predominate (hence the isoelectric point within the acid range). If some of the positive centers are "eliminated" by the shampoo, the negative charge on the hair surface so strongly predominates that all the hairs, which now carry a negative charge, mutually repulse each other and are very hard to manage. This effect can even be noticed on the hands; if they are rubbed together after using certain shampoos, a peculiar kind of resistance can be experienced, although they are quite clean and not sticky. [Schwartz and Knowles (95) describe physical measuring methods for the effects of friction on the hair surface.]

When a cationic solution is used for rinsing, the cations occupy negatively charged centers of the keratin molecules, thus causing an equilibrium between the charges and thereby reducing the electrostatic repulsion and making the hair smooth and manageable.

Cationic substances as a rule are used in 1% solutions. Sometimes conditioners (lanolin, glycerol monostearate, alkylolamide fatty acid condensation products etc.) are added. Apart from these substances, the previously discussed amphoteric materials are also suitable for rinsing preparations.

Rinses are marketed as clear (possibly colored) solutions or creams (similar to cream shampoos). In any case, consumers should be warned of the risk to the eyes which always exists when cationic substances are applied [96].

## CLEANSING OF THE TEETH

It is the function of dentifrices to keep the surface of the teeth as clean and shiny as possible, to preserve the health of the teeth and gums, to inhibit the formation of unpleasant odors in the oral cavity, and to freshen the user's breath.

To appreciate how dentifrices can best achieve these purposes we first examine the structure of teeth and the nature of the undesirable processes that occur within the oral cavity.

## ANATOMY OF THE TEETH AND PHYSIOLOGY OF THE ORAL CAVITY

We distinguish between the free-standing *crown*, the more slender *neck*, which is covered by the gingiva (gums), and the *root* which is embedded in the jaw and has one or more branches. Inside each tooth is the pulp cavity which is filled with dental pulp (nerves, lymph, bloodvessels, and connective tissue) and connected with the point of the root by one or more root channels through which blood vessels and nerves enter the tooth.

The crown is covered by very hard *enamel* which consists of densely packed, calcium-rich prisms. At the surface it is surrounded by the "Nasmith membrane," which consists of an organic substance (presumably similar to

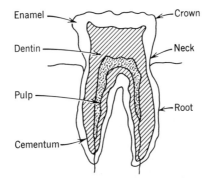

Enamel — Crown

Dentin — Neck

Pulp —

Root

Cementum —

FIGURE 7 STRUCTURE OF A HUMAN TOOTH.

keratin). The body of the tooth is formed by the bonelike *dentin*, which contains innumerable fine tubes. The roots are covered by the equally bonelike *cementum*, which is particularly thick at the point and tapers off toward the neck. The *periodontal membrane* covers the exterior of the root and merges at the edge of the tooth socket (alveolar bone) into the gingiva (Figure 7).

From a cosmetic point of view we are merely interested in that part of the tooth that is visible and exposed to exterior influences, that is, the enamel that represents the uttermost layer on the crown. It is true that an inadequate supply of nutrients during its formation weakens the tooth and has an adverse effect on its appearance or that caries starting at the outside may also penetrate to the deeper layers. These, however, are no longer cosmetic problems.

The surface of the normal sound tooth is smooth. The gingival tissue firmly encloses the neck of the tooth. Food remnants that adhere to or between the teeth are removed from all accessible surfaces by the continuously circulating saliva; saliva circulation is also maintained by the movements of lips and tongue. Hard ingredients in food polish the dental surfaces.

If there are no rough constituents in the food, a plaque forms on the surface of the teeth which consists mostly of degradation products of organic substances in saliva. This plaque is a good culture medium for bacteria and probably helps to form calculus, also called tartar, and develop caries. Wherever the surfaces of the teeth are uneven, or at the points of contact between the teeth, and wherever the gingivae do not closely surround the necks of the teeth, congestions of saliva or an accumulation of food remnants may lead to the proliferation of bacteria and enzymes. An enzymatic degradation of calcium-rich substances in saliva may result in the formation of insoluble calcium compounds that precipitate on the teeth. It is not yet certain whether this precipitation is produced by a chemical degradation reaction or a colloidal chemical process. One thing does seem certain, that various microorganisms, in particular leptotrichaea and actinomyces, play an important part [97]. Bacteria, food remnants, and sometimes blood corpuscles are usually included in calcium-rich deposits, and this is the origin of dental calculus.

Within the first 12 hours of being deposited the calculus is still relatively soft and can easily be removed by brushing. Later it hardens and can then be removed only by scraping with sharp instruments. This cleaning process must be done by a dentist or technician. The surfaces of the teeth will never again recover their original smoothness and the unevenness promotes a renewed formation of calculus; this is not only esthetically undesirable but it may cause deleterious side effects. Calculus deposits near the neck or between the neck and the gingival tissue may lead to gingivitis or gingivosis, which result in the loosening of the teeth (paradentosis) [98]. This condition may also develop when food remnants lodge between the neck of the tooth and the gingiva.

Hofmann [99] and Harnisch [100] found that nearly all patients suffering from paradentosis had tartar deposits.

The influence of bacteria on food remnants may cause an unpleasant mouth odor which is attributed mainly to the formation of ammonia and amines, hydrogen sulfide, and mercaptans, aldehydes, and ketones during the degradation of protein, fat, and carbohydrate molecules. Occasionally food remnants by themselves, even without bacterial action, cause unpleasant odors (onions, garlic) and sometimes bad breath is a symptom of some organic disorder (larynx, tonsils, stomach). Often, however, it is due to the bacterial decomposition of food remnants.

The reason for dental caries is also the bacterial decomposition of food remnants or on near the dental surface. This condition which strikes nearly everybody at one time or another in their lives was defined by a group of investigators [101] as "a disease of the dental hard tissues caused by acids developed through the effect of microorganisms on carbohydrates. It is characterized by the decalcification of the inorganic substance and the simultaneous or subsequent decay of the organic constituents." A similar description was given by Miller [102] as early as 1891. Caries has recently been linked to the bacterium *streptococcus mutans*. Animals that do not harbor this species, do not develop caries; certain racial groups, such as the American Indians, the Eskimos, and the Sikhs in India, were not affected by caries before the invasion of the white race [103].

The etiology of caries is still a highly controversial matter. The idea that the first step in the decomposition of dental substance is a process of decalcification would certainly be in accord with certain recent findings. We know today that during the enzymatic degradation of carbohydrates a whole series of polybasic organic acids develop (hydroxy and keto acids) and that these acids are able to bind calcium ions in water-soluble complexes and accelerate the dissolution of salts of very low water solubility. These acids (citric, malic, oxalosuccinic, α-ketoglutaric) usually occur only in very low concentrations because they are transformed into other compounds immediately after developing. It is possible, however, that under abnormal conditions (e.g., inhibition of the activity of certain enzymes which participate in the reaction) one or more of these substances will accumulate and then affect the dental tissue in comparatively high concentration. The mechanism of the enzymatic degradation of carbohydrates, the so-called Krebs cycle, is discussed in all modern textbooks on biochemistry and physiology. For calcium complex formation see Willems [104].

The hypothesis that the first step toward dental caries consists in the decalcification of the enamel and dentin and that the active acid in this process derives from the decomposition of carbohydrates is not universally accepted. According to Pincus [105], the acid is liberated by enzymes from the dental tissue itself. Other investigators believe that caries begins not with decalcification but with the degradation of organic substance through proteolytic bacteria [106].

### Preparations

In the preceding section we discussed the undesirable external dental symptoms that start with an accumulation of food remnants and bacteria or enzymes at or near the dental surface. The killing of certain microorganisms or the inhibition of enzymatic activity may, of course, help to prevent these symptoms, but the principal method of daily dental care should consist in mechanically cleaning the dental surfaces and in removing accumulated food remnants, bacteria, and freshly developed tartar.

Toothbrushes and dentifrices are used for this purpose. Regular brushing of the teeth is particularly important for civilized man who has carefully eliminated from his food all hard constituents, crusts, etc., and who uses his knife rather than his teeth to separate his food into manageable pieces, so that the food itself no longer contributes to the polishing of his teeth. The purpose of cosmetic dentrifices is mainly to strengthen the scouring and cleaning effect of tooth brushes, and in this context they may be regarded as polishing agents. They are available as pastes, powders, or in solid form (dental soaps).

**Tooth Powders.** In terms of structure tooth powders are the simplest tooth cleansers. Formerly they consisted for the most part of finely ground calcium carbonate (whiting, ossa sepia powder) and were often not even flavored. Even today they consist sometimes only of two ingredients: an abrasive and a surfactant with an addition of a sweetening agent and flavor.

*Abrasives.* To have a scouring effect the materials used as abrasives must be powdered and hard but not so hard that they scratch the enamel. They must, of course, not be toxic nor should they have an unpleasant taste. They are usually water-insoluble, although recently some experts have advocated the use of water-soluble abrasives. Apart from the degree of hardness and the chemical structure, the abrasive action of the various substances also depends on the particle size and purity of the material. The particle size in any given grade of abrasive is never uniform; the particle diameter varies to a certain extent. The higher the amount of large particles, the stronger the abrasive effect. This is substantiated by the data published in *Accepted Dental Remedies* (1939, p. 103), which established the loss in weight of antimony plates after scouring with different grades of precipitated chalk under standardized test conditions.

| Grade | Particle Size (diameter) | Loss in Weight |
|---|---|---|
| Sturge "50" | Under 3 $\mu$ | 0.8 mg |
| Sturge "100" | 3–15 $\mu$ | 2.3 mg |
| Sturge "130" | 3–20 $\mu$ (71.5% in the 12–20 $\mu$ range) | 4.1 mg |

The enormously important part played by the degree of purity (even small quantities of hard admixtures may increase the abrasive effect considerably) is demonstrated by the data published by Wright and Fenske [107]. They established the abrasive effect of various grades of tricalciumphosphate on teeth and found the following relative values:

| Grade | Relative Abrasive Effect |
|---|---|
| ADR* | 38 |
| "Chemically pure" | 91 |
| USP | 229 |
| Technical | 1143 |

* Specifications according to *Accepted Dental Remedies.*

Since the abrasive action varies with the respective grades used, the lists of degrees of hardness of the most important toothpaste ingredients, which appear in many publications, are somewhat irrelevant unless the grades are specified. The following abrasives are used in tooth powders as well as toothpastes and dental soaps:

*Precipitated chalk* (calcium carbonate) is still the most commonly used. It is available in different grades that vary in density (particle size) and crystalline structure. Very light grades are usually incorporated in toothpastes because pastes based on them do not harden, whereas for tooth powders heavier grades are used which do not easily pulverize.

*Dicalcium phosphate* (CaHPO$_4$) and *tricalcium phosphate* [Ca$_3$(PO$_4$)$_2$] are very mild abrasives, if they are absolutely pure, and are used extensively in the United States. Insoluble sodium metaphosphate (Na$_4$P$_4$O$_{12}$) and other insoluble metaphosphates are highly suitable ingredients for dentifrices according to Phillips and van Heusen [108] who found that chalk gave no gloss to a very dull dental surface and that even highly polished teeth lost their gloss after being brushed with precipitated chalk. The macroscopic observation was confirmed microscopically when these authors found that the dental surface was riddled with grooves after being brushed with chalk. In similar tests they found that di- and tricalcium phosphates had a neutral effect: the gloss of dull teeth was only slightly increased and that of shiny teeth only slightly diminished. A mixture of calcium phosphate and sodium metaphosphate proved to be the most efficient in these tests.

*Calcium sulfate*, in a pure state, has a very mild abrasive action. Even small amounts may considerably affect the consistency of toothpastes.

*Talcum* is rough and should be used very sparingly.

The effect of *kaolin* depends largely on the grade used. Although coarser grades which were formerly widely used in tooth powders (they are avoided at present because of their earthy taste) had a very drastic abrasive effect, colloidal kaolin is reportedly so mild that it even reduces the effectiveness of other abrasives.

*Surfactants.* Apart from one or more abrasives, most dentifrices also contain small amounts of surfactants which are added to facilitate the wetting of the powder particles (in tooth powders) or to disperse the particles in toothpastes. The surfactants should enable the aqueous suspension of polishing agents which develops during brushing to penetrate into fine cracks and fissures, contribute to the wetting and loosening of the foreign matter, and facilitate the subsequent rinsing of this matter together with the polishing agent, and finally impart a certain foaming effect to the dentifrice. Although the latter is not linked to cleansing, it is generally required by the public.

Since the surfaces in question are easily wetted, since no degreasing need be feared, and since no particular demands are made on the foam properties many surfactants are suitable. On no account can they be toxic in low concentrations or irritating to the mucosa [109], or taste unpleasantly; if other active ingredients apart from abrasives are also used, the surfactants must obviously be compatible with these and, if they are to be incorporated in tooth powders, they must be available in powder form.

According to Tainter [110], sulfonated surfactants reduce the abrasive effect of toothbrush and abrasives by about 50%. Other surfactants possibly act similarly. Braus and Herberholz [111] state that strongly wetting additives in dentifrices loosen the gums and are therefore undesirable; but this opinion is shared today by only a few cosmetic chemists. It is, of course, hard to prove such questions either way.

Formerly the surfactant most widely used was soap, but many other substances are in use today, with sodium lauryl sulfate probably heading the list. Harry [112] also mentions sodium lauryl sulfo acetate (I) and "sulfocolaurate" (II).

$$\underset{\text{I}}{C_{12}H_{25}O-\overset{\displaystyle O}{\overset{\|}{C}}-CH_2SO_3Na} \qquad \underset{\text{II}}{C_{11}H_{23}-\overset{\displaystyle O}{\overset{\|}{C}}-O-CH_2CH_2NH\overset{\displaystyle O}{\overset{\|}{C}}-CH_2SO_3K}$$

*Others.* Alginates and gum tragacanth are occasionally added to thicken the slurry which develops during brushing. Many other additives with different functions have also been recommended: oxidizing, disinfectant, deodorizing, antitartar, acidbinding, and caries prophylaxis. These functions are discussed in the next section.

The following formulations for tooth powders have been taken from some more recent publications:

|                                      | 75    | 76    | 77    | 78   |
|--------------------------------------|-------|-------|-------|------|
| Precipitated chalk, medium weight    | 92.09 | 63.66 |       |      |
| Calcium sulfate extra                |       | 31.36 |       |      |
| Dicalcium phosphate                  |       |       | 61.13 |      |
| Tricalcium phosphate                 |       |       | 33.00 | 7    |
| Sodium metaphosphate, insoluble      |       |       |       | 89.5 |
| Titanium dioxide                     | 2.00  |       |       |      |
| Soap powder                          |       | 3.44  | 3.25  |      |
| Sodium lauryl sulfate                |       |       |       | 1.5  |
| Sodium lauryl sarcoside              | 2.97  |       |       |      |
| Sodium alginate                      | 1.90  |       |       |      |
| Gum tragacanth                       |       | 1.42  | 1.50  |      |
| Fragrances                           | 1.00  | 1.00  | 1.00  | 1.9  |
| Saccharine                           | 0.13  | 0.12  | 0.12  | 0.1  |

REMARKS

75–77. Keithler, *The Formulation of Cosmetics and Cosmetic Specialties*, pp. 356–358.

78. Janistyn, *Riechstoffe, Seifen, Kosmetika*, II, p. 285.

The preparation of tooth powders is very simple: fragrance, sweetener, and coloring (if any) are ground with one of the powder ingredients or part of it, and the balance of the powder ingredients is then mixed thoroughly with the first part and passed through a sieve (usually 0.30-mm mesh).

**Toothpastes.** Toothpastes contain the same active ingredients as tooth powders; they are much more expensive in use and more complicated to prepare than powders. However, consumers prefer them, possibly because they are more conveniently spread on the toothbrush in easily measured quantities, without loss through spillage, because they are available in tubes, and, possibly, because their consistency is more attractive. Tainter [113] established that beyond a certain minimum quantity the amount of cleanser used in brushing the teeth is not really important. A sevenfold increase of chalk concentration in a chalk suspension yielded only a 20% increase of the abrasive action. The action is, of course, strongly reduced if the amount of abrasive is too small. Over and above the general requirements any tooth cleanser must meet—that it must clean the dental surface without scratching, that it must not be toxic, and that it must have a pleasant refreshing flavor—a few technical demands are added to the desirable qualities of toothpastes.

1. It must be soft enough to be easily squeezed out of the tube and to be spread on the toothbrush, but not so soft that it sinks into it. This consistency must remain almost stable within a temperature range of 5–35°C (actually the temperature range depends on the climate of the country in which the product is used) over a considerable period of time.

2. Even if the tube is left open, the toothpaste must not dry to a hard crust at the opening.

3. It must not interact with the tube material.

Toothpastes are a suspension of abrasives in glycerol, a glycerol substitute or a glycerol/water mixture. Surfactants act as dispersing agents for the polishing agents and support the cleansing action of the preparation. Gum tragacanth, methylcellulose, carboxymethylcellulose, alginates, gum karaya, carageen, and other mucins thicken the paste, and their protective colloidal effect stabilizes the suspension of the solids. Occasionally small amounts of mineral oil (about 1%) are added to increase the slip of the preparation. Sweeteners are required to give the paste a pleasant taste, and the flavoring conveys to the user the very important sensation of freshness. Occasionally red pigments are added, particularly phloxin, carmine, erythrosine or "eosine."

In addition to these ingredients which occur in nearly all toothpastes (with the exception of mineral oil and pigments), there are also some special substances that are meant to give toothpastes particular antibacterial, antitartar, and other effects. These are discussed in the following section.

TOOTHPASTES

| | 79 | 80 | 81 | 82 | 83 | 84 |
|---|---|---|---|---|---|---|
| Precipitated chalk, super fine | 15 | 34 | 30 | 24.0 | | |
| Dicalcium phosphate | | | | 9.0 | 51.8 | 51.45 |
| Tricalcium phosphate | | 12 | | | | |
| Magnesium carbonate, very light | | | 3 | | | |
| Magnesium silicate | | | | 18.0 | | |
| Colloidal kaolin | 9 | | | | | |
| Magnesium hydroxide | | | | 4.5 | | |
| Glycerol | 21.75 | 24.5 | 58.8 | 32.0 | 45.0 | 10.0 |
| Propylene glycol | | | | | | 20.0 |
| Ethyl alcohol | 0.15 | 5.0 | | | | |
| Water, dist. | 23.5 | 18.8 | | 13.72 | | 14.0 |
| Gum tragacanth | 0.075 | 1.0 | | 0.28 | | |
| CMC, high viscosity | | | | | | 0.8 |
| Carbopol C-934 | | | | | 0.5 | |
| Tallow soap, pure | 9.0 | 4.1 | 1.0 | 3.0 | | |
| Sodium lauryl sulfate | | | 0.7 | | 1.8 | |
| Saccharose monophalmitate | | | | | | 2.5 |
| Mineral oil | | | | | | 1.0 |
| Saccharin sodium | 0.0075 | 0.1 | | | | 0.05 |
| Flavoring | 2.25 | 0.5 | 3.0 | | 0.9 | 1.0 |
| Methyl-p-hydroxy benzoate | | | | | | 0.2 |

REMARKS

79. Rothemann, *Das grosse Rezeptbuch der Haut- und Körperpflegemittel*, 3rd ed., p. 737. Alcohol and 0.75 pts glycerol (28°Bé) are poured over the gum tragacanth and left to stand for one hour and then worked into a smooth mucilage with 0.75 pts water (70°C). The balance of glycerol (28°Be) and soap are stirred in a mixer with 22 pts of water under heating. Evaporating water must be replenished so that the total amounts to 45 pts (i.e., 25 pts water). The gum tragacanth mucilage is then added, followed by the saccharin solution in 0.75 pts water, the flavoring ground into the colloidal kaolin, and, finally, under constant stirring, the chalk. Stirring of the warm mass is continued until a uniform consistency has been reached and a sample taken to check it. If the paste is too thin, some colloidal kaolin is added, if it is too thick, some water is stirred in. Finally the completed toothpaste is left to mature in earthenware vessels for 5–6 days, stirred once again, and filled into zinc or aluminum tubes. (In our opinion the flavor and soap concentrations appear rather high and that of the polishing agent is on the low side.)

80. Chilson, *Modern Cosmetics*, New York, 1934, p. 132. Mix gum tragacanth and alcohol. Add hot water, glycerol, soap, saccharin, and flavoring. Mix for 1–1/2 hr. Mix and sieve the dry constituents and add slowly to the liquid. Mix until the paste is smooth; mill it.

81. Rothemann, *op. cit.*, 3rd ed., p. 739. The freshly prepared magnesium hydroxide is heated with 25.5 pts glycerol and thoroughly stirred. Heat the soap powder with the balance of glycerol (possibly 50% sorbitol) and sodium lauryl sulfate and stir until dissolution is complete. Both heated mixtures are combined and introduced into a mixer, the solids are stirred in, and, if required, a red pigment solution may then be added, with the flavoring, until the color turns pink. Stirring is continued until the required consistency has been reached and checked with a sample of the cooled paste; it may be necessary to add more chalk. After the mass is completely cold it is put through a three-roller mill.

Rothemann observes that this product must be anhydrous to avoid a reaction between magnesium hydroxide and soap under formation of insoluble magnesium soaps.

82. Harry, *Modern Cosmetocology*, 4th ed., p. 320. Two methods may be used: (a) Mix dry gum tragacanth and soap and add water and glycerol or (b) prepare a 2% tragacanth mucilage and add the mixture of soap and glycerol. Subsequently (if possible, *in vacuo*) the mixture of dry substances is blended in. Flavoring is added at the end of the mixing process. The completed product is milled or homogenized. In this formulation the gum tragacanth may be increased to about 1% and the glycerol content may be reduced.

83. Cohen, *Soap chem. Spec.*, **32** (12), 51 (December 1957). Dissolve Carbopol in glycerol and add sodium hydroxide until the pH of the mucilage is 7. Stir in the solids. (Although this and the preceding formulation do not provide for a sweetener, some should be added.)

84. Osipow, Marra, and Snell, *Drug Cosmet. Ind.*, **80**, 313 (1957). The solution of methyl-*p*-hydroxybenzoate, saccharin, and saccharose palmitate in water (85–90°C) is added to the mixture of CMC, glycerol, and propylene glycol. Heat while stirring until the whole mass is homogeneous. Cool to room temperature, add mineral oil and flavoring, and slowly stir in the dicalciumphosphate through a sieve.

Although most of these formulations do not mention a preservative, it is advisable to add one. Preparing a good toothpaste in practice is certainly not quite so simple as it might appear from the procedures given. Not only first-class raw materials and good equipment are required but also a certain know-how which is the result of experience.

## Various Active Ingredients

The dental cleansers discussed in the foregoing only contain abrasives and surfactants as active ingredients. They are relatively simple preparations; this type of product has been known for many years. If they are expertly prepared from good raw materials, they will meet all the requirements we have enumerated as the main purposes of dentifrices: they support the action of the toothbrush in removing foreign matter from the surface of the teeth and polishing them and their flavor freshens the oral cavity.

New ingredients are constantly being recommended; obviously their purpose is always to improve on certain aspects of effectiveness. Frequently, the producers of dentifrices have enthusiastically fastened onto these new ingredients, partly because they actually expected them to improve their products and partly because of their publicity value.

The market for dental cleansers, particularly toothpastes, is very large in all modern countries. Whenever products of different manufacturers do not vary fundamentally in composition, effect, flavoring, and presentation, it becomes the task of advertising to persuade the consumer to use one product rather than another. Innovations in packaging, consistency, and flavor do not generally promise much success because the public seems to be satisfied with preparations that are still what they have been for 30 years, but new special ingredients fulfill the ardent wish of the copywriter: for something that will differentiate a certain toothpaste from competitive products! The new ingredient is strongly emphasized in advertisements and announced prominently on the package. There is no objection to such advertising techniques in the short run as long as the new ingredient is not harmful in any way, but, taking a longer view, this procedure (we have witnessed it several times during the last 20 years) in our opinion carries certain risks for two reasons:

First, the public is promised more of a new ingredient than it can fulfill. This may be successful for some time but not forever. If this game is repeated too often, consumers will finally lose confidence in all scientific innovations in this field even if they should happen to be valuable.

Second, by stressing one particular ingredient the impression is created that the quality of the toothpaste depends to a considerable extent on its presence or absence. The principal active ingredients (polishing agents, emulsifiers, etc.) are not mentioned. The public is thus conditioned to an erroneous attitude that can only be harmful to the healthy development of oral hygiene.

We do not mean to imply that all new special ingredients have neither purpose nor effect. We only warn of the risks inherent in a disproportionate relationship between advertising claims and the actual value of the additives.

In the following we discuss briefly the more recent special ingredients:

**1. Ingredients affecting the microorganisms of the oral cavity.** As already mentioned, bacteria play a part in most of the undesirable processes in the mouth; in the formation of tartar they are notably leptotrichaea and actinomyces. In the opinion of many investigators caries is caused by acid formation from carbohydrates through enzymes deriving from bacteria (lactobacillus acidophilus, etc.). Swelling and inflammation of the gums are due in particular to staphylococci and streptococci penetrating small cuts. Unpleasant mouth odors may be caused by diseased internal organs or residual food, but they usually develop only with bacterial decomposition of the latter.

With its temperature, degree of moisture, and wealth of organic substances, the oral cavity is an excellent culture medium for many microorganisms. According to Braus and Herberhols [114], saliva contains about 10 billion germs per cubic centimeter. A complete extermination of these microbes is neither possible nor desirable; at best, a disinfectant may reduce their number. In selecting a disinfectant, the following questions arise:

Can the active ingredient have an effect in the proposed concentration and the expected period of contact with the germs? Here it should be taken into account that on being applied to the teeth the toothpaste is diluted with water, and the effect of the active ingredient may be reduced by adsorption onto the abrasives in the toothpaste or complexing with proteins in saliva. The period of contact is usually short (1–2 minutes), unless the disinfectant can be anchored to the dental surface by adsorption. Harry [115] remarks that a disinfectant in a toothpaste may be useful even if it does not notably reduce the germ count in the oral cavity because it disinfects the toothbrush. Natural bristle toothbrushes usually carry a large quantity of germs. An adsorbed disinfectant film on the bristles might disinfect the toothbrush when it is not in use.

Is the disinfectant effective against the microbes assumed to be harmful? The microbic flora in the oral cavity is usually in a very finely adjusted equilibrium in which growth of every single species is checked by the presence of other species. An inhibition of the growth of certain species destroys this equilibrium, and it might happen that one substance, by inhibiting the growth of certain germs, would create favorable conditions for another species. To put it differently, the incorrect selection and dosage of one disinfectant might leave certain harmful germs completely undisturbed or even promote their growth. The following disinfectants have been suggested for use in tooth pastes:

*Potassium chlorate* ($KClO_3$). The antiseptic and deodorant effect of this salt is based on molecular and atomic oxygen which is released under the influence of certain enzymes in the oral cavity. This results in an oxidative degradation of residual food and microorganisms. Moreover, potassium chlorate reportedly stimulates the salivary glands and oxygen increases the resistance of the gums [116]. It must be used cautiously because it may have harmful side effects in higher concentrations. Dry mixing of potassium chlorate with organic substances (e.g., sugar) may lead to severe explosions.

Another oxidant used in toothpastes because of its disinfectant effect is *sodium perborate* ($NaBO_3 \cdot 4H_2O$). Its use is not recommended because it easily leads to injuries and inflammations of the oral mucosa [117] if it is not completely removed after brushing.

Sodium persulfate and magnesium peroxide have also been suggested. Apart from their disinfectant and deodorant action, oxidizing agents were also expected to have a lasting beneficial effect on the enamel but it is rather doubtful that this is the case. They occur only rarely in the newest tooth cleansers.

*Phenols and essential oils containing phenol* have only a mild disinfectant action in the oral cavity in the concentrations permissible (taste, solubility, and toxicity dictate the admissible maximum concentrations). They may contribute to the disinfection of the toothbrush or the preservation of the toothpaste. Hexachlorophene has recently been used in several leading toothpastes.

*Benzoic acid, salicylic acid, and esters of p-hydroxy benzoic acid* are used only as toothpaste preservatives, mostly in the form of sodium salts.

*Quaternary ammonium salts* in concentrations of approximately 0.25% have been suggested for toothpastes [118]. It should first be established, however, that the concentrations which would make these compounds effective in the oral cavity have no toxic or mucosa-damaging side effects.

Another possibility might be *penicillin* and other antibiotics. It has definitely been established that dentifrices containing penicillin reduce the germ count in the oral cavity considerably and counteract the development of caries [119]; nevertheless, there have also been emphatic warnings from various sides that antibiotics should not be used in these (or any other) cosmetic products [120]. We have listed the reasons for this opposition in Chapter 3.

**2. Special deodorizing agents.** The most notable substances of this group are *water-soluble chlorophyllins*. They are prepared by alkaline hydrolysis of chlorophyll, the green pigment of plants. Fundamentally, deodorizing substances in toothpastes can act in two ways: they might inhibit the action of bacteria causing the decomposition of food residue or interreact with the volatile substances responsible for the unpleasant odor and inactivate them. Chlorophyllins reportedly act in both ways.

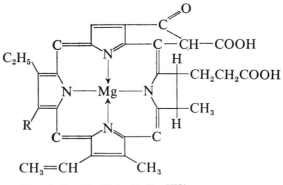

Chlorophyllin a (R=CH$_3$) and b (R=CHO).
The metal ion in the center may also be Cu.

Gruskin [121] reported in 1940 that to a certain extent chlorophyllins eliminate the putrid odor of some wounds and also accelerate their healing. This observation has since been confirmed by many practitioners [122]. Westcott [123] found that chlorophyllins *in vitro* are capable of reducing the malodorousness of certain amines and mercaptans. When these facts became known, it seemed logical to try to incorporate water-soluble chlorophyllins into toothpastes. In spite of the many publications that have appeared since 1950 in this connection, no agreement has yet been reached about the success of these attempts.

Partisans of the use of chlorophyllins in toothpastes point out that these substances inhibit proteus bacteria in such a way that they no longer decompose proteins to malodorous amines and mercaptans but to odorless amino acids, that chlorophyllins suppress the action of the acidic phosphatase which contributes to the development of tartar, and that they have a bactericidal or bacteriostatic effect on lactobacillus acidus, which is responsible for caries [124]. Chlorophyll also has been alleged to have a therapeutic effect on inflammations in the oral cavity. Other authors [125] emphasize that the tests establishing the bactericidal action of chlorophyllins were carried out under conditions that deviate considerably from those of normal tooth cleaning. The chlorophyllin concentration in toothpastes (usually 0.3–0.5%) is too low; moreover they are inactivated by adsorption to the abrasives, and the period of contact is too short to have a notable bactericidal effect. In addition, chlorophyllins are suspect as cosmetic materials because no methods are known to produce them in the pure state or to measure their degree of purity and because it is not yet known whether their use is harmful in the long run.

The actually disinfectant or deodorant effect of chlorophyllins in toothpastes can obviously never be established by argument but only in careful clinical tests. Here, as well, the data are contradictory. Harnisch [126], for instance, established that the lactobacilli and streptococci count in the mouths of boys who had been using a toothpaste with 0.3% chlorophyllin for 10 weeks had been reduced by 48–60%. In a series of tests Barail [127] compared the intensity of mouth odors of 50 persons who had used a toothpaste containing 0.1% chlorophyllin or an identical product without chlorophyllin. He came to the conclusion that the chlorophyllin had considerably weakened the mouth odors and delayed their recurrence after brushing. Other investigators did not arrive at the same results. Perhaps these contradictions are due to an observation by Birman, Kantorowitz, and van Steenis [128] that only chlorophylls fluorescent in the presence of light are capable of inhibiting the enzymatic activity in saliva. In any case, it would now appear certain that the great expectations of an almost magic effect on the public when "chlorophyll toothpastes" were first introduced—partly because of the exaggerated publicity—have not been fulfilled. Even so, it is quite possible that chlorophylls, considered objectively and realistically, may still turn out to be useful additives for tooth-cleaning preparations.

**3. Anticaries ingredients.** *Ammonium salts.* The introduction of "ammoniated" toothpastes is another example of exaggerated publicity for a new active ingredient, forgotten a few years later. The basis for the incorporation of ammonium salts in toothpastes was Kesel's [129] discovery that more ammonia developed in the saliva of caries-resistant persons after incubation than in the saliva of persons with caries. Ammonium nitrogen inhibited the activity of acid-forming bacteria such as *lactobacillus acidophilus*. It is easier to introduce ammonium ions into toothpastes in the form of diammonium phosphate, although the salty taste is an objection. On the strength of clinical tests a toothpaste containing 5% diammonium phosphate and 3% urea was patented, produced, and sold on a large scale.

Several investigators are of the opinion that diammonium phosphate is effective only as a buffering agent and that other salts which bring the saliva pH briefly to more than 7.8 have the same effect [130]. Jenkins, Wright, and Miller [131] also established that urea, not ammonium salt, has the strongest bacteriostatic action on lactobacilli and pointed out that in any case the part played by this bacillus in the pathogenesis of caries has not yet been proved. Later tests made it appear doubtful whether ammonium phosphate and urea in toothpastes really have any caries-inhibiting effect at all [132].

*Sodium-N-lauryl sarcosinate* [$CuH_{23}CO$—$N(CH_3)$—$CH_2COONa$]. Starting with the idea that the plaque is the carrier of most enzymes operative in caries formation and that it is also able to bind carbohydrates and acids in proximity to the dental surface, Fosdick [130] searched for substances that would anchor in the plaque and there act as antienzymes. Among 381 compounds tested he found two—sodium-N-lauroyl sarcosinate and sodium dehydroacetate—to be effective and satisfactory in terms of compatibility, nontoxicity, taste, and color. At a later date [133] he published the results of large-scale test series that showed a considerable reduction in the incidence of caries by using a toothpaste containing sodium-N-lauroyl sarcosinate. According to Fosdick, the antienzyme agent remains effective for more than 24 hours and need therefore be used only once a day.

Fosdick's reports as well have not remained free of criticism. He used pH values at the dental surface as a measurement of the effectiveness of the antienzyme agents. Forscher and Hess [134] as well as Brudevold, Little, and Rowley [135] question the value of this method by pointing out that the effectiveness of these substances is apparently not uniform at various locations of the dental surface and that it is already inactivated after two hours just between the teeth where caries most frequently originates.

*Fluorides.* Fluorine dental therapy is based on the discovery that a high resistance against caries was found in persons whose dental enamel is mottled and that their dental tissue has a particularly high fluorine content. Large-scale experiments in the United States and Great Britain in which water-soluble fluorides were added to drinking water in concentrations of 0.5–1.5 : 1,000,000 in certain regions, point to some success in fighting caries in this way. Dabbing the teeth with fluoride solutions has also had some success. The dental tissue is able to take up fluorine from outside by absorption [136] and, as long as it is still growing, also from the bloodstream. This hardens the enamel and makes it less easily soluble in acids.

Dental enamel consists of prisms of hydroxylapatite $Ca_3(PO_4)_2 \cdot Ca(OH)_2$ [137] which are linked by very small amounts of a keratinlike substance. Tests by Perdok [138] have shown that the absorption of fluorine by the enamel leads to a modification of hydroxyl-apatite into fluoroapatite and that this strengthens the linkage between the apatite chains and the keratinic substance from which the enamel acquires a greater mechanical and chemical resistance. The protective effect of fluorine is probably due to the increased acid resistance.

It is possible (but not proved) that through the action of acids part of the fluorine returns into solution as salts, and these fluorides may kill the bacteria that are responsible for the acidic action on teeth, thereby counteracting caries [139]. Based on the fact that fluorides are able to diffuse from outside in dental tissue, tests with fluorides in toothpastes have been carried out; some of these gave excellent results: Muehler, Radike, Nebergall, and Day [140] found a considerably reduced incidence of caries in children between 6–15 after using (over a period of six months) a toothpaste containing 0.1 % fluorine and 0.32 % tin. On the strength of these and similar favorable results, a large American company marketed a tin-fluoride toothpaste in 1955 (141); other manufacturers in the States and other countries followed suit; and at present, fluorides must be considered as the most important caries-inhibiting agents.

*Amino acid derivatives.* Needleman, Fosdick, and Blackman [142] report that various amino acid derivatives, such as phthaloyl phenylananin, inhibit the acid-forming enzymes of the plaque and may therefore be considered as caries prophylactic agents. Among the tested compounds only those with a free carboxyl group were effective.

**4. Calculus-loosening agents.** It has been variously suggested that substances be added to toothpastes that might help to remove calculus (tartar) before it has completely hardened. It is not easy to find substances that will attack tartar without impairing the enamel because they are similar in their chemical composition: tartar consists of 60–65 % calcium phosphate, 8–10 % calcium carbonate, smaller components of other salts (partially water-soluble), and 15–20 % organic substance. The best results achieved so far are a loosening of the tartar by certain additives to the toothpaste which facilitates their subsequent mechanical removal.

Tartar may be attacked in two ways: by dissolving the calcium salts or by degradation or emulsification of its organic components. Acids such as citric or amidosulfonic acids certainly degrade the calcium salts of tartar, but they affect those of the enamel at the same time. This also applies to sequestrants (polyphosphates, trilons, etc., U.S. Patent 2,019,142), and ion exchange resins [143].

Carbon dioxide also has a certain tartar-loosening effect but it is weaker than that of organic acids. According to Holtkamp [144], the effect is due to the conversion $CO_2 + CaCO_3 + H_2O = Ca(HCO_3)_2$. Bicarbonate is more easily water-soluble in an acid environment than carbonate. The oldest so-called tartar-releasing toothpastes contained "Karlsbad salt" (44% $Na_2SO_4$, 2% $K_2SO_4$, 18% NaCl, and 36% $NaHCO_3$) [145] or "Ems salt" (70% $NaHCO_3$, 28.5% NaCl, 1% $K_2SO_4$, 0.5% $Na_2SO_4$) [146]. The action of these salts is probably due to the bicarbonate content that releases carbon dioxide in the dental cavity.

*Sodium sulforicinoleate* [147] belongs to the tartar-releasing substances that affect its organic components. This substance is probably active because it promotes the wetting of the tartar and emulsifies or disperses the organic matter. A toothpaste containing 6% sodiumsulforicinoleate is reported also to reduce the germ count and to inhibit fermentation. Similar favorable results are also reported for unsulfonated sodiumricinoleate [148].

**5. Additives stimulating salivation.** Common salt and other alkaline water soluble salts stimulate the salivary glands. Increased salivation counteracts the accumulation of food residue and bacteria around the teeth and prevents the development of localized high acid concentrations. This effect may be utilized in toothpastes and 10% salt is added. It is questionable, however, whether the stimulation of the salivary glands lasts long enough after brushing the teeth to be of real value. Potassium chlorate also stimulates the salivary glands.

**6. Other special ingredients.** The following ingredients have been suggested for incorporation in toothpastes: substances neutralizing acids (e.g., magnesium hydroxide, sodium bicarbonate), astringents (aluminum salts, drug extracts containing tannic acid), and vitamins. The addition of vitamins to toothpastes is of doubtful value because it is improbable that the gums, if they are at all able to absorb vitamins from the outside, will be able to do so within the short period of contact during tooth cleaning.

Occasionally enzymes which have a protein-dissolving or fermentation-promoting effect are added to dentifrices. It is doubtful whether they are able to develop any effectiveness in the short period of contact.

Some new patents cover additives intended to form a protective film on the dental surface that will oppose the adhesion of food residue, tobacco tar, etc. (silicones [149], nonionic surfactants such as ethylene oxide polypropylene condensation products [150]), or facilitate the subsequent removal of a tar layer (polyvinylpyrrolidone [151]).

**Dental Soaps (Solid and Liquid).** In addition to tooth powders and toothpastes, there are two other types of tooth-cleaning preparation: solid and

liquid dental soaps. Solid dental soaps are milled from a mixture of 50–80 %
abrasives and 20–50 % soap chips. We do not discuss these products in detail
because their use is restricted at present and they do not offer the advantages
of tooth powders or pastes.

Liquid dental soaps consist of aqueous solutions of surfactants with an
addition of thickening agents and possibly other ingredients. They do not
contain abrasives and their action on the dental surface is therefore particularly
mild, which, in the view of some authors, is an important advantage. On the
other hand, their cleansing effect is, of course, much slighter than that of
toothpastes [152].

LIQUID DENTIFRICES

| | 85 | 86 | 87 |
|---|---|---|---|
| Sodium myristyl sulfate | 4 | | |
| Sodium lauryl sulfoacetate | | 3.00 | |
| Tween 20 (Atlas) | | 3.25 | 4.5 |
| G-2160 (Atlas) | | 1.01 | |
| Methylcellulose | 4 | | |
| Alginate | | 1.9 | |
| Gum tragacanth | | | 1.5 |
| Sodium cuprum chlorophyllin | | 0.10 | |
| Sodium lauroyl sarcosinate | | | 1.5 |
| Sodium dehydroacetate | | | 2.03 |
| Saccharin sodium | 0.1 | 0.12 | 0.125 |
| Flavoring | 0.3 | 1.5 | 1.5 |
| Amaranth | | | 0.09 |
| Glycerol | 5 | 11 | 16 |
| Sorbitol syrup (85 %) | | 5 | |
| Alcohol | 10 | 19 | 18.5 |
| Water | 85.4 | 54.12 | 54.225 |

REMARKS

85. Janistyn, *Riechstoffe, Seifen, Kosmetika*, II, p. 288. In Janistyn's formulation part
of the water consists of aromatic lotions (sage, rose, cinnamon water) which is the reason
for the low flavoring content. The preservative is 0.2 % sodium-*p*-oxybenzoic acid isopropyl
ester.

86. Keithler, *The Formulation of Cosmetics and Cosmetic Specialties*, p. 363. The alginate
used is the Seaplant Chemical Corp.'s "SeaKem Type 4." Tween 20 is polyoxyethylene
sorbitan monolaurate. Emulsifying Agent G-2160 is polyoxyethylene propylene glycol
monostearate. (In this product Janistyn's observation that in toothpastes chlorophyll is
inactivated by adsorption to the abrasive does not apply.)

87. Keithler, *op. cit.*, p. 363. This is an example for an "antienzyme" tooth-cleaning
preparation. The red dye is Amaranth.

**The Flavoring of Dentifrices.**   Nothing new can be said in this connection. The user of a dentifrice does not require an original sophisticated flavor but just one that is refreshing and stimulating and leaves the sensation after brushing that the mouth is really clean and freshened [153]. In the United States spearmint oil is the main flavoring ingredient of most toothpastes. In Europe peppermint oil remains the principal component of most dentifrice flavors. Aniseed oil is also an important ingredient of many compounds. Spicy flavors (methyl salicylate, cinnamon oil, clove oil, eucalyptus oil) are popular in the English-speaking countries. The introduction of new special dentifrice flavors has been tried repeatedly but without much success. Fruit flavors proved acceptable only to a certain degree in toothpastes for children. From time to time there have been toothpastes with a whisky flavor, surely the perfect example of an aberration in taste. Needless to say that these trials were unsuccessful. It is certainly true that the quality of the flavor is one of the decisive factors in the success or failure of dentifrices. It is difficult even in strictly controlled tests to establish statistically whether a given product significantly reduces caries and intensity of mouth odors, but every user of a dentifrice can decide without trouble whether he likes a certain flavor.

**The Evaluation of Dentifrices.**   We have already mentioned that tooth powders and pastes are abrasives, and there is a risk that the continued use of these preparations will impair the dental enamel. A good dentifrice should clean and polish the teeth as thoroughly as possible but affect the enamel as little as possible.

To develop such preparations methods are required to measure the abrasive action on dental tissue as well as the gloss of the dental surface. Unfortunately no completely satisfactory methods are available at present.

**1. Measuring the abrasive effect.**   The abrasive action of polishing agents or dentifrices has often been tested on metal plates (copper, silver, or antimony). Several investigators [154] have shown, however, that the test results on metal plates are not comparable with those on teeth. To illustrate this point we list the results established by Wright and Fenske [154] in Table 5-3.

These tests demonstrate that the metal plate test is not very suitable for comparing various substances in their abrasive effect on dental tissue but is certainly useful for comparison of different grades of the same abrasive. Sonder and Schoonhofer [155] evaluate the abrasive effect on newly extracted teeth and the gloss resulting after cleaning the dental surface by direct microscopic examination. This method has the disadvantage that the results cannot be expressed numerically. The so-called interference method by Tekenbroek and Ehrhardt [156] is very interesting because it measures the depth of the grooves that appear after polishing, even if they are very shallow, up to 0.0003 mm. The principle of this method cannot be explained in a few

TABLE 5-3

| Material | Comparative Abrasive Effect on | |
|---|---|---|
| | Teeth† | Antimony Plate |
| Precipitated chalk, USP | 1.00 | 1.00 |
| Ground chalk | 2.16 | 2.72 |
| Magnesium carbonate | 1.48 | 0.94 |
| Magnesium oxide | 1.21 | 5.72 |
| Dicalcium phosphate C.P. | 1.34 | 6.66 |
| Dicalcium phosphate ADR* | 0.76 | 0.39 |
| Tricalcium phosphate USP | 2.28 | 2.47 |
| Tricalcium phosphate, technical | 11.43 | 21.83 |
| Tricalcium phosphate C.P. | 0.91 | 1.78 |
| Tricalcium phosphate ADR* | 0.37 | 0.39 |

* ADR: meeting "Accepted Dental Remedies" specifications, United States, 1939.

† Using newly extracted teeth, the authors determined the reduction of layer thickness of enamel, dentin, and the enamel/dentin intermediary layer and calculated the average abrasive effect from these three values.

sentences and we must therefore refer the reader to the original publication of Tekenbroek and Ehrhardt.

There is a simple test to determine whether a certain abrasive contains small admixtures of a strongly grating substance [157]: a small amount of the test substance is placed on a standard glass slide and rubbed over with a metal disk. The glass slide is rinsed first with warm diluted nitric acid, then with water, and examined microscopically. If the glass is scratched, the material is not suitable for dentifrices. (In a blank test the metal disk without abrasive must, of course, cause no scratches.) This test traced 0.0037% of the finest sand in chalk. Unfortunately glass is not suitable for quantitative measuring of the abrasive effect.

The so-called "crunch" test is even simpler. Take some of the test powder between the front teeth; if there is a crunching sensation when the teeth are ground against each other, this points to coarse admixtures. It is striking how well this primitive test works and that its results are reproducible even if carried out by different persons.

**2. Measuring the polishing effect.** Different metering devices that are able to measure the gloss of the dental surface are now available. The difficulties in measuring gloss physically are due to the lack of accuracy about what is

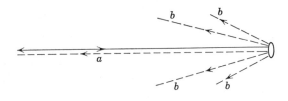

FIGURE 8   LIGHT REFLECTION.

meant by "gloss." It is certainly not the intensity of reflected light because strongly yet diffusely reflecting surfaces are not experienced as glossy. Gloss might rather be defined as the relation between the intensity of direct reflected $a$ or diffuse reflected $b$ rays (see Figure 8). Harry states that the only criterion in comparing the polishing effect of different toothpastes is to have a group of intelligent unbiased people determine whether they can see a difference after using various products.

**3. Measuring the consistency.**   To be successful a toothpaste must have a suitable consistency, quite apart from the requirements of cleaning and not scratching, and the consistency must remain stable for extended periods, even under fluctuating temperatures. To measure the cohesion, a small "ladder" is frequently used in which the distance between individual rungs increases. A band of toothpaste is squeezed from a tube over the whole length of the horizontal ladder. This band remains unbroken over the close rungs, but breaks between the rungs that are farther apart. The greatest distance over which the paste remains intact is the measure of its cohesion.

**4. Shelf-life control.**   Keithler (158) suggests a test at 40–50°C over 10–12 days. Any tendency of the solids to precipitate from the suspension will usually be established under such conditions.

Reactions of the paste with the tube may lead to gas formation that makes the tube swell and even explode. It may also develop localized spotty corrosion, possibly enabling the contents to leak out. If the paste tends to darken because of the presence of iron traces, sequestrants that are able to bind iron may be added. Special products based on ethylene diamine tetra acetic acid are most suitable for this purpose because they do not react with calcium and do not affect the teeth.

The tube should also be checked to determine whether the paste forms a dry crust around the opening if it is exposed to dry air at room temperature.

**Denture Cleaners.**   Similar to natural teeth, dentures may develop plaques and deposits of tartar; food residue may decompose and cause an unpleasant mouth odor and brown spots may develop from heavy smoking. If dentures are not adequately cleaned, it may lead to an inflammation of the gingivae underneath.

Dentures are cleaned by placing them overnight (or for at least 30 minutes) in a glass of water containing a special cleansing agent. These cleansers usually consist of the following substances or groups of substances:

1. Chemically active substances that degrade the organic components of plaque and tartar (mostly oxidizing agents such as sodium hypochlorite, sodium perborate, and urea peroxide).

2. Surfactants that facilitate the wetting of the denture and the impurities on it and contribute to their removal (for this purpose all surfactants with good cleansing properties even in low concentrations are suitable).

3. Disinfectants (here, as well, there is a wide range available; oxidants themselves have a certain disinfectant effect).

4. Flavors (as with tooth pastes) and possibly dyes.

These preparations also often contain common salt which acts as a filler and promotes the precipitation and removal of proteins in the impurities. Alkaline salts (trisodium phosphate, sodium carbonate, etc.) support the action of surfactants.

Special ingredients are occasionally incorporated; for example, protein-degrading enzymes (but they are quickly inactivated in solution if they are combined with strong oxidizing agents), chlorophyll derivatives, etc. If an organic acid is used with sodium carbonate, the preparation that results is effervescent.

Denture cleaners are always marketed as dry powders or tablets. It is important that they remain dry till they are used because otherwise they may become unattractive and lose their effectiveness. They should also dissolve quickly in water and give clear solutions.


## CLEANSING OF THE NAILS

Because of the unique conditions and problems involved in the use of nail cleansers (usually described as lacquer removers), these preparations deviate considerably from the composition of skin and hair-cleansing preparations. There is only one type of "soil" they have to remove: nail lacquer. The surface to be cleaned (the nails) is smooth and highly resistant to chemical action. In contrast to hair-cleansing agents which might equally well be described as scalp-cleaning preparations, lacquer removers hardly come in contact with the surrounding skin.

Fundamentally, all lacquer removers consist of substances that dissolve nail lacquer. The solvents should not be too volatile or they would evaporate during application. They must not irritate the skin surrounding the nails. A nail lacquer remover should not leave nails fatty or sticky nor should it have a strong degreasing effect that would make the nails brittle. It should have no unpleasant or obtrusive odor.

## Raw Materials

**Solvents.** *Acetone* has an unpleasant odor and strong degreasing action but is nevertheless an important ingredient of many lacquer removers because it dissolves it more easily and quickly than nearly all other solvents. Slightly higher molecular ketones, for example, methyl ethyl ketone, are also used.

*Ethyl acetate, ethyl butyrate* and many similar low molecular aliphatic esters are less degreasing but do not dissolve the lacquer so easily; they also have a particularly obtrusive odor. On the other hand, the *esters of dibasic acids*, for example, dibutyl phthalate and dioctyl adipate, are odorless or have only a very faint odor. They are quite frequently used in modern nail-lacquer removers. *Liquid alkyl esters of higher acids*, for example, butyl stearate, isopropyl myristate, are also used occasionally. They are not very volatile and almost odorless.

*Butyl, propyl,* and *amyl alcohols* may also be used as additional solvents.

*Monoalkyl ethers of dihydric alcohols*, for example, methyl and ethyl ethers of ethylene glycol and monoethylether of diethylene glycol (Carbitol), are also suitable. They are good solvents that are odorless and not too volatile.

**Fatting Agents.** Most lacquer solvents have a strong drying effect and in order to avoid it some fat is usually added to the remover. Vegetable oils, lanolin and lanolin derivatives, fatty alcohols, etc., are suitable additives for this purpose.

**Perfume.** If a lacquer remover contains large amounts of acetone or low molecular aliphatic esters, it is difficult to mask the obtrusive odor of the solvents. The easiest way to overcome this problem consists in adding considerable quantities (about 10%) of inexpensive volatile fragrances (orange oil terpenes, terpineol etc.) which also act as solvents.

## Preparation

The mutual solubility of solvents and fats permits the preparation of clear solutions without any difficulty. The only manufacturing problem is caused by the volatility and combustibility of the solvents; good ventilation and caution with open flames are essential.

SOME FORMULATIONS FOR NAIL LACQUER REMOVERS

|  | 88 | 89 | 90 | 91 | 92 | 93 |
|---|---|---|---|---|---|---|
| Acetone | 19 | 35 |  |  | 5 |  |
| Methyl isobutyl ketone |  |  |  | 80 |  |  |
| Ethyl acetate | 40 | 28.5 |  |  | 40 |  |
| Butyl acetate |  |  | 10 |  |  | 15 |
| Amyl acetate |  |  |  |  | 5 |  |
| Ethylene glycol diacetate |  |  |  | 10 |  |  |
| Dibutyl phthalate |  | 15 |  |  |  |  |
| Isopropyl myristate | 5 |  |  |  |  |  |
| Butyl stearate |  |  |  |  | 5 |  |
| Isobutyl stearate |  |  |  | 10 |  |  |
| Industrial ethyl alcohol 95% |  |  |  |  | 40 |  |
| Diethylene glycol monoethyl ether | 35 |  | 85 |  |  |  |
| Ethylene glycol monoethyl ether |  | 15 |  |  |  | 80 |
| Propylene glycol ricinoleate |  |  |  |  |  | 5 |
| Lanolin | 1 |  |  |  |  |  |
| Olive oil |  | 6.5 |  |  |  |  |
| Castor oil |  |  |  |  | 5 |  |
| Oleic alcohol |  |  |  | 5 |  |  |
| Perfume |  |  |  |  | 1 |  |

REMARKS

88. Keithler, *The Formulation of Cosmetics and Cosmetic Specialties*, p. 445. Heat and dissolve the lanolin in isopropyl myristate. Cool the solution, add ethyl acetate, diethylene glycol monoethyl ether, and acetone in this order.

89. Keithler, *ibid.*, 445.

90, 91. Janistyn, *Riechstoffe, Seifen, Kosmetika*, II, p. 241.

92. K. Rothemann, *Das grosse Rezeptbuch der Haut- und Körperpflegemittel*, 3rd ed., p. 730.

93. M. G. De Navarre, *The Chemistry and Manufacture of Cosmetics*, p. 578.

# REFERENCES

[1] Neis, *Aesth. Med.*, **11**, 347 (1962).

[2] *Aesth. Med.*, **13**, 343 (1964).

[3] *Parfum. Kosmet.*, **37**, 253, 305 (1956).

[4] *Parfum. Kosmet.*, **39**, 25 (1958).

[5] Stüpel and Szakall, *Die Wirkung von Waschmitteln auf die Haut*, Dr. A. Hüthig Verlag, Heidelberg, 1957.

[6] *Aesth. Med.*, **12**, 146 (1963).

[7] *Fette Seifen*, **52**, 3, 171 (1950); **53**, 285, 399 (1951).

[8] Vermeer, De Jong, and Lenstra, *Dermatologica*, **108**, 88 (1954).

[9] *J. Am. pharm. Ass.*, **29**, 251, 254 (1940).

[10] *Kolloid Zeitschrift.*, **117**, 42 (1950).

[11] Czetsch-Lindenwald and Schmidt-La Baume, *Salben, Puder, Externa*, 3rd ed., p. 457 et seq.

[12] *J. gen. Physiol.*, **24**, 399 (1941).

[13] Jones and Mecham, *Archs. Biochem.*, **3**, 193 (1943).

[14] *J. invest. Derm.*, **21**, 199 (1955).

[15] *Brit. J. Derm.*, **67**, 1 (1955).

[16] *Fette Seifen*, **55**, 178 (1953); Nelson, *Am. Perfumer*, **75** (3), 32 (March 1960).

[17] *Arch. Gewerbepath. Gewerbehyg.*, **9**, 276 (1938).

[18] Stüpel, *Chem. Z.*, **77**, 756 (1953).

[19] *Fette Seifen*, **44**, 298 (1937).

[20] *J. Am. pharm. Ass.*, **29**, 251, 254 (1940).

[21] Lane and Blank, *Archs. Derm. Syph.*, **56**, 419 (1947).

[22] Czetsch-Lindenwald and Schmidt-La Baume, *Die äusseren Heilmittel*, 1950–1955, p. 118.

[23] *J. invest. Derm.*, **4**, 69 (1941).

[24] *Parfum. Kosmet.*, **37**, 125 (1956).

[25] *Parfum. Kosmet.*, **37**, 305 (1956).

[26] Burckhardt, *Dermatologica*, **81**, 3 (1940).

[27] Greither and Kleinschmitt, *Fette Seifen*, **54**, 272 (1952).

[28] Ruf, *Parfum. Kosmet.*, **37**, 305 (1956).

[29] Schwartz, U.S. Public Health Repts., **56**, 1788 (1941); Lane and Blank, *Archs. Derm. Syph.*, **43**, 435 (1941); **44**, 999 (1941).

[30] *Soap chem. Spec.*, 49 (December 1957).

[31] Stüpel, *Chem. Z.*, **77**, 756 (1953).

[32] *Fette Seifen*, **53**, 552 (1951).

[33] See [31].

[34] *J. Am. pharm. Ass.*, **29**, 251, 254 (1940).

[35] *Fette Seifen Anstrichmittel* **61**, 965 (1959); **65**, 958 (1963).

[36a] Personal communication, Dr. H. Bober.

[36b] *Arch. Derm. Syph. Vienna*, **158**, 290 (1929).

[37] Swanson, *J. Am. med. Ass.*, in *Int. Perfumer*, **6** (11), 4 (1956).

[38] Bergwein, *Kosmetik-Parf-Drog.*, 56 (1955).

[39] *Dt. med. Wschr.* 91 (1949).

[40] *Zblt. Hautkrkh.*, **7**, 9, 333 (1949).

[41] *Berufsdermatosen*, **3**, 14 (1955).

[42] *Ind. Med.*, **17**, 421 (1948).

[43] *Chem. Z.*, **77**, 782 (1953).

[44] *SÖFW*, **83**, 99 (1957).

[45] Janistyn, *Riechstoffe, Seifen, Kosmetika*, II, Hüthig Verlag, Heidelberg, 1950, p. 80.

[46] German Patents DRP 565–461, 686,906, 745,637.

[47] Willems, *Parfum. Kosmet.*, **37**, 590 (1956) et seq.

[48] *SÖFW*, **82**, 569 (1956); U. S. Patent 2,875,153 (Colgate Palmolive); *Schimmel Briefs*, **296** (November 1959).

[49] *J. Am. med. Ass.*, in *Int. Perfumer*, **6** (11), 4.

[50] Snell, *Ind. Engng. Chem.*, **48**, 38A (1956).

[51] Mannek, *SÖFW*, **83**, 330 et seq., 556 et seq. (1957); Hiller, *SÖFW*, **84**, 29, 55 (1958).

[52] DWP 1902, Kl. 23e.

[53] French Patent 884,561.

[54] German Patent DRP 743,942.

[55] Snell, *loc. cit.*

[56] *SÖFW*, **82**, 581 (1956).

[57] Franz, *SÖFW*, **82**, 664 (1956).

[58] Schuster, *SÖFW*, **83**, 51 (1957).

[59] See [57].

[60] *Am. Perfumer*, **76** (11), 37 (1961).

[61] Harry, *Modern Cosmetocology*, 4th ed., Leonard Hill, London, 1955, p. 127.

[62] *Ibid.*, 118.

[63] de Navarre, *The Chemistry and Manufacture of Cosmetics*, 1st ed., Van Nostrand, Princeton, New Jersey, 214–215.

[64] Rothemann, *Das grosse Rezeptbuch der Haut- und Körperpflegemittel*, 3rd ed., Hüthig Verlag, Heidelberg, 1962, p. 514.

[65] Lohmann, *SÖFW*, **84**, 154 (1958).

[66] Sidi, *Verträglichkeit der Kosmetika*, p. 70.

[67] *Proc. scient. Sect.* Toilet Goods Ass., 1 (May 1952).

[68] Martin, Draize, and Kelley, *Drug Cosmet. Ind.*, **91**, 30 (1962), *Proc. scient. Sect.* Toilet Goods Ass., **37**, 2 (1962).

[69] Scholz, *Aesth. Med.*, **12**, 343 (1963); Kay and Calandra, *J. Soc. cosmet. Chem.*, **13**, 281 (1962); Russell and Hoch, *Proc. scient. Sect.* Toilet Goods Ass., **37**, 27 (1962); Batista and McSweeney, *J Soc. cosmet. Chem.*, **16**, 119 (1965).

[70] Barnett and Powers, *Drug Cosmet. Ind.*, **78**, 174 (1956); Powers, *ibid.*, **79**, 616, 768 (1956).

[71] Treon, *Proc. scient. Sect.* Toilet Goods Ass., **40**, 40 (1963).

[72] See [68].

[73] *J. Soc. cosmet. Chem.*, **1**, 335 (1949).

[74] Gaunt and Harper, *J. Soc. cosmet. Chem.*, **15**, 209 (1964).

[75] *Schimmel Briefs*, **260** (November 1956).

[76] *Drug Cosmet. Ind.*, **78**, 819 (1956).

[77] *SÖFW*, **78**, 619 (1953).

[78] Freese and Andersen, *Am. Perfumer*, **71**, 37 (March 1956).

[79] *Schimmel Briefs*, **270** (September 1957); Mannheimer, *Am. Perfumer*, **72** (4), 69 (1958).

[80] Mannek, *SÖFW*, **82**, 649 (1956); Hoffmann, *SÖFW*, **83**, 691, 720 (1957).

[81] Kroll and Lennon, *Drug Cosmet. Ind.*, **79,** 186 (1956).

[82] *Drug Cosmet. Ind.*, **78,** 239 (1956).

[83] Kroll and Lennon, *loc. cit.*

[84] Willems, *Parfum. Kosmet.*, **37,** 590 (1956) et seq.; Walker, *SÖFW*, **82,** 699 (1957).

[85] Hoch and Russell, *Proc. scient. Sect.* Toilet Goods Ass., **38,** p. 51 (1962).

[86] U. S. Patent 1,094,336, Colgate Palmolive Co.; *Schimmel Briefs*, **253** (April 1956); *Schimmel Briefs*, **274** (1958); *Parfum. Kosmet.*, **39,** 233 (1958); *Kosmetik-Parf-Drog.*, **5,** 7 (1958).

[87] Bryce and Smart, *J. Soc. cosmet. Chem.*, **16,** 187 (1965).

[88] Rothemann, *op. cit.*, 484; Janistyn, *op. cit.*, II, 122.

[89] *Schimmel Briefs*, **248.**

[90] *Drug Cosmet. Ind.*, **78,** 322 (1956).

[91] British Patent 674,896, Marchon Products Ltd.

[92] *Chem. Courant*, **55,** 225 (1956).

[93] Harry, *op. cit.*, 431.

[94] Willems, *Parfum. Kosmet.*, **38** (January 1957).

[95] Schwartz and Knowles, *J. Soc. cosmet. Chem.*, **14,** 455 (1963).

[96] Thomson, *Am. Perfumer*, **75** (4), 41 (April 1960).

[97] Bullied, *Br. dent. J.*; Citron, *J. dent. Res.*, **24,** 87 (1945). a.o.

[98] Kluczka, *Zahnärztl. Welt*, **111** 105 (1951).

[99] *Zahnärztl. Welt*, 357 (1948).

[100] *Ibid.*, 1948, p. 2.

[101] *J. Am. dent. Ass.*, **36,** 3 (1948).

[102] *Dent. Cosmos*, **33,** 689, 789, 913 (1891).

[103] Shohl, "Mineral Metabolism," in Harry, *op. cit.*, 289.

[104] Willems, *Parfum. Kosmet.*, **37,**790 (1956).

[105] Harry, *op. cit.*, 289.

[106] Jenkins, Wright, and Miller, *Nature*, **164,** 606 (1950).

[107] *J. Am. dent. Ass.*, **24,** 1889 (1937).

[108] *Am. Perfumer*, **63,** 33 (January 1948).

[109] Lammers, *Fette Seifen AnstMittel*, **63,** 628 (1961).

[110] Janistyn, *op. cit.*, II, 294.

[111] *J. med. Kosmetik*, **12,** 341 (1956).

[112] Harry, *op. cit.*, 305.

[113] Tainter, *Proc. scient. Sect.* Toilet Goods Ass. (January 26, 1944).

[114] *J. med. Kosmetik*, **12,** 341 (1956).

[115] Harry, *op. cit.*, 322.

[116] Vossnacker, *Dt. dent. Z.*, **6,** 233 (1952).

[117] *Pharm. J.*, **11,** 600 (1953); *J. Am. med. Ass.*, **5,** 445 (1937).

[118] Harry, *op. cit.*, 321.

[119] Zander, *J. Am. dent. Ass.*, **40,** 569 (1950).

[120] Report of Council on Dental Therapeutics of American Dental Association, in *Drug Cosmet. Ind.*, **71,** 517 (November 1952).

[121] *Am. J. Surg.*, **49**, 49 (1940).

[122] Czetsch-Lindenwald, *Apotheker-ztg.*, **93**, 24 (1953).

[123] *N.Y. St. J. Med.*, **50**, 698 (1950).

[124] Hafer, *Apotheker-ztg.*, **96**, 392 (1956).

[125] Janistyn, *Parfum. Kosmet.*, **34**, 289 (1953).

[126] *Profilassi Cari dentale*, First Intern. Symposium (1955).

[127] *J. Soc. cosmet. Chem.*, **3**, 1 (March 1952).

[128] Birman, Kantorowitz, and van Steenis, *Meded. Medinos-Prodent-Res.*, **14** (1956).

[129] *J. dent. Res.*, **27**, 44 (1948).

[130] *J. dent. Res.*, **32**, 486 (1953).

[131] Jenkins, Wright, and Miller, *Nature*, **164**, 606 (1950); Lammers, *Dt. zahnärztl. Z.*, **13**, 6 (1950).

[132] Davies and King, *J. dent. Res.* (October 1951).

[133] Bull. Northwestern Univ. Med. School Dent. Res., **54**, 3 (1953); *Am. Perfumer*, **71**, 50 (August 1956).

[134] *J. Am. dent. Ass.*, **48**, 201 (1954).

[135] *Ibid.*, **50**, 18 (1955).

[136] Volker and Volker, *J. biol. Chem.*, **134**, 543 (1940).

[137] Thewlis, *The Structure of Teeth as Shown by X-ray Examination*, London, 1940.

[138] Perdok, *Meded. Medinos-Prodent-Res.*, **11**, 1952.

[139] Haldwick, *Br. dent. J.*, **114**, 222 (1963).

[140] *J. dent. Res.*, **33**, 606 (1954).

[141] *Chem. Engng. News*, **1022**, 4797 (1955).

[142] Convention of American Chemical Society, New York, 1957; *Chem. Engng. News*, **35**, 63 (September 23, 1957).

[143] British Patent 332,142 and German Pat. 378,010.

[144] *Dt. dent. Wsch.*, 421 (1943).

[145] Hermann, in Bauer and Klawik, *SÖFW*, **83**, 273 (1957).

[146] Rosenthal and Heymann, *Zahnärztl. Rdsch.*, **34**, 265 (1925).

[147] Urbantschitsch, *Wien. med. Wschr.*, 1343 (1932).

[148] Mead, *J. dent. Res.*, **16**, 41 (1937); Harry, *Cosmetic Materials*, London, 1948, p. 305.

[149] British Patent 686,429.

[150] Swiss Patent 295,246.

[151] French Patent 1,075,782.

[152] Manly, *J. dent. Res.*, **6**, 479 (1943).

[153] Jellinek, *Die psychologischen Grundlagen der Parfümerie*, 2nd ed., Hüthig Verlag, Heidelberg, 1965, pp. 46, 178.

[154] Wright and Fenske, *J. Am. dent. Ass.*, **24**, 1889 (1937); Epstein, *J. Am. dent. Ass.*, **31**, 400 (1944); Tainter, *Proc. scient. Sect. Toilet Goods Ass.*, 27 (January 26, 1944).

[155] *J. Am. dent. Ass.*, **30**, 1725 (1943); **31**, 1579 (1944).

[156] *Tijdschr. Tandheelk.* (December 1947).

[157] Sonder and Schoonhover, *J. Am. dent. Ass.*, **24**, 1817 (1937).

[158] De Navarre, *op. cit.*, 216 et seq.

[159] *Am. Perfumer*, 60 (June 1956).

# CHAPTER 6

# Deodorant and Anti-Perspirant Preparations

## BODY DEODORANTS

In Chapter 5 we pointed out that the first and most essential requirement of personal hygiene is cleanliness. To this may be added another, equally important: the suppression of body odor. The ancients, and, in particular, the Romans, who made a cult of hygiene, were just as conscious of the second as they were of the first. In seventeenth-century France (in which hygiene had not been greatly developed) people of means used large quantities of toilet water whenever body odor became too obtrusive and at least succeeded in masking the unpleasant odor with another more pleasing. Although this is not a particularly elegant solution to the problem from a scientific-cosmetic point of view, it is of historic significance because the lotions of modern times are based on the toilet waters of the seventeenth century which were applied for the same purpose as today's deodorants. If preparations that do not just mask body odor but reduce its intensity considerably are now known, it is because of the knowledge acquired of the physiology of sweat and the development of body odor. We discuss these points before enlarging on modern preparations.

## PHYSIOLOGY OF SWEAT [1]

Humans lose moisture through the skin in two forms: *perspiratio insensibilis*, that is, the *unnoticeable* evaporation of vapor through the skin; *noticeable sweating*, that is, the excretion of an aqueous fluid through the sweat glands. Both forms are physiologically important, but from a cosmetic point of view we are interested only in *noticeable* perspiration. The main purpose of this physiological function is probably the regulation of temperature. In addition, part of the lactic acid that develops during muscular activity is excreted with sweat. The sweat glands of palms and soles keep these skin areas constantly moist and thus facilitate grasping and walking.

An adult human has about 2 million sweat glands which are divided into two groups: eccrine and apocrine [2].

Eccrine glands occur all over the body, with the exception of the edges of the lips and parts of the sexual organs. The glands lie in the corium, from which fine coiled tabules lead to the skin surface and end in funnellike orifices with a diameter of less than 0.03 mm. These glands secrete a clear acid (pH 4.0–6.8) fluid with the following average composition [3]:

| | |
|---|---|
| Water | 99.0200 % |
| Sodium chloride | 0.7000 % |
| Acetic acid | 0.0096 % |
| Propionic acid | 0.0062 % |
| Caprylic and capronic acids | 0.0046 % |
| Lactic acid | 0.1000 % |
| Citric acid | 0.0400 % |
| Ascorbic acid | 0.0400 % |
| Urea and uric acid | traces |

The composition of sweat may actually vary within a rather wide range. It depends on the diet, on muscular activity or inactivity during perspiration, and many other factors. Robinson and Robinson have published a survey of data regarding the composition of sweat [4]. Traces of potassium, calcium, magnesium, iron, copper, manganese, carbonate, phosphate, sulfide, iodide, bromide, fluoride, succinic acid, glutaric acid, various amino acids and vitamins of the B group, and the enzyme alkaline phosphatase have been found [5].

The apocrine glands are larger than the eccrine and usually do not terminate at the skin surface but in the hair follicles. They occur only in a few locations of the body: the axillae, around the nipples and the navel, and in the ano-genital area. They develop in puberty, are more numerous in females than in males, and may be regarded as secondary sexual characteristics.

It may be that in an earlier stage of human development (and perhaps unconsciously, even today) these glands served the purpose of stimulating sexual attraction through the odor developing from sweat [6].

The secretion of the apocrine glands is cloudy because apart from the constituents found in eccrine sweat it contains fat and cellular fragments. The content of nitrogenous compounds is higher than in eccrine sweat. Bacterial decomposition of apocrine sweat therefore soon results in an alkaline reaction which results from formation of ammonia and amines.

Fresh perspiration has a very faint and not unpleasant odor. The character-istic odor of perspiration develops only after bacteria have acted on apocrine sweat. In the main it must be attributed to the presence of fatty acids ($C_4$–$C_{10}$, butyric to capric acid), ammonia and amines, mercaptans, and other sulfurous substances derived from the degradation of sulfurous proteins. The experiments of Killian and Panzarella [7] show that the action of bacteria is really of great importance. A mixture of eccrine and apocrine sweat develops an unpleasant odor if it is left standing for some time. If fresh perspiration is immediately filtered so that the bacteria are eliminated, this odor does not develop. Shehaden and Kligman [8] proved that axillary odor is due to the effect of gram-positive and not gram-negative bacteria. That the odor arises from apocrine and not eccrine sweat is also demonstrated by the test results of Shelly, Hurley, and Nichols [9]. It is also well known that the typical perspiration odor does not occur in children before puberty, that is, before the maturing of apocrine glands.

## PRINCIPLE OF EFFECTIVENESS

Based on the fact that unpleasant body odors are caused by the effect of bacteria on apocrine sweat, five methods may be formulated to reduce or prevent them.

1. Perspiration may be inhibited. The activity of the sweat glands is regulated by the central nervous system. Certain drugs (e.g., atropin and its analogs [10]), if taken orally, affect the central nervous system in such a way that the activity of the sweat glands is restricted. All the substances known at present carry the risk of undesirable side effects and, at least for the time being, this method should not be considered.

According to Zupko [11], these substances are locally effective if they are incorporated in an unguent base and applied externally and are not the cause of side effects. In this form the anticholinergic drugs (Banthine, Probanthine, Prantal, etc.) may offer interesting possibilities.

2. Perspiration may be prevented from reaching the skin surface. This method might sound dangerous, since it must lead to sweat congestion within the ducts. Actually the antiperspirant substances used in cosmetics do act in this way. Microscopically noticeable inflammatory symptoms may indeed occur [12] and in rare instances there are some incompatibility effects, but most people use these preparations without ill effect. The low incidence of complications is probably due to the sweat flow being only partly stilled and to the activity of the sweat glands presumably stopping as soon as there is congestion in the ducts.

3. Perspiration may be removed on reaching the skin surface. This method

belongs to the subject "skin cleanliness" and has already been fully discussed in Chapter 5.

4. The bacterial decomposition of sweat may be prevented by removing, killing, or inhibiting the growth of the responsible bacteria; most body deodorants act in this way.

5. The substances responsible for the unpleasant odor of perspiration may be destroyed immediately after they have developed or their evaporation may be prevented so that their odor cannot be noticed.

6. A further method, already mentioned, consists of masking unpleasant body odors with pleasant ones. This method is no longer used by itself, but the fresh fragrance of modern deodorants probably plays its part in the masking effect.

## Active Ingredients

In the following section we discuss the most widely used ingredients and some less fully explored developments and also deal with the question whether these substances act along the lines of method 2, 4, or 5.

**Aluminum Salts.** The salts most frequently used today are aluminum salts of strong acids (aluminum chloride, sulfate, phenolsulfate, sulfamate [13]), complex salts such as aluminum hydroxychloride $[Al_2(OH)_5Cl]$ [14], sodium aluminum chlorohydroxy lactate $[Na_3Al_2(OH)_5Cl(CH_3CHOHCOO)_3]$ [15], and aluminum alcoholate chloride $[Al(OR)Cl_2, Al(OR)_2Cl, Al_2(OR)_5Cl]$ [16]. Aluminum alcoholates are also suitable in deodorants [17].

Alums, for example, potassium alum, $AlK(S_4O)_2 \cdot 12H_2O$, are now rarely being used. The aluminum salts of weak acids (aluminum acetate, lactate, etc.) themselves lack strong antiperspirant action but are used in combination with other ingredients.

One difficulty in using the aluminum salts of strong acids is the highly acidic reaction (pH 1.5–4) of their aqueous solutions. This may lead to skin irritations and damage to fabrics, particularly linens and cotton. Various attempts have been made to overcome these difficulties by adding buffering agents of different types (basic aluminum formate, acetamide, urea, etc.) [18]. Aluminum salts of weak acids and complex salts in aqueous solution do not show the same strongly acid reaction and therefore do not damage clothes.

It is widely believed today that aluminum salts act (at least in part) by preventing perspiration from reaching the skin surface. Experiments by Killian [19], Brun and Manuila [20], Richardson and Meigs [21], Hopf et al. [22] all point in this direction even if there are certain contradictions in details. If we accept that aluminum salts stem the flow of perspiration to the skin surface, a further question arises: how is this effect achieved?

One hypothesis that has many adherents assumes that aluminum salts precipitate skin proteins at the mouths of the sweat ducts and in this way block them. The protein-precipitating effect of aluminum salts is generally known [23]. However, an observation by Brun and Manuila [24] that other protein-precipitating substances such as tannin and sulfosalicylic acid have no sweat-inhibiting effect seems to contradict this hypothesis.

Sulzberger and co-workers [25], on examining skin areas that had been treated with aluminum salts in solution, could find no blocking of sweat-duct mouths. Whenever sweat secretion had been reduced, however, they found microscopically visible inflammations.

In explaining these results, the authors emphasize the significance of the electrical potential of the skin in the physiology of sweating. The charge at the edge of the sweat duct ostia is normally negative, which can be shown by selective coloring with certain dyes. Sulzberger assumes that an intraductal potential gradient is responsible for the outward movement of the sweat from the glands to the skin surface. Treatment of the skin with substances that have an electropositive reaction with cellular tissue should cancel the potential and therefore impede the outpouring of sweat. Such substances (cationic surfactants, electrolytes like lithium rhodanide, lithium salicylate, and lithium, sodium, and potassium iodides) did indeed have a certain sweat-inhibiting effect, often accompanied by skin eruptions. Aluminum salts may also tend to cause a positive charge on the skin surface through the triple positive charge of the cation and their antiperspirant effect might be explained in this way.

Apart from their sweat-impeding action, aluminum salts also have a considerable antibacterial effect [26] which contributes to the prevention of body odor. The (acid) solutions of aluminum salts also bind ammonia and amines in the form of nonvolatile and consequently odorless salts. It follows that aluminum salts act in three ways: they impede the flow of sweat from the glands to the skin surface, they kill some of the bacteria that are responsible for the decomposition of sweat, and they bind certain malodorous substances that are liberated through the decomposition of sweat.

Occasionally a fourth method of effectiveness is mentioned in some publications: aluminum salts may constrict blood capillaries and in this way reduce the secretion of the sweat glands. This hypothesis is hard to substantiate by experiments.

**Zirconium Salts.** The use of zirconium oxide, hydroxide, and certain zirconium salts in antiperspirant and deodorant powders had already been patented by Weiss in 1911 [27], but it is only within the last decade that zirconium salts have been used more extensively in cosmetics.

One zirconium salt that is mentioned in a number of publications is sodium zirconium lactate. According to Kalish [28], this salt has a deodorant effect

PRINCIPLE OF EFFECTIVENESS

in neutral or weakly alkaline solution (pH 6.5–10.5), probably by forming nonvolatile complexes with various organic compounds (e.g., fatty acids and amines) [29].

According to a British patent [30], antiperspirant preparations can be made with sodium zirconium lactate (and/or another relatively water-soluble zirconium salt such as sodium zirconium glyconate or gluconate) in combination with one or several relatively insoluble salts (from the group zirconium lactate, glyconate, and gluconate); the recommended pH for these preparations is 2.5–5.5.

Zirconium salts may also be used in combination with aluminum salts. U. S. Patent 2,734,847 covers the use of sodium zirconium lactate and related salts in combination with aluminum salts. It is reported that the antiperspirant effect of this combination is superior to that of aluminum salts only, whereas skin irritation and the attack on fabric is less frequent. A similar report is given by Helton, Daley, and Erwin [31] about 50/50 mixtures of zirconium oxychloride and aluminum oxychloride at pH 4.0.

These authors also report that zirconium oxychloride has only very slight oral toxicity and, on the basis of very limited experience, claim better skin compatibility in patch tests than most other commercially available antiperspirants. Reports by Weber and co-workers [32] and Rubin and co-workers [33] suggest that zirconium salts are not tolerated by everybody [34].

**Salts of Rare Earths.** Tests by Christian and co-workers [35] show that sulfamates and methionates of various rare earths (Lanthanum, Cerium, etc.) are suitable ingredients for antiperspirants. Lanthanum and cerium salts are actually even more effective than the corresponding zinc and aluminum salts.

**Cationic Surfactants.** Quaternary ammonium salts are efficient disinfectants and create a deodorant effect by reducing or preventing the bacterial decomposition of sweat (see Chapter 3). In addition, they act as antiperspirants according to Sulzberger's hypothesis [36] by neutralizing the negative charge at the mouth of sweat ducts. They deserve to be used more extensively in cosmetic practice than they have been up to now.

**Other Disinfectants.** Hexachlorophene is probably the most widely used ingredient in this group, but all other bactericides mentioned in Chapter 3, and in particular those that have proved satisfactory in soaps, may be used. Substances with good adhesion to the skin are especially suitable because their action lasts longer and one daily application is sufficient.

Antibiotics occupy a special place in this category, but most of them cannot be used in cosmetics for reasons previously discussed (see Chapter 3).

According to Baker [37], Tyrothricin and the related, still more active Gramicidin, Neomycin, and Bacitracin may well be suited to cosmetic application,
either free or in the form of certain derivatives. Ferguson [38] found that 3 %
Chlorotetracyclin or Neomycin in creams can suppress axillary odor. Shelley
and Cahn [39] report good results with Neomycinsulfate (0.35 % in creams or
liquid preparations).

In spite of Baker's arguments, the opinion prevails today that it is not
advisable to use antibiotics in deodorants so long as there are other effective
substances with less inherent risks.

**Chlorophyll.**   Around 1950, after the deodorant effect of chlorophyll on
malodorous wounds had become generally known [40], expectations ran high
regarding results to be achieved with these substances in the cosmetic field.
Chlorophyll derivatives were found to reduce the odor of diallyl sulfide,
garlic extract, or mercaptans in direct contact *in vitro* [41] and to possess a
bacteriostatic and inhibiting effect on certain enzymes in the putrefaction
process. Hafer [42] and Birman, Kantorowitz, and van Steenis [43], however,
could establish an antienzyme effect only for fluorescent chlorophyll derivatives in the presence of light. Westcott [44], and Montgomery and
Nachtigall [45] reported a remarkable effect of chlorophyll, namely, that
certain chlorophyll fractions taken orally reduce or eliminate axillary perspiration odor. In the years after 1950 a number of investigators tried to substantiate these reports experimentally [46] but none of them could confirm
them.

As far as localized external application of chlorophyll derivatives is concerned, Barail [47] reports that if concentrations are high enough to be
effective they leave green stains on clothes. For this reason chlorophyll
derivatives cannot be considered suitable for body deodorants in spite of the
great stir they caused initially.

**Enzyme Inhibitors.**   The  inhibiting  effect  on  fermentation  enzymes
claimed for chlorophyll cannot be utilized for cosmetic practice; nevertheless,
the idea of looking for substances that would not entirely destroy the
microflora of the skin but only suppress the action of the enzymes responsible
for these undesirable processes is certainly worth pursuing. Starting from this
basis, Rosenberg and Konzales [48] investigated the sweat-inhibiting effect of
malonates. As a matter of fact, considerable activity of the enzyme succinic
acid-dehydrase had been observed in the ducts of active eccrine sweat glands,
and this activity was known to be suppressed by the salts of malonic acid. It
was subsequently established that malonates have an antiperspirant effect
which is at least equal to that of aluminum salts. Metal chelates of $\beta$-
dicarbonyl compounds also block the enzymatic decomposition of proteins
in sweat [49].

**Ion Exchange Resins.** In 1952 Thurmon and Ottenstein [50] reported that certain ion exchange resins were able to absorb lactic acid, ammonia, and urea from sweat *in vitro*. Based on Thurmon's investigations, a patent was developed [51] to cover the use of cation exchange resins with water-soluble aluminum salts of organic acids in a hydrophilic base as an antiperspirant and deodorant. In such a preparation the aluminum salt inhibits the flow of sweat to the skin surface (alone these salts are rather weak, but the presence of ion exchange resins is supposed to strengthen their effectiveness); the ion exchange resin then binds the malodorous sweat constituents and regulates the acidity of the treated skin area. The patent claims that this preparation is highly effective without being irritating or affecting fabrics [52].

Ikai [53] tested various ion exchange resins for their deodorant effect. According to his results, both cation and anion exchange resins have a certain deodorant effect, but a combination of both types works best.

The effectiveness of ion exchange resins is mainly due to the binding of volatile substances that cause the odor of perspiration. (According to the claims made in Thurmon's patent, certain cation exchange resins absorb amino acids from sweat and thus prevent their bacterial decomposition.) In themselves these resins do not affect the intensity of sweating nor the bacterial count on the treated skin area.

## Preparations

Deodorants are commercially available as liquid preparations, sticks, creams, jellies, powders, soaps, and aerosols. We have already dealt with deodorant soaps (Chapters 3 and 5) and now discuss the other preparations.

**Liquids.** Liquid body deodorants, marketed in polyethylene spray bottles, are the most uncomplicated products in this group as far as formulation and preparation is concerned. In principle, they may consist of an aqueous solution of an aluminum salt. Their effectiveness is due mainly to their content of aluminum salts. Occasionally bactericides are also added, either alone or in combination with aluminum salts.

The solvent is usually not water but diluted alcohol, which is a better solvent for perfumes. It has a better wetting effect on the skin, evaporates faster (so that it is less likely to run off) and, if the concentration is sufficiently high, has a disinfectant property of its own. Small additions of glycerol or propylene glycol counteract the drying effect of such lotions on the skin. If aluminum salts of strong acids are used, buffering agents are often added to act as protectives for skin and textiles (see formula 2). [British Patent 967,591 (Colgate-Palmolive) covers the use of nitrogenous substances such as N(lauroylcholamino-formyl-methyl)pyridinium chloride as fabric-protecting additives in antiperspirants.] An addition of film-forming substances intended to make the antiperspirant salt adhere to the treated skin area has been mentioned in certain patents (see formula 4).

Deodorants are also available as pads (absorbent fabric soaked in liquid deodorant) but this form is not very popular. Another presentation is the roll-on type. The slightly viscous preparation is packed in a bottle with a ball inserted in the neck (about 1 in. in diameter). This ball rolls as it is applied to the skin, thereby constantly depositing certain quantities of the preparation, in what amounts to the same principle as that of a ballpoint pen. To make this method work, the consistency of the preparation must be carefully adjusted.

|                                  | 1    | 2   | 3   | 4   | 5   | 6      |
|----------------------------------|------|-----|-----|-----|-----|--------|
| Aluminum chloride                | 15   | 15  |     |     |     |        |
| Aluminum phenol sulfate          |      |     | 10  |     |     |        |
| Aluminum sulfate                 |      |     |     | 4   |     |        |
| Sodium zirconium lactate         |      |     |     |     | 15  |        |
| Alkyl dimethyl benzyl ammonium chloride |  |  |     |     |     | 0.0002 |
| Urea                             |      | 5   |     |     |     |        |
| Polyacrylic acid (25%)           |      |     |     | 24  |     |        |
| Glycerol                         | 3    |     |     |     | 5   | 3      |
| Propylene glycol                 |      |     | 7.5 |     |     |        |
| Alcohol 95%                      |      |     | 60  | 40  | 20  | 7      |
| Water                            | 81.5 | 80  | 21  | 32  | 60  | 90     |
| Perfume                          | 0.5  |     | 1.5 |     |     |        |

REMARKS

1. Chilson, *Modern Cosmetics*, 1934, p. 170. A very simple aqueous lotion.

2. Klarmann, *Drug Cosm. Ind.*, **81,** 178 (1957). Similar to (1) but with a buffering agent added.

3. Klarmann, *ibid.*, 176. Example of an alcoholic lotion.

4. *Drug Cosmet. Ind.*, **80,** 804 (1957). On drying, polyacrylic acid forms a water-resistant film that can easily be removed with water and soap. A 25% aqueous solution of polyacrylic acid is marketed by B. F. Goodrich under the trade name "K-702 Solution." The aluminum salt content of this formulation (4%) is very low; it is restricted by the solubility of the salt in about 60% alcohol.

5. Kalish, *Drug Cosmet. Ind.*, **78,** 763 (1955).

6. Keithler, *The Formulation of Cosmetics and Cosmetic Specialties*, p. 391. *Drug Cosm. Ind.* 1957.

**Sticks.** Some time ago sticks were the most popular form of applying deodorants: they are compact and handy. The product does not run off (as in lotions) nor leave greasy stains on clothes (as in creams). Some consumers, however, object to the unavoidable friction during application.

|  | 7 | 8 | 9 |
|---|---|---|---|
| Hexachlorophene | 0.25 | | 0.25 |
| NaAl-chlorohydroxy lactate (40%) | | 50 | |
| Stearic acid | 22.00 | | 22.00 |
| Potassium hydroxide | 1.00 | | 1.00 |
| Sodium stearate | | 6 | |
| Glycerol | 1.00 | | |
| Propylene glycol | | 3 | |
| Sodium alginate | | | 0.75 |
| Alcohol 95% | 71.25 | 42 | |
| Water | 4.00 | | 72.60 |
| Isopropylmyristate | | | 3.00 |
| Cetyl alcohol | | | 0.05 |
| Perfume | 0.50 | q.s. | 0.25 |
| Preservative | | | 0.10 |

REMARKS

7. Keithler, *The Formulation of Cosmetics and Cosmetic Specialties*, Drug Cosm. Ind. 1957 p. 385. Alcohol and hexachlorophene are mixed in a container with reflux condensor and heated to 60°C. Add glycerol, then potassium hydroxide dissolved in water. Stir the mixture for one minute, add the stearic acid heated to 85°C, and stir for another two minutes. The temperature of the mixture should be about 80°C. A sample of the mass should have a pH value of 9.2–9.6. If the pH is too low, potassium hydroxide is added; if it is too high, it can be adjusted by adding a small amount of salicylic acid. When the correct pH value is reached, perfume is added and the product poured into molds.

8. Kalish, *Drug Cosmet. Ind.*, **79**, 318 (1956). Propylene glycol may be replaced by glycerol and 6 pts sodium stearate by 5.25 pts stearic acid and 0.75 pts sodium hydroxide (dissolved in 2 pts water). The procedure is not given but it could be as follows: alcohol and propylene glycol are heated at the reflux condenser almost to the boiling point. Sodium stearate is added in small portions and the mixture heated until total solution. Cool slightly, add the heated solution of the aluminum complex salt, stir well, perfume, and pour into molds.

9. Keithler, *op. cit.*, 385. Dissolve the potassium hydroxide in the minimum quantity of water. Prepare a mucilage from the remaining water and sodium alginate, heat it to 75°C, and stir in the potassium lye. Add this mixture with vigorous stirring to the fat melt (75°C) in which the hexachlorophene has been dissolved. Stir until the emulsion has cooled to 50°C, perfume, and pour into molds.

In composition sticks closely resemble alcoholic lotions. An addition of alkali stearate gives the product a solid form. In most available deodorant sticks the active ingredient is a bactericide such as hexachlorophene (see formula 7). Initially, aluminum salts could not be used in sticks because they are effective only in acid solutions, whereas alkali stearates remain stable only in neutral or alkaline environment.

The introduction of a complex salt such as sodium aluminum chloro-hydroxy lactate, which is also effective in an alkaline environment, opened up new possibilities (see formula 8). Aluminum alcoholates may be added to alkaline preparations.

Descriptions of deodorant sticks of a nonalcoholic type can be found in various publications (based on petrolatum and cocoa butter or solid emulsions; see formula 9) but they have almost disappeared from the market. They are always slightly sticky and are made unattractive by adhering impurities or hair. Their preparation is complicated because it is difficult to give them a smooth and attractive shape; moreover, they usually do not retain their shape because they are too soft.

**Creams.**    Although deodorant creams with low or no water content at all are mentioned in the literature, the only form that has proved widely acceptable is the washable O/W type. Glycerol monostearate with an acid-resistant emulsifying agent (sodium laurylsulfate, etc.) has proved particularly satisfactory as a base. Alkali stearate creams are ruled out if the active ingredient is an aluminum salt which is effective only in an acid environment. According to Sulzberger [54], anionic surfactants promote perspiration. It may well happen therefore that a cream will be less effective than a lotion with the same concentration of identical ingredients.

Creams containing a phenolic bactericide should not be prepared with nonionic emulsifiers belonging to the polyoxyethylene condensation products group because they reduce the effectiveness of the bactericide (see Chapter 4).

REMARKS

10. Klarmann, *Drug Cosmet. Ind.*, **81**, 176 (1957).

11. French Patent 1,096,011 (Colgate-Palmolive, 1955), in *Schimmel Briefs*, **254** (May 1956). Glyceryl monostearate, spermaceti, mineral oil, and preservative (propyl-*p*-hydroxy-benzoate) are heated together to 85°C. The emulsifying agent (monoglyceride monosulfate) dissolved in 31.25 pts water (85°C) is stirred in.

The emulsion is heated to 91–93°C and polypropylene glycol and titanium dioxide are stirred in. The mixture is cooled with constant stirring to 43°C and a solution of aluminum sulfamate and urea in 22 pts water, as well as the perfume oil, is added. At 38°C the emulsion is passed through a colloid mill. According to this French patent, glycerol monostearate emulsions with a high content of astringent salts are not very stable and polypropylene glycol is intended to increase stability.

12. Formulation of Atlas Chemical. Melt stearic acid, wax, mineral oil, and the emulsifying agents together (70°C), stir in the solution of preservative in water (85°C), cool to

| | 10 | 11 | 12 | 13 |
|---|---|---|---|---|
| Mineral oil | | 0.7 | 1 | |
| Paraffin wax (light) | | | | 13.5 |
| Spermaceti | 5 | 4 | | |
| Beeswax | | | 2 | |
| Cetyl alcohol | | | | 13.5 |
| Glyceryl monostearate (acid resistant) | 20 | 13 | | |
| Stearic acid | | | 14 | |
| Turkey red oil | 5 | | | |
| Na-Salt of monosulfated coconut fatty acid monoglycerides | | 2.5 | | |
| Sodium lauryl sulfate | | | | 0.54 |
| Polyoxyethylene stearate (Myrj 52) | | | 5 | |
| Polyoxyethylene oxypropylene stearate (Atlas G 6162) | | | 5 | |
| Aluminum sulfate | 25 | | | |
| Aluminum sulfamate | | 18 | | |
| Aluminum chlorohydrate | | | 22 | |
| Aluminum phenol sulfate | | | | 13.5 |
| Cation-exchange resin, powdered | | | | 22.5 |
| Urea | | 5 | | |
| Polypropylene glycol 2025 | | 2.5 | | |
| Titanium dioxide | | 0.8 | | |
| Water | 42 | 53.25 | 51 | 20.0 |
| Ethyl alcohol 95% | | | | 9.0 |
| Glycerol | 3 | | | |
| Propylene glycol | | | | 6.5 |
| Perfume | q.s. | 0.15 | q.s. | |
| Preservative | q.s. | 0.1 | q.s. | 0.27 |

35°C with constant stirring, and add aluminum chlorohydrate. Continue stirring until the salt is completely dissolved, add perfume, and fill jars.

13. German Patent 955,092 (Thurmon for Roehm & Haas). Dissolve aluminum phenolsulfate in alcohol. Mix this solution and the finely powdered cation exchange resin (metacrylic acid divinylbenzene copolymer) with the completed emulsion of the other ingredients. The preservative is a mixture of equal parts of methyl- and propyl-p-hydroxybenzoate.

**Jellies.** According to *Schimmel Briefs*, **245** (1955), an addition of borax or boric acid to aqueous solutions of aluminum oxychloride results in gellike product in which the aluminum salt has retained its full effectiveness. An addition of ethyl alcohol prevents such products from becoming too soft at higher temperatures, and additions of glycerol or propylene glycol protect them from hardening at low temperatures.

**Powders.** Astringent powders have never been so popular as liquid preparations, creams, and sticks, although theoretically they are not inferior to the other products. They may not be so easy to apply. Strongly absorbent substances such as colloidal kaolin are useful because they absorb excessive perspiration.

|                          | 14 | 15 | 16 |
|--------------------------|----|----|----|
| Sodium aluminum sulfate  | 2  |    |    |
| Sodium zirconium lactate | 5  |    |    |
| Salicylic acid           | 5  |    |    |
| Boric acid               | 5  |    |    |
| Chloramin                |    |    | 1  |
| Colloidal kaolin         |    | 15 | 30 |
| Zinc oxide               |    |    | 14 |
| Talcum                   | 78 | 50 | 40 |
| Corn starch              | 10 |    |    |
| Calcium carbonate        |    | 25 |    |
| Magnesium carbonate      |    |    | 5  |
| Zinc stearate            |    | 5  |    |
| Magnesium stearate       |    |    | 10 |

REMARKS

14. Klarmann, *Drug Cosmet. Ind.*, **81**, 176 (1957).
15. Kalish, *ibid.*, **78**, 763 (1955).
16. Janistyn, *Riechstoffe-Seifen-Kosmetika*, II, Hüthig Verlag, Heidelberg, 1950, p. 233.

**Aerosols.** Technically speaking, it is possible to present liquid, cream, and powder deodorants in aerosol form.

If aluminum salts are to be added to such preparations, a number of technical problems arise: aluminum salts are completely insoluble in propellants and tend to precipitate. Moreover, the acid reaction of the solutions gives rise to more or less serious corrosion problems. Valuable data on the solubility of aluminum chloride, aluminum chlorohydrate, and aluminum sulfate in aerosol systems and the extent of corrosion in different metal containers appear in "Freon" Bulletin No. 2 (p. 688 ff), prepared by E. I. Du Pont de Nemours. Glass and plastic containers with valves without any metal parts are probably best suited to products of this kind.

Published formulations for aerosol deodorants are based mostly on disinfectants because of the difficulties of incorporating aluminum salts. Here are some examples:

| 17. | Isopropyl myristate | 2.20 |
| | Silicone 555 | 0.06 |
| | Lanogene | 0.06 |
| | PVP-VA (70–30), 50% | 0.32 |
| | Hexachlorophene | 0.06 |
| | Perfume oil | 0.10 |
| | Isopropyl alcohol | 7.20 |
| | Freon 12 | 18.00 |
| | Freon 114 | 72.00 |
| | | 100.00 |

Formulation of Sun-Lac Inc. PVP-VA is a copolymer of polyvinylpyrrolidone and vinyl acetate in proportion 70:30 (weight).

| 18. | Isopropyl myristate | 0.20 |
| | Dipropylene glycol | 4.50 |
| | Actamer | 0.25 |
| | Perfume oil | 0.50 |
| | Ethyl alcohol 95% | 44.55 |
| | Propellant | 50.00 |
| | | 100.00 |

Formulation of Dodge & Olcott ("The Aerosol Story," p. 34). No details are given about the propellants or their characteristics. The vapor pressure of the preparation is given as 21 psi.

| 18a. | Aluminum chlorohydrate | 3.5 |
| | Distilled water | 3.5 |
| | Isopropyl myristate | 0.7 |
| | Dipropylene glycol | 3.1 |
| | Tartaric acid | 0.35 |
| | Hexachlorophene | 0.2 |
| | Perfume oil | 0.35 |
| | Ethyl alcohol 100% | 58.3 |
| | Freon 12/114 (40:60) | 30.0 |
| | | 100.00 |

di Giacomo, *Am. Perfumer*, **70** (5), 45 (1957).

| 18b. | Aluminum hydroxychloride | 15.0 |
| | Water | 17.0 |
| | Denatured anhydrous ethyl alcohol | 60.0 |
| | Tween 80 (Atlas Chemical Co.) | 2.0 |
| | Arlacel 80 (Atlas Chemical Co.) | 1.3 |
| | Freon 12 | 4.7 |
| | | 100.00 |

M. J. Root, *Am. Perfumer*, **71** (6), 63 (1958). Pressure-filling essential. Propellant-in-ingredient emulsion.

18c.   Aluminum chlorohydrate        12.5 ⎫
       Water                         12.5 ⎬ A

       Emcol 14 (Emulsol Corp.)       2.5 ⎫
       Glyceryl monostearate          2.5 ⎬ B
       Isopropyl myristate            1.0 ⎭
       Freon 12/114 (15:85)          69.0
                                    ——————
                                    100.00

Root, *Am. Perfumer*, **71** (6), 63 (1958). Add A to B and finally the propellant (pressure filling). Active ingredient-in-propellant emulsion.

## EVALUATION

### Effectiveness.

The testing method selected depends on the effectiveness required of the particular preparation. In antiperspirants the reduction of perspiration intensity must be measured. Laboratory tests *in vitro* (e.g., determining protein precipitation) are unreliable, and animal or human experiments are necessary. Sweat secretion can be made visible at the duct mouths by painting the skin with a diluted alcoholic iodine solution and dusting it with powdered starch after drying. Wherever water is secreted through the sweat ducts, the iodine-starch reaction will cause a violet spot on the skin [55]. Takahashi and Wada [56] describe another method in which powdered starch is replaced by a plastic foil coated with starch; this can be pulled off the skin and preserved. Another test consists in painting the skin with a diluted alcoholic solution of ferric chloride and dusted with tannic acid. Where water is exuded dark spots appear [57]. Perspiration beads can also be made visible through the reversible color changes of a silver-mercury iodide complex salt [58].

Methods determining the quantity of secreted sweat at a defined body area are more complicated. Such methods have been described, for example, by Killian [59], Richardson and Meigs [60], Hopf [61], and Fredell and Read [62].

If the deodorant action of a preparation is due to the inhibition or destruction of bacteria, the testing method must determine the germ count in the axillary fossae before and after using the preparation. For details of this method the reader is referred to professional publications [63]. The test may be carried out, for example, by having the test subjects wear patches in the axillae, treating one and leaving the other untreated. After a definite period the patches are removed and the bacteria transferred to an agar agar culture medium where count and species may be determined. Alternatively, one hair each from the treated and untreated axillae may be examined for its resident bacteria [64]. Finally, the prime function of body deodorants, their odor-preventing action, must be tested.

Initial tests may be made *in vitro* by letting the test product act on solutions of fatty acids (butyric, caproic, etc.), ammonia and amines, mercaptans, and onion juice or by treating isolated human sweat. Ultimately, only the *in vivo* test will be decisive.

In the matter of judging the intensity of odor we still know only one instrument: the human nose. The final test in many absolutely serious evaluations of body deodorants consists in smelling the treated and untreated axillae of the testees and comparing the odor [65]. Several authors have described "osmometers": these are instruments intended to eliminate certain sources of error inherent in direct olfactory tests and to define the measurements quantitatively by establishing the minimum concentration that can be discerned [66]. The most suitable osmometer appears to be that devised by Barail [67], but the instrument that registers the odor still remains the human nose. Recent developments of gas chromatography promise an objective instrumentalized measurement of axillary odor in the near future.

## Skin Compatibility

There is a very real risk, particularly with antiperspirants, of skin irritations. Impeding the flow of sweat from the sweat glands to the skin surface is, after all, quite a radical interruption of a natural function. The production and flow of sebum are also affected, since sebum and sweat are physiologically closely related [68].

In people who perspire heavily the corneal layer in the axillary fossae may be swollen by constant moisture and the alkaline reaction of degraded sweat, and consequently have little chemical resistance so that preparations tolerated by other persons or by other skin areas may cause lesions. This applies not only to antiperspirants but to deodorants as well.

There is another, indirect risk connected with the use of these preparations: by preventing axillary odor they may cause the user to neglect washing these parts of the body properly. Because the deodorant is applied daily, it would accumulate (possibly be partly decomposed) and, although it would be tolerated in normal usage, might in the circumstances still cause lesions. Practical experience has shown that, without too much difficulty, antiperspirants and deodorants that are tolerated by most people can be formulated. Nevertheless, all products must be carefully tested before they are marketed.

## Fabric Compatibility

Preparations with an aluminum salt of a strong acid as the active ingredient may have a damaging effect on textiles, particularly linen, cotton, and viscose rayon. This effect is related to their acid reaction and may be reduced by adding certain buffering agents. The most damaging situation for the fabric (ironing without previous washing) probably does not occur very often in practice, but even normal use may weaken fabrics under the arms to such an extent that they will rot after a comparatively short time. Bien [69] published a detailed study of the effect of antiperspirants on fabric in which he also describes a method to determine the textile-corroding effect of newly developed preparations.

## Shelf Life

Body deodorants based on aluminum salts are generally rather complicated products. There is a risk of precipitation in liquid preparations: aluminum salts if the alcohol concentration is too high, perfume and other organic components if it is too low. In creams certain constituents may decompose and endanger the stability of the emulsion. According to one patent [70], glycerol monostearate is not very stable, but this is easily explained, since it is an ester. Metal containers may corrode (creams in lead or tin tubes and aerosol preparations). Unless the perfume has been especially composed for acid antiperspirants, the acid reaction always presents a risk for all types of preparation. Very careful storage tests are therefore indicated for all these products.

## OTHER DEODORANTS

The purpose of the preparations discussed so far in this chapter is to check the odor originating in the axillary fossae. In addition, there are preparations that check the development of unpleasant odors in other parts of the body: foot deodorants, mouthwashes, and preparations for feminine hygiene. We do not discuss the latter because they do not belong to the realm of cosmetics. We shall, however, briefly discuss foot deodorants and mouthwashes.

## Foot Deodorants

In his book *Modern Cosmetocology* [71] Harry observes, justifiably, how surprising it is that podiatry has been so generally neglected. Although feet are supplied with innumerable sweat glands (in similar density found only on the palms), they are first enclosed in socks or stockings and then in nearly impermeable shoes. Sweat accumulates and its organic components provide an almost perfect culture medium (35°C and a high moisture content!) for all kinds of microorganisms. The decomposition of sweat makes the environment inside the shoe alkaline and promotes the growth of two germs responsible for the development of malodorous degradation products, *bact. graveolens* and *bact. foetidum* [72]. Socks and stockings are changed regularly but bacteria remain in the shoes and clean socks and stockings are immediately reinfected.

The most suitable and most widely used form of disinfectant and deodorant foot preparations is powder. These preparations act not only as disinfectants and deodorants but also through their absorbent properties. They may be used for the treatment of the feet as well as shoes.

Here are some suggested formulations:

|  | 19 | 20 | 21 | 22 |
|---|---|---|---|---|
| Thymol | 1 | | | |
| Phenol | | | 0.5 | |
| Dichlorophene | | | 3.2 | |
| Disinfectant | | | | 0.5 |
| Boric acid | 10 | 20 | | 5.0 |
| Alum, powdered | | 20 | | |
| Zinc oxide | 20 | | 5.3 | |
| Kieselgur, extra | | 20 | | |
| Talcum | 69 | 20 | 58.8 | 93.0 |
| Precipitated chalk | | 20 | | |
| Magnesium carbonate | | | 16.5 | |
| Zinc stearate | | | 9.1 | |
| Polyethylene glycol 400 | | | | 1.0 |
| Menthol | | | 0.6 | |
| Perfume oil | | | | 0.5 |
| Alcohol | | | 6.0 | |
| Propellant | | | | 900.0 |
|  | 100 | 100 | 100.0 | 1000.0 |

REMARKS

19. Lehmann, in Harry, *Modern Cosmetocology*, 4th ed., Leonard Hill, London, 1955 p. 582. During World War II this powder was adopted by the U. S. Army. The high talcum content provides a good slip. Zinc oxide has a mild astringent effect (antiperspirant). Boric acid, a disinfectant that also attacks the alkaline reaction inside the shoes, is a widely used ingredient in foot powders.

20. Janistyn, *Riechstoffe-Seifen-Kosmetika*, II, 219. The high alum content has a sweat-inhibiting effect; diatomaceous earth is absorbent, boric acid a disinfectant.

21. Keithler, *The Formulation of Cosmetics and Cosmetic Specialties*, p. 461. Menthol and dichlorophene are dissolved in alcohol, and this solution is mixed with magnesium carbonate. After 24 hours the "impregnated" magnesium carbonate is passed through a large sieve and mixed with the other ingredients. Dichlorophene is particularly active against fungi. Menthol has a cooling effect. Zinc stearate imparts better adhesion to the powder.

22. Dodge & Olcott, "The Aerosol Story," p. 33. An aerosol powder. Mix talcum and boric acid thoroughly. The perfume is first mixed with a small amount of the powder and constantly increasing quantities of powder are then added. The disinfectant (according to manufacturers' choice) is incorporated in a similar manner. The powder is poured into aerosol containers and the propellant finally added. No mention is made of the propellants used—only that pressure in the container should be about 30 psi. Polyethylene glycol provides better skin adhesion to the preparation.

Lotions and creams have also been suggested for foot deodorants but in our opinion are not so effective as powders. Orbocki [73] suggests the following aerosol foot deodorant:

| | | |
|---|---|---|
| 23. | Bactericide | 1.0% |
| | Perfume oil | 0.5% |
| | Isopropyl alcohol | 28.5% |
| | Freon 11/12(50:50) | 70.0% |

## Mouthwashes

It may seem arbitrary to discuss toothpastes and mouthwashes in different chapters: toothpastes as cleansing preparations and mouth washes as deodorants. As a matter of fact, all toothpastes and tooth powders also act as deodorants: they assist in the removal of food residues which, when decomposed, cause mouth odor; they are effective in removing oral bacteria and, if they also contain bactericides, they contribute toward inhibiting bacterial activity. With their fresh fragrance they mask unpleasant odors. On the other hand, the cleansing effect achieved by the use of mouthwashes should not be underestimated; even rinsing with water alone removes water-soluble or loose deposits from the oral cavity and the surface of teeth.

If, nevertheless, we discuss toothpastes and mouthwashes in different chapters, we do so because the main active ingredients in toothpastes (quantitatively in any case) are polishing agents or substances that remove impurities, whereas in mouth washes disinfectants and fragrances play the most important part. Although their functions overlap those of dentifrices, mouthwashes certainly have their own raison d'être: they reach not only dental surfaces but the entire oral cavity. Their use is also much easier (no toothbrush required, no splashing of the face) and there is therefore more opportunity to use them also during the day, after meals.

The most important active ingredients in mouthwashes are the following:

1. *Flavors.* Peppermint oil, menthol, aniseed oil, anethole, fennel, eucalyptus, clove, and cinnamon oil, and methyl salicylate. Some flavors (fennel and clove oils and some others) also act as disinfectants. Usually saccharin or some other sweetening agent is added, but not sugar.

2. *Disinfectants.* Salicylic acid, quaternary ammonium compounds (these must be used very cautiously because in higher concentrations they are toxic and irritate the mucosa), oxyquinolinsulfate, thymol, and p-chloro-m-cresol.

Some authors believe that there is no point in using disinfectants in mouthwashes because of their strong dilution and the short period of contact. In our opinion this is not correct because many disinfectants are known to be absorbed by oral mucosa and can therefore continue to act for some considerable time after the mouth is rinsed. The situation here is more favorable than with the use of disinfectants in soaps because little or no surfactant need be present in mouthwashes. Bactericides in mouthwashes are not, after all, intended to sterilize the oral cavity completely but only to impede bacterial activity or possibly cause partial destruction of oral bacteria.

3. *Drug Extracts.* If these extracts are rich in tannins (e.g., tinctures of myrrh or cinchona), they act as astringents and stimulants. With their bitter taste they are also occasionally flavor components. Sometimes tinctures (e.g., benzoic tincture) are used to give the diluted preparation a milky appearance. The solvent is mostly ethyl alcohol, sufficiently concentrated to give a clear solution of the active ingredients. In recent publications there has also been mention of formulations with little or no alcohol in which a solubilizer such as Tween 20 is responsible for a clear solution of flavors and bactericides. In our opinion such formulations are not so favorable. If an alcoholic mouthwash is diluted with water just before use, flavor and disinfectants precipitate, a desirable effect because they adhere all the better to the oral cavity and their action is prolonged. If solubilizers are used, all ingredients remain dispersed in water and precipitate in the mouth to a smaller degree. If, moreover, surfactants of the polyoxyethylene condensation type are used, care must be taken that they do not form complexes with phenolic disinfectants and inactivate them.

Small amounts of surfactants are occasionally added to mouthwashes that are not intended to act as solubilizers but as wetting agents; they increase the detergent effect of the preparation.

Mouthwashes are often colored with vegetable dyes (saffron, carmine, phloxine, erythrosine) which have no effect on the action itself.

Here are some suggested formulations:

24. Essential oils                         7
    Triethanolamine lauryl sulfate         3
    Tincture of rhatany                    2
    Alcohol 80%                           88
                                         ———
                                         100

Janistyn, *Riechstoffe, Seifen, Kosmetika*, II, p. 282. Tincture of rhatany acts as an astringent and a red dye. According to Janistyn, the purpose of the surfactant here is the fine dispersion of the essential oils when diluted with water; a milky emulsion develops. With no emulsifier the essential oils would separate in large drops that would irritate lips and mucosa. A compromise must be found between complete insolubility and complete solubilization of flavors and active ingredients when the solution is diluted for use.

25. Benzoic acid                         1.0
    Cetyl triethylammonium bromide       0.5
    Resorcinol                           1.0
    Thymol                               0.1
    Methyl salicylate                    0.4
    Eucalyptol                           0.2
    Menthol                              0.1
    Alcohol                             21.0
    Water                               75.7
                                       ———
                                       100.0

Keithler, *The Formulation of Cosmetics and Cosmetic Specialties*, p. 367. To avoid clouding in such preparations with low alcohol content the best procedure is to dissolve the water-soluble ingredients (in this instance ammonium salt and benzoic acid) in water, the others in alcohol, and then to mix the two solutions. This mixture is left to mature for a few days at least and cooled to about 5°C; after 24 hours the clear liquid is pumped off from above and filtered. The remaining liquid with the sediment may be filtered separately.

26. Tincture of myrrh        1.5 ml
    Benzoic tincture         1.0 ml
    Tincture of iris         1.0 ml
    Flavor                   7.5 ml
    Saccharin sodium         3   gr
    Alcohol 96%             71.5 ml
    Water                   25   ml
                           ———
                           100   ml

Rothemann, *Das grosse Rezeptbuch der Haut- und Körperpflegemittel*, 3rd ed., Hüthig Verlag, Heidelberg, 1962, p. 741. A mouthwash without specific disinfectants.

## REFERENCES

[1] Fiedler, *Der Schweiss*, Editio Cantor, Aulendorf i. Wuertt., 1955; Reller, *J. Soc. cosmet. Chem.*, **15**, 99 (1964).

[2] Montagna, *J. Soc. Cosmet. Chem.*, **14**, 641 (1963); Dobson, *ibid.*, **14**, 619 (1963).

[3] Peck, Rosenfeld, Leifer, and Biermann, *Archs. Derm. Syph.*, **39**, 126 (1939).

[4] Robinson and Robinson, *Physiol. Rev.*, **34**, 202 (1954).

[5] Loewenthal and Politzer, *Nature (London)*, **195**, 902 (1962).

[6] Jellinek, *Die physiologischen Grundlagen der Parfümerie*, Hüthig Verlag, Heidelberg 2nd ed. 1965. p. 33, 52.

[7] *Proc. scient. Sect. Toilet Goods Ass.*, **7**, 3 (1947).

[8] *J. invest. Derm.*, **40**, 61 (1963); Meyer-Rohn, *Aesth. Med.*, **13**, 247 (1964).

[9] *Archs. Derm. Syph.*, **68**, 430 (1953).

[10] Klarmann, *Kosmetik-Parf-Drog.*, **4**, 165 (1957); **5**, 12 (1958).

[11] *Am. J. Pharm.*, **126**, 194 (1954).

[12] Sulzberger, Hermann, Keller, and Pisha, *J. invest. Derm.* **14**, 91 (1951).

[13] U. S. Patent 2,736,683, Colgate Palmolive Co.

[14] Govett and Rubino, *Am. Perfumer*, **70**, 21 (April 1955).

[15] De Navarre, *Am. Perfumer*, **71**, 25 (August 1956); Kalish, *Drug Cosmet. Ind.*, **79**, 318 (1956).

[16] German Patent DBP 1,005,690. *Schimmel Briefs*, **218** (May 1958).

[17] German Patent Anm. R 16212/30 h.

[18] Klarmann, *Drug Cosmet. Ind.*, **81**, 177 (1957).

[19] *J. Soc. cosmet. Chem.*, **3**, 20 (1952).

[20] *Dermatologica*, **104**, 267 (1952).

[21] *J. Soc. cosmet. Chem.*, **3**, 308 (1951).

[22] *J. med. Kosmetik*, **1**, 6 (1955).

[23] Govett and De Navarre, *Am. Perfumer*, **51**, 365 (1947; Christian and Jenkins, *J. Am. pharm. Ass.*, Sci. Ed., **39**, 663 (1950).

[24] *Dermatologica*, **100**, 304 (1950); **104**, 267 (1952).

[25] *Archs. Derm. Syph.*, **60**, 404 (1949); *J. invest. Derm.*, **14**, 91 (1950).

[26] Blank, Moreland, and Dawes, *Proc. scient. Sect. Toilet Goods Ass.*, **27**, 24 (1957); Meyer and Vischer, *Archs. Surg.*, **47**, 468 (1943); Klarmann, *Drug Cosmet. Ind.*, **81**, 246 (1957).

[27] German Patent 237,624.

[28] *Drug Cosmet. Ind.*, **78**, 763 (1955).

[29] U. S. Patent 2,498,514 (1950).

[30] British Patent 735,681 (1955); U. S. Patent 2,790,747 (1957).

[31] *Drug Cosmet. Ind.*, **80**, 170 (1957).

[32] *J. Am. med. Ass.*, **165**, 65 (1956).

[33] *Ibid.*, **165**, 953 (1956).

[34] *Schimmel Briefs*, **279** (1958).

[35] Collins and Christian, *J. Am. pharm. Ass.*, **47**, 25 (1958); Mantsavinos and Christian, *ibid.*, **47**, 29 (1958).

[36] Sulzberger, Hermann, Keller, and Pisha, *J. invest. Derm.*, **14**, 91 (1950).

[37] *Drug Cosmet. Ind.*, **80**, 458 (1957).

[38] *J. invest. Derm.*, **24**, 567 (1955).

[39] *J. Am. med. Ass.*, **159**, 1736 (1955); Shehaden and Kligman, *J. invest. Derm.*, **40**, 61 (1963).

[40] Gruskin, *Am. J. Surg.*, **49**, 49 (1940); Bowers, *ibid.*, **73**, 37 (1947).

[41] Killian, *J. Soc. cosmet. Chem.*, **3**, 20 (1952); Mitchell, *Soap, Perfum. Cosm.*, **24**, 1235 (1951); Westcott, *N.Y. St. J. Med.*, **50**, 698 (1950).

[42] Hafer, *Apotheker-ztg.*, **96**, 392 (1956).

[43] Birman, Kantorowitz, and van Steenis, *Meded. Medinos-Prodent Res.*, **14** (1956).

[44] *N.Y. St. J. Med.*, **50**, 689 (1950).

[45] *Postgrad. Med.*, **8**, 401 (1950).

[46] Killian, *J. Soc. Cosmet. Chem.*, **3**, 20 (1952); Shelley, Hurley, and Nichols, *Archs. Derm. Syph.*, **68**, 430 (1953); Brocklehurst, *Br. med. J.*, **1**, 541 (1953); Hopf, *J. med. Kosmet.* **1**, 6 (1955).

[47] *J. Soc. cosmet. Chem.*, **4**, 1 (1953).

[48] *J. invest. Derm.*, **29**, 251 (1957).

[49] Kellner, *Aesth. Med.*, **13**, 251 (1964).

[50] *J. invest. Derm.*, **18**, 333 (1952).

[51] U. S. Patent 2,653,902 (1953); German Patent DBP 955,092 (1956).

[52] *Am. Perfumer*, **76** (9), 30 (1961).

[53] *J. invest. Derm.*, **23**, 411 (1954).

[54] *J. invest. Derm.*, **14**, 91 (1950).

[55] Kuno, *The Physiology of Human Perspiration*, London, 1934, p. 30.

[56] Takahashi and Wada, *J. invest. Derm.*, **38**, 197 (1962).

[57] Silverman and Powell, *War Med.*, **7**, 178 (1945).

[58] J. Sivadjian, *Parfum. Kosmet.*, **46**, 162 (1965).

[59] *J. Soc. Cosmet. Chem.*, **3**, 20 (1951).

[60] *Ibid.*, **3**, 308 (1951).

[61] *J. med. Kosmet.*, **1**, 6 (1955).

[62] *Drug Cosmet. Ind.*, **79**, 468 (1956).

[63] Pillsbury and Nichols, *J. invest. Derm.*, **7**, 365 (1946); Killian, *op. cit.* [46]; Blank, Moreland, and Dawes, *op. cit.* [26].

[64] Shelley, Hurley, and Nichols, *J. invest. Derm.*, **20**, 285 (1953).

[65] Gee and Seidenberg, *Soap chem. Spec.*, **30**, 42 (1954).

[66] Moncrieff, *The Chemical Senses*, London, 1951, p. 108 et seq.

[67] Barail, *J. Soc. cosmet. Chem.*, **2**, 14 (1950).

[68] Sulzberger, *Perfum. essent. Oil Rec.*, **46**, 379 (1955).

[69] *Proc. scient. Sect. Toilet Goods Ass.*, **4**, 8 (1945); *J. Soc. cosmet. Chem.*, **1**, 2 (1947).

[70] French Patent 1,096,011; *Parfum. Kosmet.*, **37**, 379 (1956).

[71] Harry, *Modern Cosmetocology*, 4th ed., Leonard Hill, London, 1955 Chapter 33.

[72] Marchionini and Cerutti, *Arch. Derm. Syph.*, **166**, 354 (1932).

[73] *SÖFW*, **83**, 6663 (1957).

# CHAPTER 7

# Protective Preparations

One of the main purposes of cosmetics is to keep the skin healthy; another is to protect it. Cleansers protect the skin by removing impurities that might obstruct the follicle mouths as well as microorganisms and foreign matter that may affect the epidermal tissue. Brittle and cracked skin is easily attacked by microorganisms; to some extent emollients therefore act as skin protectors. Disinfectants protect the skin by destroying noxious bacteria and fungi. In addition to these preparations, there are others with a protective effect in a narrower sense: they act prophylactically by isolating the skin from harmful contacts. Typical skin protectors are applied before skin is exposed to such contacts; they do not affect the epidermal tissue in any way; they merely form a thin elastic film on the skin surface. If perfect, they act as an invisible sheath completely impenetrable to harmful contacts.

We differentiate between the following types according to their specific purposes: preparations with protective action against chemical agents (caustic chemicals, detergent solutions, decomposed urine); preparations with protective action against dust and soils, tar, and lubricants; preparations with protective action against physical agents (ultraviolet rays and heat); preparations with protective action against mechanical injuries (lubricant and massage preparations) and insect repellents.

## PREPARATIONS WITH PROTECTIVE ACTION AGAINST CHEMICAL AGENTS

In this field cosmetics are still in the initial stage of development; 30 years ago such preparations were not even mentioned in books on cosmetics [1]. Even today barrier creams have not yet been accepted by the general public. There is no doubt, however, that we are in the middle of a lively development: In the United States and Western Europe various preparations of this

311

type are commercially available, publications about problems related to skin protection in industry and the home are on the increase, and even the new supplements to various pharmacopoeiae include formulations for barrier and protective ointments and creams. It may be expected that in these circumstances this type of preparation will gain more importance within the next few years. Their development was probably not only initiated by the steadily growing industrialization of society nor by the introduction of synthetic detergents to household use, since these hardly damage the skin any more than the old soap-based preparations (see Chapter 5). Rather, the impetus may have been found in war and postwar sociological development. In 1942–1945 women entered heavy industry for the first time; and millions of women whose mothers would never have dreamed of washing dishes and laundry every day—which was the duty of the domestic help—are doing just that at present. Even if hardly any women in the western world are still working in heavy industry, industrial workers today have different values than they once had. The rough and calloused hands of industrial laborers and the red chapped hands of laundresses, formerly considered the normal and unavoidable consequences of social position, have today become a cosmetic problem. The requirements that a good barrier preparation must meet may be summarized as follows:

It must prevent any contact between skin and the harmful substance; that is, it must form a continuous film impenetrable by the substance or its solution. The preparation should remain active for a reasonable time; the film must not be too easily rubbed or peeled off the skin; it must neither evaporate nor be absorbed by the skin and must not become brittle even under prolonged mechanical stress. The preparation must not be a primary irritant or have a sensitizing effect on the skin (see Chapter 1). Preferably the film should be removable without too much scrubbing or the use of strongly degreasing solvents (acetone, benzine, etc.) It must not disturb the wearer in his work and should be easy to apply and pleasant to use (nongreasy, nonsticky, and elastic).

There is no universal barrier cream; every preparation is effective only against specific substances. The most important types of this kind of protective cream are the following:

### Preparations with Protective Action Against Aqueous Solutions

These products may have a wide variety of applications. They protect the skin of babies against urine which acts as a skin irritant, especially when it begins to decompose. Since baby skin is particularly tender and these preparations are used on large skin areas over extended periods, the first requirement is a complete absence of all irritating action. Baby creams and oils combine a water-repellent effect with protection against mechanical injuries (friction from clothing, bed sores, etc.). Housewives use barrier creams to protect their hands from the degreasing effect of warm soap and detergent solutions in household chores. Here the main technical difficulty consists in making the cream adhere to the skin even when it is affected by the solutions that are actually formulated to emulsify and remove water-insoluble substances (including the barrier cream!). On the other hand, it should also be easily removed after use. With such contrasting requirements some compromise must be made. In practice pleasant use and easy removability are essential; effectiveness must come second because no preparation that is unpleasant in application will be used voluntarily even if it fulfills its actual task perfectly.

Industrial workers may require protection against strongly acid or alkaline solutions of toxic or irritating substances. Here it may sometimes be essential to eliminate nearly completely any contact of the skin with the solution. The emphasis is on the complete impermeability of the protective film. Water-repellent barrier creams should also be used by hairdressers who work regularly with cold-wave solutions, hair dyes, etc.

**Anhydrous Preparations, W/O Emulsions, and Dual Emulsions.** The simplest product that meets the requirements of a water-repellent barrier cream is pure petrolatum. To smear petrolatum around the nostrils during colds (as a protection against mucus, which acts as an irritant, in particular when the skin has been rubbed sore with handkerchiefs) is an old domestic remedy. Petrolatum is also still being used for baby skin protection. By itself it is rather viscous and sticky, but these properties may be offset by adding about 18 % zinc oxide or other fillers. Zinc oxide also reduces heat congestion through petrolatum. Tronnier [2], however, found that petrolatum without any additives has the best covering effect against aqueous solutions. In his tests even an addition of silicone oils reduced the protective action.

REMARKS

1. Bergwein, *SÖFW*, **82**, 59 (1956).
2. *Guide to Cosmetic and Pharmaceutical Formulation*, Atlas Chemical Co., 1953. First melt castor oil, lanolin, and Tween 61 together, then add ceresine, and finally petrolatum.
3. Janistyn, *Riechstoffe-Seifen-Kosmetika*, II, Hüthig Verlag, Heidelberg, 1950, p. 379.
4. Conrad, in Lesser, *Drug Cosmet. Ind.*, **75**, 172 (1954). Add water (68°C) to the fat melt (68°C) and stir vigorously; continue stirring until cool; homogenize.

314                    PROTECTIVE PREPARATIONS

Here are a few more sophisticated formulations [3].

|  | 1 | 2 | 3 | 4 W/O | 5 Dual |
|---|---|---|---|---|---|
| Paraffin oil | 50 |  | 15 | 20 | 41 |
| Petrolatum, white | 10 | 40 | 50 |  |  |
| Ceresine |  | 5 |  |  |  |
| Astrolatum |  |  |  | 15 |  |
| Silicone oil, 400 cst |  |  |  |  | 10 |
| Isopropyl palmitate | 7 |  |  |  |  |
| Castor oil |  | 25 |  |  |  |
| Hydrogenated peanut oil |  |  | 10 |  |  |
| Beeswax | 10 |  |  |  | 2.5 |
| Spermaceti |  |  |  |  | 6.5 |
| Lanolin, hydrogenated | 15 | 25 | 15 | 10 |  |
| Amerchol L 101 |  |  |  | 15 |  |
| Cetyl alcohol | 3 |  | 2 |  |  |
| Stearic acid |  |  |  |  | 6.5 |
| Tween 61 |  | 5 |  |  |  |
| Water |  |  |  | 40 | 38.4 |
| Triethanolamine |  |  |  |  | 0.8 |
| Glycerol or Sorbitol (liquid) |  |  |  |  | 2.0 |
| Borax |  |  |  |  | 0.8 |
| Boric acid | 2 |  | 1 |  |  |
| Zinc oxide | 3 |  | 7 |  |  |
| Talcum |  |  | 7 |  |  |
| Preservative |  |  |  |  | 0.2 |

5. Ernst, *SÖFW*, **82,** 575 (1956). Melt the fats. Heat the aqueous solution of glycerol (or sorbitol syrup), borax, and preservative to the same temperature and stir slowly into the fat melt. Continue stirring until cool. A light, white, and fatting cream. This dual emulsion represents a transition to the O/W type. Because of their strongly pronounced hydrophilic character, preparations of this kind might be expected to have a lower protective effect; but the highly water-repellent silicone oil counteracts it.

In these preparations the hydrocarbons (paraffin oil, petrolatum, etc.) are the actual active ingredients; they form a water-impermeable film on the skin. Isopropyl palmitate (formula 1) improves film smoothness, silicone oil (formula 6), the water repellence.

Vegetable oils (formulas 2 and 3) give the preparations more skin affinity and fatting characteristics; beeswax and spermaceti stiffen them. The use of lanolin and related products in almost all the formulas given is very interesting. Paraffinhydrocarbons alone produce a film that is completely impermeable to sweat and will consequently be loosened by perspiration accumulating from inside. In addition, the strictly nonpolar character of hydrocarbons is responsible for rather poor adhesion to the skin. Lanolin improves the skin affinity and adhesion of the preparation and in its emulsifying capacity prevents sweat congestion. On the other hand, it obviously reduces water impermeability and consequently the protective action of the preparation.

We have dealt with anhydrous, W/O, and dual emulsions at the same time because their composition is similar. An advantage of anhydrous preparations may be the higher "concentration" because here water is an inactive ingredient. Emulsions have the advantage of more attractive appearance and possibly better consistency.

Barrier creams of this type have a good protective action and after use can easily be removed with soap and water.

**O/W Emulsions.**    Although O/W (i.e., "washable") emulsions may appear completely unsuitable at first glance as protectors against aqueous solutions, most of the formulas published in recent years belong to this type. Their water-repellent effect is due to their silicone oil content (see Chapter 4). Since they also have the attractive appearance and the nongreasy, nonsticky characteristics of "regular" O/W creams, it is not surprising that most of the commercially successful products are of this type.

It is not yet clearly understood what processes make a water-miscible cream develop a water-repellent film on drying; one thing is certain: a number of these preparations have indeed a protective effect against aqueous solutions. Silicone oils are, of course, not miracle products, and no complete protection can be expected from formulations that provide for the addition of 5% or less of silicones. High percentages of these materials in commercial products are ruled out because of their high price. As usual, the problem has to be solved by compromise.

The composition of these preparations may vary from a simple silicone oil-in-water emulsion to the traditional dry creams with silicone oil added. From the wealth of published formulas we have selected a few that are typical.

REMARKS

6. Sluis, *Chem. Courant*, **55,** 312 (1956). "Pola Wax" is a polyethylene glycol stearyl ether. (This is a simple silicone oil-in-water emulsion with a high silicone oil concentration).

| | 6 | 7 | 8 | 9 | 10 | 11 | 12 | 13 | 14 | 15 |
|---|---|---|---|---|---|---|---|---|---|---|
| Paraffin oil | 5 | | | | | | | | 2 | |
| Isopropyl palmitate | | | | 2 | | | | | | |
| Silicone oil DC 200 350–400 cst | 30 | 25 | 25 | 20 | | 10 | | | | 10 |
| Silicone oil DC 200 1000 cst | | | | | 10 | | 10 | | | |
| Silicone oil DC 555 | | | | | | | | | 2 | |
| Silicone oil AW (Wacker) | | | | | | | | 5 | | |
| Synthetic Japan wax | | | | 2 | | | | | | |
| Cetiol V | | | | | | | | 5 | | |
| Beeswax | | | 2.5 | | | | | | | |
| Spermaceti | | | | | | 5 | | | | |
| Lanolin | | | | | | | | | 1 | |
| Amerchol L-101 | | | | | | | 3 | | | |
| Cetyl alcohol | | | | | | 15 | | | 0.7 | |
| Glycerol monostearate self-emulsifying | | 7 | | | | | 10 | | 6 | |
| Diethylene glycol monostearate, self-emulsifying | | | | | | | | | | 1.5 |
| Glycerylmonomyristate | | | | | | | | 24 | | |
| Propylene glycol monomyristate | | | | | | | | 10 | | |
| Stearic acid | | | 15 | 10 | 15 | | | | | |
| Oleic acid | | | | | | | | | | 0.75 |
| "Pola Wax" (Croda) | 2.5 | | | | | | | | | |
| Brij 30 (Atlas) | | | 3 | | | | | | | |
| Brij 35 (Atlas) | | | 3 | | | | | | | |
| Sodium lauryl sulfate | | | | | | 2 | | | | |
| Fatty-alcohol sulfate | | | | | | | 2.5 | | | |
| Water | 62.5 | 67.7 | 46.35 | 67.5 | 53.7 | 61.6 | 77 | 50 | 82 | 61 |
| Glycerol | | | 3 | | | 5 | | | | |
| Sorbitol syrup 88% | | | | | 18.3 | | | 2.9 | 1.4 | |
| Propylene glycol | | | | | | | | | | 25.25 |
| Potassium hydroxide | | | | | 0.5 | 1.0 | 1.0 | | | |
| Triethanolamine | | | 2 | | | | | 0.9 | 0.9 | 0.5 |
| Gum tragacanth | | | | | | | | | | 1.0 |
| Lactic acid | | | | | | 1.2 | | 0.1 | | |
| Preservative | | 0.25 | 0.15 | 0.04 | | 0.2 | | 0.1 | | |
| Perfume | | | 0.05 | | | | | | | |

7. Currie and Francisco, *Am. Perfumer*, **69**, 421 (December 1954). Heat the solution of glyceryl monostearate in water to 80°C, add preservative (methyl-*p*-hydroxybenzoate) and silicone oil and stir rapidly; continue stirring to 50°C, add perfume, and pour.

8. Bergwein, *SÖFW*, **82**, 59 (1956). A stearic acid cream with high silicone-oil content, emulsified with nonionic emulsifiers. The preservatives are methyl (0.1%) and butyl-*p*-hydroxybenzoate (0.05%).

9. Plein and Plein, *Bull. Am. Soc. Hosp. Pharm.*, **13**, 38 (1956). Resembles the preceding formula but has potassium stearate as an emulsifier. Synthetic Japan Wax is a solid, easily hydrolized triglyceride. The preservatives are 0.025% methyl and 0.05% propyl-*p*-hydroxybenzoate.

10. Lesser, *Drug Cosmet. Ind.*, **72**, 616 (1953). Stir the aqueous phase (82°C) into the oil phase (80°C). (A classical stearate cream with silicone added).

11. Ernst, *SÖFW*, **82**, 575 (1956). Melt fats and lauryl sulfate together; dissolve the other ingredients in about half the water, heat to about 60°C, and stir in slowly; emulsify and incorporate the solution heated to about 50°C. (The high cetyl alcohol content provides an emollient effect.)

12. Conrad in Lesser, *Drug Cosmet. Ind.*, **72**, 616 (1953). Add the water (75°C) to the fat melt (75°). (In principle, similar to formula 7, but because of the addition of Amerchol and the lower silicone content the emphasis here is on skin conditioning rather than on a protective effect.)

13. Nowak in Rothemann *Das grosse Rezeptbuch der Haut und Körperpflegemittel*, Hüthig Verlag, Heidelberg, 1962, 3rd ed., p. 614. The preservative is sodium-*p*-hydroxy-methylbenzoate. The addition of Cetiol (a blend of cetyl alcohol and homologous alcohols) and 0.5% vitamin F as well as the low silicone content emphasize the conditioning rather than the protective effect.

14. Keithler, *The Formulation of Cosmetics and Cosmetic Specialities*, Drug and Cosmetic Industry, New York, 1957, p. 76. Add the solution of Sorbitol syrup in water (90°C) to which triethanolamine has been added in the last moment, to the fat melt (90°). Agitate mechanically in a stainless steel container. (This very light cream of the stearate-glyceryl monostearate dual type is also described as a protective cream!)

15. Currie and Francisco, *Am. Perfumer*, **69**, 421 (December 1954). Prepare a gum tragacanth mucilage in 49 pts. water. Dissolve triethanolamine, oleic acid, diethylene glycol stearate, and 14.75 pts. propylene glycol in the balance of the water, heat this solution to 80°C, and add first the silicone oil, then the tragacanth mucilage, and finally the remaining propylene glycol, stirring rapidly. [This is a peculiar kind of product in which, apart from water itself, a moisture-binding substance (propylene glycol) and a water-repellent agent (silicone oil) are the main ingredients!]

**Alcoholic Lotions.** Alcoholic lotions can be prepared with silicone oils of the type DC 555 (Dow Corning) which, after evaporation, leave a water-repellent film on the skin. A simple formulation is suggested by Currie and Francisco [4]:

| | |
|---|---|
| Silicone oil DC 555 | 5.0 |
| Ethyl alcohol, 95% | 94.7 |
| Perfume | 0.3 |
| | 100.0 |

Sunscreen lotions can be prepared on this basis by adding suitable active ingredients.

**Invisible Gloves.** Preparations of this type are used wherever maximum impermeability is required, for example, in industrial protection against work with caustic or toxic solutions; they contain substances that form a water-insoluble film which is completely resistant to mechanical stress. The disadvantages of these preparations are:

(a) they completely prevent the evaporation of perspiration; if it is heavy, the film will be loosened internally.

(b) Since they are completely water-insoluble, they can be removed only with organic solvents, benzene, acetone, etc., which have a strong degreasing effect on the skin. If these "invisible gloves" are used regularly, an emollient cream is highly advisable to restore the lost lipids.

Hopkins suggests the following formulations [5]:

16. Benzoin          5.0
    Beeswax          1.5
    Lanolin          7.5
    Mastic           2.0
    Ethyl alcohol   84.0
                   ------
                   100.0

17. Ethyl cellulose      4
    Mastic               6
    Castor oil         1–2
    Acetone (benzene) 88–89
                      ------
                        100

The Swedish plastic-based product "Nobecutan" is also interesting. It is available as an aerosol spray or a standard lotion and is reported to coat the skin with a durable elastic film that acts as a barrier against detergent and caustic aqueous solutions but does not prevent sweat from evaporating. TMTD (tetramethylthiuram disulfide) is added as a disinfectant and reportedly also acts as a sunscreen [6].

## Preparations with Protective Action against Organic Solutions and Solvents

Organic solvents (acetone, benzene, toluene, kerosene, alcohol, turpentine, etc.), which are used in innumerable industrial applications, may cause skin irritations in repeated or prolonged contact not only because of their strong degreasing effect but also because of certain toxic properties. Preparations that act as barriers to these solvents are therefore important auxiliaries in industrial safety programs. Most of these preparations belong to the "invisible-glove" type, which provides good protection, and, since the preparations need be impermeable only to organic solvents but not to aqueous solutions, they may be formulated so that they will have no perspiration-inhibiting effect and can easily be washed off with water. Suitable film formers are triethanolamine or sodium alginate, cellulose ether, polyacrylates, gum tragacanth, and gelatin. Many types of preparations in this group are covered by patents.

Here are some typical formulations:

| | 18 | 19 | 20 | 21 | 22 |
|---|---|---|---|---|---|
| Gelatin | 4 | | | | |
| Sodium polyacrylate | | 10 | | | |
| Cellulose ether (Polyfibron) | | | 4 | | |
| Triethanolamine alginate | | | | 25 | |
| Sodium water glass | | | | | 22.65 |
| Sodium stearate | | | | | 7.2 |
| Citric acid | | | | | 0.025 |
| Glycerol | 33.3 | 30 | 30 | 2 | 28.875 |
| Water | 62.5 | 60 | 66 | 73 | 41.25 |
| | 100 | 100 | 100 | 100 | 100.0 |

REMARKS

18, 19, 20. Czetsch-Lindenwald, *Fette Seifen*, **53**, 751 (1951).
21. Schwartz, *Ind. Med. Surg.*, **15**, 175 (1946). The dry alginate content of the "triethanolamine alginate" is 20%.
22. U. S. Patent 2,021,131.

Some formulations are less simple than the preceding; for example,

| 23. | Polyvinyl alcohol | 2.0 |
|---|---|---|
| | Starch glycolate | 3.0 |
| | Gelatin | 2.0 |
| | Sodium carboxylmethylcellulose | 8.0 |
| | Hexane triol | 5.0 |
| | Glycerol | 6.0 |
| | Talcum | 1.5 |
| | Titanium dioxide | 0.5 |
| | Water | 71.8 |
| | *p*-chloro-*m*-cresol (as sodium salt) | 0.2 |
| | | 100.0 |

GDR Patent 11595 (Schwarzkopf, 1956). This formulation illustrates the use of a combination of film formers and solid fillers.

| 24. | Stearic acid | 12.0 |
|---|---|---|
| | Sorbitol liquid | 5.0 |
| | Sodium hydroxide | 1.4 |
| | Sodium waterglass solution | 30.0 |
| | Water | 51.6 |
| | | 100.0 |

Keithler, *The Formulation of Cosmetics and Cosmetic Specialties*, p. 79. The solution of Sorbitol and sodium hydroxide in water (75°C) is stirred into the melted stearic acid

(75°C). When an uniform emulsion has formed, the waterglass solution is slowly stirred in. (This formula is an example of an emulsified solvent-protective preparation. The oil phase, stearic acid in this instance, does not contribute to the protective action but improves appearance and consistency of the preparation.)

## TESTING CHEMICALLY PROTECTIVE PREPARATIONS

Czetsch-Lindenwald [7] describes tests in which a paper membrane is coated with the test ointment to evaluate its resistance to solvents. Strongly colored membranes are recommended because they provide an opportunity for visual examination of the film thickness of the ointment. Such primitive tests cannot, of course, substantiate the effectiveness of a preparation under typical usage conditions but they are useful for the screening out of unsuitable products.

To gain greater certainty tests must be made on living skin. For ointments and creams the Carriè and Lotz method [8] may be used. Patch tests with the substance against which the cream is supposed to protect the skin are made on cream-coated and unprotected skin areas of the same person. The effectiveness of the preparation can be estimated from the different skin reactions at the two locations.

Kärcher and Schmidt-La Baume [9] dissolved fluorochromes (fluorescent substances) in various solvents against which the protective preparations were intended to be effective. Rhodamin B proved satisfactory in a test with fats, fat solvents, and lacquers; salicylic acid with lubricating oil; Auramin O, Acridin orange, and Rivanol with water, acids, and alkalies. Certain skin areas (usually the outer surfaces of the fingers) are coated with the protective ointment, dipped into a solution, and vigorously moved. After removal of solutions and protective ointments, the skin surface is photographed under a fluorescent light. This test is almost too sensitive, for traces of dyes were found in the capillary spaces of the skin surface even when preparations that had been found satisfactory in practice were used.

Finally, the only reliable test, as with all cosmetic preparations, is the usage test. Many preparations that seemed absolutely satisfactory in laboratory tests are unsuccessful in practice (e.g., because they are too sticky). Others that seemed to have only partial protective action in tests may be successful in practice if in addition to this action they also have a conditioning effect that is an advantage in practical use.

## PREPARATIONS WITH PROTECTIVE ACTION AGAINST DRY SOILS

If the hands are continually in contact with dry soils, dust, highly viscous oils, or tars, solid or viscous particles lodge in the fine skin folds and hair follicle mouths (pores). If they are not removed promptly, they may cause tissue reactions and lead to skin lesions by obstructing the sebaceous gland ducts. If dirt has penetrated deeply, it is often not easy to remove completely and this may have to be done with soap solutions and vigorous brushing or scrubbing. Such drastic treatment may in turn lead to rough and degreased skin and cause secondary damage: a dry cracked skin runs a higher risk of infections. Often the prophylactic use of preparations acting as a barrier against dirt avoids many difficulties and complications. These preparations are particularly useful for three consumer groups: industrial workers in the detergent, bleaching powder, or cement industries, mechanics, and housewives who want to avoid the deeply penetrating soil of household or garden chores.

The technical requirements of these preparations are more easily met than those of the protective creams discussed in the preceding section, and it is not difficult to produce a preparation that is both effective and pleasant to use. The product is supposed to cover the skin and block the pores; it should be nongreasy, nonsticky, and easily removed.

Creams of the washable O/W type, in which a certain content of inert fillers protects the pores, are often used. Occasionally water-soluble film-forming substances are also added:

REMARKS

25. British Codex Revision Committee, in Czetsch-Lindenwald and Schmidt-La Baume, *Die äusseren Heilmittel 1950–1955*, p. 139. (A light stearate cream; casein and sodium alginate form the dirt-repellent film.)

26. Harry, *Modern Cosmetocology*, 4th ed., Leonard Hill, London, 1955, p. 631. Stir the aqueous phase (70–75°C) into the oil melt (70–75°C) and then add kaolin and stir; continue stirring until the mixture has cooled to 30°C. Add perfume (if any) at 45°C. Homogenization (at 33–35°C) is also recommended. (A stearate cream with skin affinity—lanolin, cetyl alcohol; kaolin covers the pores.)

27. Downing, Ohmart, and Stoklosa, *Archs Derm. Syph.*, **47**, 436 (1944). Stir the aqueous phase (80°C) into the oil phase (80°C) and add talcum when emulsification is completed. Homogenize.

28. Cumming and co-workers, *Br. J. ind. Med.* **4**, 237 (1947). (A dual emulsion with a high paraffin hydrocarbon content. The nature of the solids is not specified. Probably paraffin wax and petrolatum are essential to the protective action. The product is not easily washed off.)

29. *Drug and Cosmetic Emulsions*, Atlas Chemical Co. (The protective effect is achieved by the combination of cellulose ether and the adhesive pore-covering zinc stearate.

30. Keithler, *The Formulation of Cosmetics and Cosmetic Specialties*, p. 82. Heat all ingredients with the exception of zinc stearate to 90°C, stir until the emulsion is uniform. Stir in zinc stearate in small portions. Homogenize if required. [The cream combines an emollient effect (cetyl and stearyl alcohols) with a good protective action (high solids content).] In similar formulations zinc stearate is sometimes replaced by magnesium or aluminum stearate or aluminum hydroxide.)

| | 25 | 26 | 27 | 28 | 29 | 30 |
|---|---|---|---|---|---|---|
| Mineral oil | | | | | | 3.0 |
| Petrolatum | | 2 | 4.5 | 40 | | |
| Paraffin wax | | | | 20 | | |
| Beeswax | | | 2 | | | |
| Lanolin | | 3 | | | | |
| Cetyl alcohol | | 3 | | | | 8.0 |
| Stearyl alcohol | | | | | | 6.0 |
| Lanette wax S | | | | 10 | | |
| Stearic acid | 10 | 6 | 10 | | 15 | |
| Span 60 | | | | | 2.0 | |
| Tween 60 | | | | | 1.5 | |
| Triethanolamine lauryl sulfate | | | | | | 1.0 |
| Water | 76.75 | 67.35 | 54 | 15–25 | 46.5 | 54.0 |
| Glycerol | 6 | | 8 | | | |
| Sorbitol liquid | | | | | 5.0 | |
| Propylene glycol | | | | | | 2.0 |
| Polyethylene glycol (mol wt 4000) | | | | | | 8.0 |
| Sodium alginate | 2 | | | | | |
| Casein | 3 | | | | | |
| Methylcellulose mucilage (4%) | | | | | 25.0 | |
| Triethanolamine | 1.55 | | 1.5 | | | |
| Sodium hydroxide | | 0.65 | | | | |
| Phenol | 0.5 | | | | | |
| Chlorocresol | 0.2 | | | | | |
| Kaolin | | 18 | | | | |
| Talcum | | | 20 | 5–15 | | |
| Zinc stearate | | | | | 5.0 | 18.0 |

# PREPARATIONS WITH PROTECTIVE ACTION AGAINST ULTRAVIOLET RADIATION

## Physiological Effects of Ultraviolet Rays

Sunlight reaching the surface of the earth contains, in addition to *visible rays* (with wavelengths between 4000 and 7400 Å; 1 Å = 1/10,000,000 mm), others with longer and shorter wavelengths. The rays with the longer lengths

(7500–53,000 Å), the *infrared,* are heat rays; shortwave rays (2800–4000 Å) are designated as *ultraviolet.* Ultraviolet rays with lengths below 3200 Å, are responsible for most of the therapeutic as well as noxious effects that we attribute to sunlight.

It is important that this biologically highly effective segment of solar radiation, which, incidentally, amounts to less than 0.2 % of the total solar light energy in temperate climates, is most subject to atmospheric influence. When rays fall obliquely on the earth, that is, when they must travel a long way through the atmosphere, those under 3200 Å wavelengths are largely absorbed by the atmosphere. In the temperate zone these rays reach the earth only in summer, between 8 A.M. and 4 P.M. in any appreciable quantity. Obviously the intensity is higher in the mountains than at sea level. Windows, dust, and soot in the atmosphere block these biologically effective rays. Their scarcity is one of the reasons for the considerable attention paid to open air and sunlight in countries of the temperate zone.

These rays stimulate blood circulation in the derma, cause the development of vitamin D from provitamins contained in skin fat, and are also supposed to shift the redox potential of the epidermal tissue toward more intensive reduction, which, in turn, is believed to lead to an activation of various vitamins, hormones, and enzymes and a favorable effect on the visceral nervous system [10]. Subjective results of radiation are increased well-being and activity. Clinically, sunlight has been found to have a favorable therapeutic effect in skin and bone tuberculosis as well as ricketts (through vitamin D formation); it also reduces the susceptibility to infections [11].

On the other hand, the identical ultraviolet rays are damaging in the case of excessive exposure. They may cause sunburn with symptoms of mild irritation to serious inflammations. It may also be regarded as certain that excessive solar radiation not only leads to a disposition to cancer but to skin cancer itself [12]. Excessive radiation also destroys vitamin D in skin fat, modifying it to toxic steroids (which probably have nothing to do with the carcinogenic properties of ultraviolet rays), and in the long run causes the connective tissue of the corium to degenerate which is manifested in a coarsening of the skin relief and the formation of wrinkles.

The discovery of the therapeutic effect of sunlight at the turn of the century has resulted in sun worship that may be justified to a certain extent but is often exaggerated. The beneficial effects of exercise and fresh air have all too often been ascribed to the sun, and tanning, a defense mechanism of the body, has been regarded as an achievement of health and beauty.

It is interesting that other defense mechanisms of the skin, for example, strong callous formation on the hands or tough leathery facial skin, are regarded as cosmetically undesirable because these symptoms are associated with manual work and exposure to inclement weather. On the other hand, suntanning which is associated with sports and vacations, appears to be so desirable that many people do not lie in the sun because they love it but only to achieve a rich tan.

Cosmetic preparations should protect the skin as effectively as possible from the noxious effects of radiation without reducing the beneficial action, particularly tanning. (Protection against ultraviolet rays is also occasionally required in industry, medicine, mountaineering, and the armed forces. It is not a selective action that is required here but an absorption that is as complete as possible over a wide range of wavelengths 2000–4000 Å.) To determine whether any selective action is at all possible we have to examine the modifications shown by the skin under the influence of sunlight [13].

## Effect of Ultraviolet Rays on Epidermal Tissue

According to Blum [14], the primary effect of ultraviolet rays on the skin is the degradation of proteins in the prickle cells. Various substances generated in this process cause erythema and edema and stimulate the basal cells to greater activity in the formation of new cells; also developed are melanin (the brown skin pigment) and promelanin (a colorless substance that, under certain conditions, may be oxidized to melanin). This first passive reaction of the skin tissue, which becomes noticeable a few hours after radiation has started, is followed after about 24 hours by an active reaction; that is, the epidermal tissue develops a defense against continued radiation. Melanin bodies, usually present in the germinative layer, migrate to the skin surface and assist in protecting the corneal cells. The increased activity of the basal cells eventually results in a thickening of the corneal layer; in persons constantly exposed to strong sunlight, the thickened horny layer is the most important protective agent of the skin. Perspiration also provides a certain amount of protection because it contains substances that act as screens [15], since they show strong absorption within the wavelength range below 3100 Å. Zenisek identified one of these substances as urocaninic acid (imidazol acrylic acid). Degradation of prickle cell proteins and the subsequent skin reactions occur with greatest intensity under the influence of rays with a wavelength of 2800–3200 Å. Rays with shorter wavelengths have a similar effect, but they no longer occur in sunlight when it reaches the surface of the earth and may therefore be ignored. Rays with wavelengths of 3200–4000 Å cause identical but less intense reactions [16]. Erythema and edema as well as melanin develop only after more prolonged periods of radiation by longer wave UV rays than by those of the medium range (2800–3200 Å).

It was formerly held that UV rays could be divided into "erythemal" (wavelength below 3200 Å) and "melanogenic" (3200–4000 Å) rays. According to today's opinions, erythemal and melanogenic effects cannot be separated from one another; both are caused primarily by medium rather than long UV rays.

In addition to causing protein degradation, rays of 3200–4000 Å have another effect. In the presence of oxygen they accelerate the transformation of colorless promelanin into brown melanin. (Probably promelanin develops simultaneously with melanin during the degradation of spinous cell proteins and can also occur in the outer layers of the epidermis through the bleaching of melanin). Contrary to melanin synthesis, which becomes apparent only after about 24 hours or longer, this tanning effect is already noticeable about one hour after radiation [17].

## PRINCIPLE OF EFFECTIVENESS OF SUNSCREENS

The fact that the exposure of unprotected skin to sunlight not only produces the desired therapeutic effect but (particularly if exposure is prolonged) also results in sunburn and subsequent peeling of the corneal layer is a cosmetic problem. In principle, this problem can be treated in different ways:

1. The skin can be provided with a protective layer that does not permit UV rays to reach it by absorbing or reflecting them. Some of the materials used in powders do indeed reflect a certain amount of UV rays and are occasionally incorporated into suntan preparations. In this context zinc oxide is more effective than titanium dioxide [18]. Preparations which reflect UV rays may be very effective and are used by people who find themselves frequently exposed to an excess of UV radiation: mountaineers, the armed forces, etc.; for regular use, however, these preparations have the disadvantage of eliminating the beneficial rays as well as the harmful ones.

2. Biologically effective substances may be used that would prevent symptoms of inflammation without reduction of tanning. Since the skin reaction to sunburn is similar to that occurring when the protein degradation product histamine is liberated in the tissues, attempts have been made to avoid inflammation by using substances with antihistamine effects. It became apparent that although some antihistamines have an inflammation-reducing effect, it is not due to the histamine binding action but to the absorption of ultraviolet rays [19].

Because of their anti-inflammatory action, hydro- and fluorocortisones may be useful in treating sunburn but their use in suntan preparations cannot be recommended; inflammation (increased blood circulation, stimulation to cellular division) is an important skin reaction and the introductory stage in the healing process. It is possible that the elimination of this reaction with continuing radiation might result in far-reaching destruction of the epidermal cells.

It is not impossible, of course, that biologically effective suntan preparations will be developed in the future. Today our knowledge of skin-tissue processes is still too limited.

3. Substances that cause or accelerate tanning of the skin can be applied. Dioxyacetone [20] belongs to the first type: it forms a brown complex with the keratin of the corneal layer. Skin-tanning agents of this type appeared on the American market some years ago and enjoyed great but brief popularity. There is only one step from products of this type to brown make-up.

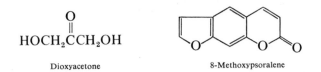

$$O$$
$$\parallel$$
$$HOCH_2CCH_2OH$$

Dioxyacetone                    8-Methoxypsoralene

8-Methoxypsoralene has a quite different action. If a dose of about 10–20 mg is taken internally two hours before exposure to the sun, this substance is reported to accelerate tanning to a considerable extent and to avoid sunburn at the same time [21].

4. A final possibility is to incorporate substances in suntan preparations which "filter" the sunlight by absorbing ultraviolet rays of the medium range (2800–3200 Å) but letting rays of greater lengths pass. Based on the preceding observations, the result is the following:

A strong reduction in the erythema and edema effects of sunlight. On the other hand, melanogenesis and thickening of the epidermis (the natural defense mechanisms of skin) are also reduced.

Retention of a certain amount of tanning effect after sunbathing caused by oxidation of promelanin.

All modern suntan preparations are based on this principle. They are capable of protecting the skin adequately even over extended periods of exposure to sunlight and permit a certain amount of tanning but can never, as is sometimes claimed in their advertising, accelerate tanning.

### Active Ingredients

The first requirement that must be met by any substance being considered for sunlight protection is its capacity to absorb the majority of rays in the 2800–3200 Å range while transmitting those in the higher range [22]. The absorption capacity of any substance in the ultraviolet range is measured with an UV spectrophotometer. This instrument measures the screening capacity of the substance (usually not pure but in dilute solutions) for any wavelength; that is, the ratio of the incident and transmitted ray intensity. By presenting the respective values of different wavelengths in a graph (Figure 9) the absorptive capacity of the test substance is illustrated for the UV range.

Every substance is characterized by the shape of the curve and the wavelength at which maximum absorption is reached; occasionally there are several maximum values. The kind of solvent used also plays a certain part. The intensity of absorption is determined not only by the type of substance used but also by its concentration in solution and the thickness of the layer. Absorption is subject to Lambert-Beer's law, that is,.

$$D^+ = 10^{-c \cdot d \cdot \epsilon},$$

where $D^+$ is the transmittance at a definite wavelength, $c$ is the concentration of the active substance, $d$ is the layer thickness in centimeters, and $\epsilon$ is a constant characteristic of the substance and dependent on the wavelength. Figure 9 shows that transmittance is a function of the concentration of the active substance.

Even if graphs of this kind give some information about the suitability of a material as a sunburn preventive (to be suitable, a substance must have little transmittance below 3200 Å and high transmittance above this point), they

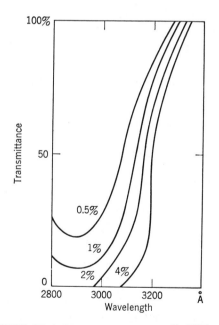

FIGURE 9   TRANSMITTANCE OF A SUNBURN PREVENTIVE (1:1000) CONTAINING VARIOUS CONCENTRATIONS OF $p$-AMINOBENZOIC ACID ($d = 1$ cm). IT IS IMPORTANT TO DEFINE THE UNITS IN WHICH THE CONCENTRATION IS EXPRESSED (WEIGHT, MOLE PER LITER, ETC.), SINCE THE NUMERICAL VALUE OF C, AND CONSEQUENTLY OF $D^+$ DEPENDS ON THE UNIT CHOSEN. UNFORTUNATELY THIS IS NOT ALWAYS DONE IN THE LITERATURE.

have an important disadvantage in practical application, as pointed out by Masch [23]: the diagram can be read accurately only to about 1%, and Figure 9, for example, does not show whether the transmittance of the preparation containing 4% p-aminobenzoic acid amounts to 0.1 or 0.001% at 3050 Å. The presentation is inaccurate just within the important medium range where the activity is highest. Masch therefore suggested the use of extinction (E) rather than transmittance of the substance. This is defined as follows:

$$E = -\log D^+ = c \cdot d \cdot \epsilon.$$

The advantages of the use of E (see Figure 10a) consist in the fact that it clearly shows the differences between various solutions exactly in the important range of slight transmittance; in addition, extinction is directly proportionate to concentration and to layer thickness, as can be seen from the diagram. If extinction graphs for the same substance at different concentrations or layer thicknesses are drawn on logarithm paper, the curves will cover each other by simple shifts in the direction of the ordinate (see Figure 10b). The shape of the curves will then no longer depend on concentration and layer thickness but only on the characteristics of the substance. For this reason extinction curves recorded in this way are particularly suitable for identifying active ingredients in sunburn preventives.

Masch suggests that in the physical testing of sunscreens the "critical film thickness," that is, the film thickness that will transmit 10% of the incident radiation, should be used as the measure of effectiveness.

The factor 10% has been adopted for very realistic reasons. According to Luckiesh and Taylor [24], normal unprotected skin around noon on a sunny day in midsummer in a country of the temperate zone will begin to show erythema symptoms after about 20 minutes. Preparations that would increase this delay tenfold, that is, to 3–4 hours, would therefore meet all normal requirements.

The critical film thickness (S in $\mu = 1/10,000$ cm) can be calculated for each wavelength from E (extinction) by using the formula

$$S = \frac{10}{E}.$$

Since E changes with the wavelength, S is also a function of it. The critical film thickness is most usefully determined at a wavelength in the center of the erythemally most effective range (3050 Å). As we can see in Figure 10b, the critical thickness for a preparation with 1% p-aminobenzoic acid would be $10\mu = 0.01$ mm. With twice the concentration of active ingredients, S would be $5\mu = 0.005$ mm.

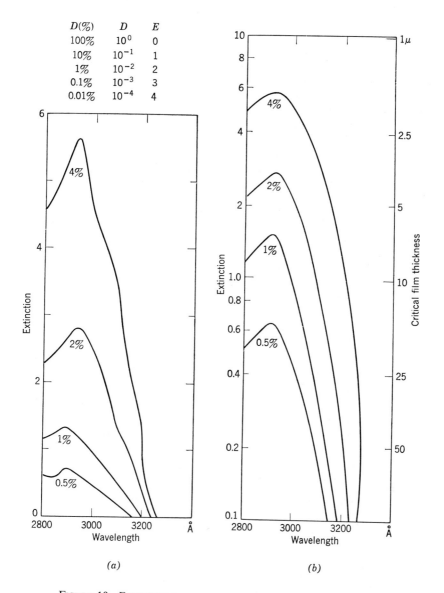

| $D(\%)$ | $D$ | $E$ |
|---------|-----|-----|
| 100% | $10^0$ | 0 |
| 10% | $10^{-1}$ | 1 |
| 1% | $10^{-2}$ | 2 |
| 0.1% | $10^{-3}$ | 3 |
| 0.01% | $10^{-4}$ | 4 |

(a)

(b)

FIGURE 10   EXTINCTIONS OF THE SAME PREPARATION $(d = 1\ \text{cm})$.

329

Absorption and extinction graphs are not only helpful in determining whether a material is suitable as an ingredient in a sunburn preventive, they also give important data about the use of the particular substance. Producers of sunburn preventives may calculate which active ingredient concentration is required for their preparations. We demonstrate the method of calculation on the basis of a practical example.

A sunburn preventive based on p-aminobenzoic acid which should protect the skin from 95% of the radiation around 3000 Å is to be marketed. The vehicle has been selected and it is only a matter of deciding on the concentration of the active ingredient.

First of all we establish the film thickness that would result from practical application by having a number of test subjects spread the preparation in the normal way on skin areas with known surface measurements. The weight of the preparation used up in this way is determined and the volume calculated (the specific gravity of the preparation must of course be known for this purpose). If, for example, the average use is 1 ml preparation for 1600 cm$^2$ skin surface, the average film thickness is 0.0006 cm = 6$\mu$.

The graph (Figure 10$b$) for a preparation containing 1% p-aminobenzoic acid shows that at a wavelength of 3050 Å, $E = c \times d \times \epsilon = 1$. Here $c = 10^{-5}$ (because we are dealing with a 1:1000 dilution of a 1% preparation), $d = 1$ cm, therefore

$$\epsilon = \frac{1}{10^{-5} \cdot 1} = 10^5.$$

The intended preparation must screen 95% radiation, that is, transmit 5%; $D = 0.05$ and $E = -\log D = 1.3$. As we have seen, $d = 6 \times 10^{-4}$ cm, $\epsilon$ is constant for every substance at a given wavelength (here $10^5$). According to the equation $E = c \times d \times \epsilon$, we find $1.3 = c \times (6 \times 10^{-4}) \times 10^5$. The required concentration is therefore $c = 1.3/60 = 0.022 = 2.2\%$.

In this section we have dealt with absorption within the UV range on which the effectiveness of any sunburn preventive is based. When selecting substances for cosmetic application, the following requirements must also be taken into consideration:

The substance must have no primary irritant action and should also act as a sensitizer only in very rare cases, if at all. This is an important stipulation because sunburn preventives are regularly applied to large parts of the skin surface, frequently in areas whose resistance has been lowered by exposure to sun, cold, wind, or water.

The substance must retain its sunburn preventive effect on the skin for several hours. It must not be subject to chemical modification under the influence of UV rays, water, or perspiration that might reduce its protection or cause irritation to develop. During this period it should also remain on the skin surface, that is, it should neither evaporate nor be resorbed by the skin.

Finally, the substance should have no unpleasant odor in the concentration used nor cause any discoloration of the skin or have any other esthetically undesirable properties.

The cosmetic industry today knows of many substances with suitable absorption curves which also meet the other known requirements; and new ones are being added every year. It would be impossible to list all of these materials. Janistyn [25] and Klarman [26] list suitable materials.

We want to mention very briefly one group of new subscreen agents because they represent an interesting type. These are the silicone oils (see Chapter 4) whose end groups are esterified with salicylic acid:

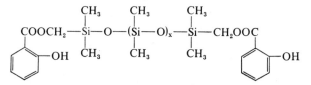

Substances in which $x = 4$, 8, and 12 have been described [27]; $x = 4$ has the highest efficiency per gram and $x = 12$ is most effective if the concentration is expressed in moles per liter. These substances show a maximum absorption at 3050 Å; here the critical film thickness of a 1% solution of $x = 4$ is 0.03 mm. "Silicone-salicylates" are soluble in silicone oils, 99% isopropyl alcohol (not 70%!), isopropyl myristate, and miscible with glyceryl monostearate, stearyl alcohol, and stearic acid; they are insoluble in water, 95% ethyl alcohol, propylene glycol, and glycerol.

The investigations of Christensen and Giese [28] regarding the changes in effectiveness caused by UV rays in widely used sunburn preventives are of great interest. The authors supply the following table:

| Group | Compound | Effect of Two Hours of Radiation on Absorption |
|---|---|---|
| p-Aminobenzoic acid ester | Ethyl-p-aminobenzoate | Strong increase |
|  | Ethyl-p-dimethylamino-benzoate | Slight change |
| Salicylic acid ester | Menthyl | Slight change |
|  | Homomenthyl | Slight decrease |
|  | Isoamyl | Slight change |
|  | Amyl | Strong increase |
|  | Phenyl | Slight increase |
|  | Benzyl | Part increase, part decrease |
| Anthranylic acid ester | Menthyl | Increase |
|  | Homomenthyl | Decrease |
| Acetophenones | Benzyl | Strong decrease |
| Naphthol sulfonic acids | 2-Naphthol-6-sulfonic acid | Strong increase, loss of specific absorption |
| Tannins | Tannin | Increase |
| Quinine salts | Sulfate | Slight decrease |
| Phenols | Phenol | Increase |

The authors observe that light susceptibility may change considerably in the presence of other substances (in particular antioxidants, because radiation effects often involve oxidation).

## Preparations

We distinguish between three types of sunburn preventive: anhydrous, emulsions, and greaseless preparations.

**Anhydrous Preparations.** Here liquid suntan oils occupy the most important place. A specific advantage of oily preparations is their water resistance which leaves them unaffected by perspiration during sunbathing or swimming. The lubricant effect (mechanical protection) is also considered helpful. Vegetable oils are employed in sunburn preventives because they have a certain absorption in the critical UV range [29]. This is particularly pronounced in sesame oil which is therefore widely used. Vegetable oils are also better solvents than mineral oils for most oil-soluble sunburn preventive agents.

Good results are obtained by incorporating 10–15% inert powders into oil preparations. These substances impart a stiffer consistency to the preparations and diminish stickiness. Some solids, in particular zinc oxide, have a considerable screening effect against UV rays which is not restricted to around 3000 Å but extends over the whole range.

The tacky feeling on the skin is most noticeable when the vegetable-oil content is high. It can be avoided by using low viscosity oils (or is the operative factor here the surface tension of the oils?), such as low-viscosity mineral oil, isopropyl myristate or palmitate, or silicone oils.

It should be borne in mind that the effectiveness of any sunburn preventive agent of a given concentration depends on the film thickness, which again depends on the viscosity of the preparation: the higher the viscosity, the thicker the film.

As far as the concentration of the active ingredient is concerned, many differing data appear in the published formulas: in those given here it fluctuates between 2 and 10%. The concentration selected depends primarily on the substance itself or, more exactly, on its extinction in the range around 3000 Å. In addition, the film thickness and the desired degree of screening are also important.

In evaluating ingredient costs more than the price per unit weight of sunscreen agents must be taken into account: the concentration required to achieve the desired effect is just as important.

This may be the place to consider the advantages of aerosol formulations for these products. The cosmetic effectiveness of these preparations hardly differs from that of traditional oils. A more uniform film thickness can perhaps be obtained by spraying than by manual application. On the other hand, the process of manual application guarantees a minimum film; with aerosol products there is the risk of spraying too sparingly so that the film does not provide adequate protection. Manufacturers can affect spraying speed and film thickness obtainable in a given time by selecting suitable valves and should tell the user in the directions on the package just how long each skin area should be sprayed to achieve the desired results.

One important potential advantage of aerosol packs is the avoidance of greasy hands; unfortunately this is not fully realizable, since to protect the eyes the face must not be sprayed, and the hands must be used anyway. Outside contamination of the container can, of course, be avoided with aerosol packs and the well-known unpleasant problem of having to pack a sticky, greasy, half-empty container with clothes and towels is ruled out.

Whether the higher prices of aerosol products are considered worthwhile depends largely on the buying power of the public.

| | 31 Oil | 32 Oil | 33 Oil | 34 Oil | 35 Jelly | 36 Aerosol | 37 Aerosol |
|---|---|---|---|---|---|---|---|
| Mineral oil | 60 | 70 | abt. 50 | | | 47 | 26 |
| Ceresine | | | | | 15 | | |
| Silicone oil 300 cst | | | | 10 | | | |
| Isopropyl palmitate | | | | 88 | | | |
| Isopropyl myristate | | 4 | 43 | | | | 1.1 |
| Sesame oil | 36.5 | | | | | | |
| Olive oil first pressing | | 25 | | | | | |
| Coconut oil deodorized | | | | | 75 | | |
| Lantrol | | | | | | | 0.6 |
| Acetylated lanolin | | | 5 | | | | |
| Vitamin F | | 1 | | | | | |
| Menthyl anthranylate | 3.5 | | | | | | |
| Sun protector (Dr. K. Richter) | 1 | | | | | | |
| Glyceryl p-amino-benzoate | | | | 2 | | | |
| Menthylsalicylate | | | | | 10 | | |
| Filtrosol A (Schimmel) | | | | | | 2.5 | |
| 2-Ethylhexylsalicylate | | | | | | | 2.0 |
| Perfume | | | | | | 0.5 | 0.3 |
| Genetron 101 | | | | | | 50 | |
| Freon 12 | | | | | | | 14 |
| Freon 114 | | | | | | | 56 |

REMARKS

31. De Navarre, *The Chemistry and Manufacture of Cosmetics*, p. 613. Dissolve menthyl anthranylate in sesame oil, add pigment, perfume, and antioxidants as required, and finally mix in mineral oil. This preparation is claimed to absorb 93% of the radiation between 2900 and 3200 Å.

32. Rothemann, *Das grosse Rezeptbuch, der Haut- und Körperpflegemittel*, 3rd. ed., p. 643. Dissolve the sunscreening agent in slightly warmed olive oil and add the other ingredients. Olive oil may be replaced by peanut oil and isopropyl myristate, by Eutanol G. The perfume is 0.2% lavender essence absolute.

33. Conrad and Motiuk, *Am. Perfumer*, **71**, 35 (April 1956). Acetylated lanolin may be replaced by acetylated lanolin alcohols. The type of sunscreen agent is not specified; its concentration depends, of course, on its characteristics. (Lanolin derivatives impart skin affinity to the preparation and avoid viscosity and stickiness which occur when pure lanolin is used. The preparation has no tacky feeling because of the absence of vegetable oils.)

34. Bergwein, *SÖFW*, **82**, 60 (1956). (This is also a nongreasy, low-viscosity product whose water-repellent effect is due to silicone oil. The film thickness of this preparation must surely be very small, and the low concentration of active ingredient is therefore somewhat surprising.)

35. De Navarre, *op. cit.*, p. 614. Dissolve the ingredients, strain while hot, and fill. The preparation has a firm gel-like consistency. (The film thickness must be greater here than in the preceding formulation, and the active ingredient dosage would therefore appear to be very high.)

36. *Schimmel Briefs*, 195–196. (An example of a simple aerosol preparation. The composition is based on the same principle as traditional oils.)

37. Personal communication. Sun-Lac Inc. [Lantrol (Maalstrom Co.) is a lanolin derivative that is clearly soluble in mineral oil.]

**Emulsions.** All kinds of emulsions, nongreasy O/W, semigreasy dual, and fatty W/O, have been used as sunburn preventives; those with a high fat content obviously resemble oils; those that are nongreasy are similar to aqueous preparations.

As usual, the advantage of emulsified products is their attractive appearance and pleasant consistency which facilitates application. There is no risk of spillage by overturning the bottle (with the exception of liquid emulsions) and the products may be packed in the ever-popular and handy tubes. Creams may be formulated as aerosols but hardly offer any advantage. The sunscreen agents for O/W emulsions are water-soluble and for W/O emulsions, oil-soluble; in dual emulsions a combination is sometimes used.

Polano [30] made the interesting observation that the water-soluble active ingredients tannin, altrazeozone, and Cibazol only show a protective effect on O/W emulsions but not in W/O emulsions.

|  | 38 | 39 | 40 |
|---|---|---|---|
| Petrolatum |  |  | 40 |
| Isopropyl palmitate | 1 |  |  |
| Sesame oil |  | 5 |  |
| Peanut oil |  |  | 10 |
| Yellow beeswax |  |  | 2.5 |
| Lanolin, anhydrous |  |  | 5 |
| Cholesterol |  |  | 1.2 |
| Cetyl alcohol |  |  | 1.2 |
| Propylene glycol ricinoleate |  | 15 |  |
| Propylene glycol monostearate |  | 6.5 |  |
| Stearic acid | 15 |  |  |
| Oleic acid |  | 3 |  |
| Span 60 |  | 2 |  |
| Tween 60 | 1.5 |  |  |
| Sunscreen agent | q.s. |  | q.s. |
| β methyl umbelliferone |  | 5 |  |
| Water | 78 | 64 | 40 |
| Triethanolamine |  | 1.5 |  |
| Sorbitol liquid | 2.5 |  |  |
| Perfume |  |  | 0.2 |

REMARKS

38. Harry, *Modern Cosmetocology*, 4th ed., p. 264. Add the melt of stearic acid, isopropyl palmitate and emulsifying agents (90°C) to the aqueous solution of Sorbitol sunscreen agent (not specified) and preservative (95°C) with vigorous stirring. Add perfume at 50°C. Continue stirring occasionally and fill after 24 hours. (A typical example of a nongreasy liquid cream.)

39. De Navarre, *The Chemistry and Manufacture of Cosmetics*, p. 614. Dissolve the β-methyl umbelliferone in propylene glycol ricinoleate, add propylene glycol monostearate, triethanolamine, and water, and heat to boiling. Cool to 60°C and stir in the mixture of sesame oil and oleic acid (60°C). Stir for 5 minutes and again for 5 minutes after 15 and 75 minutes, respectively. Add perfume and pigment, and let the mixture stand overnight before filling. [This is an O/W cream which is somewhat greasy because of the sesame oil. The extended and strong heating of triethanolamine (to boiling!) recommended in the formulation appears undesirable.]

40. Rothemann, *Das grosse Rezeptbuch der Haut- und Körperpflegemittel*, 3rd ed., p. 642. Petrolatum, cholesterol, beeswax, and lanolin are melted together (not above 65–70°C; any commercial absorption base may also be used instead of this mixture); stir in the solution of the sunscreen agent (e.g., "6653" Merck) in peanut oil. At 50°C water is gradually stirred in; perfume (lavender type) is added when the cream is almost cold and it is finally homogenized. (Example of a W/O sunscreen cream.)

**Greaseless Preparations.**   Compared with suntan oils, these preparations have the advantage of being neither greasy nor sticky and therefore pleasanter in use. They can be subdivided according to their high or low alcohol content; there is no sharp distinction because many preparations with a medium alcohol content fall between the two groups.

Certain oily materials (isopropyl myristate, silicone oil DC 555, etc.) are often incorporated into products based on concentrated alcohol; after the alcohol has evaporated, they leave a water-repellent film on the skin. Possible disadvantages of these preparations are their high alcohol content which might cause skin irritations, particularly if the skin has already been sensitized by exposure to wind, salt water, or sun; also the low viscosity and consequently thin film necessitate a relatively high concentration of active ingredients. Ethyl alcohol is often replaced by isopropyl alcohol in these preparations; it is a better solvent for many substances, less expensive than ethyl alcohol, and has the additional advantage in the case of aerosol products of being less corrosive to metal containers. The unpleasant odor of isopropyl alcohol is a disadvantage, but it can be masked by a suitable fragrance. Thickening agents (see Chapter 4) are often added to products with low alcohol content, since a firmer consistency results in increased film thickness, and ease of application is also improved by such additives. Glycerol and sorbitol have a similar effect. Higher concentrations of these substances should be avoided because they make the film on the skin sticky. Increasing the thickening agent component yields jellies that may be packed in tubes.

The main disadvantage of aqueous and low alcoholic preparations is their water solubility: they lose their effectiveness in strong perspiration or in water. The same applies to nongreasy O/W creams.

There may be water-soluble sunburn preventives with strong affinity for skin proteins that, once applied, cannot easily be washed off the skin; these substances would, of course, be very interesting. It may be that some of the suntan preparations known today have this effect, but to my knowledge nothing has yet been published on this subject.

Greaseless sunburn preventives have also been marketed in aerosol form. Most published formulations refer to two-phase aerosols on the basis of concentrated alcohol (usually isopropyl alcohol). Aqueous sunburn preventives can be formulated as three-phase aerosols.

| | Aerosols | | | | | | Jellies | |
|---|---|---|---|---|---|---|---|---|
| | 41 | 42 | 43 | 44 | 45 | 46 | 47 | 48 |
| Mineral oil | | | 2.4 | | | | | |
| Silicone oil DC 555 | 5 | | | | | | | |
| Sesame oil | | 2.75 | 2.4 | | | | | |
| Isopropyl alcohol 99% | | 33.75 | 17.2 | | | | | |
| Ethyl alcohol 95% | 94.45 | | | 60 | 45 | 10 | | |
| Water | | | | 30 | 47 | 80.5 | 73 | 95 |
| Glycerol | | | | | | 2 | 10 | |
| Sorbitol liquid | | | | | | | | 5 |
| Propylene glycol | | | | | 5 | | | |
| Dipropylene glycol | | | 17.2 | | | | | |
| Methylcellulose | | | | | | 0.5 | | |
| Gelatin prime grade | | | | | | | 2 | |
| Carrageenan | | | | | | | | 5 |
| Dipropylene glycol salicylate | 0.25 | | | | | | | |
| Isobutyl-*p*-amino-benzoate | 0.75 | | | | | | | |
| *p*-amino benzoic acid | | 0.75 | | | | | | |
| Glyceryl-*p*-amino-benzoate | | | 0.8 | | | | | |
| Ethylene glycol monosalicylate | | | | 5 | | | | |
| Quinine oleate | | | | 5 | | | | |
| Solprotex Hydro (Firmenich) | | | | | 3 | | | |
| Filtrosol B (Schimmel) | | | | | | 7 | | |
| Triethanolamine β-methyl umbelliferone acetate | | | | | | | 5 | 3 |
| 2-Ethylhexanediol-1,3 | | 10 | | | | | | |
| Perfume | 0.3 | | | | | | | |
| Freon 11/12 (50:50) | | 50 | 60 | | | | | |

REMARKS

41. Currie and Francisco, *Am. Perfumer*, **69** 421 (December 1954). The ingredients are dissolved together. (With the low film thickness that can be expected for this product, the dosage of sunscreen agents seems rather small.)

42. Private communication. (The 2-ethylhexanediol-1,3 gives this preparation an insect-repellent effect as well.)

43. Private communication.

44. Keithler, *The Formulation of Cosmetic Specialties*, p. 420. Allow the solution to mature for 7–10 days, cool for 24 hours to 0°C, filter, and fill.

45. Janistyn, *Riechstoffe, Seifen, Kosmetika*, II, p. 195.

46. *Schimmel Briefs*, 205, April 1952. (Methylcellulose serves to increase the viscosity of this low-alcohol preparation.)

47. Janistyn, *Op. cit.*, II, p. 396.

48. Rothemann, *Das grosse Rezeptbuch der Haut- und Körperpflegemittel*, 3rd ed., p. 640. Carrageenan is heated with 50 pt water (with preservative) for 3 hours to 90°C with frequent stirring; the mucilage is passed through a fine cloth (muslin or batiste). Stir in sorbitol syrup, then the solution of sunscreen agent (which may be replaced by others) in the remaining water. Scent with 0.2% absolute lavender essence and 0.02% fennel oil.

## EVALUATION OF SUNBURN PREVENTIVES

As we have already stated, the selection of a sunscreen in the development of a new sunburn preventive as well as the determination of the required concentration is made on the basis of extinction curves of various test substances. Finished products may also be evaluated with the help of spectrophotometer readings. The critical film thickness within the range of 3000 Å can be determined, and a comparison with the experimentally established film thickness in "normal" use will show whether the preparation will give the necessary protection. Such spectrophotometric examinations of sunburn preventives and their active ingredients will provide valuable guidelines; nevertheless, positive results will not guarantee the effectiveness of a preparation in practical application. Wiskemann and Zinnermann [31] list nine factors that may be responsible for differences between effectiveness expected according to physical measurements:

1. The film thickness may fluctuate within a wide range (0.001–0.03 mm); in addition to composition and method of application, it also depends on temperature.

2. The absorptive capacity may be lost through chemical modifications of the sunscreen under the influence of the UV rays.

3. After evaporation of the solvent the sunscreen may crystallize, which would inactivate it.

4. With emulsified products, changes in the emulsion pattern on the skin may reduce the effectiveness of the preparation.

5. The sunscreen may diffuse into the skin.

6. Evaporation of the solvent may cause the protective film to become brittle and cracked.

7. Mixture with skin secretions changes the composition as well as the pH of the sunscreen film and may alter its effectiveness.

8. Water-soluble preparations may be washed off by perspiration or water.

9. The preparations may act as irritants or sensitizers and thus accelerate rather than prevent erythema.

For these reasons biological tests are essential when evaluating sunburn preventives. There are two different kinds of test: the strict clinical test under reproducible conditions and the usage test, which is less controlled but essential to the definitive evaluation of a product.

Descriptions of clinical testing methods have been given by De Navarre [32], Klarman [33], Schulze [34], and Tronnier and Klussmann [35]. Daniels [36] suggests the quantitative determination of the degree of erythrozythene formation by black and white photography and gray-scale intensity measurements.

Since in many countries the sun is an unreliable and changeable source of radiation, ultraviolet lamps with suitable filters that eliminate radiation below 2800–2900 Å (these are not present in sunlight) are used in these tests.

Tests can be made by exposing adjoining skin areas that have been treated with the test substance for different periods: one strip for 2 minutes, the next for 4, etc., so that five skin strips, for example, have been exposed to radiation for 2, 4, 6, 8, and 10 minutes respectively. A blank test should be made with a symmetrical skin area on which untreated skin strips are exposed for 1, 2, 3, and 4 minutes, respectively. A comparison of the periods of radiation required to cause erythema just visible after 10 hours on both treated and untreated areas determines the effectiveness of the preparation. If after 8 minutes the protected skin area develops erythema of the same intensity as untreated skin after 1 minute, it means that the preparation transmits only about 12% of the most active rays. This test design cancels out individual differences between test subjects by simultaneous blank tests with each person, but even so it is advisable to carry out these tests with several persons with different types of skin.

Unfortunately, the biological testing method also has some weaknesses:

1. The test period is usually less than half an hour, whereas in practice radiation lasts for several hours. Slow chemical modifications or slow penetration of the substance into the skin would therefore not become apparent in clinical tests but might play an important part in practice.

2. The light of even the best ultraviolet lamp does not equal solar radiation. The intensity of shortwave rays (2800–3200 Å) in proportion to the total intensity of radiation is much higher for lamps than for the sun. The infrared rays of the sun are almost entirely absent in UV lamps. According to Stambovsky [37], these rays act as sensitizers for UV rays.

3. In the practical use of sunburn preventives there may be conditions that are absent in clinical tests. Heavy perspiration, or activities in and near the water may make the skin wet. The water may then partially or entirely remove the sunburn preventive or it may increase the UV sensitivity of the skin [38]. The protective film may also become brittle or be rubbed off.

As can be seen, these cosmetic preparations, like all others, must be tested under normal conditions before a definite statement regarding their suitability and usefulness can be made.

## PERFUMING OF SUNBURN PREVENTIVES

The perfume to be selected depends on the image that the manufacturer wishes to give his product. If in naming and advertising it he emphasizes the athletic aspects of being in the sun, he should select a fresh, dry fragrance type, such as lavender or citrus. If, on the other hand, the product is linked to glamor on the beach, a heavier, more sultry or sophisticated fragrance is appropriate. In other cases an unobtrusive, neutral, perhaps mildly floral scent may fit the product best. Very sweet perfumes should be avoided because they attract insects.

In any case, it is important that the perfume used contains no primary irritants or materials that cause dermatoses through the chemical modifications they undergo under the influence of solar radiation (oil of bergamot, celery seed oil, angelica root oil, etc.).

The perfume must, of course, also mask any unpleasant odor the preparation itself may have.

The requisite dosage depends on the type of product. Suntan oils based on vegetable oils often require additions of perfume of 1% and more, whereas with aqueous and weakly alcoholic preparations 0.1–0.3% is usually sufficient: here Tween 20 or another solubilizer must be added to the perfume.

## PREPARATIONS WITH PROTECTIVE ACTION AGAINST MECHANICAL STRESS

### Lubricating and Massaging Preparations

One of the natural life processes is the continuous sloughing off of the corneal layer which is offset by its normal regeneration. Even though modern man accelerates constant corneal abrasion by more or less sophisticated cleansing processes (washing, bathing, brushing), the healthy organism does not normally show skin lesions. Abnormal conditions, however, may well cause an excessive wastage of the corneal layer. This happens particularly in situations in which the corneal layer swells and softens under the influence of water or an aqueous liquid (perspiration, urine) and is simultaneously or subsequently exposed to strong mechanical stress.

With bedridden patients the stress on the corneal layer is further increased because it is swollen and softened by perspiration which cannot evaporate under covers. The tender corneal layer of babies is particularly prone to soreness in the areas covered by diapers. Bathing softens the skin over the entire body, and it therefore must be protected with baby oil and powder.

Even healthy adults may experience soreness of the skin that is exposed to excessive stress, and if foreign matter or bacteria penetrate into irritated areas, they may lead to inflammations. We have only to think of the martyr-dom (quite apart from muscular pains!) undergone by inexperienced horse-back riders. Massage as well strains the corneal layer rather more than normally; massaging oils, creams, and powders derive their function from this fact.

The effectiveness of protective preparations is quite mechanical; they may be described as "skin lubricants." Oils can be compared with lubricating oils, powder with graphite. These preparations can also reduce the swelling of the skin: oils (consisting mostly of mineral oil, isopropyl palmitate, and other water-repellent substances) keep aqueous liquids away from the skin; powders absorb them.

In theory, it would be advantageous if these skin protectors could adjust the pH of the skin surface to about 5 or help to maintain it, because at this point the tendency to swell is lowest. In practice, however, this requirement cannot be met by oils or powders. It would not be difficult to obtain this pH value in creams, but it is quite a different and more complicated matter to prepare a cream that not only has this pH itself but also imparts it for an extended period to the skin.

## Skin Oils and Fats

|  | 49 | 50 | 51 | 52 | 53 | 54 | 55 | 56 |
|---|---|---|---|---|---|---|---|---|
| Mineral oil | 90 | 75 | 80 | 59.9 | 20 |  |  |  |
| Petrolatum |  |  |  |  | 60 |  | 50 |  |
| Ethyl stearate | 4 |  |  |  |  |  |  |  |
| Isopropyl palmitate |  | 21.9 |  |  |  |  |  |  |
| Ispropyl myristate | 3 |  |  |  |  |  |  |  |
| Cetiol V |  |  |  |  |  | 9 |  |  |
| Olive oil |  |  |  | 40 |  |  |  |  |
| Peachkernel oil |  |  |  |  |  | 90 |  |  |
| Neatsfoot oil |  |  | 10 |  |  |  |  |  |
| Cocoa butter |  |  |  |  | 10 |  |  |  |
| Hydrogenated cottonseed oil |  |  |  |  |  |  |  | 100 |
| Hydrogenated lard |  |  |  |  |  |  | 50 |  |
| Lanolin, liquid | 3 | 3 |  |  |  |  |  |  |
| Cetyl alcohol |  |  |  |  | 5 |  |  |  |
| Vitamin F concentrate |  |  |  |  |  | 1 |  |  |
| Hexachlorophene |  | 0.1 |  |  |  |  |  |  |
| Oxyquinoline sulfate |  |  |  | 0.1 |  |  |  |  |
| Water |  |  |  |  | 5 |  |  |  |

49. Lower, *Perfum. essent. Oil Rec.*, **47**, 403 (1956). (Liquid lanolin increases the skin affinity of the preparation and makes it slightly water-permeable which avoids sweat buildup.)

50. Keithler, *The Formulation of Cosmetics and Cosmetic Specialties*, p. 406. First dissolve lanolin (standard purified lanolin may also be used), then hexachlorophene in heated isopropyl palmitate. Add the solution to the mineral oil and stir until the mixture is uniform.

51. Janistyn, *Riechstoffe, Seifen, Kosmetika*, II, p. 201. A massage oil.

52. Keithler, *loc. cit.* Heat while mixing until the quinoline salt is dissolved and the mixture is clear. Oxyquinoline sulfate may be replaced by chlorothymol.

53. Rothemann, *Das grosse Rezeptbuch der Haut- and Körperpflegemittel*, 3rd ed., p. 619. A massage cream. (In spite of the water content, this preparation resembles the others to a considerable extent); 5 pts petrolatum may possibly be replaced by an equal amount of lanolin. Perfume: 0.1–0.15%.

54. Rothemann, *ibid.*, p. 619. A skin oil, free from mineral ingredients.

55. De Navarre, *The Chemistry and Manufacture of Cosmetics*, p. 273. Melt petrolatum and fat with antioxidants, add perfume, strain through a coarse sieve, and fill into pre-heated jars to three quarters of their capacity; allow to cool (the surface will show a funnel formation) and top off.

56. De Navarre, *ibid.*, p. 273. Thoroughly mix the antioxidant/perfume oil solution into fat which has been heated sufficiently to make it malleable but not to such an extent that the air dispersed in it can escape, since it will give the mass a creamlike consistency. Fill when cold.

In most cases mineral oil is the main ingredient in these preparations. The opponents of the use of mineral oils in cosmetics usually suggest formulations based on vegatable oils (e.g., No. 6). Care must be taken that the preparation does not penetrate the skin too quickly, since its lubricant effect will remain only as long as it stays on the skin surface.

Additions of isopropyl palmitate and similar substances facilitate application of the product, reduce its tackiness, and act as solubilizers between lanolin and mineral oil.

Additions of lanolin, cetyl alcohol, or other W/O emulsifying agents increase the adhesion of the preparation and help to avoid congestion of heat and perspiration because through them the protective film acquires a certain water-permeability.

Disinfectants are occasionally added to baby oils but dosage must be kept low in order to avoid skin irritations.

These preparations can be made in liquid or solid form but the solids must be formulated in such a way that they melt immediately on application and can be spread evenly and without friction.

## Body and Baby Powders

As with oils, the effect of body or baby powders is based on their physical characteristics and not on some kind of interaction with the skin. Smooth and neutral talcum is therefore the main, in some powders even the only, ingredient. The talcum used must be thoroughly sterilized to ensure the absence of tetanus spores.

Additions of zinc or magnesium stearates make the powder more adhesive; colloidal kaolin makes it absorptive. Body powders should not have too high a content of absorptive ingredients since they make the powder excessively drying. Carbonates lighten powders; German formulators tend to be cautious with calcium carbonate (precipitated chalk) because it reportedly causes an alkaline skin reaction; however, it amounts to 20–40% of the total weight in British and American formulations.

Starch is also occasionally added and sometimes it is even the main (see formula 62) ingredient of a body powder. On moist skin, however, starch shows an undesirable swelling and it should therefore not be used in baby or body powders for use in hot climates.

| Body Powders | 57 | 58 | 59 | 60 | 61 | 62 |
|---|---|---|---|---|---|---|
| Talcum | 90 | 85 | 56 | 44 | 25 | 10 |
| Zinc stearate | 5 | 3 | 4 | | | |
| Magnesium stearate | | | | 3.4 | | |
| Magnesium carbonate | 5 | 2 | 35 | | 10 | 20 |
| Calcium carbonate, light | | | | 38.6 | | |
| Colloidal kaolin | | | | | 30 | |
| Rice starch | | | | 10 | | 50 |
| Corn starch | | | | | | 20 |
| Wheat starch | | | | | 10 | |
| Boric acid powder | | 10 | 4 | 3.0 | | |
| Perfume | | | 1 | 1 | | |

REMARKS

57, 58, 61, 62. Janistyn, *Riechstoffe, Seifen, Kosmetika*, II, p. 217.

59, 60. Keithler, *The Formulation of Cosmetics and Cosmetic Specialties*, p. 124. (In No. 60 the high content of calcium carbonate is remarkable.)

Among disinfectants boric acid is the most important ingredient; in body powders it is used in quantities up to 20%. Following reports in the United States of serious, even fatal cases of poisoning of children after the use of boric acid powders [39], its incorporation in baby powders has been legally prohibited in this country. Today the U.S. medical profession seems to hold that boric acid is harmless when used on sound skin; greater caution has nevertheless been exercised. Fisher [40] found no increase in the boron level of the blood after external application of boric acid on healthy skin [41].

| Baby Powders | 63 | 64 | 65 | 66 |
|---|---|---|---|---|
| Talcum | 63.63 | 58.5 | 50 | 50 |
| Zinc stearate | 5 | | | |
| Magnesium stearate | | 3 | 5 | 5 |
| Magnesium carbonate | | | | 5 |
| Calcium carbonate, light | 5 | 14 | 10 | |
| Silica gel, superfine | | | 2 | |
| Cab-o-sil | | | | 5 |
| Colloidal kaolin | 20 | 11.5 | 30 | 25 |
| Zinc oxide | | 6 | | |
| Boric acid | 6 | 7 | | |
| Oxyquinoline sulfate | 0.12 | | | |
| Lycopodium | | | | 10 |
| Anhydrous lanolin | | | | 1 |
| Vitamin F (250,000 units/g) | | | | 0.2 |
| Superfatting agent | | | 3 | |
| Perfume | 0.25 | | | |

REMARKS

63. Chilson, *Modern Cosmetics*, New York, 1934, p. 305.
64. Keithler, *The Formulation of Cosmetics and Cosmetic Specialties*, p. 129.
65. Janistyn, *Riechstoffe, Seifen, Kosmetika*, II, p. 218. The superfatting agent consists of 60% paraffin oil, prime grade, 20% cetyl alcohol extra, 10% anhydrous lanolin, and 10% glyceryl monostearate, prime grade.
66. Rothemann, *Das grosse Rezeptbuch der Haut- und Körperpflegemittel*, 3rd ed., p. 676. Stir together 2.5 pts magnesium carbonate and 0.5 pt lavender oil; then add 10 g

(1 pt) anhydrous lanolin dissolved in a volatile solvent (caution! work only with open windows or in circulating air!). Mill the solution with the remaining magnesium carbonate and Cab-o-sil and Vitamin F, and spread the mass at an open window or in other ventilation until dry. Finally mix in the remaining ingredients. The mixture is sieved first through mesh V, then through mesh VI.

## Massage Creams

In some textbooks O/W "rolling" creams (see Chapter 5) are recommended as massage creams.

## INSECT-REPELLENT PREPARATIONS [42]

Insect-repellent preparations belong to the kind of products that became generally acceptable only after World War II. Certain essential oils (citronella, eucalyptus, clove, lavender, and sassafras) were formerly used for this purpose; quite apart from the fact that they sometimes cause skin irritations and, being volatile, do not maintain their effect for any length of time, their strong odor not only repels insects but also disturbs people.

During World War II the armed forces in the Pacific urgently demanded efficient insect repellents. Many thousands of substances were tested in this search for ingredients that had to meet the following requirements: They had to repel insects (mosquitoes, flies, etc.) before they alighted on the skin or at least before they stung. They had to maintain this effectiveness for several hours, that is, they should not evaporate too quickly nor penetrate the skin, and were preferably water-insoluble. They also had to remain effective under the influence of skin fluids or ultraviolet radiation. They should not be irritating or sensitizing (not even with simultaneous ultraviolet radiation) and even in small amounts should not be toxic. They should have no unpleasant odor, nor should they color the skin or show any deleterious effect on the clothes.

Eighteen substances were found that met these requirements adequately; among them were [43]

dimethyl phthalate, 2-ethylhexandiol-1,3, di-isopropyltartrate, cyclo-hexylaceto acetate, hexahydrophthalic acid diethyl ester, piperonyl butoxide.

Keithler [44] also mentions

butylmesityl oxalate, dibutyl malate, diethyl malate, benzyl lactate, tetra-hydrofurfuryl oleate and lactate, diethylene glycol monobutyl, monobenzyl, and monophenyl ethers, diethylene glycol butyl benzyl ether, ethylene glycol monophenyl and mono eugenol ethers, "Indalon," (*a,a*-dimethyl-*a'*-carbobutoxy-dihydro-*γ*-pyrone U. S. Industrial Chemicals Inc.).

It is not yet known on which specific properties the effectiveness of these substances is based [45], but it is remarkable that in most instances they are esters of dibasic acids (hydroxy or ketonic acids) or ethers of bihydric alcohols.

The most widely used substances from those mentioned above are probably dimethyl phthalate [46], and 2-ethylhexandiol-1,3 [47] which act not only against flies, mosquitoes, and horseflies but also against fleas.

According to Nabokov [48], anabin sulfate (an alkaloid salt in 5% aqueous solution) has an insect-repellent effect that lasts for 10 hours.

U.S. Patent 2,724,677 (McCabe, November 1955) covers the use of o-ethoxy-N,N-diethylbenzamide insect repellents. Swiss Patent 304,461 (Citag Ltd.) of the same year refers to mixtures of N-acetyl-N-(1-cyano-cyclohexyl)-alkylamine with aromatic N,N-dialkylamides. New patent applications for insect repellents appear almost every month; many of the above mentioned substances are also covered by patents.

Diethyl-m-toluamide [49] is widely used because of its many excellent qualities. (The technical grade contains several other isomers in addition to 75% diethyl-m-toluamide.) It has a long-lasting and intensive effect, in particular against mosquitoes, and is tolerated by the skin. It causes no unpleasant sensations and is not easily rubbed off. It is only slowly resorbed. Insects do alight on skin treated with the amide but they do not sting.

Pyrethrum extract prevents insects from stinging and acts as an insecticide [50].

According to Pijvan and co-workers [51], certain hydrated naphthol derivatives and hydrated diphenyls (e.g., 2-phenylcyclohexanone, 1,2,3,4-tetrahydro-2-naphthyl acetyl glycin ester) are also good insect repellents.

"Indalon" acts as an insect repellent as well as a sunscreen and is therefore suitable for preparations that are required to combine both actions. According to the manufacturer, the sunscreen effect can be considerably increased by an addition of 0.25% butyl cinnamoylpyruvate. Indalon is stable only in preparations with a water content below 10%.

Since a combination of protection against radiation and insects offers interesting possibilities, other pairs of sunscreen and insect-repellent agents have already been incorporated in one preparation.

The *dosage* of insect-repellent ingredients in the finished product is generally high (20–70%) because the timespan of effectiveness depends on the concentration of the active ingredient. The film thickness on application, as well as the temperature and perspiration intensity, certainly plays a part. The protective effect of any substance differs for different insects. For this reason combinations of various ingredients are often used; for example, dimethyl phthalate, 2-ethylhexane-1,3-diol, Indalon (at a ratio 6:2:2) has proved highly satisfactory.

| | 67 | 68 | 69 | 70 | 71 | 72 | 73 | 74 | 75 |
|---|---|---|---|---|---|---|---|---|---|
| Dimethyl phthalate | 89.5 | 67 | | 55.8 | 30 | | | 20 | 18.2 |
| 2-Ethylhexandiol-1,3 | | | 66.7 | 18.5 | 5 | 30 | 30 | | 18 |
| Indalon | | | | 18.6 | | | | 4 | |
| Benzyl lactate | | | | | 4 | | | | |
| Diethyl malate | | | | | 3 | | | | |
| Diethylene glycol monobutyl ether | | | | | | | | 10 | |
| Isopropyl palmitate | | | | | 4 | | | | |
| Glycerol monostearate, self-emulsifying | | | | | 9 | | | | |
| Propylene glycol monostearate | | | | 2.0 | | | | | |
| Stearic acid | | | | | 7 | | | | |
| Zinc stearate | | 23 | | | | 20 | 20 | | |
| Magnesium stearate | | 10 | | | | | | | |
| Triethanolamine lauryl sulfate | | | | | 1 | | | | |
| Span 80 | | | | | 0.5 | | | | |
| Tween 80 | 10 | | | | | | | | |
| Tween 60 | | | | | 2.5 | | | | |
| Tween 20 | | | | | | | | 10 | |
| Isopropyl alcohol 91% | | | | | | | | | 31.5 |
| Ethyl alcohol 96% | | | 13.3 | | | | | 40 | |
| Water | 0.5 | | | | 34 | 20 | 43.4 | 16 | 4.7 |
| Potassium hydroxide (41%, aqueous) | | | | | | | 1.8 | | |
| Glycerol | | | 13.3 | | | | | | 12.1 |
| Sodium stearate | | | | | | | | | 21.3 |
| Ethyl cellulose | | | | | 2.7 | | | | |
| Cellulose acetobutyrate | | | | | 2.7 | | | | |
| Polyethylene glycol 4000 | | | | | | 30 | | | |
| Phenolphthaleine (10% in alcohol) | | | 6.7 | | | | | | |
| Perfume | | | | | | | | | 1.2 |

67, 69, and 74 are liquid; 68 and 70, jellies; 71, a cream; 72 and 73, pastes; and 75, a stick.

REMARKS

67. Janistyn, *Riechstoffe, Seifen, Kosmetika*, II, p. 436.

68. Scottish Scient. Advisory Comm. [*Manuf. Chem.* 437 (October 1950)]. Heat the ingredients until a gel develops. (The stearates are intended to make the film emollient and water-repellent.)

69. U. S. Patent 2,496,270, in *Am. Perfumer*, **65**, 36 (July 1950). Sodium carbonate added to the preparation (a viscous liquid) gives it an intensely red color which disappears shortly after application. (The indicator prevents the omission of certain skin areas during application. This is important because insects attack unprotected skin areas even if they are surrounded by treated skin.)

70. Dreyling, U. S. Patent 2,404,698, in Harry, *Modern Cosmetocology*, 4th ed. p. 592.

71. Keithler, *The Formulation of Cosmetics and Cosmetic Specialties*, p. 479. Heat all ingredients together to 95°C, stir, let cool to room temperature, and add perfume.

72, 73. General Metallurgical and Chemical Ltd., in Harry, *op. cit.*, p. 51.

74. Keithler, *op. cit.*, p. 480. Add water to the oil/Tween mixture and finally stir in alcohol. Continue stirring until the solution is clear.

75. Harry, *op. cit.*, p. 493. Mix active ingredients with isopropyl alcohol and add sodium stearate, glycerol, water, and dye solutions, if any. Heat the mixture, stirring occasionally, to 81–82°C. Remove from heat when the mixture has clarified (usually after 7–10 minutes), cool to 60°C, add perfume, and pour into molds.

Various types of preparation are feasible. The most widely used are probably (a) preparations in which the active ingredient accounts for the major part (60–90%) of the total quantity and the other substances merely improve the consistency of the product or the properties of the film; (b) active ingredients in water emulsions; (c) hydroalcoholic lotions in which the active ingredient is in clear solution; (d) solid preparations in stick form (similar to eau de cologne sticks) which are made by adding sodium stearate to hydro-alcoholic lotions; and (d) aerosol preparations.

**Perfuming Insect Repellents.**   Perfume should be fresh and discreet, just strong enough to mask any possible odor of the preparation itself. The requisite dose will therefore vary according to the type of product. Sweet and distinctly floral fragrances should be avoided, since they seem to attract insects.

**Evaluating Insect Repellents [52].**   To evaluate the effectiveness of an insect repellent against mosquitoes the forearm is treated with 1 ml of the test preparation and introduced into a cage with a few hundred to a few thousand mosquitoes. The period elapsed to the first sting or the average number of stings per 30 seconds is determined. Some sources of error in this test are (a) possible differences between various batches of the ingredient; (b) the effect of the diluent (which may be synergistic or antagonistic); (c) if several tests are made with the same group of mosquitoes, the insects may be fatigued, but if different groups are used this may also be a source of error because the insects may show different behavior (e.g., depending on age); (d) the test is affected by temperature and atmospheric humidity and some substances are known to be affected by perspiration (e.g., dimethyl phthalate and ethyl hexandiol).

## REFERENCES

[1] Winter, *Handbuch der gesamten Parfümerie und Kosmetik*, 3rd ed., Springer Vienna 1942; De Navarre, *The Chemistry and Manufacture of Cosmetics*, Van Nostrand, New York 1941.

[2] Tronnier, *Z. Haut u. GeschKrankh.*, **32**, 9 (1961).

[3] *Schimmel Briefs*, 298, January 1960, *Soap, Perf. Cosm.*, **33**, 474 (1960).

[4] *Am. Perfumer*, **69** 421 (December 1954).

5] *Mfg. Chem.*, **18**, 389 (1947).

[6] Weber, paper read at the 23rd Convention of the German Dermatological Association, Vienna, May 1956, in *Kosmetik-Parf-Drog.*, **3/4**, 36 (1956).

[7] *Fette Seifen*, **53**, 10 (1951).

[8] Carrié, *Fette Seifen*, **56**, 32 (1954).

[9] Czetsch-Lindenwald and Schmidt-La Baume, *Die äusseren Heilmittel 1950–1955*, p. 132.

[10] Schulze, *Parfüm. Kosmet.*, **37**, 310 (1956).

[11] Schulze, *op. cit.*; Klave, *Internat. Z. prophyl. Med. soz. Hyg.*, **1**, 98 (1951); *Parfüm. Kosmet.*, **39**, 28 (1958).

[12] Gartmann and Reimers, *Dermat. Wschr.*, **136**, 1123 (1951); Harry, *op. cit.*, 235.

[13] E. Klarmann, *Am. Perfumer*, (July/August 1949); Ippen, *J. Soc. cosmet. Chem.*, **14**, 566 (1963).

[14] *Physiol. Rev.*, **25**, 483 (1945).

[15] Zenisek, Hain, and Kral, *Biochem. biophys. Acta*, **12**, 479 (1953); Zenisek, *Parfüm. Kosmet.*, **37**, 350 (1956); Vandenbelt et al., *Science*, **119**, 514 (1954); Everett, Anglin, and Bever, *Archs. Derm.*, **84**, 717 (1961); Zenisek and Kral, *Parfüm. Kosmet.*, **46**, 196 (1965).

[16] Luckiesh and Taylor, *Gen. elect. Rev.*, **42**, 274 (1939); Klarmann, *Am. Perfumer*, 33 (July 1949).

[17] Pathak, Riley, Fitzpatrick, and Curwen, *J. invest. Derm.*, **39**, 435 (1962); *Nature* (London), **193**, 148 (1962).

[18] Grady, *J. Soc. cosmet. Chem.*, 17 (July 1947).

[19] Barmak, *Am. Perfumer*, **75** (3), 57 (March 1960).

[20] Flesch and Esoda, *Proc. scient. Sect.*, *Toilet Goods Ass.*, **34**, 53 (1960); Goldman and Blancy, *Archs. Derm.*, **85**, 730 (1962).

[21] *SÖFW*, **82**, 660 (1956); Sulzberger and Lerner, *J. Am. med. Ass.*, **167**, 2077 (1958); Trabaud, *Industrie Parfum.*, **11**, 369 (1956); Imbrie, Bergeron, and Fitzpatrick, *Archs. Derm.*, **82**, 617 (1960); Ali and Agarwala, *J. scient. ind. Res.* (New Delhi), Sect. C 21, 321 (1962); *Parfüm. Kosmet.*, **45**, 199 (1964).

[22] Lasser, *J. Soc. cosmet. Chem.*, **14**, 577 (1963).

[23] *Parfüm. Kosmet.*, **37**, 609 (1956); *J. Soc. cosmet. Chem.*, **14**, 585 (1963).

[24] Klarman, *Am. Perfumer*, **64**, 126 (August 1949).

[25] Janistyn, *Riechstoffe, Seifen, Kosmetika*, I, 251; II, 393.

[26] *Am. Perfumer*, **64**, 126 (August 1949).

[27] Currie and Gergle, *J. Soc. cosmet. Chem.*, **7**, May 1956.

[28] *J. Am. pharm. Ass.*, Sci. Ed., **39**, (1950).

[29] Orelup, *Am. Perfumer*, (May 1936).

[30] *Dermatologica*, **91**, 297 (1945).

[31] Schulze, *Parfüm. Kosmet.*, **37**, 370 (1956).

[32] De Navarre, *op. cit.*, 604.

[33] *Am. Perfumer*, **64**, (August 1949).

[34] *Parfüm. Kosmet.*, **37**, 310, 356 (1956); *J. Soc. cosmet. Chem.*, **14**, 544 (1963).

[35] *Z. Haut-u. GeschKrankh.*, **21**, 43, 75, 96 (1956).

[36] *J. Soc. cosmet. Chem.*, **15,** 709 (1964).

[37] Klarman, *Am. Perfumer*, **64,** (August 1949).

[38] De Navarre, *op. cit.*, 587.

[39] Brooke, *Gen. Practnr.* (Kansas), **7,** 43 (1953); *Excerpta med.*, Sect. XIII, **8,** 238.

[40] Fisher, *Archs. Derm.*, **73,** 336 (1956).

[41] *Food, Cosmet. Toxicol.*, **1,** 249 (1963).

[42] Bergwein, *Parfüm. Kosmet.*, **38,** 619 (1951).

[43] Draize, Alvarez, and Whitesell, *J. Pharmacol.*, **93,** 26 (1948).

[44] Keithler, *The Formulation of Cosmetics and Cosmetic Specialties*, p. 478.

[45] Peters, *Z. angew. Zool.*, 1–75 (1956).

[46] *Br. med. J.*, 703 (May 19, 1945).

[47] *Chem. Engng. News*, **22,** 416 (1944).

[48] *A. Rev. Soviet Med.*, **2,** 449 (1945); *Drug Cosmet. Ind.*, **57,** 4 (October 1945).

[49] *Chem. Engng. News*, **35** (10), 90 (1957).

[50] Holden and Findlay, *Trans R. Soc. trop. Med. Hyg.*, **38,** 199 (1944); Hornby and French, *ibid.*, **37,** 41 (1943).

[51] Dethier, *Chemical Insect Attractants and Repellents*, Blakistone, Philadelphia, 1947, p. 211 et seq.

[52] Dethier, *op. cit.*, 209 et seq.

CHAPTER 8

# Emollients

## PHYSIOLOGICAL PRINCIPLES

The preceding chapters have dealt with preparations intended to protect the skin from harmful contacts or to remove foreign matter from its surface; in this chapter and the next we consider preparations which have the purpose of correcting minor disturbances of a healthy skin and maintaining a youthful appearance as long as possible. Cosmetics deal with two different types of skin lesion: superficial damage to the corneal layer and degeneration and senescence in the deeper strata. The preparations aimed at the deeper layers are discussed in Chapter 9; we now consider products for the care of the corneal layer.

As the outermost layer of the skin, the *stratum corneum* is exposed to all the impacts of the outside world. Even if it is amazingly resistant, damage cannot always be avoided in view of the manifold and often far from natural exposures to which the skin is subjected. Any serious damage must be subject to medical treatment. There are, however, two frequently occurring types of lesion that are relatively harmless and can be successfully countered by purely cosmetic means: the *degreasing* and the *drying out* of the corneal layer. Although these symptoms often occur simultaneously, they differ in character.

### Degreasing of the Stratum Corneum

Normally there is a very thin lipid layer on the skin surface. The most important functions of skin lipids are probably the smoothing of the surface and the prevention of dirt particles and microorganisms from penetrating the corneal layer; they also, if indirectly, are a protection against dehydration (see below).

Thorough washing with soap or repeated exposure to soap and detergent solutions removes part of the skin lipid layer. A considerable amount of surface fat is also removed with, for example, cleansing cream in removing make-up. The degreasing effect is even more drastic when the skin is washed or rubbed with organic solvents (concentrated alcohol, ether, benzene, etc.) Spoor [1] describes a method for determining experimentally the amount of degreasing caused by different treatments.

The damage resulting from degreasing can easily be deduced from the above mentioned functions of the surface lipid layer. When the surface fat is removed, the protruding edges and ridges of the corneal disks emerge on the surface. Although each disk is invisibly minute, their accumulation produces a rough surface on which bacteria and dirt particles can easily lodge and makes the skin look dull.

These bacteria and dirt particles can then penetrate into the corneal layer and possibly reach deeper layers where they may cause inflammation. The risk is even greater when the *stratum corneum* is not only degreased but also dehydrated.

Removal of the surface lipid layer often results secondarily in dehydration of the *stratum corneum*.

### Dehydration of the Stratum Corneum [2]

The water content of the corneal layer is normally low (about 10%), but this small amount of moisture is very important. Investigations by several teams of dermatologists (in particular, I. H. Blank and his collaborators) have demonstrated that the softness and flexibility of the corneal layer do not, as was previously assumed, depend on its fat content but entirely on its moisture content. Flesch [3] summarizes the functions of water in the softening of the epidermis. Blank and Shappirio [4] found that a corneal disk, stored in a dry atmosphere, becomes hard and brittle. It could not be softened with petrolatum, lanolin, or olive oil but only by treating it with water. Peck and Glick [5], who measured the hardness of keratin on living skin with a new instrument, the "tonometer," also found that water softens dried keratin, whereas anhydrous lanolin, mineral oil, soyabean oil, and glycerol have no emollient effect in the absence of water.

That the elasticity of the *stratum corneum* is a function of its moisture content is easily explained from its structure. The *stratum corneum* consists of keratin disks and a waxlike cement that fills the spaces between them. Keratin (see Chapter 1) is composed of long-chain molecules linked by salt or hydrogen bonds. The smaller the amount of water between the chains, the stronger the bonds and the lower the elasticity of the keratinic tissue. The cement between the horny disks normally also contains water, probably bound as a W/O emulsion to the fat. It is quite possible that the consistency of this substance depends on the water content and that, with a low moisture content, the cement stiffens, like, for example, anhydrous lanolin.

Whereas the *stratum germinativum* and the layers underneath are protected from drying out by Rein's membrane, the horny layer is directly exposed to all atmospheric influences. Healthy skin is protected from drying out by its content of water-soluble, partly hydroscopic substances: amino acids, purins, pentoses, choline, and phosphoric acid derivatives. The total amount of these substances accounts for 20% of the weight of the corneal layer. They bind the water it requires [6].

These water-soluble substances could be removed from the skin by perspiration or washing if they were not protected by the lipid layer that covers the skin surface with a water-insoluble film. If the skin lipids are removed, the water-soluble substances are exposed and subsequent water treatment flushes them out, leaving behind tissue that has partly or completely lost its hydrophilic character and elasticity [7]. Thus degreasing of the skin also leads to its dehydration.

Prolonged or repeated contact of the hands with soap and detergent solutions is particularly unfavorable in this connection. Here, the surface fat is first emulsified and the hydrophilic components of the corneal layer dissolved. As soon as the hands are again exposed to air, the corneal layer easily dries out and becomes rough and fissured. This is a special risk for laundry personnel, certain industrial workers, kitchen workers, and, of course, every housewife.

Powers and Fox [8] investigated the effect of different detergents on the loss of moisture from the corneal layer. One forearm of the test subject was thoroughly brushed with warm water and detergent, rinsed with warm water, brushed again, rinsed again, and then left to dry for $\frac{1}{2}$ hour. A desiccator was then applied to the treated and an untreated skin area. Powers and Fox found that the loss of water was accelerated by triethanolamine alkyl aryl sulfonate, sodium lauryl sulfate, and a coconut fatty-acid diethanolamine condensation product. The drying effect was even stronger with a cationic detergent, whereas soap had a much weaker drying action (here the loss in moisture of the treated skin area was even below that of untreated skin). The authors quote figures, but since the tests were made with only one person, these values are not very meaningful. Gaul and Underwood [9] found that dry-skin symptoms occur with seborrhoea subjects as well as with representatives of the dry-skin type and that there is no difference between fair and dark types, male or female. The operative factor was always that the people in question had frequent or prolonged exposure to detergent solutions.

The surface lipid layer of the skin protects the *stratum corneum* from dehydration in other ways as well. Although the fat layer is not water-impermeable, it delays evaporation of water from the corneal layer and thus acts as a kind of buffering agent in fluctuations of atmospheric humidity. In addition, when there is no fat film, the surface of the *stratum corneum* is rough and consequently larger than if it were smoothly covered by a fat film; the larger the surface, the quicker the evaporation.

In summary it is important to recognize that skin owes its water impermeability to Rein's membrane and that the lipid layer protects only the top skin (the corneal layer) from drying out.

The influence of weather on corneal dehydration is known. If relative air humidity is low, the risk of drying out is great.

Absolute humidity is the weight of water contained in a definite volume of air. The ratio of absolute humidity to the maximum quantity the air could absorb at the given pressure and temperature is described as the relative humidity, 30% relative humidity, for example, means that the atmosphere contains 30% of the water it requires for saturation; in this instance it is rather dry, since it can still absorb more than twice its water vapor content. Only the relative humidity index shows whether the air is actually "humid" or "dry."

In warm weather the corneal layer will not dry out so quickly as in cold, even if the relative humidity is rather low, because at higher temperatures the sweat glands continually supply the skin surface with water. If there is no air movement, the air immediately surrounding the skin has a higher humidity than the air farther away because it is constantly being humidified by the skin. When it is windy, however, the more humid air is continuously blown away and evaporation from the skin surface is accelerated.

In cold weather the elasticity of the corneal layer is still further reduced because the skin wax (the cement between the corneal disks) becomes harder and tougher in low temperatures. In addition, a low skin temperature results in decreased sebum secretion. As shown by Ikai, Sugie, and Nitta [10], the activity of skin sebaceous glands does not depend on the sweat glands but directly on the temperature of the skin.

### The Anatomic Picture of Dry Skin

When the corneal layer loses its elasticity through dehydration, the horny disks no longer slide over one another in skin folds or with mechanical stress. They stick together and when the skin is bent, cracks appear which have been described by Jäger [11] as V-shaped fissures. Microorganisms may penetrate into these fissures and are then not easily removed by water. Dirt particles, soap residue, etc., accumulate so that the V-fissures become potential seats of infection.

When bacteria or irritants penetrate the V-fissures below Rein's membrane, another type of skin lesion, incomplete and abnormal keratinization, may develop, according to Blank [12]. The *stratum germinativum* reacts to irritants by increased cellular division. The resulting unusually quick outward migration of cells leads to a thicker corneal layer in which the cells are only partly keratinized. The composition of the corneal cement also deviates from normal. One of the results is an agglomeration of corneal cells to coarser flakes, often visible to the naked eye, instead of the normal microscopically small disks. When the flakes work loose, relatively deep fissures form which further facilitate the entry of microorganisms and dirt particles.

Generally speaking, minor lesions of the corneal layer may under unfavorable conditions give rise to more serious disturbances. If V-fissures develop and foreign matter penetrates, degreed skin may lead to irritations and inflammations or abnormal keratinization may occur which would further weaken the skin.

On the other hand, skin is a biologically active tissue with excellent regenerative properties under favorable conditions. After removal the surface-fat film is quickly renewed by the continuous activity of the sebaceous glands, although this renewal occurs less quickly in people with dry skin than in those of the seborrhoic type. Loss of water from the corneal layer is soon compensated, since water vapor in small quantities is transmitted through Rein's barrier. The situation is more serious, however, when the hydrophilic components are removed from the corneal layer, because it is then no longer capable of retaining the amount of water required. In living skin this generally occurs only in the top layers. Provided there are no disturbances, the situation reverts to normal quite soon through a new supply of hydrophilic substances.

## PREPARATIONS

As we have shown in the preceding section, slight lesions of the corneal layer easily occur in the course of normal living conditions. Such lesions (degreasing and dehydration) soon heal by themselves under favorable conditions but may under less favorable conditions give rise to unpleasant and cosmetically undesirable complications. Preparations for the care of the corneal layer are intended to create such favorable conditions wherever lesions may occur and to promote the intrinsic healing processes of the skin.

Applying a fat cream on degreed skin, for example, is not intended just to replace the surface lipids of the skin; it should protect the skin from dehydration and the invasion of foreign bodies until sufficient new fat has developed and the corneal layer has returned to normal. For this reason it is not especially important whether a fat cream resembles natural skin lipids in all its properties. It must merely fulfill its purpose during the limited period it is needed by the skin.

This opinion is not shared by all experts. Statements are found in various publications that a certain cream is particularly good because it comes close to human skin fat in both chemical composition and physical properties. In our opinion the repertory of cosmetic chemists is unnecessarily limited by the demand that skin creams be as similar to natural skin lipids as possible often coupled with the request for the exclusive use of natural raw materials. This attitude would completely eliminate such valuable raw materials as silicone oils and polyethylene glycols.

The effect of emollients is based primarily on their capacity to leave a thin film on the skin with limited water permeability or static hygroscopicity. Products with a high moisture content also supply the corneal layer with water by external application but this is not absolutely essential for an emollient effect.

Testing numerous substances for their capacity to form water-impermeable films, Weizel, Fretzdorff, and Heller [13] found that water permeability is inhibited by straight-chain fatty acids with more than 15 carbon atoms, their ethyl esters and glycerides, and petrolatum. Branched chains and some unsaturated fatty acids (particularly of the *cis*-series) and their glycerides have a much greater permeability. De Navarre [14] recalls experiments to prevent water evaporation from reservoirs and swamps by covering the surface with a monomolecular layer of some chemical substance. Cetyl alcohol showed the greatest effectiveness. Powers and Fox [15] investigated the effect of various cosmetic raw materials and emulsifying agents on the dynamic hygroscopicity of living skin. The forearms of the test subjects were treated with these materials and small calcium chloride desiccators (1 in. in diameter) were attached to this part and to an adjoining untreated skin area; the increase in weight of the desiccators was then determined after two hours (Table 8-1).

Here the high effectiveness of petrolatum and the comparatively low one of silicone oil is remarkable; the latter was no more effective than mineral oil or isopropyl palmitate. It is because of the test method used that glycerol, the main ingredient in many skin emollients, had a pronounced dehydrating effect here. Glycerol can absorb water from skin tissue or the surrounding atmosphere and release it in whatever direction (outward or inward) the relative humidity is lowest. It acts as an emollient when the "outside" (i.e., the skin surface and the air layer above it) is moist, if it is applied with water on a preferably moist skin surface; but when anhydrous glycerol is applied on dry skin in extremely dry surroundings (the interior of a desiccator!) a strong attraction of water from the skin is not surprising.

Flesch [16] found, in apparent contradiction to Powers and Fox, that glycerol inhibits the diffusion of water vapor through human skin *in vitro;* this contradiction may be due to differences in experimental methodology of the authors. Laden [17] tested corneal disks moistened with glycerol and found that the water absorption simply totaled the absorption by the components; thus in this list, glycerol affects hydration of the skin through the process of its own hydration.

Shelmire [18] investigated the effect of emulsions on the elasticity of isolated corneal disks and established that an adequate covering action depends on a certain minimum viscosity of the oil phase.

The smoothness of the skin may be judged by its resistance to friction.

Table 8-1

| Material | Effect on Dynamic Hygroscopicity* (%) |
|---|---|
| Petrolatum USP | −48 |
| Anhydrous lanolin | −32 |
| Light mineral oil, technical grade | −28 |
| Lanolin alcohols, 25% in mineral oil | −28 |
| Isopropyl palmitate | −28 |
| Silicone oil | −26 |
| Squalene | −23 |
| Trioleine | −23 |
| Lanolin oil, free of wax | −22 |
| Sorbitan sesquioleate | −17 |
| Polyoxyethylene glycol 200 mono-oleate | 0 |
| Polyoxyethylene glycol 600 mono-oleate | 0 |
| Polyoxyethylene glycol 400 monostearate | 0 |
| Glyceryl mono-oleate (90% monoester) | 0 |
| Safflower oil fatty acid monoglyceride (40% monoester) | 0 |
| Oleylsarcosinate | 0 |
| Polyoxyethylene sorbitan monolaurate | +5 |
| Diethylene glycol mono-oleate | +9 |
| Polyoxyethylene sorbitan mono-oleate | +13 |
| Polyoxyethylene oleyl ether (15–20 oxyethylene groups) | +22 |
| Polyoxyethylene oleyl ether (5–10 oxyethylene groups) | +25 |
| Anhydrous propylene glycol | +35 |
| Anhydrous glycerol | +43 |

\* − signifies a reduction and + an increase in dynamic hygroscopicity.

Appeldorn and Barnett [19] developed an apparatus for a quantitative determination of the reduced friction resistance caused by cream bases between a rubber ball (used as a substitute for skin) and a steel roller.

H. Tronnier [20] investigated the effect of bases and active ingredients on the static hygroscopicity of the skin on the back of the hand by measuring resonance frequencies. He found that O/W as well as inverted emulsions are able to cause reductions in water evaporation from the skin without complete covering. Among the tested active ingredients a steroid-free ovary extract and some hygroscopic substances (glycerol, etc.) showed a humectant effect.

We may distinguish between two types of emollient: preparations based on fats or preparations based on glycerol and similar humectants. The first type is particularly suitable for correcting the degreasing process and is mostly used for facial skin. Nearly all hand jellies and hand lotions belong to the glycerol type. These preparations counteract dehydration symptoms. The two types are discussed separately.

## Preparations Based on Fat

Preparations of this type are often named "moisturizers" or "moisturizing creams." The effect of these creams is due to the formation of a thin fat film which covers the skin surface, makes it smooth, and probably slightly delays the evaporation of water. The viscosity of the fat must not be too low because the film would then be too thin for easy and even spreading. It should, at least partly, remain on the surface of the corneal layer, cover the sharp edges of the corneal disks, and prevent the penetration of foreign matter, but it should not make the skin too greasy or sticky. The fat film should delay the evaporation of water from the corneal layer but not prevent it altogether because this would lead to a congestion of perspiration and, possibly, heat. These, like any other cosmetic preparations, must obviously have no primary irritating effects nor should they contain ingredients that have been observed to act as sensitizers. According to Sidi [21], skin irritations caused by these preparations have only rarely been noted.

**Basic Materials.** It is hardly a coincidence that fats known as skin emollients (lanolin, wool fat alcohols, higher fatty alcohols and lanette wax, and glycerol monostearate etc.) are all W/O emulsifying agents. These substances play an important part in all emollient creams. We are still not absolutely sure how their effect is achieved. The surface fat of the skin contains sterols (as does lanolin) and is itself a W/O emulsion. However, this by itself would not explain the effect of cetyl alcohol. Perhaps these substances act as dispersing agents in the corneal cell/skin lipids dispersion of the corneal layer. In addition to emollients, these creams also contain a wax/oil mixture that is formulated to give the preparations a suitable consistency both on the skin and in the container. Vegetable oils are probably more suitable here than mineral oils because they mix more readily with skin lipids and wax, are better able to penetrate between the corneal cells, and have better adhesion. Mineral oils just remain on the skin surface. It is probable, however, that additions of lanolin, cetyl alcohol, and similar materials which enormously increase the static hygroscopicity of mineral fats and oils, also improve their skin affinity. In German and French publications the use of mineral oils in these preparations is not recommended, yet they appear regularly in British and American formulations. (It is important to distinguish between the preparations discussed here and creams with depth effect. In the latter the use of mineral oils and fats is certainly inadvisable.)

Preparations of the dual or O/W emulsion type also contain O/W emulsifiers. Because of their skin compatibility, nonionic emulsifying agents are probably most suitable here. Triethanolamine soaps are also often recommended. Their alkaline reaction in the presence of water is less strong than that of sodium soaps and they should have a better skin compatibility.

In addition, O/W creams always contain humectants (glycerol, sorbitol syrup, etc.). These probably contribute to the emollient effect but their main purpose is to prevent or at least delay the drying of the cream in the jar.

The water used in creams for skin care should be distilled or desalted with ion-exchangers. Traces of iron and copper are very harmful because they accelerate fat rancidity.

Because of their high content of vegetable oils, many of these preparations are prone to rancidity. An addition of antioxidants is therefore essential. It is best to mix antioxidants into the various oils as soon as they are received As all cosmetic preparations, these creams must also be protected from bacterial decomposition and mold formation by preservation.

**The Type of Emulsion.** Fat-based emollients may take any forms, beginning with anhydrous fat creams, through W/O creams, dual emulsions, and fat-rich O/W creams to liquid O/W emulsions with more than 80% water. We have already discussed the advantages and disadvantages of the individual types in Chapter 4. Fat-rich W/O, dual emulsions, or anhydrous fat creams appear more suitable for night creams, whereas less fatty solid or liquid O/W emulsions are preferred for day preparations.

## Anhydrous Emollient Creams, W/O and Dual Emulsions.

|  | 1 | 2 | 3 | 4 | 5 | 6 |
|---|---|---|---|---|---|---|
| Mineral oil |  | 9.5 |  | 54 |  | 29.8 |
| Ceresine |  | 2 |  |  |  |  |
| Microcrystalline wax |  |  |  |  |  | 2 |
| Paraffin wax |  |  |  |  |  | 3 |
| Isopropyl myristate |  | 30 |  |  |  |  |
| Almond oil (sweet) | 80 | 20 |  |  | 61 |  |
| Avocado oil |  | 20 |  |  |  |  |
| Olive oil |  |  | 18.75 | 8 |  |  |
| Sesame oil |  |  |  |  |  | 30 |
| Beeswax | 10 |  | 4 |  | 18 | 5 |
| Spermaceti | 10 |  | 1 |  |  | 4 |
| Anhydrous lanolin |  |  | 37.5 | 4 |  | 2 |
| Liquid lanolin |  | 20 |  |  |  |  |
| Cetyl alcohol |  |  |  | 4 |  |  |
| Stearyl alcohol |  |  |  | 2 |  |  |
| Glyceryl monostearate |  |  |  | 6 |  |  |
| Oleic acid |  |  |  |  |  | 1 |
| Triethanolamine |  |  |  |  |  | 1.5 |
| Borax |  |  | 0.25 |  |  |  |
| Sodium lauryl sulfate |  |  |  | 1 |  |  |
| Water |  |  | 37.5 | 19 | 20 | 19.9 |
| Allantoin |  |  |  |  |  | 0.2 |
| Perfume oil |  | 0.5 | 0.5 |  | 0.1 | 0.4 |
| Butyl-p-hydroxybenzoate |  |  |  |  |  | 0.2 |

REMARKS

1. Cold cream from the Italian Pharmacopoeia, in Rothemann, *Das grosse Rezeptbuch der Haut- und Körperpflegemittel*, 3rd ed., Hüthig Verlag, Heidelberg, 1962, p. 559. A simple anhydrous cream.

2. *Riechst. Aromen.*, **7**, 10 (1957). A semiliquid anhydrous product. "Fluilan" (Croda Ltd., London) may be used as the liquid lanolin constituent. Orange blossom is recommended as a scent.

3. Rothemann, *op. cit.*, p. 561. Spermaceti may be replaced by cetyl alcohol and olive oil, by peanut oil. The "water" is triple rose water. Stir the solution of borax in rose water (45°C) into the fat melt (45°C). The perfume oil (rose type) is added at the end. (This is a W/O cream with a high lanolin content.)

4. Keithler, *The Formulations of Cosmetics and Cosmetic Specialties*, Drug and Cosmetic Industry, New York, 1956, p. 58. A W/O or dual emusion with a very high mineral oil content.

5. Cold cream from the British Pharmacopoeia. The "water" is rose water, the perfume oil rose oil. The difference between cold creams for cleansing and cold creams for skin conditioning is the partial or whole substitution of mineral oils in cleansing creams (see Chapter 5) by vegetable oils. With this modification all cold creams mentioned in Chapter 5 can be turned into skin conditioners. The emollient effect of creams of this type is, however, considerably less than that of lanolin-rich creams such as formula 3 as well as formulas 2 and 4 in this table.

6. Mecca, *proc. Scient. Sect.*, Toilet Goods Ass., 8 (May 1955). Dissolve Allantoin in the aqueous phase, and butyl-*p*-hydroxybenzoate in the oil phase. Allantoin is intended to stimulate cellular proliferation in the *stratum germinativum* and promote the degradation of worn out corneal cells. (A dual emulsion in which, in addition to the beeswax/borax emulsifier system, lanolin as a W/O emulsifier and triethenolamine as O/W emulsifier are also present.)

Shelmire [22] observed that O/W emulsions are more effective than oils alone or W/O emulsions in preventing the dehydration of isolated corneal layer sections. Such sections can, however, not really be compared with living skin because they are deprived of the constant internal water supply.

REMARKS

7. Rothemann, *Das grosse Rezeptbuch der Haut- und Körperpflegemittel*, 3rd ed., p. 595. A superfatted lanolin cream. Nipagallin is a gallate, serving as antioxidant.

8. Keithler, *The Formulation of Cosmetics and Cosmetic Specialties*, p. 85. Add the aqueous solution of propylene glycol and trilauryl sulfate (85°C) to the fat melt (80°C) with continuous stirring. A hand cream.

9. Skin conditioning cream of the British Pharmacopoeia Revisions Committee, in Janowitz, *SÖFW*, **82**, 111 (1956). This cream is solid in spite of its high water content.

10. Conrad and Motiuk, *Am. Perf.*, **71**, 35 (April 1956). Stir the aqueous phase (85°C) into the oil phase (85°C). Continue stirring slowly until cool, leave overnight, and stir once again next morning. An all-purpose cream. (Acetylated lanolin and acetylated lanolin alcohols are less sticky on the skin than lanolin but lack the same emollient effect.)

| | 7 | 8 | 9 | 10 | 11 |
|---|---|---|---|---|---|
| Almond oil (sweet) | 10 | | | | |
| Cetiol V | 10 | | | | |
| Isopropyl palmitate | | 4 | | | 2 |
| Polyethylene glycol 400 distearate | | | 11 | | |
| Acetylated lanolin alcohols (liquid fraction) | | | | 10 | |
| Acetylated lanolin | | | | 2 | |
| Wool wax alcohols | | | 6 | | |
| Cetyl alcohol | | 8 | | 0.5 | |
| Stearyl alcohol | | 4 | | | |
| Oleyl alcohol | | | 3 | | |
| Lanette N | 15 | | | | |
| Diethylene glycol monostearate | | | | 2 | |
| Glyceryl monostearate (self-emulsifying) | | | 10 | | 3.2 |
| Stearic acid | | | | 2 | 2 |
| Oleic acid | | | | | 2 |
| Triethanolamine | | | | 1 | 1 |
| Triethanolamine ricinoleate | | | 1 | | |
| Triethanolamine lauryl sulfate | | 1.2 | | | |
| Water | 60 | 59.8 | 83.8 | 82.5 | 83.7 |
| Alcohol | | | | | 4 |
| Glycerol | 5 | | 6 | | |
| Propylene glycol | | 12 | | | |
| Sorbitol syrup | | | | | 2 |
| Nipagin (a $p$-hydroxybenzoate) | 0.1 | | | | 0.1 |
| Chlorocresol | | | 0.2 | | |
| Nipagallin | 0.1 | | | | |
| Perfume oil | 0.4 | | | | |

11. Keithler, *op. cit.*, p. 302. Heat all ingredients, with the exception of alcohol and perfume oil, to 95°C. Stir until emulsification is complete and continue stirring until cool (caution: do not stir in any air). Add perfume, dissolved in alcohol, at 45°C. A hand lotion. (In this cream the fats are again the main active ingredients, even if they account for only 5.2% of the total. The comparatively high stearic acid and oleic acid content imparts a matting effect. Alcohol causes the cream to dry faster on the skin and is intended to reduce its stickiness.)

## Preparations Based on Glycerol and Similar Active Ingredients

These preparations dry on the skin to a hygroscopic film which retains moisture and remains on the skin surface. They make the skin look smooth and prevent further dehydration of the corneal layer.

The traditional glycerol/rose water represents the simplest type; its formulation 50:50 glycerol:rose water is probably only of historical interest.

This high glycerol concentration has an irritating effect on the skin; today, concentrations of 10–20% glycerol are preferred.

In these products glycerol may be wholly or partly replaced by sorbitol syrup or propylene glycol. Carbitol (diethylene glycol monoethyl ether) is less suitable because it causes beads of perspiration to form on the skin.

Mucins or gel-forming agents are usually incorporated in modern formulations which impart a pleasanter consistency to the preparations. Various consistencies may be obtained, depending on the thickening agents selected and their levels. In the United States viscous preparations are preferred; jellies are popular in Europe. Nearly all thickening agents mentioned in Chapter 4 may be used. The only materials to be avoided are adhesives such as gum arabic and those that on drying form a resistant film (e.g., polyvinyl pyrrolidone and polyvinyl alcohol). An emollient effect is attributed to some of these thickening agents. As far as we are aware, it has never been determined whether an effect on the corneal layer is involved here or merely the application of a smooth coating.

Liquid and solid polyethylene glycols are also suitable for these preparations. They give a more substantial film on the skin, yet without a greasy feeling. In addition, low molecular weight polyethylene glycols are hygroscopic.

Alcohol in small quantities is occasionally added to accelerate the drying of the preparation on the skin. It is also meant to reduce the tackiness of the film. Small amounts of partly saponified stearic acid are frequently added to American liquid preparations. This gives the preparation a milky effect or mother-of-pearl luster and produces a matting effect on the skin.

Preparations containing appreciable quantities of fats, such as glyceryl monostearate or lanette wax, achieve the emollient effect in two ways: with the hygroscopic substances and with fats.

Some modern hand creams also contain silicone oils in addition to the usual ingredients. Thus they combine their emollient effect with protection against aqueous solutions. However, this protective effect comes into play only if the cream is applied before contact with the dehydrating medium (e.g., detergent solution), and the emollient effect, if it is applied subsequently.

Next to glycerol, honey used to be the most important humectant in skin jellies and creams. It is still occasionally being used today.

Fruit juices are sometimes incorporated in skin jellies and lotions (lemon juice, cucumber juice, etc.) Their main value probably lies in their acid reaction. The question is whether such reaction is actually desirable in preparations that are meant to cause a certain softening and swelling of the epidermal keratin.

Small additions of antiseptic agents, such as boric acid, may be indicated. In any case hand jellies and lotions must be adequately preserved, particularly if they contain natural mucins such as gum tragacanth and quince seed mucilage because these provide good culture media for many bacteria and fungi. De Navarre [23] found some commercially available products of this type with pH values between 3.5 and 4.5, an indication that bacterial decomposition had led to the formation of acids.

Floral waters or water-soluble perfume compounds are the fragrances most commonly used for these preparations. In emulsified preparations water-insoluble compounds may also be used. Perfume may emphasize or suggest the presence of certain basic materials; the scent of almonds will cause an association with almond oil, the scent of honey, which incidentally blends particularly well with rose type perfume, recalls honey. The type of perfume to be selected for a lemon cream is obvious.

## Hand Lotions and Jellies.

|  | 12 | 13 | 14 | 15 |
|---|---|---|---|---|
| Almond oil (sweet) |  |  | 0.3 |  |
| Glyceryl monostearate |  |  | 0.3 |  |
| Stearic acid |  |  | 1.2 |  |
| Ricinoleic acid |  |  | 0.3 |  |
| Triethanolamine |  |  | 0.3 |  |
| Glycerol | 20 | 20 | 6 | 14.5 |
| Honey | 5 |  |  |  |
| Sorbitol liquid | 5 |  |  |  |
| Gelatin | 4 |  |  |  |
| Quince seed mucilage ($2\frac{1}{2}\%$) |  |  | 50 |  |
| Gum tragacanth |  |  |  | 1 |
| Sodium alginate |  | 2 |  |  |
| Calcium citrate |  | 0.2 |  |  |
| Water | 65 | 78.5 | 38.6 | 75 |
| Alcohol | 2.5 | 3.0 |  | 8 |
| Boric acid |  |  |  | 1 |
| Nipagin (a $p$-hydroxybenzoate) | 0.2 |  |  |  |
| Perfume oil | 0.3 | 0.1 |  | 0.5 |

REMARKS

12. *Riechst. Aromen*, **7**, 141 (1956) a hand jelly: 4 pts gelatin and 10 pts cold water are left to swell overnight; about 20 pt rose water (described as water in the formulation) are then added and the mass heated until it becomes homogeneous. Dissolve the honey separately in the remaining water, add glycerol and sorbitol, and heat and stir in the gelatin solution. Finally add perfume oil and preservative dissolved in alcohol and stir thoroughly.

13. Rothemann, *Das grosse Rezeptbuch der Haut- und Körperpflegemittel*, 3rd. ed., p. 607. Alginate is dissolved in the major portion of water (distilled, preserved!) with stirring. The calcium citrate suspension in the remaining water is then stirred in until a gel has formed. (Rothemann prescribes 1.5–3.0% alginate. The exact quantity must be

determined in preliminary tests because various commercial grades of sodium alginate behave differently. The requisite quantity of calcium citrate is also not fixed; it depends on the quantity and quality of the alginate. Sufficient citrate must be added for the jelly to show a weakly acid reaction—pH 6.4–7.) Stir in glycerol and finally perfume oil.

14. De Navarre, *The Chemistry and Manufacture of Cosmetics*, 291. (An emulsified viscous preparation with an addition of partly saponified stearic acid and very low content of fats.) Shortly before use quince-seed mucilage is prepared as follows: pour 1 pt preserved water (60–65°) over 1 pt quince seed and leave overnight. Pass the mucilage through a sieve. The remaining seeds are again soaked for 12 hours in 1 pt water (60–65°C). This mucilage is also strained and both portions combined.

Add the aqueous solution of glycerol and triethanolamine (72°C) to the fat melt (70°C), stirring quickly. Stir in quince-seed mucilage when the mass is cooled to 60°C. Leave for 24 hours and then add perfume and preservative dissolved in alcohol. Pass the cream through a sieve and homogenize, possibly in a colloid mill.

15. Keithler, *The Formulation of Cosmetics and Cosmetic Specialties*, p. 312. Heat the solution of glycerol and boric acid in water to 90°C and pour it over the gum tragacanth/ alcohol mixture. Stir until the gum is completely dispersed and no lumps are left, cool to room temperature, and stir in perfume.

## REFERENCES

[1] Spoor, *Drug Cosmet. Ind.*, **80**, 42 (1957).

[2] Buettner, *J. Soc. cosmet. Chem.*, **16**, 133 (1965).

[3] Flesch, *Proc. scient. Sect.* Toilet Goods Ass., **40**, 12 (1963).

[4] *J. invest. Derm.*, **8**, 433 (1952).

[5] *J. Soc. cosmet. Chem.*, **7**, 530 (1956).

[6] Flesch, 3rd Annual Cosmetics Seminar, Society Cosmetic Chemists, New York, 1956.

[7] Blank and Shappirio, *J. invest. Derm.*, **25**, 391 (1955).

[8] *Drug Cosmet. Ind.*, **82**, 234 (1958).

[9] *J. invest. Derm.*, **19**, 9 (1952).

[10] Ikai, Sugie, and Nitta, *Arch. Derm. Syph.*, **88**, 734 (1963).

[11] Jaeger in Czetsch-Lindenwald and Schmidt-La Baume, *Salben, Puder, Externa*, 3rd ed., Springer Verlag, 1950, p. 457 et seq.

[12] Blank, *Am. Perfumer*, **71**, 35 (May 1956).

[13] *Z. physiol. Chem.*, 301, 26 (1955).

[14] *Am. Perfum.*, **70** (6), 10 (1957).

[15] *Drug Cosmet. Ind.*, **82**, 32 (1958).

[16] Flesch, *Proc. scient. Sect.* Toilet Goods Ass., **35**, 1 (1961).

[17] K. Laden, *J. Soc. cosmet. Chem.*, **13**, 455 (1962).

[18] *J. invest. Derm.*, **26**, 105 (1956); *Schimmel Briefs*, 258 (1956).

[19] *Proc. scient. Sect.* Toilet Goods Ass., **40**, 28 (1963).

[20] *Arch. Biochem. Cosmetol.*, **4**, No. 46, 12 (1962); *Parfum. Kosmet*, **42**, 513 (1962).

[21] E. Sidi, *Tolérance aux Produits Cosmétiques*, p. 57.

[22] *J. invest. Derm.*, **26**, 105 (1956).

23] De Navarre, *The Chemistry and Manufacture of Cosmetics*, Van Nostrand, New York, 1941 1st ed., p. 294.

CHAPTER 9

# Preparations with Depth Effect

Here we are dealing with the most controversial subject in modern cosmetics.

*Author's note:* This sector of cosmetics has received far more attention on the European continent than in Great Britain and the United States. Neither the "gullible idealists" nor the "charlatans" have had much influence in the English-speaking countries. However, the Continental perspective from which the German edition of this book was written has been retained in the translation. It may prove of some interest to English-speaking readers.

This is a field in which medicine and cosmetics overlap to a certain extent and in which dedicated physicians have done valuable research. At the same time gullible idealists as well as charlatans have been more active in it than in any other and have caused considerable confusion. We shall try to remain critical and unprejudiced. First of all the nature of the problems involved must be defined.

## PROBLEMS

Cosmetics in depth deals mainly with two kinds of problem: first with the aging and degeneration of the skin in all its manifestations and second with certain common disorders in the physiology of the scalp such as seborrhoea, dandruff, and loss of hair. We shall discuss these problems briefly.

### Senescence and Degeneration of the Skin

Skin, as the protective organ of the human body, is exposed to many external agents. It is quite capable of resisting most of their effects without much difficulty; this, after all, is its function. Some influences, however, the skin cannot tolerate without the aid of cosmetic preparations. Contact with irritating and toxic substances or detergent solutions, excessive solar radiation may cause lesions which, if the contact is prolonged or repeated, may lead to chronic degeneration of the epidermis: the skin becomes rough, and pigmentation and keratinization disorders occur. Once these symptoms have

365

fully developed they can hardly ever be reversed. Their onset may be delayed, however, and even prevented by conditioning, hygiene, and regular care.

Even the most carefully conditioned, best looked after skin does not retain a fresh and smooth appearance forever. As the whole body ages, so does the skin. Physiological senescence of the skin develops earlier in some people than others; the difference is largely due to genetic factors. In women it usually begins between 35 and 45. An advanced stage of senescence has the following external characteristics: the skin becomes pale to yellowish-brown (marked by occasional small dark or red spots due to hyperpigmentation and dilation of the blood vessels, respectively), dry, flabby, creased, and wrinkled. The skin becomes thin, the subcutaneous lipid layer disappears, and the veins are more clearly visible. Skin can be lifted in large folds and in some areas of the body it hangs down loosely.

Microscopic observation shows that the epidermis as well as the collagenous connective tissue of the corium have narrowed and that the fat patches of the subcutis have also withered. Whereas in young skin the papillary bodies of the corium penetrate the *stratum germinativum* deeply, they are now flattened and the elastic fibrils have to a large extent been dissolved. Hair follicles and sebaceous glands are atrophied, but sweat glands and hair-follicle muscles are usually sound; the number of sweat glands, however, does diminish with advancing age [1].

Apart from senescence and the degeneration of the epidermis caused by external factors, there is a third phenomenon: the degeneration of the corium. This is caused primarily by disorders of the skin metabolism. Microscopically, it becomes apparent in the loss of structural integrity of the fibrous tissue, with only shapeless debris of lumps, crumbs, and granules left. This colloidal degeneration starts in the elastic fiber bundles of the papillary bodies and the upper third of the cutis and gradually extends to collageneous fibers and deeper layers of the cutis. The external appearance of "colloidally degenerated" skin is usually somewhat tougher and fleshier than that of typical "aged skin."

The most important aspects of aging skin changes have been summarized by Weybrecht [2]. Chemical changes in the corium caused by aging and solar radiation are thoroughly covered by Smith and Finlayson [3]. Ippen and Ippen [4] describe some prophylactic measures against skin aging. A good summary of current knowledge of this subject, with contributions by Flesch, Harber, and Bjorksten, has also been published in *Proc. scient. Sect., Toilet Goods Ass.*, **41** (1964).

## Disorders in Scalp Physiology

Modern man suffers from three types of scalp disease: seborrhoea, dandruff, and baldness. According to Kumer [5], seborrhoea is an excessive and pathologically altered secretion of the sebaceous glands due to genetic factors. It is not necessarily restricted to the scalp, for it may occur wherever these glands occur in the body. Seborrhoea has different forms: on the scalp it is predominantly *seborrhoea oleosa* (the skin fat is oily and the hair becomes shiny and fatty), or *seborrhoea sica* (an admixture of solid cellular elements often inherited and strongly affected by metabolism and hormone level, this disorder cannot really be cured by external application; only the symptoms can be alleviated. The most important treatment is the removal of the excess fat and maintenance of a clean scalp.

Formation of dandruff frequently accompanies seborrhoea of the scalp. When the skin is healthy, the corneal layer is constantly renewed from inside and flakes off on the surface in microscopically small disks. In functional disorders these small disks may not slough off but may stick together on the scalp in flakes which can easily be discerned by the naked eye. It is not known whether dandruff is a result of seborrhoea or whether both are due to the same cause.

Apart from seborrhoea, other diseases of the scalp may also lead to dandruff. According to Vanderwyk and Roia [6], dandruff may be inhibited by attacking the microbic flora of the skin which suggests causation by microorganisms.

According to another hypothesis, dandruff and loss of hair often occur with seborrhoea because a seborrhoic scalp is an excellent culture medium for many microorganisms. Both seborrhoea and dandruff may cause unpleasant pruritus. Laden [7] found that dandruff cells in comparison to normal cells had a lesser capacity to bind water, a smaller content of ninhydridrin positive substances, and a higher content of sulfhydryl groups and pentoses. This points to accelerated and incomplete keratinization.

The third disorder is often described as loss of hair, but this is not really correct. A certain loss of hair (up to 40 hairs a day) is normal even in persons whose scalps are healthy. New hair grows simultaneously in other places. Loss of hair is only pathological if it really exceeds 40 hairs a day or when the hair no longer grows back on parts of the scalp.

Pathological loss of hair may be due to different causes. Rothemann [8] lists the following:

1. Following infectious diseases, such as influenza, typhus, scarlet fever, tuberculosis, diabetes; also after pneumonia and certain stages of syphilis.

2. Accompanying or following skin diseases, such as seborrhoea and psoriasis.

In this connection Flesch postulated that loss of hair is triggered off by various unsaturated substances contained in skin fat. A survey of Flesch's investigations and other studies of the relation between the composition of skin fat and hair growth is given by Harry in *Modern Cosmetocology*, 4th ed., p. 361 et seq.

3. Following disorders of the central nervous system.
4. Following functional disorders in internal secretion.

5. Following disturbances in diet, digestion, or metabolism.

6. An inherited disposition (*alopecia premature*), that is, "family baldness."

7. An attack by microorganisms (fungi, spores, cocci) or parasites (lice).

8. Accompanying premature senescence (*alopecia parasenilis*).

9. Natural symptom of aging (*alopecia senilis*).

10. Following poisoning (thallium, arsenic, lead, or mercury), after the continuous use of strong medication and sedatives, the excessive consumption of alcohol and nicotine, the influence of chemical solutions or vapors (industrial diseases), and mercury cures.

11. Through radiation; for example, after X-ray treatment of hairy parts of the body.

12. Following continuous mechanical pressure in the absence of air and light, by constant wear of headscarfs, uniform caps, or steel helmets.

When loss of hair has occurred more or less suddenly as a result of illness, poisoning, or infection, the hair usually grows again when the cause of the disorder has been removed. As long as the roots of the hair remain healthy, it can grow back. Cases are complicated when a degeneration of the hair papillae has occurred, in particular if baldness is inherited or caused by premature or normal aging. It is unfortunate that the people who suffer from these types of hair loss are the main users of biological hair lotions because for them no effective therapy has yet been discovered.

### FUNCTION OF COSMETICS

The cosmetics that we have discussed so far in this book are intended to protect, cleanse, and condition the epidermis. Sensible application of these preparations will prevent epidermal degeneration by harmful external forces. Cosmetic science is not content, however, with the fine results achieved in this area; it also wants to control and delay the degeneration of the corium and senescence.

This is a new field with completely new requirements. The preparations discussed so far develop their effectiveness where there are applied: on the surface of the skin. Preparations intended to affect deeper epidermal layers and the corium must transmit their active ingredients through the external skin layer. They must act in depth.

There is another even more significant difference: the corneal layer is dead, and processes occurring there may be explained according to physical and chemical laws. The *stratum germinativum* and the corium, on the other hand, are living cellular tissues. To understand what happens in these layers we must draw on physiology.

The traditional knowledge of the cosmetic formulator, his chemical and technical experience are no longer sufficient; in this sector he is no longer an expert. For this reason he often adopts the attitude that "cosmetics with depth effect" are really over-rated, that it will, of course, do no harm to add a few vitamins to skin creams (the public likes that!), that hormones must be treated with utmost care because they may have undesirable side effects, and that actually no single cosmetic preparation will give eternal youth to the skin.

On the other hand, we also have the opposite view: every new active ingredient reported to be effective is adopted with alacrity. It is widely publicized and perhaps added to new products before any clinical evidence of its effectiveness has been provided.

Cosmetic chemists should never forget that in the field of biologically effective substances they are really laymen and that neither exaggerated skepticism nor blind enthusiasm will lead to a development of cosmetic science. What is needed here is close collaboration between physicians and physiologists on the one hand and cosmetic chemists on the other. Dermatologists and physiologists must suggest new materials and chemists must blend them into useful and stable preparations; finally they must be tested by dermatologists for their effectiveness and absence of harmful ingredients.

This kind of collaboration can actually be found in many companies and universities. The entire field is still young, and we must not overestimate its achievements. In terms of quantity, biologically effective preparations account for only a very small fraction of the total sales of cosmetics, but, if collaboration between medicine and cosmetics as we know it today continues to expand, this area is bound to gain in importance. Results already achieved with female sex hormones and certain organic extracts surely warrant optimistic expectations.

## Active Ingredients

The active ingredients of biological cosmetics could be predetermined only if we were fully aware of all important processes in the living organism; that is, if we knew exactly which physical and chemical modifications cause degeneration and senescence of the skin. So far we lack this complete knowledge and active ingredients are found more or less empirically. The impetus for using vitamins in cosmetics came, for instance, from the observations made in many laboratories that dermatoses are caused and hair growth impaired by a deficiency of certain vitamins and that this damage is repaired as soon as these vitamins are added to food.

It has been known for many years that shifts in the hormone equilibrium affect the appearance of the skin and the growth of hair. The frequent occurrence of acne in puberty and the fact that castrates are never bald, are definite signs that the health of the skin and growth of hair are affected by hormones. On the basis of these observations it was logical to test the suitability of certain vitamins and hormones in cosmetic preparations. If such a method is properly understood, there can be no objection to it. Almost all biologically active ingredients of modern cosmetics have been found in this manner, but we should never lose sight of the fact that the physiological effect of a substance (vitamin or hormone) only furnishes the *occasion for testing* its effectiveness on skin tissue, if applied percutaneously, but must never be taken as *evidence* of such effectiveness.

It would, for example, be quite erroneous to say that a cream containing the vitamin B complex must effect the skin *because* vitamin B deficiency in the diet leads to dermatoses and impaired growth of hair or that turtle oil, because it is derived from turtles which reach a great age, carries rejuvenating properties. It is not at all ruled out that vitamin B and turtle oil have indeed some cosmetic advantage, but this can never be established by theoretical considerations or romantic comparisons but only in exact clinical tests.

There is another important reason for stressing the fact that physiological action of a substance only furnishes the occasion for testing its effectiveness on skin tissue: often, when cosmetic and dermatological effectiveness of vitamins or hormones was tested, the results obtained pointed to a very loose connection between vitamin or hormone effect and cosmetic effect. The dermatological effectiveness of vitamin D, for example (cure of skin tuberculosis by massive doses of vitamin D taken orally [9]), is not in any known way connected with the action of the vitamin (regulation of bone and tooth formation). In cosmetics vitamin E is used as an antioxidant; vitamin K, in dermatology, as an antimycotic. Vitamin A actually does have the cosmetic effect which is expected in view of vitamin A deficiency symptoms, but, according to Flesch [10], certain chemically related substances show similar cosmetic action, although they do not counteract diet deficiencies. Something similar probably also applies to polyunsaturated fatty acids ("vitamin F").

A number of natural and synthetic female sex hormones (estrone, estradiol, and stilbestrol) resemble each other in their hormone as well as their skin action. Here as well the connection between the effect on the skin and the effect on the entire organism is only a loose one, as proved by the fact that related substances, some of which are inactive as sex hormones ($\beta$-estradiol and androstenediol [11], pregnenolone [12], and others [13]), and some of which are male sex hormones (testosterone [14]) act in the same manner on the skin.

With some exaggeration we might say that we are looking for cosmetically active ingredients among vitamins and hormones for historical and not for biological reasons. Many vitamins and hormones are uninteresting as active cosmetic ingredients. On the other hand, we will surely find many substances that will act exclusively on skin tissue.

Biologically active substances that develop their effectiveness underneath the skin surface produce observable results only after some time, and even then the results are not clearly defined. It is much easier for the user to determine whether a hand cream or lipstick has the desired effect than to decide whether a hormone does actually rejuvenate the skin as promised.

Biological ingredients combine a hardly discernible action with strong suggestive power: what could be more appealing to a woman who has just discovered her first wrinkles than the idea of a skin-tightening, nourishing, rejuvenating, biologically highly active substance?

It is understandable that the temptation is great to try substances that are alleged to produce certain results highly desirable to the formulator and the public but whose effectiveness and harmlessness have not really been established by careful clinical tests. We must advise against the use of such unproved materials for several reasons.

The indiscriminate use of new ingredients leads to a market flooded with preparations of doubtful value. The use of new impressive-sounding ingredients may have a certain transitory advertising success, but if the product does not come up to expectations in use it will not hold its own in the long run. This kind of publicity often leads to an all-too-justified distrust of the manufacturer who produces it, of the "new ingredients," or of whole groups of cosmetic preparations.

The saying "if it does not help, neither will it do any harm" unfortunately does not apply in all cases. Absolute proof of the complete harmlessness of a preparation in constant use may only rarely be feasible; nevertheless, no product must on any account be marketed before controlled tests have shown that it causes no undesirable side effects on the human skin.

Because we hope to develop cosmetics into a science, we must consciously adopt a critical attitude toward all raw materials, active ingredients, and methods. We must not employ a substance just because somebody—possibly the producer—has made claims of "body affinity" or "high biological activity," nor must we reject it because it is synthetic or alien to body chemistry. The decision that a substance is suitable for cosmetic preparations can be made only on the strength of carefully controlled experiments.

It is neither necessary nor possible for every cosmetic manufacturer to carry out these tests himself. He must rely on data published in recognized medical, dermatological, and cosmetic literature, which must, of course, be supported by exact descriptions of experimental methods and observations and not restricted to vague phraseology.

With this critical attitude it is probably unavoidable that substances will be rejected even when they are effective if this effectiveness has not been established by clinical tests. Such losses have to be accepted if we want to achieve a wholly responsible cosmetic science. Dermatological research should be done on substances for which specific cosmetic properties are claimed and the results published.

In the following we discuss a few active ingredients and complexes that have been used in modern cosmetics and dermatology. Because of the great number and variety of recommended materials, it is impossible to give a complete summary, all the more so since new materials are being added every month.

### Individual Ingredients

**Vitamins.**  The cosmetic and physiological effects of vitamins and hormones (or substances resembling them) do not run parallel and it is therefore illogical and even misleading to retain this classification in cosmetics when it is justified only in physiology. I have nevertheless used it in this chapter for purely practical reasons: any reader looking for active ingredients will do so under the name of the respective vitamin or hormone.

According to the definition of Randoin and Szent-Györgyi, vitamins are "substances which the normal organism with only few exceptions is not able to synthetize, of which minimum amounts are absolutely essential for the development, maintenance, and functioning of the organism, and whose absence results in characteristic disorders and damage." Since vitamins are quickly degraded and excreted, a regular supply from external sources is essential; normally it is furnished in the food.

We are now certain that some vitamins (in particular the B group) form essential constituents of certain enzymes (ferments) which are catalytic in specific vital processes inside the cells (i.e., they accelerate reactions that would be extremely slow without them). Other vitamins (A, C, E) may have similar catalytic action, either alone or in relatively simple compounds. Vitamins must be present in individual cells in their physiologically active form, that is, possibly linked with several other molecules and atom groups to chemically highly complicated enzymes.

It is obvious that the presence of vitamins is of particular importance in cellular tissue with strong biological activity. In adult humans the *stratum germinativum* and the groups of cells responsible for the growth of new hair belong to the most active tissues of the body. Therefore disturbances in the vitamin supply often become noticeable first in the appearance of the skin and hair.

As already mentioned, vitamins are absorbed in the main from food. They are transmitted to the bloodstream by resorption through the intestinal walls and then transported to the different tissues in which they perform their function. Somewhere (in the blood, liver, or other tissues) each vitamin must be converted from the form in which it occurred in food to the form active in animal tissue. Vitamin-deficiency symptoms may occur either when food contains insufficient vitamins or if resorption through the intestine or conversion into the active form is impaired. Often the presence of other vitamins or certain hormones is required for normal resorption or conversion. The action of vitamins in the organism involves an extremely complicated process based on the synchronization of many factors. We are at present only beginning to disentangle this complex, and so far our knowledge of the function and effectiveness of individual vitamins has thrown light on only a few isolated aspects. Even so we are already able to draw certain practical conclusions from this restricted knowledge; big developments in this field are surely still reserved for the future.

Even with vitamin-rich food, normal resorption, and conversion to the active form, certain tissues may be short of vitamins: this shortage occurs when blood circulation in these tissues is inadequate and the supply of vitamins and other vital substances is not sufficiently rapid. Bad circulation is also a factor in certain diseases of the scalp: substances or methods (massage, radiation) that stimulate circulation may have a favorable effect in these cases. Although vitamins are normally taken orally (in the diet), they may also be injected or absorbed percutaneously (by application to the skin). If we were to include in the definition of cosmetics everything that pertains to the health of the skin, we would have to discuss all routes of vitamin supply and certainly the diet. This book is limited to a discussion of cosmetic preparations; that is, those preparations that are applied to the surfaces of the skin, hair, nails, or teeth.

The application of vitamin-rich preparations to the skin is, of course, useful only when the vitamin in question is resorbed by the skin. In general we must differentiate between three possibilities in the resorption of active ingredients by the skin. The ingredient may pass through the skin into the blood without particularly affecting the tissue that serves as the transmitter (e.g., mercury). It may also penetrate the tissue and be completely absorbed by it (e.g., sulfur). Finally, part of it may be absorbed by the skin and part may pass through into the blood.

It is generally useful to apply an active ingredient externally only if it is absorbed, at least in part, by the skin and if it exerts some action on the skin tissue. If the epidermal tissue is able to utilize an ingredient only if it is supplied by the blood (i.e., after the ingredient has been converted into its active form somewhere in the body), it is usually better to provide the substance in the diet.

There are, however, certain exceptions in which a substance must not be given orally either because it would have a toxic effect or because it is degraded in the stomach or the intestines. In these instances the substance is usually injected.

*Vitamin A.*   When referring to vitamin A in this section, we mean vitamin $A_1$, which is so important to human nutrition. Not much is known about the cosmetic properties of vitamin $A_2$; vitamin A plays a large part in normal keratinization [15]. Deficiency leads to abnormally increased keratinization (hyperkeratosis). The color of the skin fades as the corneal layer thickens. If the corneal layer proliferates over the hair-follicle mouths, sebum builds up under the skin surface: the comedones (blackheads) that develop may in turn become infected (acne). In addition, the skin may become dry and flaky, hair loses its luster and falls out, wrinkles may develop, and the risk of infections increases.

Although vitamin A deficiency diseases are comparatively rare today, slight vitamin A avitaminoses are much more frequent, according to Lehmann and Rappaport [16]. The symptoms frequently become noticeable on the skin before other organs (eyes and mucous membrane) are affected [17].

It has been confirmed by Kimmig [18] and Sobel [19] that vitamin A can enter the bloodstream through the skin. Although it was formerly assumed that this vitamin is active only after it has reached the bloodstream and therefore oral administration is more economical than percutaneous application [20] even in skin lesions, Kimmig as well as Sobel could demonstrate localized effects. Skin lesions caused by vitamin A deficiency will heal after external treatment, but other areas will remain unaffected. According to Sobel, with identical doses 5 to 10 times as much vitamin A is absorbed in the blood if taken orally than when applied percutaneously. In cases of vitamin A deficiency the skin will transmit less vitamin A to the blood from the surface than the skin of nondeficient individuals. These observations may also point to absorption of vitamin A by the epidermal tissue. The addition of vitamin A to cosmetic preparations is justified by the evidence of its localized effectiveness. If, however, there is a general vitamin A deficiency, oral administration of the vitamin, possibly supported by vitamin ointments, is essential. The dosage suggested by Rothemann [21], namely, 100,000 IU (60 mg) per kilo of finished product, seems reasonable. With this dose the possibility of damage to the skin or health in general is completely ruled out.

The cosmetic effect is smoother and softer skin and tightening of the tissue tension. In dermatology, as well, vitamin A has been used successfully in certain keratinous disorders (e.g., acne), but such applications are no longer considered cosmetological.

One difficulty of using vitamin A cosmetically has been its sensitivity to oxidation. The standard form of the vitamin (vitamin A alcohol) has limited stability in contact with the air. The esters of the alcohol are more stable, and usually the vitamin is administered in that form. Preparations containing vitamin A must be protected from light and air as much as possible and during production the preparations should be heated as little as possible.

According to Flesch [22], the inhibiting effect of vitamin A on keratinization is shared by various substances which have similar structures but which lack vitamin properties. Gerhard [23] attributes a cosmetic effect to carotenes but without adducing any experimental evidence (carotenes are yellow vegetable pigments; the animal organism forms vitamin $A_1$ from $\beta$-carotene).

There seems to be some connection between vitamins A and E; vitamin E helps to store vitamin A in the body, particularly in the liver (Kimmig, *op. cit*). According to Sobel (*op. cit.*), when vitamin A is applied locally, vitamin E also promotes its storage in the body. Perhaps this interrelation is due to the oxidation sensitivity of vitamin A, whereas vitamin E is a good antioxidant.

*The Vitamin B Complex.* This complex includes $B_1$ (aneurine and thiamine), $B_2$ (lactoflavin and riboflavin), the $B_6$ group (pyridoxinehydrochloride, pyridoxal, and pyridoxamine), folic acid, $B_{12}$, nicotylamide, pantothenic acid, biotine (vitamin H), *p*-aminobenzoic acid (vitamin H'), and various other substances. The vitamins in this group are all water-soluble and stable against heat and oxidation. Only very few data are available regarding skin resorption of vitamin B. Villeia [24] reportedly has observed skin resorption of pyridoxine. According to Weis [25], nicotinic acid derivatives are resorbed. Although disorders of the skin and hair have been observed because of a deficiency of nearly all vitamins in this group, at present no clinical observations have been made that would warrant the cosmetic use of these vitamins.

Roccheggiani [26] has suggested the use of pyridoxine tripalmitate (the oil-soluble tripalmitate ester of vitanim $B_6$). According to Yashuda [27], a study of 162 patients revealed that lotions containing 0.02% pyridoxine-3,4-dipalmitate were effective against dandruff and pruritus in about 80% of the cases.

It is quite possible that one or several of these vitamins will in the future prove to be cosmetically useful. According to the principle that no substance should be incorporated into cosmetic preparations if its purpose is not absolutely clear, we must for the time being advise against the addition of these vitamins. Perhaps an exception may be made for pantothenic acid. Animal tests (with rats, dogs, and foxes) clearly show that a lack of pantothenic acid in the diet causes the hair to turn gray [28]. In addition, various animal dermatoses have been cured with pantothenic acid.

Several investigators also report good results from the treatment of humans with pantothenic acid [29]. In many cases grayness was prevented or reversed, and the development of certain scalp diseases and loss of hair connected with increased sebum secretion (seborrhoea) were temporarily and often permanently eliminated. A combined therapy in which calcium pantothenate is given internally and panthenol (the alcohol of pantothenic acid) or calcium pantothenate (both in 2.5% solution in diluted alcohol) applied topically is reported to be especially effective. Some investigators [30] nevertheless remain skeptical of the treatment of scalp diseases and grayness with pantothenic acid in spite of the positive results published; in their opinion many of the experiments made so far have not been sufficiently controlled nor correctly interpreted.

In any case, pantothenic acid (either in the form of calcium pantothenate or its derivatives panthenol and bepanthene) is the only vitamin of the B group that is applied cosmetically on a large scale today. Future studies may show how effective it actually is.

U. S. Patent 2,791,534 (1957) recommends the use of nicotinic acid amide in a hormone cream. The vitamin is supposed to stimulate circulation. Ethyl nicotinate penetrates the skin much more rapidly than the free acid.

*Vitamin C (ascorbic acid)*. This vitamin is also water-soluble. That vitamin C can be absorbed by the skin was demonstrated by Kashara and Kawashina [31] who applied a 30% solution of ascorbic acid to the breasts of lactating women and subsequently found that the vitamin C content of their milk had increased. This vitamin plays an important part in the healing of wounds but it is usually administered orally. This does not rule out a percutaneous effect, although so far nothing is known about it. Vitamin C can hardly be considered for addition to cosmetic preparations because in solution in contact with the air it is quickly oxidized and inactivated. Fruit juices in cosmetic preparations are probably justified because of their acidity and not because of their vitamin C content.

*Vitamin D*. At the time of writing there are no indications that vitamin D applied to the skin surface would have any cosmetic effect.

*Vitamin E (d-tocopherol)*. A good summary of the significance of vitamin E in dermatology is given by Nikolowski [32]. Vitamin E deficiency causes disturbances of the metabolism and sexual function and decreased capillary circulation. Nothing has been proved for percutaneous application. Certain concentrates of active ingredients with a high vitamin E content (e.g., cold-pressed wheat germ oil) have shown good cosmetic results, but it is in no way established that they are due to vitamin E as such.

Vitamin E is an effective antioxidant and is occasionally used for this purpose in cosmetic preparations. In wheat-germ oil and other complexes vitamin E is probably useful because it protects oxidation-sensitive ingredients from being inactivated by oxygen.

*Polyunsaturated Fatty Acids ("Vitamin F")*. Much that is contradictory has been written in the last 25 years about the significance of these substances in dermatology, diet, and cosmetics. A summary of the importance of these fatty acids in the diet is given by Franzke [33] and we refer the reader to his article for a bibliography of original publications.

The principal nutrients required by humans are carbohydrates, fats, and proteins. Although carbohydrates and fats differ considerably in their chemical composition, they play a similar part in nutrition. This is illustrated by the fact that some populations (e.g., the Chinese) have a carbohydrate-rich diet almost completely devoid of fats, whereas others (e.g., Eskimos) remain healthy on a fat-rich diet with hardly any carbohydrates.

The relationship between fats and carbohydrates in nutrition had been known for a long time when Burr proved with experiments on young rats (1930) that these animals did not thrive on a diet without fat. Their growth was stunted and the skin showed keratinous disorders and dermatites. When Burr fed the rats suffering from these symptoms with individual fatty acids that normally occur in their diet, he found that only linolenic and arachidonic acid reversed the growth and skin abnormalities, whereas linolenic acid alone removed growth damage.

$$CH_3(CH_2)_4CH\!\!=\!\!CHCH_2CH\!\!=\!\!CH(CH_2)_7COOH$$
Linolenic acid (9,12 unsaturated)

$$CH_3CH_2CH\!\!=\!\!CHCH_2CH\!\!=\!\!CHCH_2CH\!\!=\!\!CH(CH_2)_4COOH$$
Linolenic acid (9,12,15 unsaturated)

$$CH_3(CH_2)_4CH\!\!=\!\!CHCH_2CH\!\!=\!\!CHCH_2CH\!\!=\!\!CHCH_2CH\!\!=\!\!CH(CH_2)_4COOH$$
Arachidonic acid (6,9,12,15 unsaturated)

None of the other naturally occurring acids could remove the damage nor could the isomers of linolenic acid with conjugated double bonds. (A growth stimulating effect was found later in some rare or purely synthetic fatty acids, all of which had several nonconjugated double bonds similar to that of linolenic acid. It was determined subsequently that only a definite steric form of linolenic acid is effective as "essential fatty acid." Essential fatty acids have been grouped under the designation "vitamin F," although it is doubtful whether these substances should be regarded as vitamins.

It is generally assumed that these fatty acids are also important in human nutrition, but the daily requirement is not yet known. There is a close inter-relation between essential fatty acids and various vitamins, notably E and $B_6$ and probably $B_{12}$: these substances increase one another's effectiveness in the animal organism.

As for the importance of essential fatty acids in cosmetics, a few years after Burr had described his experiments Shepherd [34] found that certain isomers of linolenic acid (substances that do not act as essential fatty acids in the diet!) have a beneficial, frequently therapeutic effect on exzema, dry skin and hair, and diseases of the scalp. Subsequently, other investigators reported success in the treatment of wounds, hyperkeratoses, and exzema following the application of essential fatty acids (present in appreciable amounts in cold pressed wheat germ oil and poppyseed, sunflower seed, linseed, and sesame oils) and polyunsaturated higher fatty acids (which occur in cod-liver oil) [35]. The esters and glycerides of polyunsaturated acids are also reported to have a similar therapeutic effect.

According to some investigators, the effect of these substances is due to their ability to form unstable peroxides with atmospheric oxygen which is then released in the deeper skin layers [36]. Perhaps this effect is akin to that of vitamin A which is also highly unsaturated and has antikeratinous action.

All polyunsaturated fatty acids (in particular those with conjugated double bonds, the free acids more than the esters and glycerides) are, in any case, oxidation-sensitive and must therefore be protected from oxidation if they are to be used in cosmetic preparations. The use of vitamin E as an antioxidant is recommended in this connection and is also indicated because this vitamin is frequently present with the unsaturated fatty acids in natural oils.

A critical evaluation of the cosmetic significance of polyunsaturated fatty acids is unfortunately not yet possible, for the extensive literature is full of contradictions. Confusion arose when unsaturated fatty acids with an anti-keratinous effect were referred to as "vitamin F" by some authors, whereas other investigators used this designation only for essential fatty acids (linoleic, linolenic, and arachidonic). This confusion grew when Shepherd and Linn [37] attributed skin and scalp lesions, which are cured by un-saturated fatty acids, to a "vitamin F deficiency." In addition, the methods used in the tests of "vitamin F" on the skin are quite inadequate in many cases and consequently the results obtained are unreliable; nevertheless they were often cited by other authors and thus gained a permanent place in the literature. In reading the literature, the impression is created that poly-unsaturated fatty acids have wound-healing and keratinization-inhibiting (skin-emollient) effectiveness in certain cases. Whether this effectiveness becomes apparent in healthy skin, which fatty acids are the most helpful, and how they are best processed cannot be answered with any certainty. Further critical investigations must be carried out in order to gain assurance that the fatty acids and not some other substances are responsible for the effect observed. Both conjugated and unconjugated fatty acids should be investi-gated, and, at least temporarily, the idea should be disregarded that certain acids of this type also play an important dietary role, since a relation between the dietary and the cosmetic effects has never been convincingly demon-strated.

*Vitamin K.* The use of these vitamins in the treatment of the skin has little to do with their action as vitamins: they are antimycotics [38]. They also have antibacterial action, in particular against gram-positive cocci, and may be used in external therapy in skin diseases [39]. Vitamin K has also proved to be effective against chilblains.

**Hormones.** Hormones might be described as "chemical messengers." They are organic substances that originate in certain glands and then enter the blood. They fulfill their function in one or several specific organs or tissues by stimulating or inhibiting their activity.

Many different hormones act simultaneously in the animal organism: they regulate the metabolism, the sex life of the individual, and the growth of individual tissues. No hormone acts alone, and certain hormones stimulate or inhibit the secretion of still other hormones. A complex interaction of all hormones not only directs the physiological processes of the organism but also decisively affects its psychological make-up and character.

It would be beyond the scope of this book to elaborate here on the rich field of endocrinology. The points of contact between this science and cosmetics are still rather limited. We mention only a few facts that are fundamentally important to the use of hormones in cosmetics.

Like vitamins, hormones are effective in small amounts. They are also used up very slowly by the body. In any case, if any disturbance in the hormone equilibrium is to be counteracted by the external administration of a hormone, it must not be given only once but in regularly repeated doses. In many instances the action of hormones is not limited to one organ. Sex hormones, for instance, also have considerable influence on the condition of the skin.

Many hormones are not specific to one animal species but sometimes act in species zoologically far removed from one another; for example, an often-used test for the effectiveness of male sex hormones employs cockerels! The chemical composition of most hormones is now known. When produced for therapeutic purposes, many are no longer derived from animal organs or the products of elimination, in which they were first discovered and isolated, but are prepared synthetically or semisynthetically, that is, starting from chemically related and more abundantly available natural products.

*Sex Hormones.* It has been known for some time that sex hormones also affect the condition of the human skin and hair [40]. During puberty the drastic changes in the hormone balance of the body are often accompanied by skin disorders (acne, seborrhoea). Women usually develop wrinkles and loss of skin tension when the production of sex hormones begins to diminish. During pregnancy the blood has an unusually high content of certain female hormones, and the skin of expectant mothers is often especially smooth and fresh. Men whose gonads have been inactivated in early youth by sickness, accident, or surgery hardly ever become bald. If male sex hormones are regularly administered, many of these men will begin to lose their hair [41]. The activity of the sebaceous glands and keratinization are also affected by sex hormones: male sex hormones promote keratinization and stimulate the sebaceous glands to increased activity; estrogens have an inhibiting effect.

(The literature contains many contradictory reports in this connection; according to Goldzieher [42a] there is a similarity of effect between the male sex hormone testosterone and female sex hormones. As with vitamins, the discovery of the effect of sex hormones in the blood on the condition of the skin was no proof of the usefulness of hormones in cosmetics but only provided the impetus for testing cosmetic applications. In particular, estrogens, the female sex hormones, showed great promise and were thoroughly examined.

The three principal female sex hormones are estrone, estradiol, and estriol. Hormone preparations from natural sources (e.g., mare's urine, one of the most important) contain a mixture of these and other estrogenic substances, but estrone and estradiol are mainly responsible for the effect. Several synthetic organic substances with estrogen-like activity are also known: farogynol [di-(p-acetoxy-phenyl)-hexadiene], stilbestrol (also called diethyl stilbestrol), and hexestrol (dihydrodiethyl stilbestrol) differ considerably in their structures from natural estrogens but have a similar physiological effect.

The relative value of these substances is shown in Table 9.1. The inter-

TABLE 9-1   EFFECTIVENESS OF ESTROGENS

| Substance | IU per Gram (in millions) | Relative Effectiveness with External Application [42a] |
|---|---|---|
| Estradiol | 60 | 1 |
| Estrone | 10 | 1 |
| Estriol | 1 | |
| Equiline | 3.5 | |
| Equilenine | 1 | |
| Foragynol | 10 | |
| Stilbestrol | 28 | 2 |
| Hexestrol | 60 | |

national unit derived from biological tests on castrated female mice (Allen and Doisy, 1923) indicates the usefulness of the substance as a female sex hormone. A detailed description of a modification of this test, particularly in regard to the effectiveness of cosmetic preparations, is given by Levenstein [42]. However, as the table indicates, Allen and Doisy's international unit is not a good measure of cosmetic effectiveness. It would be useful to develop a reproducible biological test to measure the effect of estrogens and related substances on epidermal tissue.

Klarmann has published a summary of studies that cover clinical tests of the cosmetic effectiveness of hormone creams [43]. The skin surfaces of women (mostly over 40) were treated over periods of one to six months with creams containing 250–350 IU estrogenic substances per gram. Other women were treated simultaneously with creams containing no hormones. The results obtained by investigators did not coincide on all points, but the following observations were confirmed by several of them.

No change in the skin was observed in young women between 20 and 30 whose hormone functions and epidermis were normal. Test subjects whose skin before treatment had shown symptoms of senile atrophy produced the following changes:

1. The cell content of the epidermal cells was increased and the appearance of the *stratum germinativum* became fuller and more hydrated.

2. The base line between the *stratum germinativum* and the papillary layer became more noticeably wavy, which indicates increased cell proliferation in the *stratum germinativum*. The epidermis had increased in thickness because the number of cellular layers had increased.

3. The elastic fibrils of the papillary bodies showed regeneration, and blood circulation in the papillaries also increased.

4. Several authors saw no significant changes in the elastic and collageneous connective tissue of the lower layers of the corium; others found increased turgor.

5. The outer appearance of the skin became fresher and more youthful.

6. The above mentioned effects were entirely topical and occurred only on those skin surfaces that had been directly treated with the cream. Accordingly, the action of the hormone is an external one; the hormone does not become effective only after it has entered the circulation.

Another significant effect described by Spoor [44] is an increased lipid formation in the top and the basal cell layers which does not seem to be based on any increased activity of the sebaceous glands; according to Strauss, Kligman, and Pochi [45] estrogens (only in high dosages, however) inhibit the secretion of these glands, whereas androgens increase it. A latent period of 10–20 days was observed in the hormone cream treatment during which no changes were apparent. The maximum effect occurred after 30–50 days and lasted for the rest of the treatment. When it was discontinued, the skin reverted to its previous state. These observations refer to the treatment of aging skin with estrogen creams. In cosmetics estrogens may also be used in scalp preparations.

It has been observed repeatedly that an increase in the blood level of male sex hormones (testosterone) coincides with restricted hair growth, and occasionally with loss of hair [46]. It is possible that the female sex hormone has the opposite effect. Reiss and Cellis [47] confirmed this stimulation of hair growth in tests with rabbits [48]. Certain biological hair lotions contain estrogens or vegetable and organic extracts in which there are estrogens. Since such preparations are used mainly by men and the possibility of undesirable systemic effects can never be ruled out, only substances and complexes that are relatively ineffectual as sex hormones should be used, and their dosage should be adjusted to maximum 200 I.U. per gram.

Finally there is the possibility of treating acne with estrogens. According to Tate [49], good results have been achieved. The required estrogen dosages are so high, however, that the risk of serious functional sexual disorders (even permanent sterility) is more than academic.

*Possible Risks of Estrogen Preparations.*   In estrogen cream treatment the hormone is partly absorbed by the skin but some of it also reaches the bloodstream. This is a source of danger because even very small amounts in the blood may cause distinctly noticeable physiological and psychological changes. The effect of estrogens on women consists mainly in menstruational disorders. Increased pigmentation and swelling of the breasts (as in pregnancy) and even changes in temperament (apathy, loss of sexual drive) have occasionally been observed. Obviously such side effects must be avoided in any cosmetic treatment.

The experience of both American and European dermatologists indicates that sensible application of estrogen creams containing 250–350 IU per gram can produce favorable cosmetic results without harmful side effects, even with prolonged use. The amounts of hormone entering the circulation under these conditions is too small to cause any damage. The situation is different for certain bust preparations with high hormone dosage; they must be used only under medical supervision. Of particular interest in cosmetics are some substances which are chemically closely related to natural or synthetic estrogens (e.g., "Pregnenolone" by Ciba [50] and a number of steroids mentioned in the German Patent 1,017,748 [51]) and which have similar effects in the epidermal tissue but only weak action as sex hormones. Correct application of these substances almost rules out undesirable side effects.

Several authors have mentioned a further risk following the use of estrogen-containing preparations: a possible carcinogenic effect. Continued injection over several weeks of massive doses of estrogen derivatives has indeed caused cancer in mice. The hormone dosage required, however, was so much greater than any used in cosmetic preparations that the risk of cancer is almost nonexistent. As far as I am aware, medical literature does not mention a single case in which cancer has been related to the use of cosmetic hormone preparations.

The great number of other hormones that play an important part in the human organism need not be mentioned here; at present there is no reason to consider their use in cosmetic preparations. Hydrocortisone and fluorocortisone, chemically related to the hormones of the cortex of the suprarenal gland, are used in dermatology to reduce inflammations but have no importance in cosmetics.

**Enzymes.** Chemical reactions constantly occur in almost all tissues of the living organism. It is remarkable that the majority of these reactions, if they were conducted at body temperature *in vitro*, would either not occur at all or immeasurably slowly. That they do occur in the living organism is due to the presence of enzymes in the body tissues; these act as biochemical catalysts and thus considerably accelerate all chemical reactions that occur in the body. Kludas has summarized the significance of enzymes by saying that "wherever there is life, enzymes are present; without enzymes there is no life."

As far as the properties of enzymes are concerned, like vitamins and hormones, they act in very small amounts. Enzymes are produced by the body itself but the building stones have to be supplied in the diet. The catalytic effect of enzymes is usually specific; that is, it is restricted to one definite reaction or type of reaction. Enzymes affect not only the speed but also the direction of the reaction.

Enzymes function only under certain conditions: acidity of the environment, redox potential, and temperature must be in a certain range (different for each enzyme) or the enzyme will not display its catalytic effect. Heating beyond 60°C destroys most enzymes.

Generally enzymes are proteins or consist of a protein fragment and a nonproteinic prosthetic group. Often they are activated only if a coenzyme is present. Various vitamins, particularly those of the B group, play an important part in the composition of coenzymes.

Enzymes contribute, perhaps decisively, to the effectiveness of certain active complexes (e.g., placenta extract), but have been used hardly at all in cosmetics until recently, in either pure or almost pure form. The experimental application of ribonuclease (an enzyme that attacks and degrades ribonucleic acid, an important constituent of the cell nucleus) in face masks, as described by Mantegazza and Rovesti [52], is still in the pioneering stage. Results are reportedly favorable, particularly if ribonuclease is combined with nucleic acids: treatment of flabby skin improves circulation, increases elasticity, and makes the skin smoother. The use of lactic enzymes in cosmetic preparations suggested by Ardin [53] should also be mentioned.

The use of certain proteinases (enzyme-degrading proteins) has a different purpose: in ointments for wounds, face masks, and peeling preparations [54] proteinases break down old cellular tissue which in the treatment of wounds is the initial stage of the healing process; in the peeling cure they remove old corneal cells and expose the fresh underlying layers.

**Proteins, Peptones, Peptides, and Amino Acids.** Gerhard [55] has reported on the use of these substances in cosmetics. Large *protein molecules* (e.g., casein, a lactic protein) are not resorbed by the skin. Proteins may be used as film-forming substances (e.g., casein in certain skin-protecting creams), thickening agents of aqueous products (e.g., gelatin) wrinkle-smoothing and masking agents, or medicinal vehicles in powders but not as active biological ingredients.

*Amino acids* (cf. Chapter 1) are resorbed by the skin. They play a crucial part in the organism as building stones: protein molecules of all cells (including the epidermis) are built up from them. Amino acids are supplied to the body in the diet in the form of vegetable and animal proteins. It is possible that the epidermal tissue might be able to utilize amino acids as building stones if they were applied on the surface, but so far there has been no indication that this application offers any advantage compared with the administration of these substances in food. It may be possible that certain amino acids have specific functions in the epidermal tissue. Cysteine and cystine are the building stones of the sulfur bridges which are partly responsible for the properties of skin and hair proteins. Tyrosin is the substance from which the brown skin pigment melanin is developed in the epidermal tissue.

At present we cannot provide details of the cosmetic application of amino acids because no systematic study has yet been made and only isolated reports of the results of the treatment of certain skin diseases are available.

In this connection we may mention 5-oxytryptamine, which, although it is not a natural amino acid derived from proteins, is closely related to one of them (tryptophane); 5-oxytryptamine is found in vertebrates and mollusks in certain skin cells and is probably one of the active ingredients in skin extracts. Its effect is reported to consist mainly in stimulating the smooth muscles outside the circulatory system [56].

Amino acids are obtained by total hydrolysis of proteins, which is carried out under rigorous conditions. If the hydrolysis is carried out carefully under mild and strictly controlled conditions, the resultant mixture also contains, in addition to the individual amino acids, peptones and peptides (like proteins, they are composed of amino acids but the molecules are much smaller). Peptides contain two to about 10 amino acid residues, peptones as many as 40 or 50. Partial degradation of the protein molecule may take place either under the influence of warm dilute acid or alkali or, at body temperature, by the action of protein-degrading enzymes (trypsin, papain, etc.). For cosmetically useful products only the last method has been used. The cosmetic effect depends on the protein selected as the substrate and the size of the fragments (i.e., the conditions under which hydrolysis is performed).

Lodi and Rovesti have reported on the experimental application of various protein hydrolysates in cosmetic preparations [57] and have come to the conclusion that most of the examined protein hydrolysates have a definite therapeutic effect on atrophied skin. Each product has a specific value that depends on its derivation.

To illustrate the working method of Lodi and Rovesti we offer the following summary of their report on hemoglobin proteolysate.

Enzymatic degradation and subsequent purification of freshly prepared ox blood hemoglobin resulted in a colorless, almost odorless hydrolysate, tasting faintly of soup, which was clearly soluble in water; 2.5% of this substance was added to a cream base (see Formulation 19, p.400). The activated ointment was tested on three subjects who had been selected because of their cosmetically unattractive skin (looseness, wrinkles, etc.) The activated cream was applied on the right side of the face, and the left side was treated with cream containing no proteolysate. First the skin was cleaned, then lightly dabbed with aqueous glycerol solution, massaged with the cream for 3 to 5 minutes, and wiped off with tissue after two hours. The test results demonstrated to the authors that hemoglobin hydrolysate is an "excellent nourishing agent for undernourished and neglected skin" and "particularly suitable for healing chapped and reddened skin caused by excessive use of acne ointments." The test procedure described can, of course, in no way qualify as sufficient evidence for the authors' broad conclusions; however, some interesting possibilities may be opened up by this kind of exploration.

Fassbender [58] reports on the cosmetic application of protein hydrolysates in which the protein has been largely degraded to amino acids. The stimulating effect of these protein hydrolysates is based, at least in part, on its irritant action: the alien peptides and peptones that invade the epidermal tissue cause defense reactions and in this way produce a revitalization of the tissue.

Cameron and Spector [59] report that certain peptides which contain 8–14 amino acid residues increase the transmittance of blood capillaries and cause inflammations. There is, of course, a certain risk in this irritating action. Serious allergic reactions may occur when alien proteins and peptides penetrate into the bloodstream. In any case, if protein hydrolysates such as Lodi and Rovesti have described are to be incorporated into marketable cosmetic products, thorough tests must be carried out to prove their compatibility and effectiveness.

A product derived by the enzymatic degradation of milk protein ("Labilin," Deutsche Milchwerke, Zwingenberg/Bergstrasse [60]) has been used successfully for many years in pharmaceutical powders and creams. It is, however, a product in which protein has been only slightly degraded so that lower molecular peptides which appear to be responsible for the irritant effect are either not present or only in very small quantities.

**Chlorine, Betaine, their Derivatives and Salts, and Similar Compounds.** Hanusch (Austrian Patent 176,948, 1953) reports that weekly treatments with ointments containing choline, betaine, and salts of these substances with organic and inorganic acids or similar compounds in a resorbable base cause a "certain increase in human performance" and "improve premature aging symptoms." The effect is reportedly based on influencing the postganglionic nerve fibers of the parasympathetic nervous system.

According to Ruehs and Klein (German Patent 1,007,957, 1958), preparations that contain these ingredients, preferably in concentrations of 5 to 15%, also inhibit the loss of hair and promote the processes of regeneration.

**Sulfur and Sulfuric Ingredients.**    Even today sulfur is still one of the best and most widely used therapeutics in various types of keratin disorder. Perhaps the fact that keratin differs from most proteins because of its comparatively high content of sulfuric amino acids has something to do with this. Perhaps its effectiveness is due to its action in the epidermal tissue as an oxidating as well as a reducing agent and as a keratolytic and keratoplastic substance. In cosmetics colloidal sulfur is used in the treatment of acne, dandruff, and seborrhoea. However, sulfur cannot always be used without limitation; its application, especially over large skin areas, occasionally causes irritations. This also applies to selenium sulfide which is used in certain scalp preparations. Sulfur is often applied in the form of organic compounds; for example, polythio acids, dimethylthianthrene, triphenyl-stibin sulfide [61]. Schneider [62] recommends a thiocarbonic acid derivative "S 54" for the treatment of seborrhoic dandruff. Walker [63] reports on the use of thiodiglycollic acid, quaternary ammonium polythionates, and phenyl mercapto acetic acid.

**Irritants.**    The action of the irritants is based on the principle that the organism usually counters irritation with increased activity in the affected tissue. Circulation is increased, metabolism activated, and the proliferation of cells accelerated. For this reason irritants may be used cosmetically whenever the blemish is due to "apathy" of the epidermal tissue.

Irritants are employed only to a limited degree in cosmetics. Any irritation is always slightly damaging to the tissues and cosmetics are usually intended to prevent or alleviate such effects. The most important field of application is hair lotions: here irritants are intended to stimulate scalp activity and with it the growth of hair.

Janistyn [64] lists 15 different substances that are used in hair lotions as stimulants; among them are cantharidin, capsicin, pyrogallol, pyrogallol monoacetate, formic acid, and histamin.

**Allantoin.**    Allantoin is used in the treatment of wounds because it accelerates scarring. Because this effect is combined with good skin compatibility and nontoxicity, some authors recommend the incorporation of allantoin in small quantities in all kinds of cosmetic products [65]. Allantoin is stable in aqueous solutions at pH 4–9 and in nonaqueous solutions. It decomposes in boiling water and is destroyed by ultraviolet rays (solar radiation). In addition to the healing property, the aluminum salt of allantoin also has a deodorant effect and is recommended for body deodorants (U.S. Patent 2,761,861).

**Azulene.** Azulene, the active constituent of camomile extract, inhibits inflammations in very small doses and in larger doses heals them. Thomas and Gribou [66a] and Zorn and Kraul [66] recommend small doses with propgylactic effect in various cosmetic products. Either the synthetic guaja-zulene or natural camomile extract may be used. (According to Janku and Zita [67], however, other constituents of the extract are also responsible for the inflammation-inhibiting effect.)

### Complexes of Active Ingredients

Cosmetic complexes are preparations of vegetable or animal origin which are not chemically uniform and which owe their cosmetic effectiveness to one or more active ingredients. In some cases the individual active ingredients are known; quite often they are not.

These complexes of active ingredients have become increasingly important in cosmetics. Before discussing them individually we shall compare advantages and disadvantages between them and individual ingredients.

The most important argument in favor of complexes is that biological processes in the living organism are not directed by a single substance (one hormone, one vitamin, or one enzyme) but that various substances act together to support, inhibit, or complement one another. Cosmetics try to adjust to the biological process as much as possible. If an isolated substance is replaced by a group that occurs in vegetable and animal tissues, the effect obtained is harmonious and may be stronger or milder than that of any single substance. Certain substances, for example, compounds of metal traces (magnesium, copper, etc.), which would have no specific effect by themselves, may possibly be activated only in a natural complex.

The transfer of an active complex derived from plants or animals to the human organism naturally always carries certain risks. The fact that certain substances occur together and perhaps also act together in vegetable and animal tissues is no proof of their combined action in the same proportion in humans or of any resultant beneficial effect. Effectiveness in humans can be established only by tests with human subjects. Evidently the cosmetic effect of complexes is less one-sided than that of individual ingredients; whether it is also better will have to be determined in clinical tests in each case.

Another argument in favor of using complexes is the possibility of a certain content of active ingredients still unknown in isolation and which therefore cannot be used singly.

In addition, provided the active ingredients have not been synthetized but are derived from natural sources by isolation, the use of crude extracts or partially purified extracts (i.e., complexes) is often more economical than pure products. There is not only the difficulty of isolating the ingredient (which increases costs) but the yield in total purification is far from complete, and often some of the substances being removed could also be useful. A good case, for example, can be made for using deacidified wheat germ oil or another oil with a high content of polyunsaturated fatty acids (vitamin F) and vitamin E instead of the pure form of these substances.

Obviously the total extract is preferable only to an isolated ingredient if it causes no undesirable side effects, nor should it have an unpleasant odor, darken, or cause fast deterioration of the end product.

Working with an active ingredient or an active complex presupposes its analytical definition. It must be possible to determine the strength of the concentrate and to assess whether its effect will be maintained after addition to the cosmetic preparation and extended storage.

Basically, there are two methods of analyzing biologically active ingredients:

1. If the chemical composition is known, it can be determined according to chemical and chemical/physical testing methods. Color reactions have been established for almost all vitamins; here the intensity of the developing pigmentation, which can be measured accurately in an electrophotometer, reflects the vitamin concentration in the test product.

2. Whenever good chemical testing methods are not available or when we are faced with an unknown ingredient or mixture of ingredients, biological tests are applied. These tests usually consist in administering the active concentrate or preparation to animals whose reaction resembles that of humans and determining the minimum quantity required to cause an exactly defined reaction in the test animal.

Occasionally the effect can even be read quantitatively on the test animal; for example, that of male sex hormones in the cockerel test. The comb of a castrated cock withers but starts to grow again if the bird is fed male sex hormones. The amount of administered hormone may be measured from the surface increase of the comb.

Zenisek [68] suggests using the oxygen consumption of the skin *in vivo* as an evaluation of the effectiveness of preparations intended to increase skin metabolism. On the basis of exact measurements of a royal jelly cream, he determined that it did not, as assumed, increase the oxygen consumption of the skin but that this particular effect was due to the ointment base and that the royal jelly itself had an inhibiting effect. If it can be confirmed that the desired effect of complexes such as royal jelly is indeed based on an increase of epidermal metabolism and that Zenisek's method which measures oxygen absorption from outside and carbon dioxide elimination outward (not into the circulation) is a valid measure for the intensity of skin metabolism, a valuable method for measuring biological agents will have been found.

Wherever possible, chemical methods are preferred because animal tests take more time, are more costly, and less accurate. In many cases, however, biological tests are the only possibility.

We must emphasize again that ingredients and ingredient complexes may be used for cosmetic applications only when quantitative determination methods have been established. So long as these methods have not been proved, the producer himself can have no idea how effective his ingredients are (the quality of biological preparations is known to fluctuate even with uniform processing) and the manufacturer of cosmetics cannot tell how long the active ingredients in the end product will remain effective. If cosmetics are to progress beyond the alchemistic stage, such groping in the dark is quite inadmissible. In pharmacology it has long been mandatory that the concentration of active ingredients in any preparation be known exactly; the same requirement should apply to cosmetics.

**Vitamin-Rich Oils.** Many vegetable and animal oils contain vitamins (particularly the fat-soluble A, D, E, and F) and certain other ingredients (lecithins and estrogens). We describe a few valuable oils in this connection: Among animal oils cod-liver oil is of particular importance; it contains vitamins A and D and is rich in unsaturated fatty acids. Cod-liver oil has been used for a long time in healing ointments. Once the value of the oil was supposed to be due to its vitamin A and D content; nowadays the main stress is laid on its unsaturated fatty acids [69]. Cod-liver oil has not been found acceptable in cosmetics, probably because of the unpleasant odor of the oil when it is no longer fresh.

Among vegetable oils, avocado oil, according to Schwob [70], is rich in vitamin A and in certain B vitamins; in addition, it contains vitamins D and E, linolenic acid, sterols, and lecithin. Wheat germ oil is particularly rich in vitamin E and contains vitamins A and D, certain B vitamins, polyunsaturated fatty acids, lecithin, estrogenic substances, and other steroids.

**Placenta and Other Animal Organ Extracts.** The use of placenta as a biological stimulant is reported to have been known in China since the third century. In the cosmetic industry placenta and other organic extracts have been available only since it became possible to convert them to stable forms without loss of effectiveness.

In lyophylization, a very successful method (freeze dehydration), the substance is frozen to $-30$ to $-50°C$ and the water sublimated (i.e., converted directly from ice into vapor) in high vacuum: if dehydration is carried out at a higher temperature, the substance completely loses its biological effectiveness. The dry extract has an almost unlimited stability. Shortly before its addition to cosmetic or pharmaceutical preparations, it is dissolved in water; the solution then has the same efficacy as the fresh extract.

The individual active agents contained in placenta extract are vitamins A, C, and E, the various vitamins of the B group, $B_2$, $B_{12}$, folic acid, and biotin, and several amino acids, enzymes, and compounds of trace elements (magnesium, silicium, phosphorus, calcium, manganese, iron, and copper). The hormone content varies according to the origin; mature placenta, for example, has a high content of follicle hormone, which is barely present in placentae three and four months old.

Placenta extract stimulates circulation [71] and epidermal metabolism. Tronnier [72] demonstrated the increase of erythema formation under ultraviolet radiation and simultaneous application of placenta-extract ointment; Eschbach and Kludas [73] found an increase in cellular respiration *in vivo* (infantile mouse uteri). The reported effects have been summarized by Bureau [74]. According to Kludas [75], the effect of placenta extract is based mostly on its enzyme content. Vitamins and trace elements would then be important as active groups in enzymes or constituents in coenzymes. Following this reasoning, Benedikt [76] suggests a biological test that determines the "placenta activity" of a preparation by measuring the content of respiratory enzymes.

Benedikt describes the test as follows: "The substrate used is rat-liver homogenate. The method is based on the principle that all animal breathing consumes oxygen and develops carbon dioxide." (*Author's note:* Such "breathing" continues in the liver of a recently killed test animal; for technical reasons the liver is homogenized.) "The apparatus is constructed in such a way that the carbon dioxide is absorbed in alkali, whereas the pressure deficiency resulting from the oxygen consumption is read off the manometer. The oxygen consumption of the substrate alone is measured and in a parallel test that of the substrate together with the organ extract to be tested. The difference between both readings indicates the increase of tissue breathing caused by the test extract." Benedikt recommends this test not only for placenta but also for other organic extracts.

Benedikt's test method may be open to criticism because it is too one-sided: placenta extract has other effects that have nothing to do with cellular respiration and do not become apparent in the suggested test. Nevertheless Benedikt's test appears to be a step in the right direction. An incomplete method of determination is better than none.

Placenta extract is one of the most widely used complexes in cosmetics today. Considering the many clinical tests available, it can hardly be doubted that it achieves increased circulation and improved turgor of the skin.

In addition to placenta extract, other organ extracts are also produced for use in cosmetics. (An example is "Epidermin" Richter, G.m.b.H., Berlin) which contains active ingredients taken from the ovaries, testicles, mammae, and placenta as well as from the skin of young animals.

Rovesti and his co-workers examined the effects of various animal organ extracts and reported on the action of extracts from lyophylized mitochondria of calves' hearts and extracts from sea and land mollusks [77]. Brambilla [78] describes the composition and cosmetic applications of skin extracts from mammalian embryos.

**Extracts from Germinal Plants.**   This group of complexes has been studied in particular by Italian cosmetic chemists. Rovesti [79], following Carrel, identifies growth-stimulating substances present in embryonic sap of young plants as trephones. He produced them in highly concentrated form from brewer's yeast, fertilized plant ovaries (St. John's wort, apple and cherry trees, and tomatoes) and the juices of germinated seeds of barley, wheat, rye, cloves, and corn. Rovesti describes trephones as water-soluble, completely dializable compounds which can be precipitated with alcohol in alkaline environment. They are soluble in 90% acetic acid and are extremely sensitive to heat. Trephones have been examined for their cosmetic effectiveness by adding them to bentonite masks in different concentrations.

Comparisons were made with trephone-free masks with facial half-packs. Unfortunately, Rovesti gives no details of their effect and does not mention how many subjects were used in the tests. He generalizes about the activation of cellular metabolism of aging and atrophied skin and accelerated proliferation of cells in the epidermal tissue. Best results were achieved with trephones derived from germinated seeds, fertilized plant ovaries, and brewer's yeast.

Compared with animal embryo extracts, trephones act more slowly, according to Rovesti, but their effect is more lasting. Within the last 10 years many papers have been published, particularly in Italy, on the cosmetic application of botanical extracts (e.g., see Bigi [80] Galli and Rovesti [81]). Fayand and Rivera [82] extracted sprouting germs of various fruits and vegetables and obtained concentrates that, in addition to plant hormones, also contain vitamins and amino acids. These concentrates are commercially available under the designation "Hormo-Fruit Extracts." "Polyvitamin Concentrate L" (Keimdiät, G.m.b.H., Augsburg) is a concentrated extract of wheat germ which is particularly rich in vitamins A, B, and E [83]. According to Rothemann [84], excellent results have already been achieved with this extract in cosmetics.

The similarity, at least in effect, of plant hormones to hormones of warm-blooded animals is suggested by Rothemann's observation [85] that symptoms of pregnancy were induced in baby mice with an extract of onions; hops is also rich in estrogens.

The "aleurones" and "bialeurones" recently discussed by Avalle [86] also belong to the botanical extract group. Aleuron is a liquid secreted in wheat cells which envelops both germ and grain and stimulates and directs the growth of the germ in the first days of its independent existence.

According to Avalle, special conditions must be maintained to preserve biological action during the processing of wheat chaff. It is interesting to note that the ingredients are exposed to temperatures as high as 100°C in the isolation process without losing their effectiveness. Thermostability goes so far that aleurone, which may be distilled under normal pressure, yields a water-soluble distillate aleuronin that reportedly has a still stronger biological action. Various subsequent concentration processes are finally said to yield the highly active bialeurone.

Several chemical properties of aleurone, aleuronin, and bialeurone [87] have already been described. These products contain nitrogen but no amino acids. Aleurone, contains carbohydrates; aleuronin and bialeurone do not, but they do contain carbonyl groups and have a positive keto acid test.

In biological tests aleuronin caused accelerated growth of wheat germ and (by internal administration) rats. After experimental damage to the liver of rats it also caused accelerated regeneration of the liver and red blood corpuscles. Cosmetic tests were also carried out, but unfortunately the results were again described only in general terms as vitalization of cells, disappearance of wrinkles and aging symptoms, and rejuvenation of the tissues.

Finally, according to Filatov [88], biostimulines may be produced from various animal or vegetable tissues, which, if exposed to agents that create obstacles to the life process but do not kill them, undergo a biochemical adjustment and develop substances that support vital processes in the matrix tissue. (The conditions that cause biogenic stimulation are described in detail in Filatov's article.) If introduced into the living organism, these substances activate vital processes and increase resistance. The action is reported to be broad and unspecified. Biogenic stimulants are not, like enzymes, proteins but complexes from which dicarbonic acids, oxydicarbonic acids, unsaturated aromatic acids, and oxyacids have been isolated. Filatov himself speaks only about the injection of extracts or implantation of tissues but later authors have also considered purely cosmetic applications.

Summarizing, we may say that extracts from plant tissues offer a completely new group of complexes to cosmetics which, according to early laboratory reports, have valuable biological properties. Before they are ready for use in the cosmetic industry, wide-ranging clinical tests will have to be carried out to supply answers to the following questions:

What exactly is the effect of extracts and concentrates on epidermal tissue?

How does it differ from the effect of a "synthetic" preparation that contains identical vitamins and hormones? Are there any undesirable side effects?

Finally, chemical or biological analytical methods will also have to be developed for these active complexes.

**Condensed Fruit and Vegetable Juices.** These products are quite different from the plant-germ extracts discussed in the preceding section. The preparations referred to here are obtained by pressing ripe fruits and vegetables and condensing the juice by evaporating the water contained in it. They can be used in cosmetics only if they can be preserved without any effect on their active constituents. Rovesti [89] discusses the problems of preservation and recommends various methods. He finds that preserved juices, either pure or mixed in creams, milks, and face masks, have a beneficial effect on the skin. This he attributes to the content of vitamins, plant hormones, growth factors, and emollients.

Here again we have no clinical reports so far that describe the exact effect of these complexes on the epidermal tissue and no methods to assay the activity of any preparation.

**Royal Jelly.** Much has been written in recent years about the possibility of using royal jelly, the food of the queen bee, in cosmetics [90]. Queen bees are considerably larger than worker bees, live 10 times longer, and are incredibly fertile, whereas worker bees are sterile; the invigorating effect of the special food that causes a normal bee larva to develop into a queen has long been known. It became possible to utilize this effect in medicine and cosmetics only when the Frenchman de Belvefer succeeded in stabilizing the preparation so that it could be stored for longer periods, at least when kept in airtight ampuls without losing its effectiveness.

The composition of royal jelly is largely known. It contains a number of vitamins, particularly of the B group in which pantothenic acid predominates; there is also a rather high content of acetylcholin as well as unknown bee sex hormones whose effect is, however, quite unlike that of the steroids of warm-blooded animals. The specific effect of royal jelly has so far not been explained by its known constituents; a synthetic royal jelly which contained all the known substances in correct proportion proved ineffectual.

Butenandt and Rembolt [91] have isolated 2-amino-4-hydroxy-6-(1-erythro-1,2-(dihydroxypropyl)-pteridin (Biopterin) from royal jelly but the value of this substance is not yet fully understood.

According to all reports, the effect of royal jelly, when applied topically, consists in general rejuvenation of atrophying tissues and improved circulation [92]. In a three-month clinical study of 24 female patients, aged between 25 and 70 [93], 10 women showed an improvement, 10, no results, and four, symptoms of irritation. Whenever the effect was positive, it was similar to that of estrogens, but the dosage (about 0.5 g daily use of an ointment containing 0.3% lyophylized royal jelly) caused only two cases of increased hormonal activity in the organism.

The use of royal jelly in cosmetics is described in German Patent 1,007,956, 1958. It would be most desirable to develop a testing method to determine how long royal jelly retains its specific effectiveness in cosmetic preparations.

Active ingredients resembling those of royal jelly also seem to be present in the pollen of a number of plants. An important disadvantage of using pollen in cosmetic preparations is its tendency to cause allergic reactions. According to Luzuy [94], water-soluble protein fractions (he is probably referring to peptides) are responsible for these reactions, and their removal results in better toleration. Data available on the effect of pollen on the organism appear even less reliable than those on royal jelly.

Royal jelly is the food of queen-bee larvae; this fact gave rise to the interesting notion that the bees themselves contain this substance, in biologically processed form, and must therefore be valuable cosmetic agents. Larvae not older than four days were crushed and deacidified before use (Swiss Patent 317,697). According to Schmidt [95], the cosmetic effect is reported to be excellent but no critical studies have yet been made available.

**Botanical Extracts.**    Botanical extracts are used rather rarely in cosmetic preparations. Rothemann discusses them in detail [96], and the reader is referred to his book. Some plant extracts may be effective because of their vitamin content (e.g., nettle extract, rich in vitamin A, and extracts of fresh carrot roots which contain vitamins A, C, and certain forms of B); others contain organic sulfur compounds (onions and horseradish), some inhibit inflammations (e.g., St. John's wort oil and camomile extract), some are disinfectants (fennel oil and parsley), others are irritants (arnica tincture and jaborandi extracts), and many, rightly or wrongly, are said to have a stimulating effect on hair growth.

## Preparations

**Functions of the Base.**    Cosmetic preparations containing biological agents do not usually have more than 5% active ingredients, often considerably less. It is obvious that the properties of these preparations are not only determined by the 5% but also by the remaining 95%, or the base.

The following requirements must be met by the base:

1. It must be completely skin compatible in every respect.
2. As the vehicle for the active ingredients, it must be able to dissolve them or at least finely disperse them.
3. The base must be selected to allow the active ingredients to remain effective as long as possible.

4. The base must promote penetration of the active ingredients so that they may reach the deeper strata of the skin at which they are supposed to be active; in any case, it should not inhibit this penetration.

5. The base should enhance the effect of the active ingredient and certainly not counteract it.

For example, an emollient base would be an excellent vehicle for a vitamin A preparation that is intended to make the skin soft and supple. An alcoholic solution of vitamin A would be senseless cosmetically because the astringent effect of the alcohol is in direct opposition to the intended action of vitamin A. Zenisek and co-workers [97] described the case of a royal jelly cream designed to increase the skin metabolism but which actually seemed to inhibit it because of the base used.

6. From the consumers' point of view it should be as attractive as possible, white or light colored, preferably not sticky, and have no unpleasant odor. There is hardly any need to dwell on the first and last two requirements. The last one may seem somewhat frivolous but it is a fact that women will not use preparations that are at all unpleasant to apply unless the results are really quite extraordinary. Cosmetic products differ from pharmaceutical ones just in this respect: that users select them freely and not according to medical prescriptions. In order to be accepted, cosmetics must be attractive.

The stability of many sensitive active materials depends to a large extent on the base in which they are employed. Penicillin ointments based on petrolatum, lard, or lanolin, for instance, show a considerable loss in effectiveness, even after two to three months, whereas in suitable bases the loss amounts to no more than 20 % per year and usually less [98].

Generally the stability of active ingredients must be determined experimentally for various bases; certain considerations, however, may be helpful in selecting a suitable base.

Oxidation-sensitive ingredients, such as vitamin A or unsaturated fatty acids, are best incorporated in bases that are suitable for tube packaging. For ingredients extremely sensitive to oxidation, aerosol containers which exclude every possibility of contact with the air, should offer interesting possibilities. The base must contain no fats that become easily rancid because rancidity causes the certain destruction of oxidation-sensitive ingredients. If the base is an emulsion, it must be prepared in such a way that it does not contain any entrapped air at the time the active ingredients are added.

Alkali-sensitive ingredients must, of course, not be processed with alkaline emulsifiers (e.g., alkali soaps), nor can the acid-sensitive be processed with acidified thickening agents (e.g., alginates).

Good preservation is essential because vitamin-rich preparations or those that contain organic extracts represent particularly good culture media for microorganisms. On the other hand, the preservative must be carefully selected because many ingredients are inactivated by certain preservatives; for example, proteins, peptides, and enzymes are incompatible with phenolic preservatives or those that split off formaldehyde.

In any case it is important during the formulation and production of a preparation to determine which are the "weak spots" of the active ingredients to be used and against which agents they are particularly sensitive.

**Depth Effect and Resorption.**   We finally come to the requirement that the base should assist the active ingredient to reach that layer of skin at which it is meant to develop its effect. Much has been written about the connection between base and depth effect of cosmetic and pharmaceutical preparations. To gain a clear picture we must first define the concept of "resorption":

We speak of *resorption* of an active ingredient or a base only if the substance has *penetrated* to the epidermal strata below Rein's barrier. Certain vegetable fats, cetyl alcohol, and isopropyl myristate soon disappear after application to the skin surface. This is not a matter of resorption but merely of penetration into the top corneal layers and the hair follicles. Barail and Pescatore have demonstrated this action for cetyl palmitate [99].

It is, incidentally, not easy to measure exactly how far a certain base is resorbed by the skin. Theoretically, certain skin layers can be isolated and the absence or presence of substances contained in the base, chemically determined. In practice this normally cannot be done because of the chemically complicated composition of the epidermal tissue and the minute quantities of foreign substances that would have to be traced in it. The use of radio isotopes (e.g., $C^{14}$, an isotope of normal carbon) has offered means to mark substances chemically and to trace the minutest imponderable amounts in complicated mixtures [100]. This method, however, is applicable only to substances that can be synthetized in the laboratory, hence not to natural fats and waxes. The study by Barail and Pescatore [99] of the behavior of cetyl palmitate is an example of the application of this method to a synthetic wax.

Another method—until the introduction of radio isotopes it was the only one—that determines the penetration of bases consists in incorporating substances that act as indicators. They may be pigments that can be traced microscopically under normal light in histological sections of the skin tissue or fluorescent substances that become apparent under a fluorescence microscope. They may be substances whose presence can be demonstrated by color reactions, either in microscopic preparations or in extracts from epidermal tissue layers [102] or that, once they have penetrated beyond Rein's barrier, enter the blood capillaries and can then be traced in urine (e.g., salicylic acid). Of interest also is the use of certain alkaloids that cause easily recognizable reactions in test subjects, both animal and human; Valette and his co-workers use eserine [103]. The interval between application and reaction (for eserine, muscular contraction) was used as a measure of the penetrating capacity of the base.

Radioactive substances have also been used as indicators [104]; this method differs in principle from that of Barail and Pescatore in which one constituent of the base was marked radioactively. Harry [105] reports on a study in which several of the methods mentioned were applied side by side.

All indicator methods have one fundamental shortcoming: what is measured is not really the penetration of the base but rather that of the indicator. In many instances the authors make a close relation between both effects plausible, but the published data of different authors regarding the penetration capacity of certain bases are contradictory because results are dependent not only on the bases in question but also on the indicators used.

It is obviously a different matter if the experiments are to determine from which particular base an ingredient will best penetrate to the deeper skin layers. Here the results can be obtained directly from pigment reactions of histological sections or an assessment of the blood and urine level of the ingredient to be measured. No fundamental objections can be made in these cases. Tests of this kind are now also conducted with ingredients marked with radio isotopes [106].

Other methods that measure the resorption of active ingredients have been described by Wilson [107]: (a) determination of the inhibition of enzyme activity [108]; (b) comparison of vasodilation resulting from topical application on the one hand and intradermal injection of an identical quantity of the respective substance on the other [109]; (c) profusion method [110]; (d) application of the substance in saline solution on the conjunctiva of rats and microscopic measuring of size and shape changes of the iris.

*Transepidermal and Transfollicular Resorption.* The distinguished dermatologist Rothman was the first to emphasize that in order to understand the problems of depth effect two pathways of resorption must be clearly distinguished [111]: In one (*transepidermal* resorption) the substance migrates through the corneal layer, passing Rein's barrier, and reaches the deeper layers over the total breadth of the skin.

The other (*transfollicular* resorption) leads through the hair follicles. Once a substance has penetrated the follicles it need only pass a thin lipid layer and an equally thin corneal cell layer to reach the deeper skin tissue; Rein's barrier is absent here. From the hair follicles the substance may also reach the sebaceous glands and from there the corium. In transfollicular resorption the sweat glands probably play a minor role.

Although many details regarding resorption are still unknown and we do not yet understand which resorption route is followed by many ingredients, we can, according to Rothman, make some generally valid observations.

Substances able to penetrate Rein's barrier usually follow the transepidermal resorption route. For this route the total surface of the skin is available, whereas transfollicular resorption can start only from the relatively small internal surfaces of the follicles, which are difficult to reach, or from the walls of the sebaceous glands, which are even harder to reach.

Rein's barrier is permeated by all gases, including water vapor, and by lipid soluble substances that are miscible with cholesterol and phospholipids. It is noteworthy that free phenols and alkaloids have good penetrating capacity, whereas their salts, which are water- but not fat-soluble, cannot penetrate at all. Neither can strongly hydrophobic substances, for example, mineral oil [112].

The penetration of a substance through the corneal layer and Rein's barrier (i.e., *transepidermal* resorption) can be facilitated or impeded by the presence of certain other substances. Substances that dissolve cholesterol (chloroform and ether) or precipitate it (saponins) facilitate resorption of predominantly water-soluble substances and impede it for fat-soluble substances. Cholesterol (hence also lanolin) in the base has the opposite effect. On the other hand, Carson and Goldhamer [113] found that water from an emulsion penetrates the skin and particularly Rein's barrier 10 times more quickly if the emulsion contained Lantrol (wax-free, oil-soluble lanolin fraction). Salicylic acid, $\beta$-naphthol, and resorcinol facilitate the resorption of many substances, probably by destroying Rein's barrier [114]. For this reason these and similar substances as well as essential oils are occasionally used in dermatology to help carry the active ingredient into the deeper layers of the skin.

In *transfollicular* resorption the base must convey the active ingredient deep into the hair follicle. For this purpose the base must have a good wetting effect on the skin and must flow easily. Here emulsions are generally the most suitable bases. Several authors state that O/W emulsions are preferable to the inverted type. This may be because the emulsifying agent has to play a double part: it also acts as a wetting agent. Although the best emulsifiers are usually not the best wetting agents, the wetting effect of typical O/W emulsifying agents (fatty alcohol sulfates and soaps) is certainly much better than that of W/O emulsifiers (cholesterol).

One factor that is important in the transmission of active ingredients from the base to the skin tissue is the distribution coefficient: the ratio of the solubility of the ingredient in the epidermal tissue and the base. If it is much higher in the base than in the skin, conditions for the transmission of the active ingredient to the skin are unfavorable. A base should therefore be selected in which the ingredient in the concentration used, is soluble, though not too easily. (In those instances in which the base is an emulsion this obviously applies only to the phase in which the ingredient is dissolved). The distribution coefficient could perhaps explain the observation made by Eller and Wolff [115] that the skin absorbs sex hormones with greater facility from aqueous than from oily bases.

In this context the skin tissue may be regarded as a cholesterol phospholipid-rich mass because the active ingredients do not dissolve in keratin but in the extracellular substance.

**Penetration Capacity of Active Ingredients.** We have seen in the preceding section that the speed and extent of ingredient resorption depend on the base used, nevertheless the properties of the active ingredient itself are the most important factor.

Some substances (e.g., phenols and certain essential oils) are resorbed by the skin from all bases; others (e.g., sugar and common salt) from none. We summarize the most important facts known about the penetration capacity of individual substances. Among the vitamins the fat-soluble vitamin A and, according to Lang [116], D and K and carotene are definitely resorbed. It is doubtful if vitamins E and polyunsaturated fatty acids are resorbed. Not much is known so far about resorption of water-soluble vitamins B. According to Burler [117], panthanol, an oil-soluble derivative of pantothenic acid, can be resorbed. Apart from the report by Kashara and Kawashina [118] that the vitamin content of milk had increased after application of a 30% solution of ascorbic acid to the mammae, we do not yet know much about resorption of vitamin C.

Phenols, including salicylic acid, quickly penetrate transepidermally except when their concentration is so high that they precipitate the protein of the epidermis and are themselves bound. Many perfume aromatics, for example, oil of thyme, eucalyptus oil, eucalyptol, α-pinene, linalyl, and geranyl acetate, are also quickly absorbed [119].

Estrogenic sex hormones, testosterone, progesterone, and desoxycorticosterone are easily resorbed by the skin. That estrogens at least penetrate transepidermally is made plausible by the following observation: masseurs working with estrogenic preparations often develop disorders that may be attributed to the penetration of estrogens into the system. Contact with hormone preparations in this instance is restricted to the palms of the hands on which there are no hair follicles. Hydrocortisone acetate easily penetrates the skin, probably transepidermally as experiments by Scott and Kalz have shown [120]. Cortisone acetate is hardly resorbed at all. A number of factors of which we know little are operative in resorption.

Water and volatile organic solvents penetrate in the form of their vapor. The isotope studies of Szcesniak, Sherman, and Harris [121] are relevant.

Among inorganic elements and compounds that also penetrate are sulfur, mercury, iodine, boric acid, potassium cyanate, oil-soluble salts of mercury ($Hg^{2+}$), lead ($Pb^{2+}$), bismuth ($Bi^{3+}$), and copper. Strongly dissociated water-soluble salts such as common salt are not resorbed by the healthy epidermis.

**Preparations to Stimulate Flabby Skin.** This group includes "anti-wrinkle" creams, hormone creams, and in general all the preparations that are intended to restore a taut and youthful appearance to the aging skin of women over 40. The most important active ingredients are follicular hormones and related substances, synthetic estrogens, and complexes such as placenta liquid. Royal jelly is also recommended for this purpose. In this group we also include preparations with protein hydrolysates and enzymes.

Eller and Wolff [122] report that sex hormones are better resorbed by the skin from an aqueous than an oily base, and Gohlke [123] had the same experience with placenta liquid. Goldzieher [124] states that estrogens if applied to the skin in aqueous solution do not reach the circulation in any significant concentration. This probably indicates a far-reaching absorption of the hormone by the epidermal tissue. On the other hand, hormones penetrate to the circulation in organic solvent solutions (e.g., alcohol), and the systemic action is as strong as in oral administration. Applied in emulsions, systemic activity amounts to about $\frac{1}{7}$ to $\frac{1}{10}$ of oral introduction. For-mulations have been published in the literature for hormone and placenta preparations in a high-water-content base as well as fat-rich night creams enriched by estrogens. Examples of both types as well as a protein hydrolysate cream follow.

REMARKS

16. U. S. Patent 2,791,534 (Schaaf and Gross, Ciba, May 1957). A stearate cream, high water and low fat content. Methyl-$p$-hydroxy benzoate is recommended as the preservative.

17. Rothemann, *SÖFW*, **83,** 59 (1957). Emulsification at about 75°C. Extrapon VC is described by the manufacturer as a complex of biogenic ingredients (skin vitamins, regu-lators of fat metabolism). It may be dissolved in the fat melt. Placenta liquid and perfume oil may be stirred in only when the cream is almost cold. The preservative specified is Rokonsal B liquid.

18. Rothemann, *"Das grosse Rezeptbuch der Haut- und Körperpflegemittel* 3rd ed., p. 620. An "antiwrinkle" oil. Foragynol is dissolved in Cetiol V. Lavender absolute is recommended for perfuming.

18a. Levenstein in Sagarin, *Cosmetics, Science*, and *Technology*, p. 183. Add the water phase (75°C) with constant stirring to the oil phase (75°C) in which estrogen concentrate has been dissolved. Continue stirring to 55°C, add perfume, and fill immediately. Paraffin wax may be replaced by microcrystalline wax. This formulation differs from the others by its strikingly high content of mineral waxes which are generally not acceptable for this type of formulation. The author of the formulation holds the opinion that in order to allow

| | 16 | 17 | 18 | 18a | 19 |
|---|---|---|---|---|---|
| Paraffin wax | | | | 7.0 | |
| Petrolatum | | | | 42.5 | |
| Almond oil | 2.5 | | | | |
| Avocado oil | | | 60 | | |
| E Grandelat | | 10 | 25 | | |
| Isopropyl myristate | | | | 4.0 | 5 |
| Cetyl alcohol | 0.8 | | | 2.0 | |
| Cetostearyl alcohol | | | | | 10 |
| Cetiol V | | | 15 | | |
| Eutanol G | | 10 | | | |
| Lanette N | | 12 | | | |
| Anhydrous lanolin | | | | 4.0 | |
| Stearic acid | 20.0 | | | | |
| Pregnenolone | 0.5 | | | | |
| Placenta liquid | | 2 | | | |
| Extrapon VC | | 1 | | | |
| Foragynol | | | 0.004 | | |
| Epidermin tenfold | | | 0.2 | | |
| Estrogen concentrate | | | | 0.5 | |
| Emulgin M-8 | | | | | 3 |
| Triethanolamine | 1.8 | | | | |
| Sorbitan mono-oleate | | | | 4.0 | |
| Protein hydrolysate | | | | | 2.5 |
| Water | 69.2 | 54.5 | | 33.4 | 73.6 |
| Magnesium sulfate | | | | 0.2 | |
| Glycerol | 5.0 | | | | 5.0 |
| Sorbitol liquid | | 10 | | 2.0 | |
| Preservative | 0.2 | 0.5 | | 0.2 | 0.2 |
| Perfume | 0.2 | 0.5 | | 0.2 | 0.5 |
| | 100.2 | 100.5 | 100.204 | 100.0 | 102.5 |

hormone creams to act on the skin tissue it is important that the active ingredients be only slowly transferred from the cream to the skin. Mineral waxes that impede resorption therefore do not interfere here. Levenstein prefers W/O emulsions to the O/W type for hormone creams because they permit immediate contact between the hormone solution and the skin lipids, cover and protect the skin and do not dry like water-rich creams to a small residue with high hormone content.

19. Lodi and Rovesti, *Praktische Chemie*, symposium on the occasion of the 11th international congress for cosmetics, Vienna 1957, p. 69. The authors incorporated various protein hydrolysates in this cream. Its pH value should be adjusted to 6.

**Preparations for the Care of Brittle, Flaky, Dry Skin.**    The most important active ingredients in these preparations are vitamin A, carotene, and poly-unsaturated fatty acids. Vitamin E seems to support the effectiveness of vitamin A and polyunsaturated fatty acids, perhaps by protecting them against oxidation.

| | 20 | 21 | 22 |
|---|---|---|---|
| Olive oil, first pressing, preserved | 12.7 | 22 | |
| E Grandelat | 11 | 5.5 | |
| Spermaceti | 9.5 | 7.5 | |
| Beeswax, natural yellow | 6.4 | | |
| Sunbleached beeswax | | 9 | |
| Lanolin, pharmaceutical grade | 16 | | |
| *Adeps lanae*, anhydrous | | 8 | |
| Bleached wool wax | | 1.5 | |
| Cetiol V | | | 2.5 |
| Cetiol | 16 | | |
| Lanette N | | | 8.0 |
| Stearic acid | | | 8.0 |
| Lecithin ex ovo | 0.65 | | |
| Carotene | 10,000 units | | |
| Vitamin oil | | 11 | |
| Epidermin tenfold | | 0.1 | 0.1 |
| Isolinoleic acid ester | | | 0.4 |
| Water | 27 | 22 | 70.5 |
| Borax | 0.32 | 0.5 | |
| Triethanolamine | | | 0.4 |
| Glycerol | | | 5.0 |
| Sorbitol liquid | | | 5.0 |
| Perfume | 0.38 | 0.3 | 0.4 |
| Preservative | 0.25 | | 0.2 |
| | 100.2 | 98.4 | 100.4 |

REMARKS

20. Rothemann, *Das grosse Rezeptbuch der Haut- und Körperpflegemittel*, 3rd ed., p. 567. "Skin nourishing cream," cold cream type. Perfume oil: natural or synthetic rose oil; distilled water may be replaced by rosewater. Olive oil and E. Grandelat are stirred into the wax melt (60°C). At 55°C slowly stir in the aqueous borax solution (also at 55°C). Mix in the perfume oil shortly before the cream congeals. Homogenize the completed cream to improve appearance and internal structure.

21. Rothemann, *op. cit.*, p. 575. This cream resembles the preceding one in composition but contains other active ingredients.

22. Rothemann, *op. cit.*, p. 574. The preservative is methyl hydroxy benzoate which is dissolved in water. Rothemann's book contains many suggestions for oils and solid and liquid creams with vitamins, hormones, and active complexes. All emollient preparations based on fats (see Chapter 8) may be used as bases.

**Biological Hair Lotions.** Cosmetic hair lotions meant to act as stimulants, to provide fragrance, or to give the hair a more attractive appearance are discussed in Chapter 10. According to Rothemann, biological hair lotions should really be correctly described as scalp lotions. In this discussion we must never lose sight of one fact: preparations that stop the permanent loss of hair or make hair grow again once baldness has started do not exist. Advertisements for hair-growing preparations often contain photographs of people whose bald heads before treatment show complete growth after. These are mostly cases—not so very rare—in which the hair would also have grown again without any treatment.

This does not mean that the application of hair lotions is useless. These preparations can contribute to the removal of infection, suppress or control dandruff formation; they can eliminate pruritus and may, if treatment is started early enough, assist in delaying baldness.

Many types of active ingredients are used in biological hair lotions. A summary is given by Heald [125].

1. *Sulfur, Sulfur Compounds, and Selenium Compounds.* Pathological dandruff formation and, in a wider sense, seborrhoea may be regarded as keratin disorders.

Seborrhoea, dandruff, and baldness may be described as the results of a pathological proliferation of the epidermal tissue. Seborrhoea is the hyperactivity of the sebaceous glands. Dandruff formation may be the result of incomplete keratinization which in turn is due to hyperactivity of the *stratum germinativum*. Finally, some dermatologists are of the opinion that baldness is due to an exhaustion of the scalp following overaccelerated production of new hair [126]. It might be interesting to pursue this argument further [127].

Sulfur is the traditional treatment for such disorders. For many years colloidal sulfur has been an ingredient of hair lotions. More recently selenium sulfide [128], cadmium sulfide [129], sodium sulfacetamide [130], alkali polythionate [131] ($M_2S_xO_6$), and "S-54", a thiocarbonic acid derivative [132] have been recommended for combating seborrhoea and dandruff and are used in hair lotions. Selenium sulfide is toxic and may cause diffused loss of hair [133]; it must be applied only in very small doses. Tellurium oxide has also been used successfully [134].

The use of water-soluble selenites ($MHSeO_4$, $M_2SeO_4$) as antidandruff agents in hair preparations is covered by a German patent (DAS 1,078,590).

2. *Phenols.* Resorcinol, $\beta$-naphthol, and certain other phenols (often contained in essential oils) have been employed for many years in the treatment of skin diseases. In hair lotions they can develop fourfold action: they have a keratolytic (tanning), disinfectant, and stimulating effect and can also serve as resorption promoters for other ingredients.

3. *Other Disinfectants.* We have already stated the hypothesis that subjects with seborrhoea are inclined to dandruff formation and baldness because oily sebaceous skin provides a particularly good culture medium for microorganisms. This hypothesis is supported by the discovery that on microscopic examination scalp scales are always found with a bottleshaped microorganism: *pityrosporum ovale.* This bacterium, however, is also found frequently on healthy scalps. Although many investigators have explored this problem, the question whether *pityrosporum ovale* must be regarded as the cause of dandruff or as a harmless member of the resident flora has not yet been decided.[135].

In any case some control of the germ count of an oily sebaceous scalp, covered with scales and furrowed by fissures, may well be useful. Complete sterilization is impossible nor would it be desirable. The majority of the disinfectants mentioned in Chapter 3 may be used here. In this application quaternary ammonium salts have the additional advantage that they make the hair more easily manageable after shampooing.

Incidentally, most hair lotions act as disinfectants even if they do not contain a specific active ingredient because they are based on ethyl or isopropyl alcohol. The optimum for disinfectant action is about 70 percent for ethyl and 50% solution for isopropyl alcohol.

4. *Keratin Hydrolysates.* Shortly after World War I Zuntz [136] suggested combating premature loss of hair by administering the amino acid cystine which plays an important part in the composition of hair. The cystine was incorporated in a keratin hydrolysate intended for oral administration. Its success was doubtful. Hair growth increased wherever the roots were sound, not only on the scalp but over the entire body; nails also grew faster. On the bald head on which the function of the hair papillae was disturbed hair did not generally grow again. The preparation soon disappeared from the market but the idea of using a keratin hydrolysate persisted [137]. Certain hair lotions containing keratin hydrolysates intended for external application to the scalp have been on the market for many years and have many faithful users.

5. *Cholesterol.* Jaffé reported [138] that rubbing the scalp with ointments containing cholesterol stimulates the hair growth of rabbits. Since then cholesterol has found acceptance in many hair preparations in spite of the many skeptical and negative reports on its effectiveness.

Linser and Koehler [139] had already reported in 1928 that an ointment without cholesterol stimulated the rabbits' hair growth as much as that with cholesterol. The operative factor seems to be the massage—the mechanical stimulation. Chemical stimulation (e.g., with phenols) or physical stimulation (with ultraviolet radiation) also increases the hair growth of rabbits. The animal reacts to each kind of stimulant with increased circulation which in turn leads to an activation of the quiescent hair follicles. Experts have for a long time disagreed on whether increased hair growth in humans can be by mechanical, chemical, or physical stimulation.

6. *Irritants: Circulation-Promoting Substances.* Following a review of the literature dealing with this question [140], Flesch arrives at the following conclusion: permanently increased circulation causes with a certain number of subjects increased growth and thickened hair shafts, but there seem to be major individual differences. There is no indication that short-term increases in circulation have a lasting effect on hair growth. It has not yet been determined where the border line between "permanent" and "short-term" should be drawn.

A far more positive opinion can be found with Neumann [141]. The observation that baldness usually starts at the places at which circulation of the scalp is weakest leads him to the conclusion that bad circulation is a main factor in baldness and that treatment with preparations that stimulate circulation are promising.

Among the many substances in hair lotions, that have been recommended as circulation stimulants, we list only a few: capsicin, cantharidene, quinine, pilocarpine, and nicotinic acid benzyl ester. The protein hydrolysates which Gerhard [142] suggests for use in hair preparations also belong to this group. In this case the active agent is not, as in the keratin hydrolysates, cystine but the irritant and stimulating effect of peptides contained in protein partial hydrolysates.

7. *Hormones.* Estrogens may also be regarded as circulation stimulants (but they cannot be described as irritants). They are used for a different reason in hair preparations, which we have already discussed. The incidence of seborrhoea is much higher in men than in women, and baldness is a typical male phenomenon. Estrogen treatment of seborrhoea and baldness has indeed achieved good results. Considering that estrogens may enter the bloodstream, caution is indicated in treating male scalps with female hormones. Only those substances that have slight or no action as sex hormones may be considered and dosage must be kept low (maximum 200 IU per gram of hair lotion). Goldzieher [143] reports on experiments in which he treated the scalps of men and women with solutions of 1.5–3.0 mg estradiol, estradiol monobenzoate, or diethyl stilbestrol per 100 g of alcoholic hair lotion. These preparations were massaged into the scalp once or twice daily over a period

of four to six weeks; at the end of the period loss of hair had been stopped in 84 percent of the women and 80 percent of the men. Success with the men was only temporary.

In the light of later results we can now say that the dosage selected by Goldzieher (more than 1000 IU per gram) was much too high and that the estrogens were not the most suitable because they all have a strong sex hormone effectiveness.

A few years ago Roberts [144] reported that he had isolated one of the hormones from the frontal lobes of the hypophysis which stimulated exhausted hair papillae to renewed activity. Such reports have not been confirmed.

8. *Pantothenic Acid, Panthenol.*   Pantothenic acid is one of the vitamins of the B group. It is a component of "coenzyme A" which plays a central part in many vital processes. Panthenol, the corresponding alcohol, is easily resorbed by the skin and therefore especially suitable for external application. Juon [145] reports good results in the treatment of various skin diseases, including seborrhoic loss of hair, with high doses of panthenol. Similar favorable results are also reported by other investigators [146]. Nevertheless skepticism remains among some authors [147]. The effect is reported to be particularly good if the external application of panthenol is accompanied by oral administration of bepanthene or calcium pantothenate: the latter may also be injected intravenously. Derivatives of pantothenic acid may also be used. The German patent 966,040 (Schwarzkopf) protects the use of tetra alkylammonium pantothenates such as acetylcholine pantothenate and acetyl methylcholine pantothenate in hair preparations; German patent 955,093 (Janistyn) covers the use of condensation products of pantothenic acid (and its salts) with chlorides of amino acids (or amine alcohols derived therefrom) in skin and hair preparations.

In some animals discoloration of the hair is caused by a deficiency of pantothenic acid or $p$-amino benzoic acid: it has not yet been determined which of the two substances is operative here. For this reason these substances have been described as "antigraying" agents. Experimental evidence for the assumption that they might also be instrumental in restoring gray human hair to its original color is, however, weak [148].

9. *Pruritus-Alleviating Substances.*   The most widely used ingredient for the relief of itching is Peruvian balsam tincture. Phenols and quinine salts are also reported to be effective.

10. *Choline, Betaine, β-Amino Ethyl Alcohol.*   Properties that impede the loss of hair and stimulate regeneration are attributed, according to Ruhs and Klein (German Patent 1,007,957), to choline, betaine, and β-amino ethyl alcohol in the form of their salts, inorganic esters, or organic compounds

They may be incorporated in lotions or emulsions, preferably in concentrations between 5 and 15%.

11. *Botanical Extracts.* The oldest biological hair preparations were extracts and tinctures of herbs and their use in hair lotions has been continued into the present (eau de quinine, birch extract). The effect of the majority of the extracts used is due to stimulation. In addition, some of these active complexes also have a keratolytic (tanning) and disinfectant effect. Some also contain vitamins (nettle extract, for instance, has a high content of vitamin A), sulfur compounds, or substances with a hormone action (e.g., onion extract).

Plant extracts may be prepared by the cosmetic manufacturer and some can be bought ready made. Water- and alcohol-soluble concentrates of certain plant extracts which are especially easy to process (Extrapone special, Dragoco) have also become commercially available.

12. *Nucleic acids.* The use of sodium ribonucleate in hair products has been recommended [149]. Nothing is known so far about its cosmetic effectiveness.

SUGGESTED FORMULATIONS

23. Hair lotion with keratin hydrolysate (Janistyn, *Riechstoffe, Seifen, Kosmetika*, II, p. 149).

| | |
|---|---|
| Keratin hydrolysate hydrochloride | 1.0 |
| Colloidal sulfur | 0.5 |
| Thymol | 0.1 |
| Salicylic acid | 0.4 |
| Glycerol, 28° Bé | 1.0 |
| Alcohol 60% | 97.0 |
| | 100 g |

Glycerol helps to groom the hair, but if used in large amounts it makes the hair sticky.

24. Eau de Quinine, foaming (Janistyn, *op. cit.*).

| | |
|---|---|
| Alcohol 60% | 950 ml |
| Tincture of cinchona bark 60% | 50 ml |
| Saponin extra | 2 g |
| Tincture of saffron | 3 g |
| Archil powder | 0.1 g |
| Perfume (rose) | 5 g |
| | 1000 ml |

Saponin is a foaming agent that quickly yields an unstable foam. Physiologically, foaming is of no importance, but some consumers like it. Saffron and archil are used to color the preparation.

25. Cholesterol hair lotion (Janistyn, *op. cit.*).

| | |
|---|---:|
| Isopropyl alcohol extra | 52 |
| Ethyl polyglycol acetate (or 0.3 glycerol diethyl ether) | 2 |
| Lecithin, water soluble (from whey) | 0.3 |
| Cholesterol, technical grade | 0.3 |
| Sodium or triethanolamine cholate | 0.5 |
| Tincture of balsam peru | 1.0 |
| Perfume | 0.4 |
| Distilled water | 43.1 |
| Hexyl resorcinol | 0.05 |
| | 99.65 g |

Sodium and triethanolamine cholates are emulsifying agents for cholesterol.

26. Fat-containing hair lotion (Harry, *Modern Cosmetocology*, 4th ed. p. 385).

| | |
|---|---:|
| Resorcinol | 5 |
| Tincture of capsicum | 5 |
| Castor oil | 5 |
| Alcohol 90% | 85 |
| Perfume | q.s. |
| | 100 g |

The higher alcohol concentration than normally contained in hair lotions is required to dissolve the castor oil. This high concentration has the disadvantage of withdrawing water from the scalp and the disinfectant effect is slight.

27. Birch Lotion (formulation of Dragoco; Rothemann, *Das grosse Rezeptbuch der Haut- und Körperpflegemittel*, 3rd ed. p. 429).

| | |
|---|---:|
| Alcohol 95 weight % | 50.0 |
| Distilled water | 44.0 |
| Extrapon S birch | 5.0 |
| Perfume Oil | 1.0 |
| | 100 g |

28. Biological herbal lotion (Rothemann, *op. cit.*, p. 427).

| | |
|---|---:|
| Fine spirit 95 vol. % | 632 ml |
| Rosewater triple | 185 ml |
| Tincture of colts foot | 50 ml |
| Tincture of clove blossom | 50 ml |
| Tincture of burdock roots | 50 ml |
| Tincture of equisetum | 50 ml |
| Isolinoleic acid ester | 5 g |
| Perfume oil | 2 g |
| Possibly: perestrone 100,000–200,000 IU | |
| | abt. 1025 ml |

The perfume oil should consist of natural oils and resinoids.

# REFERENCES

[1] Salfeld, *J. Soc. cosmet. Chem.*, **16**, 269 (1965).

[2] *Parfum. Kosmet.*, **37**, 486 (1956).

[3] *J. Soc. cosmet. Chem.* **16**, 527 (1965).

[4] *Ibid.*, 305 (1965).

[5] Kumer, *Dermatologische Kosmetik*, 2nd and 3rd ed., 1953, p. 143.

[6] *J. Soc. Cosmet. Chem.*, **15**, 761 (1964).

[7] *Ibid.*, **16**, 491 (1965).

[8] Rothemann, *Das grosse Rezeptbuch der Haut- und Körperpflege Mittel*, Dr. Alfred Hüthig Verlap, Heidelberg, 1949, 3rd ed., p. 418.

[9] Charpy, *Annls. Derm. Syph.*, Paris, **3**, 331, 340 (1943); **4**, 110 (1944); **6**, 310 (1946); Dowling and Thomas, *Brit. J. Derm.*, **58**, 45 (1946).

[10] Rothman, *The Physiology and Biochemistry of the Skin*, Univ. of Chicago Press, Chicago, 1955, p. 385.

[11] Klarmann and Peck, *Practitioner*, **17**, 159 (1954).

[12] Janistyn, *Parfum. Kosmet.*, **39**, 16 (1958); U. S. Patent 2,791,534.

[13] German Patent DAS 1,017,748, *Kosmetik-Parf.-Drog.*, **4**, 173 (1957).

[14] See [11]; Goldzieher et al., *Archs. Derm. Syph.*, **66**, 304 (1952).

[15] Flesch and Escoda, *Archs. Biochim. Cosm.*, **6**, No. 52, 21 (1962); *Parfum. Kosmet.*, **45**, 18 (1964).

[16] *J. Am. med. Ass.*, **114**, 386 (1940).

[17] Pemberton, *Lancet*, **I**, 285 (1940).

[18] *Kosmetik-Parf.-Drog.*, **3**, 37 (May 1956).

[19] *Archs. Derm*, 1956, 388; *Am. Perfumer*, **71**, (6), 33 (1958).

[20] Harry, *Modern Cosmetocology*, Leonard Hill, London, 1955, 4th ed., p. 103.

[21] Rothemann, *op. cit.*, 44.

[22] *J. invest. Derm.*, **19**, 353 (1952); *Am. Perfumer*, **78** (7), 15 (1963).

[23] *Parfum. Kosmet.*, **36**, 66 (1956).

[24] *Revta bras. Biol.*, **14**, 443 (1954).

[25] *Am. J. med. Sci.*, **231**, 13 (1956).

[26] *Soap, Perfum. Cosm.*, **34**, 547 (1961).

[27] *Jap. J. Derm.*, **73**, 487 (1963); Ohta, *J. Soc. cosmet. Chem.*, **16**, 349 (1965).

[28] Mitchell, *A Textbook of Biochemistry*, McGraw-Hill, New York, 1950, p. 179.

[29] Gsell, *Schweiz. med. Wschr.*, **74**, 1171 (1944); Juon, *Dermatologica*, **91**, 310 (1945); *Parfum. Kosmet.*, **36**, 567, 621 (1955); Lebeuf., *Bull. Soc. fr. Derm. Syph.*, **56**, 76 (1949); Oesch, *Schweiz. med. Wschr.*, **76**, 6 (1946); Goldman et al. *J. Am. med. Ass.*, **132**, 570 (1946); *J. invest. Derm.*, **11**, 323 (1948); *Archs. Derm. Syph.*, **63**, 443 (1951); Glanzmann and Meier, *Z. VitamForsch.*, **16**, 322 (1945).

[30] Flesch in Rothman, *op. cit.*, 601 et seq.

[31] *Klin. Wschr.*, **16**, 135 (1937).

[32] Nikolowski, *Parfum. Kosmet.*, **37**, 425 (1956).

[33] *SÖFW*, **83**, 289 (1957) et seq.

[34] *Drug Cosmet. Ind.*, **38**, (March 1936).

[35] Grandel, *Dt. Parfumztg.* 15 (1941); Kaufmann, *Fette Seifen*, **54**, 2 (1952); Schneider and Wagner, *Medsche Klin.*, 456 (1955).

[36] Holmann, *Fette Seifen*, **53**, 6 (1951).

[37] *Drug Cosmet. Ind.*, **38**, (May 1936).

[38] Grimmer, *Zbl. Hautkrkh.*, **2**, 102 (1952).

[39] Rubisz-Brzezinska, *Przegl. derm.*, **51**, 47 (1964), in *Parfum. Kosmet.*, **45**, 264 (1964).

[40] Dodds, *J. Soc. cosmet. Chem.*, **16**, 431 (1965).

[41] Hamilton, *J. invest. Derm.*, **473**, (1942).

[42] Sagarin, *Cosmetics: Science and Technology*, Interscience Publishers, New York 1957, p. 184 et seq.

[42a] Sagarin, *op. cit.*, p. 1238.

[43] *J. Soc. cosmet. Chem.*, **1**, 406 (December 1949).

[44] *Archs. Biochim. Cosm.*, **6**, No. 61, 11 (1963).

[45] *J. invest. Derm.*, **39**, 139 (1962).

[46] Hamilton, *J. clin. Endocr.*, 570 (1941); *J. invest. Derm.* **5**, 473 (1942).

[47] *J. invest. Derm.* **12**, 159 (1949).

[48] Shappiro *J. med. Soc.*, *New Jers.*, **50**, 17 (1953); Rovesti, *Parfums Cosmét. Savons*, **5**, 491 (1962).

[49] *Practitioner*, (March 1950).

[50] Janistyn, *Parfum. Kosmet.* **39**, 16 (1958), U. S. Patent 2,791,534 (1957); Silson, *J. Soc. Cosmet. Chem.*, **13**, 129 (1962).

[51] *Kosmetik-Parf.-Drog.*, **4**, 173 (1957).

[52] *Prakt. Chem.*, Symposium for XI International Convention for Cosmetics, Vienna 1957, p. 71.

[53] Ardin, *Parfum. Kosmet.* **38**, 34 (1957).

[54] Neumann, *SÖFW*, **81**, 473 (1955).

[55] Gerhard, *Kosmetik-Parf.-Drog.*, **3**, 120 (1956); **4**, 29 (1957).

[56] Jankowitz, *Parfum. Kosmet.*, **36**, 243 (1956).

[57] Lodi and Rovesti, Papers read at the 8th Convention for Cosmetics and Beauty Care, Lausanne, 1954 [cf. *Riv. ital. Essenze Profumi;* (September 1954)]; 9th Convention, Baden-Baden 1955 [cf. *Riv. ital. Essenze Profumi* (October 1955)]; 11th Convention, Vienna 1957 (cf. *Sypm. Prakt. Chem.*, p. 69).

[58] *Parfum. Kosmet.*, **39**, 11 (1958).

[59] Cameron and Spector, *Modern Trends in Dermatology*, 2nd Series, London, 1954, p. 57 et seq.

[60] Schmidt, *SÖFW*, **82**, 497 (1956); Kuntscher, *Parfum. Kosmet.* **38**, 197 (1957).

[61] Czetsch-Lindenwald and Schmidt-La Baume, *Die äusseren Heilmittel 1950–1955*, Springer Verlag, 1956, pp. 65–66.

[62] *Drug Cosmet. Ind.*, **92**, 298 (1963).

[63] *Drug Cosmet. Ind.*, **92**, 298 (1963).

[64] Janistyn, *Riechstoffe, Seifen, Kosmetika*, II, p. 147.

[65] Mecca, *Soap Perfum. Cosmet.*, **37**, 33, 129 (1964).

[66a] *Proc. scient. Sect.*, Toilet Goods Ass., **25**, (May 1956).

[66b] *Naturwissenchaften*, **44**, 267 (1957).

[67] Janku and Zita, *Čslká Farm.*, 93 (1954).

[68] Zenesek, Fiser, Krs, Spanlangova, and Paroulkova, *Parfum. Kosmet.*, **46**, 226 (1965); Ruckebusch, *Fette, Seifen, Anstr-mittel*, **65**, 228 (1963).

[69] Fiedler, *Fette Seifen*, **52**, 12 (1950).

[70] *Perfum. essent. Oil Rec.*, **46**, 412 (1955).

[71] Burger and Weitzel, *Medsche Klin.*, 603 (1953).

[72] *Arzneimittel-Forsch.*, **4**, 627 (1954).

[73] Kludas, *Prakt. Chem.*, *op. cit.*, 72; Gohlke, *Parfum. Kosmet.*, **39**, 776 (1958).

[74] Bureau, *Am. Perfumer*, **75** (4), 37 (1960).

[75] *Medsche Kosm.*, **6**, 77 (1957).

[76] *Prakt. Chem*, *op. cit.*, 51.

[77] *Cosmetici, Profumi, Saponi*, **2**, 385 (1961).

[78] *Riv. ital. Essenze Profumi*, **45**, 573 (1963).

[79] *Prakt. Chem.*, *op. cit.*, 3.

[80] Bigi, *Riv. ital. Essenze Profumi*, **45**, 562 (1963).

[81] Galli and Rovesti, *op. cit.*, **45**, 569 (1963).

[82] *Perfum. essent. Oil Rec.*, **48**, 389 (1957).

[83] Neumann, *SÖFW*, **78**, 297, 327 (1952).

[84] Rothemann, *op. cit.*, 231.

[85] *Ibid.*, 27.

[86] *Prakt. Chem.*, *op. cit.*, 18.

[87] Volterra, *Boll. chim.-farm.*, **94**, 265 (1955).

[88] Münch, *Medsche Wschr.*, **97**, 1016 (1955).

[89] *Parfum. mod.*, **46**, 28 (1952); *Industrie Parfum.*, **12**, 305 (1957).

[90] Schmidt, *Parfum. Kosmet.*, **37**, 416 (1956); **38**, 131 (1957); *SÖFW*, **83**, 112 (1957); Kerschbaumer, *J. med. Kosmet.*, 99 (1956).

[91] *Z. phys., Chem.*, 79 (1958).

[92] Krögler, *Prakt. Chem. op. cit.*, 41.

[93] Sterba, Kvicalova, Sasko, and Danielisova, *Parfum Kosmet.*, **45**, 307, (1964).

[94] Second International Symposium Paris 1956; *Industrie Parfum.*, **12**, 42 (1957).

[95]. *SÖFW*, **84**, 16 (1958).

[96] Rothemann, *op. cit.*, 64–92.

[97] *Parfum. Kosmet.*, **46**, 226 (1965).

[98] Czetsch-Lindenwald and Schmidt-La Baume, *op. cit.*, 70 et seq.

[99] *J. Soc. cosmet. Chem.*, **5**, 277 (1951).

[100] Siess, *Parfum. Kosmet.*, **37**, 669 (1956); M. Ainsworth, *J. Soc. cosmet. Chem.*, **11**, 69 (1960).

[101] Miescher, *Dermatologica* (Basel), **83**, 13 (1941).

[102] Flesch, Satanove, and Brown, *J. invest. Derm.*, **25**, 289 (1955); Carson and Goldhamer, *Proc. scient. Sect.*, Toilet Goods Ass., **38**, 48 (1962).

[103] Valette, second International Symposium Paris 1956; *Kosmetik Parf.-Drog.*, **4**, 33 (1957).

[104] Tronnier and Wagener, *Hautarzt*, **4**, No. 5 (1953).

[105] *Brit. J. Derm.*, (March 1941); Harry, *op. cit.*, 85 et seq.

[106] Scott, *Brit. J. Derm.*, **69**, 39 (1957); Kalz and Scott, *Archs. Derm.*, **73**, 355 (1956).

[107] Wilson, *Drug Cosmet. Ind.*, **88**, 444, 521 (1961).

[108] Griesemer, Blank, and Gould, *J. invest. Derm.*, **31**, 225 (1958).

[109] Stoughton, Glendenning, and Kruse, *J. invest. Derm.*, **35**, 357 (1960).

[110] Ainsworth, *J. invest. Derm.*, **35**, 71, 75 (1960).

[111] Rothman, *op. cit.* Chapter 3.

[112] Macht, *J. Am. med. Ass.*, **110**, 408 (1938).

[113] *Proc. scient. Sect.*, Toilet Goods Ass., **38**, 48 (1962).

[114] Strakosch, *Arch. Derm. Syph.*, **47**, 16 (1943).

[115] *J. Am. med. ass.*, **114**, 1865, 2002 (1940).

[116] *Physiol. Rev.*, **26**, 510 (1946).

[117] Lomber and Zuckermann, *J. invest. Derm.*, **16**, 379 (1951).

[118] *Klin. Wsch.*, **16**, 135 (1937).

[119] Valette, *Kosmetik-Parf.-Drog.*, **4**, 33 (1957).

[120] *J. invest. Derm.*, **26**, 149 (1956).

[121] Szczesniak, Sherman, and Harris, *Science*, **113**, 293 (151); Pinson, *Physiol. Rev.*, **32**, 123 (1951).

[122] *J. Am. med. Ass.*, **114**, 1865, 2002 (1940).

[123] *J. med. Kosm.*, **7**, (1953).

[124] Sagarin, *op. cit.*, 1234.

[125] Heald, *Am. Perfumer*, **79**, (8), 23 (1964).

[126] Kumer, *Dermatologische Kosmetik*, p. 58.

[127] Maguire and Kligman, *J. invest. Derm.*, **39**, 469 (1962).

[128] Matson, *Perfum. essent. Rec.*, **47**, 139 (1956); Rihava quoted in *Parfum. Kosmet.* **38**, 220 (1957).

[129] Kirby, *J. invest. Derm.*, **29**, 159 (1957).

[130] Gould, *Perf. essent. Oil Rec.*, **47**, 139 (1956).

[131] *Schimmel Briefs*, **271**, (1958).

[132] Schneider, *SÖFW*, **82**, 493 (1956).

[133] Grover, *J. Am. med. Ass.*, **160**, 1397 (1956).

[134] Gross and C. S. Wright, *Archs. Derm.*, **78**, 92 (1958).

[135] Harry, *op. cit.*, 370 et seq.

[136] *Dt. med. Wschr.*, **46**, 145 (1920).

[137] Jansion and Brigon, *Revue. Sci. Méd.*, **4**, 85 (1951).

[138] *Klin. Wschr.*, **5**, 507 (1926).

[139] *Ibid.*, **7**, 116 (1929).

[140] Rothman, *op. cit.*, 618 et seq.

[141] *Materia medica Nordmark* **9**, 256 (1957); *Parfum. Kosmet.*, **38**, 583 (1957).

[142] *Kosmetik-Parf.-Drog.*, **3**, 120 (1956).

[143] *Dermatologica*, **93**, 31 (1946).

[144] *Proc. scient. Sect.*, Toilet Goods Ass., 40 (December 1952).

[145] *Parfum. Kosmet.*, **36,** 567, 621 (1955).

[146] Goldman and coworkers, *J. Am. med. Ass.*, **132,** 570 (1946); *J. invest. Derm.*, **11,** 323 (1948); *Arch. Derm. Syph.* **63,** 443 (1951).

[147] Flesch in Rothman, *op. cit.*, 601 et seq.

[148] Harry, *op. cit.*, 357.

[149] *Schimmel Briefs*, **315** (June 1961).

# CHAPTER 10

# Decorative Preparations:
# Preparations with Surface Effect

Decorative preparations may also be called "beauty aids," which would be shorter and certainly neater linguistically, but not really exact. After all, most cosmetic products may be regarded as beauty aids. Soaps, for instance, serve beauty directly by removing impurities and indirectly because their regular use prevents the formation of blackheads, pimples, and other blemishes. Hand creams are beauty aids because they prevent the development of rough, chapped, or even red, swollen, or inflamed skin on the hands. Antiwrinkle creams, sunburn preparations, dentifrices, and bust developers as well—all are in a sense beauty aids, even if not as their sole purpose.

On the other hand, cold-wave lotions, shaving soaps, hair lacquers, etc., are not usually called beauty aids, although we may well regard them as decorative preparations.

We include in the group of preparations with decorative action all products whose sole purpose is an alteration of the appearance (the key word here is "sole"). We also include preparations that serve as auxiliaries in purely decorative treatments (hair setting, shaving, etc.).

The maintenance or promotion of skin health was the main purpose of all products discussed thus far: cleansing, protective, emollient, and those with depth effect (with the exception of body deodorants, which in a sense are also decorative). Decorative preparations, however, relate to the health of the skin only to the extent that they must damage it as little as possible. From the point of view of skin health their use is hardly warranted; they are applied for psychological reasons. Decorative preparations are used to hide small blemishes or symptoms of aging; they are also used to create a well-groomed appearance and to demonstrate the desire not to create a bad impression on the outside world. These forms of decoration are dictated by man's herd instinct. Decorative cosmetics are also used to attract the other sex

414

and—indirectly—to imply that one would like to be noticed. The motive is always psychological: the impression to be made on others.

It is advisable to realize clearly that cosmetics have two basic principles, two roots: one dealing with the health of the skin, the other with the impression to be made on the outside world. Both motives are inherent characteristics of cosmetics, and even if some members of the medical profession scoff at the psychological side it will always, rightly or wrongly, be of outstanding importance to the consumer. Manufacturers of cosmetic preparations should always endeavor to present their skin-care products as "decoratively" as possible (pleasantly fragrant, nontacky, and nonshiny) and to make them at least harmless to skin and hair. Cosmetic decoration may consist in *surface* measures, in which the preparation is applied only to the surface of skin, nails, or hair, or in *permanent* measures that cannot be canceled by simple countermeasures. We discuss the preparations that serve as auxiliaries to surface measures in this chapter and permanent treatments in Chapter 11.


## PREPARATIONS FOR COLORING SKIN AND NAILS

Poets and satirists since time immemorial have derided women's tendency to color their hair, cheeks, lips, nails, lids, and lashes. With the same perseverance women have followed their inclination down through the ages. They must have their own very good reasons.

On examining these reasons we soon find a number of motives. Signs of aging should be hidden, graying hair dyed. The total effect should be striking (and thus attract men's attention): the color of the lips is heightened, nails are lacquered, lashes made to look darker than they are by nature, and the hair, if it is "mousy," is given a more striking color. The best features of the face are to be stressed: mascara and eye shadow accentuate the eyes, lipstick, the mouth.

Cosmetics can serve both the urge to belong (within given groups of society in any one period most women use more or less the same type of adornment; in other periods, in other groups, quite different standards prevail) and the wish to be noticed and attract a mate. It is an interesting point that we cannot draw a definite line between the two; much depends on the social environment. In a European village community, for example, a woman would be noticed even if she used only a little lipstick; in urban life lipstick is a part of being well groomed and a woman would be more likely to attract attention by its absence.

The main active ingredients in all coloring preparations are, of course, dyes. We therefore discuss them first before dealing with the individual preparations in this group.

## Coloring Agents in Cosmetics

Coloring materials in cosmetic products must meet the following requirements: They must provide the desired tone and intensity. It is an advantage if the coloring effect is strong so that the desired result can be achieved with the smallest possible amount of dye.

Tone and intensity should be as stable as possible in the preparation. According to Cole and de Navarre [1], fading may be caused by excessive sunlight, heat, oxidation, reduction, hydrolysis and microorganisms. The selection of the coloring must always depend on the conditions prevailing in the preparation (pH, redox potential). The materials should be commercially available in uniform quality and should not be too highly priced. These considerations have led to the ever-increasing replacement of natural dyes by synthetics.

Even if the preparation is used frequently over long periods of time, the coloring agents must not irritate the skin or cause symptoms of toxicity. A number of synthetic dyes belong to classes of materials in which some representatives are toxic, irritating, or carcinogenic. In many countries the use of dyes is subject to strict laws, and official lists of permissible products are published by the authorities.

Skin compatibility not only depends on the composition of the dyes but also on their degree of purity, and symptoms of incompatibility are often caused not by the dyes themselves but by small amounts of impurities they contain. Sulzberger and Hecht [2] cite a number of examples.

Although it is not possible to exclude all dyes that might lead to allergic reactions, since these reactions are inherently unpredictable, some substances give rise to symptoms of allergy only very rarely indeed and others rather more frequently. Certain dyes belong to the latter group: phenylene diamine dyes on which most modern hair coloring is based and eosine derivatives which are widely used in lipsticks and nail lacquers. These substances are not "caustic" and are easily tolerated by most people and their use is therefore permitted by law. Certain allergic reactions, particularly from hair dyes, are sufficienty frequent, however, for E. Sidi, a leading French dermatologist, to recommend patch tests on individual customers before every hair-dying job [3]. In France these preliminary tests are now required by law.

Two types of coloring agent are used in cosmetics: the soluble dyes (soluble in alcohol, water, or oil), and the insoluble pigments and lacquers. Both groups can be subdivided into synthetic and natural products.

**1. Natural Soluble Dyes.** Nowadays these dyes are used comparatively rarely in cosmetics. They may be more skin compatible than synthetic dyes (i.e., they cause fewer allergic reactions) but their coloring power is relatively weak, their light resistance not very good, and they are considerably more expensive in application. The most widely used are probably alkannin, a red dye extracted from the bark of the alkanna root (*radix alcannae*); carmine, a red dyestuff obtained from the dried bodies of the insect *coccus cacti:* and chlorophyll, the green coloring agent of leaves, also commercially available in the form of various derivatives, both oil- and water-soluble;

Henna, an extract of the leaves of *lawsonia inermis*, is used by itself or mixed with "reng," the powered leaves of *indigofera argentea*, as a hair dye (golden, red, brown, and black).

Carotene, a yellow vegetable dye, has repeatedly been suggested for use in cosmetics, but it is probably more suitable as an active ingredient in conjunction with vitamin A than as a dyestuff: it fades in light and strongly colors the skin.

**2. Synthetic Soluble Dyes.**   The first synthetic dyes were synthesized from aniline; at present benzene, toluene, anthracene, and other coal-tar isolates serve as starting products for most synthetic dyes. For this reason dyes in this group are designated as "aniline" or "coal-tar" dyestuffs. More than 1000 coal-tar dyes are known today. Only a few of them, however, can be considered for use in cosmetics.

In addition to shade and intensity, cosmetic chemists are interested in the following properties of synthetic dyes:

*Solubility.*   Depending on the preparation in which it is to be used, the dye must be soluble in water, alcohol, or oil. (For the coloring of emulsions the dye must be soluble in the outer phase: water-soluble for O/W, oil-soluble for W/O emulsions). Water-soluble dyes are almost always soluble in dilute alcohol, glycerol, and glycols; oil-soluble dyes are also soluble in benzene, carbon tetrachloride, and other organic solvents and occasionally in high-grade alcohol. No dye is ever both oil- and water-soluble.

*pH-Related Properties.*   Some dyes are soluble only in an acidic environment, others only in alkaline; some develop the desired shade within a definite pH range or are unstable in an acidic or an alkaline medium.

*Affinity to Skin or Hair.*   Dyestuffs differ considerably in their adhesion to the skin or hair. In certain applications such adhesion should be avoided as much as possible (e.g., in soaps); in others (e.g., "kissproof" lipsticks) adhesion is required to be as strong as possible. In hair dyes in which a lasting effect is required a special indirect dyeing method is used.

Generally speaking, the skin affinity of water-soluble dyes is more or less strong; that of oil-soluble dyes, rather slight.

*Toxicity.*   Dyes that are a hazard to health obviously must not be used at all in cosmetics, but there are differences in the "degree of harmlessness," even for permissible dyes. American law distinguishes between three classes of cosmetic dyestuff: those that are admitted for use in all food as well as all cosmetic preparations (F. D. & C.), those admitted for use in cosmetics only (D & C), and those that may be used in cosmetic products only for external application [i.e., not in preparations coming in contact with the lips or other mucous membrane. (Ext. D & C)]. According to United States law, no coal-tar dyes must be used in any preparations for use around the eyes. In addition, chemical and physical properties, as well as the admissible maximum content of lead, arsenic, and other impurities, are prescribed for each dyestuff.

As an illustration, we list some of the properties of various synthetic dyestuffs in Table 10-1.

TABLE 10-1   PROPERTIES OF SOME SYNTHETIC SOLUBLE DYESTUFFS

| Commercial Description | Color in Solution | Solubility | | | Resistance | | | Group |
|---|---|---|---|---|---|---|---|---|
| | | $H_2O$ | Eth | Oil | Lt | Alk | Ac | |
| Naphthol blue-black | Blue-black | S | SS | I | G | G | M | D & C |
| Indigotin | Light blue | S | S | I | M | M | P | D & C |
| Quinizarin green SS | Blue-green | I | SS | SS | M | G | G | D & C |
| Orange I | Red-orange | S | SS | I | M | M | P | F D & C |
| Amaranth | Purple | S | SS | I | G | G | G | F D  C |
| Erythrosin J | Cherry red | S | S | I | P | G | P | F D & C |
| Azoburin extra | Purple | S | SS | I | G | B | M | Ext. D & C |
| Oil red XO | Red | I | SS | S | M | M | M | F D & C |
| Tartrazine | Golden yellow | S | SS | I | G | G | G | F D & C |
| Yellow AB | Orange yellow | I | SS | S | IP | IM | IP | F D & C |

*Solubility.* $H_2O$ = water. "Eth" = 95% ethyl alcohol. S = soluble. SS = slightly soluble. I = almost insoluble.

*Resistance.* Lt = light. Alk = alkali. Ac = acid. G = good. M = moderate. P = poor. The additional letter "I" stands for insolubility in acid or alkaline aqueous solution.

**3. Natural Pigments.** These are naturally occurring earths (aluminum silicates) whose color depends mostly on the content of hydrated iron or manganese oxides [e.g., yellow ochre, Terra di Siena (brown), red bolus (brick red), umber (dark brown)]. These colors are completely harmless, provided they are pure. They play an important part in the coloring of powders, make-up sticks, and creams. Their color—as all properties of natural products—is not completely uniform and fluctuates according to the origin of the material. Strong heating of the earth colors (burning) yields pigments with new shades (burnt sienna, etc.).

**4. Synthetic Pigments.**   Today, synthetic iron oxides and synthetic ochres frequently replace natural earth colors. Their hues are more intense and brighter. There is a choice of various yellow, brown-to-red, and violet shades. White synthetic pigments such as zinc oxide and titanium dioxide belong to the most important cosmetic coloring agents. Zinc oxide, in particular, not only plays a major part in decorative products but also in many other cosmetic and pharmaceutical preparations. Occasionally bismuth carbonate is also used as a white pigment, while bismuth oxychloride is commonly used for pearly shades.

Some cobalt compounds are used as blue synthetic pigments; in particular, cobalt and ultramarine. Cobalt green is a bluish-green pigment.

Some coal-tar dyes are also classified among the synthetic pigments; they have low solubility in water, alcohol, and oil and are therefore used in finely dispersed solid form. One of the important representatives of this group is indanthrene blue.

Many synthetic pigments (e.g., cadmium sulfide and Prussian blue) are ruled out for cosmetic preparations because of their toxicity.

**5. Natural and Synthetic Lakes.**   Lakes are prepared by precipitating one or more water-soluble dyes on one or more insoluble substrates and fixing them in such a way (usually by chemical reaction) that the end product becomes a coloring agent almost insoluble in water, oil, or other solvents.

Most lakes used today are prepared from synthetic dyes. An exception is "Florentine lake," which is obtained from a precipitation of carmine and brasilin (a red vegetable dye) on aluminum hydroxide. In a similar manner a lake is prepared from alizarin red, a synthetic dye.

Lakes prepared from coal-tar dyes are the most important coloring agents in powders, lipsticks, and makeup. Brighter and deeper shades can be obtained with them than with pigments; they are also more colorfast than most of the soluble dyes and have good skin compatibility. When they are dry, they should be soft and friable.

The soluble dye or dyes used in the preparation of a lake determine its shade and intensity, the substrate, its covering effect. The most common substrates are zinc oxide, titanium dioxide, aluminum hydroxide, aluminum phosphate, barium phosphate, barium sulfate (some authors object to barium salts in cosmetics because of the toxicity of soluble barium salts), magnesium carbonate, alumina hydrates, and kaolin. Pigments such as zinc oxide and titanium dioxide have a much higher covering power than "neutral" substances such as aluminum hydroxide. The precipitation agent for acid dyes is barium chloride in presence of aluminum and/or potassium salts. Tannic acid is often used for alkaline dyes. Some alkaline dyes even precipitate without special precipitating agents on substrates containing silicic acids.

A slightly different type of lake is formed by a chemical reaction between a colorless soluble substance and an equally colorless insoluble compound, which results in an insoluble dyestuff characterized by extreme light fastness.

It is impossible within the framework of this book to give a complete or even approximately complete list of coloring agents suitable to cosmetics. The number of such substances is increasing steadily, and manufacturers of dyestuffs will be able to provide the necessary information.

## Rouges [3]

The purpose of these products is to simulate the natural reddening of the cheeks. They are occasionally applied directly to the skin, but more often on a makeup foundation. Over the years rouges have been marketed in various forms: as loose or compact powders, fat-based makeup, liquid or cream emulsions, clear liquids, or gels.

**Loose and Compact Powder Rouges.** These preparations are the simplest. They contain pigments and lakes in dry form, "diluted" with standard powder materials: for example, talcum, zinc stearate, and magnesium carbonate. According to the intensity of the pigment and the required coloring effect of the powder, the pigment content is usually 5 and 20% of the powder mass. Pigments are often wholly or partly replaced by lakes, which have a more intense color effect and may be used in much smaller quantities. Janistyn [4] lists the pigments and lakes required to obtain standard shades. In addition to insoluble coloring agents, rouges also sometimes contain water-soluble dyes. Whereas insoluble agents remain on the skin, soluble ones, in the presence of some perspiration, stain the skin tissue itself. Very strong or permanent staining is certainly undesirable.

A rouge without dye is described in German patent 1,012,729 (Wella AG, 1958). The active ingredient is nicotinic acid benzyl ester which causes hyperemea on the powdered skin area (i.e., an absolutely natural blush!) which lasts for a few hours. The powder base is tetrastearoxysilane.

Compact rouges are more popular than loose powders because they have two advantages: first, they dust less on application. Dusting is particularly undesirable in the case of rouges because their strong colors might easily stain the clothing. Second, the presence of binders makes compact rouges adhere better to the skin. We do not need to discuss the formulation and preparation of these products in detail because they are the same as those of loose and compact powders, although with much higher pigment content.

**Anhydrous Cream Rouges.** In these preparations the colors (pigments, lakes and/or oil-soluble dyes) are dispersed or dissolved in a fat-oil-wax base.

Compared with powders, anhydrous cream rouges have the advantage of forming a continuous film on the skin which appears more natural than loose powder and, in addition, is water-repellent so that the risk of perspiration making the makeup run is eliminated. The melting point of the vehicle should not be below 40°C and is often 60°C or even higher. Occasionally, these rouges are formulated as thixotropic preparations: they are solid in the container but immediately liquefy under pressure and spread easily. To obtain a thixotropic mass, high melting waxes are required to form the "skeleton," oils to fill it, and microcrystalline waxes or amorphous substances to prevent the sweating of the oils (see Chapter 4).

| | 1 | 2 | 3 | 4 | 5 | 6 |
|---|---|---|---|---|---|---|
| Ceresine | 18 | | 37.5 | 32.5 | | |
| Carnauba wax | 1 | | | | | |
| Beeswax | 7 | 15 | | | | |
| Spermaceti | 4 | | | | | 12.5 |
| Petrolatum, short fiber | 25 | 4 | | 13.5 | 40 | 11.8 |
| Castor oil, semihydrogenated | | 55 | | | | |
| Paraffin oil | 16.5 | 10 | 37.5 | 32.5 | | 37.5 |
| Isopropyl myristate | | | | | 34.5 | |
| Isopropyl palmitate | 20 | | | | | |
| Lanolin, light | | 4 | | | 5 | 16.7 |
| Adeps lanae, anhydrous | | | | | | 4.2 |
| Cholesterol CP | | | | | | 0.38 |
| Cetyl alcohol | | | 4.7 | | | 0.38 |
| Eutanol G | | | | | | 4.2 |
| Glyceryl monostearate | | | | | 12 | |
| Stearic acid | | | | 16 | | 4.2 |
| Lake | 8 | 10 | 6.1 | 5.5 | 8 | 4.5 |
| Titanium dioxide | | | | | | 1.32 |
| Eosine dyes | | | | | | 1.32 |
| Perfume | 0.5 | | 0.2 | | 0.5 | 1.0 |

REMARKS

1. Keithler, *The Formulation of Cosmetics and Cosmetic Specialities*, Drug and Cosmetic Ind., 1957, p. 166. Mix and grind the lakes together. Mix fats, oils, and waxes and heat to just above the melting point of the highest melting wax. Stir pigments into the melt and grind the mixture a few times on a heated roller mill; add perfume toward the end of the process.

2. Janistyn, *Riechstoffe, Seifen, Kosmetika*, II, Hüthig Verlag, Heidelberg, 1950, p. 245. Grind the pigments thoroughly with paraffin oil and mix the paste with melt of the remaining fats. Add soluble dyes, if any. Homogenize the mass, remelt cautiously, perfume, and fill into containers.

3. Winter, *Handbuch der gesamten Parfümerie u. Kosmetik*, 3rd ed., 1940, p. 555.

4. Janistyn, *op. cit.*, p. 245. According to Turabian. Procedure similar to formula 2.

5. Keithler, *op. cit.*, p. 167. Proceed as for formula 1.

6. Rothemann, *Das grosse Rezeptbuch der Haut- und Körperpflegemittel*, 3rd ed. Hüthig Verlag, Heidelberg, 1962, p. 695. Melt the fats, with the exception of lanolin, in a water bath at a temperature as low as possible (certainly below 80°C). Add the pigments to the melt (Rothemann prescribes 4.2–5%). Stir into the hot mass 25 ml 95% alcohol per kilo mass and immediately afterward stir in the eosine colors in small portions (0.83–2.08%). Add the finely ground titanium dioxide (0.83–2.08%) and stir thoroughly. Add perfume oil (rose type) and finally lanolin. The mass is then filtered through a fine cloth (muslin or batiste), homogenized twice in a pigment grinder or roller mill, and stirred again until completely cool.

**Emulsified Cream and Liquid Rouges.** The popularity of this type (in particular, the liquid emulsions) is due to the equally great popularity of liquid foundation makeup. Liquid powders and liquid rouges blend well, and with some practice the user can achieve very nice effects by applying liquid rouge on the still liquid foundation. From a dermatological point of view, however, these preparations are not quite so beneficial: in the presence of wetting and emulsifying agents solid dye particles easily penetrate hair follicles and possible small fissures in the skin and, if they are not soon removed, may cause an irritation. If preparations of this type are used, careful cleansing of the skin, preferably with cream, is essential. Solid as well as liquid cream rouges are complicated in composition and resemble corresponding powder creams to a large extent [5]. For a detailed discussion the reader is referred to the section on solid and liquid foundation makeup.

The great difference between rouges and powders is the color content. In addition to colored lakes and pigments, white pigments, which affect the covering power as well as the shade, are also used in rouges. Water-soluble dyes are often used to support the effect of the rouge by staining the skin. They also have a secondary purpose in liquid emulsified rouges: even if pigments settle on the bottom of the product, the supernatant liquid will not be colorless.

Insoluble pigments must, of course, be as finely dispersed as possible and should preferably be ground together after mixing to make the blend uniform. It is important to control the shade of the dry color mix because of the difficulty of adjusting it in the end product.

A few formulas for cream rouges from the literature follow.

|  | 7 | 8 | 9 |
|---|---|---|---|
| Petrolatum, white, short fiber | 30 | 20 | |
| Paraffin oil, prime grade | 16 | | |
| Isopropyl myristate | | 30 | |
| Beeswax | | 14 | |
| Lanoline, anhydrous | 2 | | |
| Cetyl alcohol | | 3 | |
| Glycerol monostearate SE | | | 4 |
| Stearic acid | | | 16 |
| Sorbitan sesquioleate (Arlacel C) | 2 | | |
| Triethanolamine lauryl sulfate | | 0.4 | |
| Borax | | 1.0 | |
| Triethanolamine | | | 0.50 |
| Distilled water | 35 | 20.95 | 67.85 |
| Glycerol, white | 5 | | |
| Propylene glycol | | 2 | |
| Sorbitol liquid | | | 2 |
| Lake | 6 | 8.0 | 8 |
| Eosine acid | 1 | | |
| Perfume | 0.5 | 0.4 | 0.5 |
| Preservative | | 0.15 | |

REMARKS

7. Water-in-oil type. Rothemann, *Das grosse Rezeptbuch der Haut- und Körperpflege-mittel*, 3rd ed., p. 697. Melt Arlacel, lanolin, paraffin oil, and petrolatum together in a water bath and heat to 90°C. Stir in the glycerol-water mixture (95°C) and add the dyes with careful stirring. Add perfume, homogenize the mixture in a three-roller mill, and fill at 45°C.

8. Dual emulsion (cold-cream type). Keithler, *The Formulation of Cosmetics and Cosmetic Specialties*, p. 170. Stir lakes and isopropyl myristate into a paste and grind. Add the aqueous phase (water, propylene glycol, "tri" lauryl sulfate, borax, and preservative) at 70°C to the oil phase (petrolatum, beeswax, and cetyl alcohol, 70°C), stirring slowly. Continue stirring for about 10 minutes and then stir thoroughly into the color paste. Grind the warm product, add perfume, and stir slowly to 50°C.

9. Oil-in-water (vanishing-cream type). Keithler, *op. cit.*, p. 168. Lakes and sorbitol liquid are mixed together and ground. Stir the aqueous phase (water and triethanolamine, 75°C) into the wax-oil phase (glycerol monostearate, stearic acid, lanolin, and preservative, 75°C). Continue stirring until the mass starts thickening at about 60°C. Stir in the pigment paste and continue stirring until cool.

**Liquid Rouges.**    These preparations consist of aqueous or hydroalcoholic color solutions. The colors selected must be highly substantive to the skin. Glycerol, sorbitol liquid, etc., give them a softer feeling during application but should be used in limited amounts because they would unduly delay drying on the skin. Gums, or mucins, impart the kind of consistency that facilitates spreading.

Here is a simple formulation as an example (Janistyn, *Riechstoffe, Seifen, Kosmetika*, II,

| | | |
|---|---|---|
| 10. | Erythrosine, 100% pure | 0.5 |
| | Propylene glycol | 20 |
| | Ethyl alcohol | 10 |
| | Rose water | 69.5 |
| | | 100 |

## Eye Shadow [6]

The purpose of these preparations is to accentuate the eyes and to make their whites look brighter. They are applied to the skin in proximity to the eyes, usually over the lids. The shades range from gray-blue to gray-green to olive green. Metal powders are occasionally incorporated (bronze, aluminum, gold) to achieve a metallic sheen.

Eyeshadow belongs to the "extreme" wing of decorative preparations. From the point of view of health the application of preparations with a high content of pigments in proximity to the eyes is hardly advisable. American regulations for dyes used in these preparations are stricter than for other cosmetic applications. Use of these preparations hardly falls in the category of "good grooming." When a woman uses eyeshadow she wants to be noticed.

The use of eyeshadow is neither new nor typical of our modern way of life. Elegant ladies in Egypt used it 4500 years ago! Some suggested formulations follow on page 425.

REMARKS

11. Harry, *Modern Cosmetocology*, 4th ed., Leonard Hill, London, 1955, p. 231.

12. Keithler, *The Formulation of Cosmetics and Cosmetic Specialties*, p. 176. Mix the dyes with half the petrolatum. Stir this color paste into the melt of the remaining fats. If required, the completed mass may once again be milled to guarantee uniform dispersion of the pigments.

13. Rothemann, *Das grosse Rezeptbuch der Haut- und Körperpflegemittel*, 3rd ed., p. 699. Mix the pigments with Eutanol or Satol. Eutanol G (Dehydag, Duesseldorf) is a mixture of saturated fatty alcohols; Satol (L. Givaudan & Cie) is an unsaturated, non-saponifiable, neutral, colorless, and odorless oily material of vegetable origin. Melt the remaining fats (75°C) and add water (80°) in a thin jet. (Rothemann prescribes rose water, triple.) Add the pigment paste, then the perfume. Continue stirring until cool.

|                            | 11   | 12  | 13   |
|----------------------------|------|-----|------|
| Petrolatum, white, viscous | 55   | 40  | 15.5 |
| Beeswax                    | 3    | 9   |      |
| Spermaceti                 | 5    |     |      |
| Cocoa butter, oderless     | 2    |     |      |
| Lanolin                    | 5    |     |      |
| Isolan                     |      | 15  |      |
| Cholesterol, purified      |      |     | 0.14 |
| Cetyl alcohol              |      |     | 2.4  |
| Eutanol G                  |      |     | 9.0  |
| Isopropyl myristate        |      | 4   |      |
| Glyceryl monostearate      |      | 20  |      |
| Triethanolamine stearate   |      |     | 18.0 |
| Lake                       | q.s. | 8   | 3.6  |
| Zinc oxide                 | 30   |     |      |
| Titanium dioxide           |      |     | 9.0  |
| Oil-soluble color          |      |     | 0.9  |
| Water                      |      |     | 49.2 |
| Preservative               | q.s. |     |      |
| Perfume                    |      |     | 0.36 |

## Mascara [6]

The use of mascara is less noticeable than that of eyeshadow and, at least in Europe, more extensive. Mascara is intended to darken lashes and occasionally eyebrows. It has the same purpose as eyeshadow: to accentuate the eyes. Mascara is really a hair dye and ought to be discussed in Chapter 11, but since their effect is so closely related to that of eyeshadow we discuss mascara and eyebrow preparations here. Mascara is available in various forms.

**Cake Mascara.**  Preparations of this type consist of a mixture of color, fats and waxes, and oil-in-water emulsifying agents. Potassium and sodium soaps, which were once used as emulsifiers, cause irritations of the eye. At present triethanolamine stearate is most commonly used.

These preparations are applied with a moistened brush, the water causes the formation of an oil-in-water emulsion on the surface of the mascara cake which is picked up by the brush. It then dries on the lashes. The manufacture of a good cake mascara is complicated and requires special equipment; it is hardly worthwhile for small-scale production.

| | 14 | 15 | 16 | 17 |
|---|---|---|---|---|
| Carnauba wax No. 1 yellow | | 15 | | |
| Paraffin wax | | | 15 | |
| Beeswax | | 5 | | 18 |
| Castor oil, first pressing | 1.7 | | | |
| Adeps lanae, anhydrous | | 10 | | |
| Lanolin | | | 8 | |
| Glyceryl monostearate SE | 3.3 | 5 | 60 | 9 |
| Stearic acid, prime grade | 64 | | | 14 |
| Oleic acid | | | | 3 |
| Triethanolamine stearate | | 45 | | |
| Triethanolamine | 27.7 | | | |
| Triisopropanolamine | | | | 4 |
| Nigrosine, 100% pure | 3.3 | | | |
| Lampblack | | 20 | 10 | 7 |
| Ultramarine | | | | 2 |
| Carboxymethylcellulose, high viscosity | | | | 1.5 |
| Water | | | | 38.5 |
| Ethyl alcohol | | | | 3 |

REMARKS

14. Rothemann, *Das grosse Rezeptbuch der Haut- und Körperpflegemittel*, 3rd ed., p. 702. Melt nigrosine (a black aniline dye; specially purified grades are suitable for mascara) in stearic acid at 75°C. Stir in triethanolamine (75°C) in a thin jet until the mass has saponified. Add castor oil and glyceryl monostearate SE.

15. Rothemann, *op. cit.*, p. 704. Grind lampblack with heated lanolin as fine as possible and add this mixture to the other melted fats. Homogenize the completed mass and fill.

16. *Drug Cosm. Ind.*, **51**, 469 (1942).

17. Keithler, *The Formulation of Cosmetics and Cosmetic Specialties*, p. 173. Wet CMC with alcohol, pour over hot water (80°C), and stir until a smooth mucilage forms. Add amine and pour the mixture into the fat melt. Stir until the mass is smooth and add the dyes. Grind the mass, fill the molds, and cool.

**Cream Mascara (anhydrous).** The composition of these preparations is similar to that of cream rouges;

| 18. | | |
|---|---|---|
| | Bees wax | 4 |
| | Spermaceti | 4 |
| | Cetyl alcohol | 2 |
| | Cocoa butter | 6 |
| | Petrolatum, short fiber | 64 |
| | Oil soluble dye (blue) | 20 |
| | Antioxidants and preservative | q.s. |

In Harry, *Modern Cosmetocology*, 4th ed. p. 229.

**Cream Mascara (emulsified).**   Here the base is usually an oil-in-water cream of the stearate or glyceryl monostearate type. The formulation in Keithler's *The Formulation of Cosmetics and Cosmetic Specialties* (p. 17) is different:

| 19. | | |
|---|---|---|
| Stearyl alcohol | 15 |
| Lanolin | 3 |
| Polyethylene glycol 400 distearate | 10 |
| Diglycol stearate | 8 |
| Triethanolamine lauryl sulfate | 1.5 |
| Dye | 8 |
| Water | 54.5 |
| | 100.0 |

Heat all ingredients, with the exception of the dye, to 90°C. Stir until a smooth emulsion has formed. Stir in the dye, homogenize, and cool.

**Liquid Mascara.**   Formulations based on aqueous mucilages of gum tragacanth, quince seed, and other mucins have been published for liquid mascara. They are not very useful, however, since they are more or less water-soluble and can easily be smudged by perspiration or tears.

Mascara based on alcohol containing rosin or other resins or ethyl cellulose form a kind of lacquer on the lashes. This kind of coating has good water resistance, but alcohol-based products have an irritating effect if they happen to get into the eyes.

Some liquid mascara is based on oil:

| 20. | | |
|---|---|---|
| Castor oil | 87 |
| Span 80 (Atlas Chemical Co.) | 4 |
| Lampblack | 9 |

Keithler, *op. cit.*, p. 175. This product does not dry quickly and has a certain glossy effect.

### Eyebrow Pencils and Crayons

The thickness and shape of the eyebrows affect the total impression of the face and at various periods women have more or less drastically changed these features. The desired shape is obtained by total or partial plucking and re-drawing according to taste with an eyebrow pencil or crayon. Mascara is sometimes used for darkening eyebrows. Crayons are hardened creams.

This can be seen from the following formulation (Rothemann, *Das grosse Rezeptbuch der Haut- und Körperpflegemittel*, 3rd ed., p. 704):

| 21. | Ozokerite, white refined, free from paraffin wax (M.P. 70–75°C) | 45 |
| | Beeswax, natural yellow | 22 |
| | Cocoa butter | 21 |
| | Petrolatum (white, viscous, free of acid, odorless) | 5.64 |
| | Paraffin oil, prime grade | 5 |
| | Satol (Givaudan) | 1 |
| | Cholesterol, pure | 0.18 |
| | Cetyl alcohol | 0.18 |
| | Lampblack | 10 |
| | Oil-soluble black or brown dye | q.s. |

Dissolve the oil-soluble dye in Satol or perfume oil by heating and then stir into the remaining melted fats. Lampblack or another black or brown covering color should finally be stirred into the hot liquid mass. Homogenize with a pigment grinder and fill into molds.

The manufacture of eyebrow pencils requires specialized technology and equipment which is the same as that for lead pencils. It is consequently hardly worth the cosmetic chemist's time to work on such products.

According to Keithler, *The Formulation of Cosmetics and Cosmetic Specialties*, p. 177, the composition of "leads" for eyebrow pencils is something like this:

| 22. | Paraffin wax | 29 |
| | Carnauba wax | 5 |
| | Beeswax | 21 |
| | Petrolatum, viscous | 21 |
| | Lanolin | 9 |
| | Cetyl alcohol | 8 |
| | Color | 10 |

## Lip Makeup

Skin on the lips is characterized by an exceptionally thin corneal layer. The *stratum germinativum* is strongly developed and the corium pushes papillae with a high blood content just below the surface. There are no sweat glands on the lips but salivary glands occur on the inner surface. Saliva keeps the lips moist. Since sebaceous glands are very sparse, the lips are almost entirely free from fat, and in cold or dry weather the corneal layer tends to dry out.

Since the corneal layer of the lips is so thin and, moreover, often cracked when dry, alien substances applied on the lips can quite easily penetrate to the *stratum germinativum*. This is of great importance to the cosmetic chemist.

It is generally known that many pigments and eosine dyes have a drying effect on the lips. Possibly they actually bind the water or the moisture-retaining substances of the labial corneal layer. In our opinion it is more probable that dyes irritate the *stratum germinativum* and initiate abnormal keratinization. The corneal layer thus formed is then erroneously called "dry."

**Lipsticks.**   An expert stated recently that there is only one way of increasing the use of lipsticks in the United States: an increase in the population. The market is not quite so saturated in other countries, but lipsticks are generally among the most widely used cosmetic products. They certainly lead in sales of decorative preparations.

Lipsticks also occupy a special position because of their composition and physical structure: they belong to the most complicated cosmetic products. Not much is known so far about the microstructure of the lipstick mass, the way in which crystalline and amorphous waxes, oils, fatty alcohols, and pigments are dispersed. Hence it is also difficult and even impossible to predetermine the behavior of a lipstick developed according to a new formula; slight shifts in the proportion of the ingredients or replacement of one by another that is similar (e.g., cetyl alcohol by stearyl alcohol) may cause completely unexpected changes in its structure and properties. Even experienced chemists are often faced with surprises. Great progress in lipstick technology will have been made once their microstructure is better understood.

**Requirements of the Consumer.**   The many requirements laid down by the consumer are not only widely divergent but often contradictory. These requirements refer to appearance and consistency of the lipstick itself, its behavior during application, and the properties of the film it deposits on the lips.

To begin with the film, it should cover the lips adequately, have some gloss, and last as long as possible. If the film is too soft and not very water-resistant, it soon rubs off at the points of contact of the lips, although it remains around the edges and in the fine creases. The result is an uneven and unattractive coating. In addition, a film that is too soft leaves undesirable traces on cups, linen and cigarettes. The film therefore must adhere firmly to the lips but must be neither brittle nor tacky. General wearing off can hardly be avoided, but during this process the color of the lips must remain unchanged.

Lipsticks should make the lips soft and certainly not dry them out. They must, of course, also be nonirritating and taste and fragrance must be pleasant. Consumers also require certain characteristics in application: this should be easy and without friction and color should be transmitted on slight pressure. The mass must not be too soft, however, because during application it must neither crumble nor lose its shape. Behavior during application must not depend on the prevailing room temperature. Finally the appearance of the product itself must be taken into account; even though, rationally speaking, this may be completely irrelevant, provided the product fulfills its purpose, the consumer is also highly critical in this respect. If a lipstick is dull and unattractive, shows particles or small punctures on its surface, exudes oil droplets, or exhibits a whitish coating, it will not sell, no matter how many good qualities it may otherwise have.

**Composition.** Coloring agents are the active ingredients in lipsticks. Modern lipsticks contain lakes as well as pigments that remain finely dispersed *on* the lips and soluble dyes that actually stain the skin. The coloring agents are incorporated in a base, the composition of which is dictated by the consumer's requirements and by the necessity that it dissolve the dyes contained in the formulation.

The second requirement is not easy to meet. It follows from the chemical composition of skin keratin (see Chapter 1) that substances intended to adhere firmly to it must contain polar groups. Substances rich in polar groups usually dissolve easily in water and alcohol but not so easily in fats or oils. We find that the same is true of dyes: those that color the skin tissue are almost always water- and alcohol-soluble but not oil-soluble; but oil-soluble dyes are essential for lipstick. We cannot use water, alcohol, or other polar solvents here or the need for a water-resistant film would not be met!

There is only one group of red dyes that comes close to meeting the twin requirements of skin affinity and oil solubility: the eosines that are universally used in lipsticks.

Wilmsmann [7] reported that free sulfonic acids of a number of azo dyes suitable for food and drugs are also well suited to lipsticks. They are adsorbed on the skin of the lips, are sufficiently soluble in 1,2-propylene glycol, isopropyl myristate, castor oil, and waxes, and yield color that cannot be obtained with eosine dyes.

Eosine dyes are not perfect, however, for they dissolve poorly in most oils and fats. The best solvent for eosine is castor oil in which the dyes are soluble at about 1%. Castor oil is still used in many lipsticks, although recent years have seen the discovery of other suitable solvents with higher solvency for eosine dyes. The most important among them are furfuryl alcohol (dissolves about 22% by weight of eosine dyes) and its esters, in particular, stearate and ricinoleate, which dissolve up to 26% dyes, and polyethylene glycols, which dissolve about 10–12% of eosine. These gycols have the disadvantage of being water-soluble. Ethers and esters of polyethylene glycols as well as polypropylene glycols have a higher water resistance and are also reported to be good solvents for eosine dyes. Some esters of sebacic acid are good solvents for eosines.

**Fatty acid alkylolamides** [8] have a lesser solvent capacity for eosine dyes than those mentioned above, but this is compensated for by the fact that certain alkylolamides, when used as vehicles for dyes, leave a highly intensive color on the skin (the intensity of coloring depends not only on the dyestuff concentration but on the solvent used).

Consumer demands that lipsticks be firm enough to retain their shape yet be applied without too much friction can be met in two ways: either by formulating lipsticks that are hard at room temperature but quickly melt at body temperature (cocoa butter shows this quality to a large extent and has therefore been much used in lipstick formulas) or by making the lipsticks thixotropic so that they liquefy on the surface under the pressure generated during application. On closer examination it is obvious that a lipstick that melts at body temperature is not suitable because it leaves a liquid or very soft film on the lips and soon wears off. A high melting thixotropic lipstick is therefore the only satisfactory solution. All modern lipsticks are actually formulated on this principle. They contain macrocrystalline waxes (carnauba, paraffin, etc.), amorphous substances or microcrystalline waxes (petrolatum, ceresine, and ozokerite), and oils.

**Waxes.**   Gloss and hardness of lipsticks are to a large extent dependent on the characteristics and quantity of the waxes used.

*Carnauba wax* increases the melting point, hardens the lipstick, and gives it an attractive luster. It can be used only in small quantities.

High melting macrocrystalline *paraffin waxes* have a similar effect; they also reduce resistance during application.

*Ozokerite* imparts toughness and nonfriability. An excess causes crumbling, however.

*Beeswax,* an important constitutent of many lipsticks, makes them firm, stabilizes the thixotropic system, and therefore counteracts oil exudation. Since beeswax contracts slightly on congealing, lipsticks containing this ingredient are easily removed from their molds. Yellow wax is slightly more tacky than the bleached variety; mixtures of both grades are often used. Too much beeswax will make the product granular and dull.

*Candelilla wax* has good oil retention similar to that of beeswax but is harder and glossier.

*Spermaceti* is occasionally added in small quantities. It is intended to give a certain soft touch on application.

Microcrystalline paraffin waxes such as *ceresine* are used because of their oil retention. They increase stability and prevent oils from separating.

**Oils.**   The constituents of the oil phase in lipsticks are selected primarily for their solvent power for eosine dyes. We have already mentioned the most important solvents for eosines. They differ considerably in their behavior in the lipstick base.

*Castor oil* is viscous and thus imparts body to the film left on the lips; it also prevents sedimentation of the pigments during preparation. A disadvantage of this high viscosity is an increased resistance during application, and the difficulty of wetting pigment lumps being added to a viscous liquid base. In modern lipstick formulations part of the castor oil is often replaced by isopropyl myristate and related substances that decrease viscosity.

*Tetrahydrofurfuryl alcohol* has a certain tendency to separate from the lipstick mass. Among the esters of this alcohol the *acetate* has the best solvent capacity but is somewhat volatile, which is certainly an undesirable quality. A volatile solvent evaporates on contact with the warmer inner surface of the lips, settles again on the cooler edges, and thus causes smudging of the outline. Furthermore, the acetate has an unpleasant taste and odor. These undesirable properties are less pronounced with the higher esters of tetrahydrofurfuryl alcohol (stearate and ricinoleate) but their solvent capacity is smaller. One disadvantage of tetrahydrofurfuryl alcohol and its esters is that they attack many of the synthetic resins, of which lipstick cases are often made.

*Fatty acid alkylolamides* have good properties as lipstick-base components: they are nonvolatile, have no unpleasant taste or odor, do not impair the stability of lipsticks but rather increase it, and have an emollient effect on the labial skin. They also promote dispersion of the pigments in the mass.

*Dihydric alcohols* as well as their *monoethers* and *monofatty acid esters* strengthen the stick, but their relatively hydrophilic characteristics may adversely affect the stability of the film on the lips.

In addition to oils and oily liquids, which are incorporated as eosine solvents, the oil phase also contains certain other basic materials:

*Isopropyl myristate, isopropyl palmitate, and butyl stearate* facilitate smooth application, have a good wetting effect on insoluble lakes and pigments because of their low surface tension, and act as mutual solvents for vegetable oils and fats, mineral oils, and waxes. The low surface tension of these synthetic oils makes them difficult to anchor in the skeleton of macrocrystalline waxes (this is how we must visualize the thixotropic mass). If there are insufficient binders in the stick mass, isopropyl myristate easily separates out. The solubility of eosine colors in these esters amounts to a maximum of 1 %.

*Paraffin oil* also acts as a lubricant on application and imparts gloss to the film. It should be used only in small amounts because larger quantities affect film adhesion to the lips. Paraffin oil also facilitates removal of the sticks from the molds after pouring. The same effect is achieved by high viscosity silicone oils; their use in lipsticks was suggested, among others, by Leberl [9]. They also produce a higher gloss on the lips, reportedly without affecting adhesion of the film, promote dispersion and wetting of pigments and lakes, and inhibit foam formation during production. Another advantage is the independence of their viscosity from temperature fluctuations.

**Fats.** In addition to the oils and waxes mentioned, lipsticks also contain a certain proportion of fats or fatlike substances. These mainly serve the purpose of giving the film on the lips more body, of smoothing the skin of the lips or of softening it (or of counteracting the "drying" effect of the eosine solvents), and of promoting the dispersion of insoluble pigments by their thickening or surfactant action. Widely used substances of this group are the following:

*Cocoa butter* was once an important constitutent of lipsticks because of its hardness, low melting point, and beneficial effect on the lips. It is rarely used today. One of the reasons is that it often causes a white rime to form on the stick surface.

Various *hydrogenated vegetable oils* (including hydrogenated castor oil) are used in modern lipsticks; an important advantage of these substances is their low tendency to turn rancid.

*Cetyl alcohol* has an emollient effect and also promotes dispersion of pigments. It must not be used in large quantities because the film on the lips then loses gloss (which may be due to the water-binding effect of cetyl alcohol, a W/O emulsifying agent). *Oleyl alcohol* has a similar effect but hardens stick and film less than cetyl alcohol. Moreover, oleyl alcohol has an appreciable solvent capacity for eosine dyes (about 1 %). One disadvantage is the fishy taste and odor of the fatty alcohol which are hard to mask. *Stearyl alcohol* has an even stronger hardening effect than cetyl alcohol. It may cause drastic hardening of the stick after a few months.

*Lanolin* and *lanolin absorption bases* also act as emollients, increase the toughness of the stick, and impede the tendency for oils to separate.

The use of **acetoglycerides** in lipsticks has also been recommended [10]. They are reported to improve thixotropic properties of sticks and even with temperature fluctuations give them an almost constant viscosity. They also improve the plasticity of the film on the lips.

Contrary to the fats and fatlike substances mentioned so far, *petrolatum* has no emollient properties. Its effect is similar to that of paraffin oil: it facilitates easy application of the stick and gives the film an improved gloss.

**Coloring Agents.**    One of the most important differences between various modern lipsticks is the ratio of pigments and soluble dyes. Some modern lipsticks (the so-called "indelible," "permanent" type) contain only comparatively small amounts of lakes and pigments in addition to relatively large quantities of eosine dyes. Others contain more than 10 % lakes and pigments and only just sufficient eosines to give the lips a faint stain. This type has a better covering and brightening effect and is less drying, but the coloring of the lips does not last so long. Among lakes only the synthetics (based on coal-tar dyes) play an important part and among pigments, only titanium dioxide. The shade of a lipstick is usually determined by the selection of these insoluble coloring agents; the direct staining of the lips is then adjusted to the shade of the stick by suitable mixture of eosine dyes. It must be borne in mind that not all eosine dyes stain the lips equally well.

It is important that pigments and lakes be thoroughly blended before they are incorporated in the base; this is usually achieved by grinding the finely dispersed colors once again after mixing. It is also important that pigments be well dispersed in the stick mass and form no lumps. Lump formation not only affects the distribution of color on the lips but also the shelf-life of the stick.

The adsorption of air or vapor on the surface of the pigment particles is a related problem [11] that leads to incomplete wetting of the particles by the oil phase. If adsorbed gas is finally liberated in fine bubbles, which migrate to the stick surface, the result may be oil separation. Experiments have demonstrated that sticks have a smoother surface and better shelf-life if pigments and lakes are blended in under vacuum rather than under atmospheric conditions. Unfortunately this procedure is costly and complicated in industrial practice.

**Surfactants** are occasionally added to the lipstick mass. They are intended to promote wetting and dispersion of solid pigment particles but such additions often adversely affect the consistency of the stick (e.g., by softening it). Insoluble colors sometimes amount to 10% or more of the total lipstick mass and therefore affect, as any powder would, the consistency of the stick. Various pigments and lakes differ considerably in density and particle size and consequently differ in the effect they have on the stick consistency. It may be therefore that by using one lipstick base for a series of different shades the completed sticks will differ in consistency and behavior during application; it is often necessary to adapt the composition of the base to the pigments and lakes. The majority of pigments, lakes and eosine dyes have a drying effect on labial skin. The content of emollients should therefore increase with increased color content.

As in all oil-fat-wax mixtures, it is a matter of course that adequate amounts of antioxidants and preservatives be added to lipsticks to prevent rancidity and deterioration. Caution is indicated because high concentrations of these substances affect taste and skin compatibility.

An important aspect for the consumer is fragrance or rather flavoring which must cover the unpleasant fatty taste and odor of the base and replace it with an odor and taste as pleasant as possible.

The perfume oil must of course be free of skin irritants. The epidermis on the lips is thin and tender, and the simultaneous presence of dyes provides an opportunity for cross sensitization. Even the best perfume oil never has a skin-conditioning effect; at best it is neutral. From the point of view of skin care it is always a liability rather than an asset. The perfume selected should therefore be as strong as possible so that it can be used in small amounts (not more than 1%).

| | 23 | 24 | 25 | 26 | 27 | 28 | 29 | 30 |
|---|---|---|---|---|---|---|---|---|
| Carnauba wax | 4 | 4.2 | 3 | 4 | | | | |
| Paraffin wax (54/56°C M.P.) | | | | | 15 | | | |
| Spermaceti | | | | | | 9.4 | | |
| Ozokerite | 12 | 8 | 3 | | 5 | 22.5 | 6 | |
| Ceresine, white | | | | 15 | 10 | | | |
| Beeswax | 14 | 4 | 7 | 10 | 12 | 2.1 | 20 | 36 |
| Candelilla wax | | | 7 | | | | | |
| Castor oil | 14 | | 55 | 22 | | | | |
| Fatty acid monoethanolamides | | 30 | | | | | | |
| Tetrahydrofurfuryl stearate | | | | | | | 22 | |
| Sebacic acid diethyl ester | | | | | | | | 10 |
| "Color solvent" | 5 | | | | | | | |
| Isopropyl myristate | | | 5 | 9 | | | | 10 |
| Eutanol G or Satol | | | | | | 12.6 | | |
| Paraffin oil | | 29.3 | | | | | 20 | 6 |
| Silicone oil (80,000–100,000 cst) | | | 10 | | | | | |
| Cocoa butter | | 5.5 | | | | | | |
| Hydrogenated palm kernel oil | | | | | | | | 23 |
| Hydrogenated castor oil | | | | | | 10 | | |
| Cetyl alcohol | | | | | 10 | 0.15 | 2 | 2 |
| Oleyl alcohol | | 7 | | | | | | |
| Lanette wax N | | | | | 6 | | | |
| Lanette wax O | | | | | 8 | | | |
| Lanolin, anhydrous | | 10 | 10 | | 7 | 1.57 | 10 | 4 |
| Wool wax | | | | | 6 | | | |
| Cholesterol | | | | | | 0.15 | | |
| Iso-Lan | | | | 27 | | | | |
| Petrolatum, white, short fibre | | | | | | 23.8 | | |
| Glyceryl monostearate SE | | | | | | 3.15 | | |
| Stearic acid, triple pressed | | | | | | 3.15 | | |
| Acetoglyceride (Cld Pt. (abt. −7°C) | 16 | | | | | | | |
| Acetoglyceride (Softening Pt. abt. 31°C) | 19 | | | | | | | |
| Lakes | 14 | 11.5 | 12 | 10 | 8 | 15.7 | 8 | 13 |
| Carmine nacarate | | | | | | 1.0 | | |
| Titanium dioxide | | | | | | | | 2 |
| Eosine acid | 3 | 4 | 3 | 3 | 6 | 2.4 | 2 | 1.5 |
| Oil soluble dye | | | | | | 1.57 | | |
| Perfume oil | | 0.5 | 1 | | 1 | 0.8 | q.s. | |
| Antioxidants | | | | | | | | 0.15 |

REMARKS

23. Ruemele, *Kosmetik-Parf.-Drog.*, **4**, 3 (1957) No details are given about the characteristics of the color solvent. Newman [12] prescribes 5% di-2-ethyl-hexyl sebacate in a very similar formulation.

24. Bergwein, *Parfum. Kosmet.*, **38**, 95 (1957).

25. Leberl, *Kosmetik-Parf.-Drog.*, **4**, 86 (1957).

26. Keithler, *The Formulation of Cosmetics and Cosmetic Specialties*, p. 159. Iso-Lan is a lanolin absorption base. The melting point of the ceresine should be around 65°C. Heat castor oil to 70°C, add eosine dye, and stir (not so vigorously that air is stirred in) until it has dissolved. The other fats, oils, and waxes are melted in a different container at a temperature as low as possible and pigments and lakes, already thoroughly blended in a grinder, are then added. The pigmented color mass is ground and mixed into the warm eosine solution. The mass is stirred until it is completely homogenous. Air introduced during the preceding operations must then be allowed to escape. This may be done by heating the mass until it liquefies and letting it stand for some time at high temperature; it is then stirred a few times and allowed to cool. However, it is better to draw the air off with a vacuum above the hot mass. When the mass has cooled to about 5°C above its solidification point, it is poured into molds. The molds are quickly cooled in a cooling chamber and the sticks removed. To give the completed sticks a smooth glossy surface a gas flame is passed over them. Addition of antioxidant is recommended.

27. Bergwein, *Parfum. Kosmet.*, **38**, 95 (1957).

28. Rothemann, *Das grosse Rezeptbuch der Haut- und Körperpflegemittel*, 3rd ed., p. 707. One part (per weight) ammonia (specific gravity, 0.935) is poured over 1 pt/wt carmine superfine, fine powder, and thoroughly stirred. Add 3 pt/wt distilled water, stir, and leave the solution overnight in cool storage (not in contact with iron!). On the following day the solution is mixed with 15.7 pt/wt melted, odorless, anhydrous lanolin.

The remaining fats and waxes (with the exception of Eutanol or Satol) are melted together on a waterbath, stirred, and then filtered through fine muslin or cheesecloth. The colored lanolin is stirred into the melt, followed by oil-soluble dye and lake. Subsequently some 95% alcohol (20 ml/kilo of mass) is stirred in and immediately followed by eosine acid (Rothemann prescribes 2.35–3.15%) which had previously been mixed with the Eutanol or Satol. Cool the mass with constant stirring and add perfume oil (0.79-1.18%) shortly before congealing. Homogenize with a pigment grinder or on a three-roller mill, heat carefully until it can be poured, and fill lipstick molds. The completed sticks are removed from the molds after cooling, which may be accelerated by cold water or freezing.

The ozokerite used must be hard, white, and free from paraffin. It may be replaced by equal parts of high-melting ceresine.

29. Harry, *Modern Cosmetocology*, 4th ed., p. 216. The original formulation does not specify individual proportions of eosine dyes and lakes. The total content amounts to 10%.

30. *The Use of Isopropyl Myristate in Cosmetics*, A. Boake, Roberts & Co. Carefully stir the antioxidants into the fat melt, add eosine (1–2%) and finally the lakes (12–14%) and pigments. Mix thoroughly, grind, melt, add perfume oil, and grind again. Melt again and pour into molds.

**Liquid and Cream Lip Makeup.** Liquid and cream preparations for coloring the lips have appeared on the market from time to time, but they have never gained the popularity of lipsticks. Cream makeup for the lips is mostly emulsified. The main disadvantage is the short life of the film on the lips.

Modern liquid makeup for lips [13] resembles nail lacquer in its composition. It consists of a film-forming substance (e.g., cellulose acetate), plasticizers, dyes, and solvents. It deposits a durable film on the lips but a drying action can hardly be avoided. Another reason for the failure of these products is the greater convenience of carrying a lipstick than a small bottle in a handbag.

A Dutch patent [14] describes an interesting product: a lipstick in the form of a ballpoint pen.

### Nail Lacquer

Today nail lacquer is as much an essential part of makeup as lipstick. So far we have not discussed the anatomy and physiology of the nails and shall deal only briefly with the subject. (A description of the structure, growth, and care of the nails is given by Achten [15].) Nails are hard keratinous tissues which are lifeless in the same sense as hair: there is no circulation in the nails, nor do they contain nerves. However, the nail matrix, situated below the nail, is richly supplied with blood capillaries and nerve ends. It has not yet been established what effect water and fat content have on the general condition of the nails. Strong alkaline solutions and prolonged contact with detergent solutions are known to make them brittle; probably the degradation of nail keratin and loss of water are involved in this process.

The nails themselves and the skin immediately surrounding them are relatively resistant to the influence of alien substances. This became most distinctly apparent in Sidi's remarkable observation that skin lesions caused by nail lacquer almost never appear on the fingers or hands but usually on other parts of the body, particularly the face (Sidi has observed only one exception in his entire practice [16]).

If nail lacquer is used, the whole nail surface is covered with a water- and air-impermeable lacquer film that is left on for days on end and finally removed with a more or less strongly degreasing solvent. Hardly any other part of the body surface would be able to support such treatment for any length of time; it is only in rare cases that complications occur in the nails. It does seem, however, that women who use nail lacquer are more prone to infections of the nail matrix than would otherwise be normal. This may be the result of swelling and softening due to moisture congestion caused by covering the nail surface.

**Requirements of the Consumer.**   As with lipsticks, consumer requirements for nail lacquers may be divided into three groups: quality demands for the lacquer in the bottle, for its behavior during application, and for the lacquer film.

To start with the latter, the film must be glossy and retain this gloss under the influence of high atmospheric humidity, light, and warm or cold detergent solutions. It must adhere firmly to the nail surface and neither chip nor rub off during normal wear. The color of the film must not rub off on clothing or stain the nails themselves.

Finally, the lacquer, must obviously not irritate the skin. There is a certain risk in the high resistance of the nails themselves and the skin surrounding them: it may be overlooked that nail lacquer, even if it causes no immediate damage to the nails and surrounding skin, may produce undesirable reactions elsewhere. This may be the reason for Sidi's observation that in 15 months of practice a comparatively high proportion (17%) of the skin lesions caused by cosmetics were due to nail lacquer [17].

During application nail lacquers must be liquid long enough for a smooth film to be applied easily, but it should also not take too long to dry because as long as it remains moist the user must remain inactive or the nails will be smudged. In addition, a lacquer that takes a long time to dry is often spread too thin. The lacquer must be thin enough for easy application but not so fluid that it will drip or accumulate at the free end of the nail. During application it should not have an unpleasant or obtrusive odor.

The consistency of the lacquer while it is still in its container is also important. It must remain homogeneous even during storage, and the pigments must not settle on the bottom; nor should the color be changed by the influence of solvents on the lakes.

It is impossible in practice to manufacture a lacquer that meets every one of these requirements. Individual differences of the nail substance and resultant variations in the behavior of the lacquer make it even more difficult to satisfy all users. In addition, the user's occupation also decisively affects the resistance of the lacquer film. There are great differences between the demands placed on the lacquer film by a housewife who exposes her hands to hot detergent solutions several times a day, by a typist, or by a woman who bathes regularly in sea water and then lies in the sun.

Boelcke [18] deals with the many problems around the question "Is there a perfect nail lacquer?"

**Composition.**   Contrary to the other preparations discussed in this chapter, coloring agents are not the most important active ingredients in nail lacquers. Film-forming substances, resins, and plasticizers are just as important; for transparent colorless preparations are very popular. Modern nail lacquers contain the following components:

**Film-Forming Substances.**   The traditional material for nail lacquers is nitrocellulose. Over the years various other substances have been suggested as film formers: cellulose acetate, cellulose aceto butyrate, ethyl cellulose, and methacrylate and vinyl resins, but none of these materials proved wholly acceptable. Nitrocellulose remains the best basic material for nail lacquer because of its unexcelled hardness, toughness, and low solvent retention.

Nitrocellulose is commercially available in various grades, but only low viscosity grades are suitable for nail lacquer. Since low viscosity nitrocelluloses are chemically less resistant than the higher viscosity grades, batches may occasionally degrade. Lacquer made with such a batch tends to turn yellowish. Nitrocellulose flocculates after longer periods, which makes the lacquer unusable. Methods for measuring stability and viscosity are described in special studies of cellulose lacquers [19]. Nitrocellulose is marketed dampened with ethyl or butyl alcohol to reduce its high inflammability.

*Plasticizers.*   Nitrocellulose solutions alone dry to a brittle dull film which easily chips off the nail because it tends to contract when dry. Plasticizers are added to the lacquer to give it the required flexibility, gloss, and adhesion and to reduce its tendency to shrink. Plasticizers should be high boiling (nonvolatile), miscible with the film former and the other constituents of the lacquer, colorless, odorless, and nontoxic. Esters of polybasic acids (dibutyl phthalate, triethyl citrate, tricresyl phosphate, and dioctyl adipate) are often used as plasticizers. Castor oil, camphor (celluloid is a nitrocellulose film with camphor as a plasticizer), urea derivatives, and monobasic acid esters such as butyl stearate may also be used for the same purpose. Keithler [20] recommends the use of chlorinated diphenylenes, marketed in United States under the trade names "Arochlor 5460" and "Arochlor 1254" (Monsanto). Selection of the plasticizer and of the quantity depend on the resin and grade of nitrocellulose used. Nitrocellulose, plasticizer, and resin must form a balanced combination.

**Resins.**   Resins are used in nail lacquer to give the film more body, depth, gloss, and adhesion. In addition, resins often act as dispersing agents for insoluble pigments and lakes.

Natural resins, such as gum damar, benzoic resin, gum copal, gum elemi, and shellac, once widely used, have to a large extent been replaced by synthetic resins. Sulfonamide-formaldehyde resins are probably the most common; in particular, a polymer made from equimolecular proportions of formaldehyde and *p*-toluene sulfonamide imparts excellent gloss, depth, adhesion, and resistance to aqueous solutions. However, formaldehyde-sulfonamide resins cause allergic reactions more frequently than other nail enamel constituents. Other synthetics which may also be considered for nail lacquers are alkyd resins, polystyrene, polyvinyl acetate, polyacrylic ester, epoxy ester, coumarone indene polymers, and copolymers of vinyl acetate and vinyl chloride. Each of these resins has characteristic properties. Polyester and polyisobutylene resins, for instance, act almost as plasticizers [21]. Glycol esters of abietic acid (main constituent of rosin) have a pronounced dispersing effect for pigments and lakes [22].

**Solvents.**    Solvents are more or less volatile organic liquids that combine all ingredients of a lacquer into a homogeneous viscous preparation. For reasons explained in the following paragraphs mixtures of solvents are used in most nail enamels. Various properties must be considered in their selection:

*Solvent Capacity for Nitrocellulose.*    We differentiate three groups according to solvent capacity:

1. "Active" solvents with a good solvent capacity for nitrocellulose: esters (butyl acetate, amyl acetate, etc.), ketones (acetone, diisobutyl ketone, etc.), glycol ethers [ethylene glycol lauryl ether, diethylene glycol ethyl ether, etc., or dimethylsulfoxide $(CH_3)_2SO$] [23].

2. "Latent" solvents which lack good solvent capacity by themselves but increase the effectiveness of active solvents in combination with them. These are mostly alcohols which are used in combination with their esters (e.g., butyl alcohol with butyl acetate).

3. "Diluents" which have almost no solvent capacity for nitrocellulose, mainly aliphatic and aromatic hydrocarbons. Diluents are intended to stabilize the viscosity of the lacquer, to contribute to solubilization of various resins, and to lessen the effect of freshly applied enamel on a previously applied lacquer film. In addition, the cost of lacquers is reduced by diluents. It may sound paradoxical, but high proportions of diluents make the lacquer viscous.

The solvent mixture must be adjusted so that it not only dissolves nitrocellulose, plasticizers, and resins while the enamel is in the container but also retains its solvent capacity as it slowly evaporates on the nail surface. If, for instance, the solvent mixture contains only volatile active solvents (acetone, butyl acetate), nitrocellulose will precipitate shortly after application, when they have evaporated, because the remaining solvents will not be able to hold it in solution. After complete drying a very uneven unsightly film will form. The quality of the film is also adversely affected when resins precipitate during evaporation of the solvent mixture.

Another property to be considered is the *rate of evaporation* of solvents. Comparisons of these rates have been made by allowing equal quantities to evaporate in open pans at constant temperature and measuring the time until evaporation was complete. Table 10-2 shows the comparative evaporation

TABLE 10-2 RELATIVE EVAPORATION RATES OF
SOME LACQUER SOLVENTS*

| | |
|---|---|
| Diethyl ether | 1.0 |
| Acetone | 2.1 |
| Petroleum ether (60–80°C) | 2.5 |
| Cyclohexane | 4.2 |
| Ethyl acetate | 4.8 |
| Methyl ethyl ketone | 5.0 |
| Ethyl alcohol | 9.0 |
| n-Butyl acetate | 12.8 |
| Amyl acetate | 13.0 |
| Xylene | 13.4 |
| n-Butyl alcohol | 34.0 |
| Diethylene glycol monoethyl ether | 45.0 |
| Ethyl lactate | 90.0 |

\* Generally, a high boiling point is linked to a fast,
and a low boiling point to a slow evaporation rate
but this relationship does not always hold.

times for some widely used solvents at 15°C, based on ethyl ether $= 1$. This table provides some useful guidelines but it must always be borne in mind that the evaporation rate of a liquid changes when it is mixed with other liquids. Generally the lowest boiling liquids in a mixture evaporate more slowly, the highest boiling more quickly than would be expected from their behavior when examined singly: there is a certain amount of leveling out.

If solvents in a nail enamel evaporate too quickly, it is difficult to apply a smooth coating on the nails. Sudden evaporation creates an "orange peel" effect. Rapid evaporation of solvents also causes local cooling and results in the condensation of fine water droplets from the atmosphere on the lacquer film. The degree of cooling not only depends on the rate but also on the heat of evaporation.

If solvents evaporate too slowly, the enamel on the nails stays liquid for a long time and in this instance as well it is difficult to apply a film of even thickness; under these conditions the film is usually too thin. In addition, the user is inconvenienced by slow evaporation.

The *odor* of nail enamel must not be unpleasant or obtrusive. For this reason the use of solvents with a strong or unpleasant odor is often restricted (amyl acetate, acetone, and butyl acetate).

Neither the liquid solvents nor their vapor should be *irritating*. Aromatic hydrocarbons such as xylene occasionally cause difficulties in this connection because some people are allergic to their vapor.

**Coloring Agents.** With soluble dyes alone the lacquer film does not acquire sufficient depth of color or intensity and for this reason pigments and lakes are used. Staining of the nail surface itself is undesirable. The lakes must of course be resistant to light and to the action of organic solvents. If solvents cause a separation of the color from the substrate, changes in shade and staining of the nails may result.

## Preparation of Nail Lacquer

Fine grinding and thorough mixing of the pigments is important. The rule of adjusting the desired color shade in the dry color mix must be observed because it is difficult to correct once the colors have been mixed with other ingredients. Occasionally solid dyes are ground with plasticizers; extended periods of grinding are essential to make the mixture homogeneous. According to French Patent 1,006,605, a favorable effect is obtained by grinding the colors with the esters of abietic acid [24].

| | 31 | 32 | 33 | 34 |
|---|---|---|---|---|
| Nitrocellulose | 4.0 | 7 | 13.1 | |
| Dibutyl phthalate | | 5 | | |
| Dioctyl adipate | | | 13.4 | |
| Triethyl phosphate | | | 6.5 | |
| Tricresyl phosphate | | | | 8.0 |
| "Arochlor 5460" | | | | 15.0 |
| Sorbitol | | | | 20.0 |
| Camphor | | | 3.0 | |
| Plasticizer | 4.0 | | | |
| Polypropyl methacrylate | 18.6 | | | |
| Polymethyl methacrylate | | | | 7.0 |
| Polyvinyl acetate | | 8 | | |
| Vinyl chloride-vinyl acetate copolymer | | | | 10.7 |
| Acetone | | | 3.0 | |
| Methyl ethyl ketone | | | | 21.5 |
| Ethyl acetate | | | | 22.3 |
| Butyl acetate | 23.9 | | | |
| Methylene chloride | | 30 | | |
| Ethylene glycol monomethyl ether | | 28 | 35.0 | |
| Diethylene glycol monomethyl ether | | 2 | | |
| Ethyl alcohol, denaturized | 25.6 | 14 | | |
| Toluene | 23.9 | | | |
| Coloring agents | | | 0.4 | 0.5 |
| Perfume oil | | 6 | | |

REMARKS

31. U. S. Patent 2,195,971 (E. I. du Pont de Nemours). A nail lacquer base without color.

32. German Patent 946,841 (Dr.-Ing. Pichlmayr). Also a base for nail lacquer in which all solvents with an obtrusive odor have been avoided. The perfume oil is dissolved in phthalate, which solution is added to polyvinyl acetate, and this mass is mixed with the nitrocellulose solution.

33. Keithler, *The Formulation of Cosmetics and Cosmetic Specialties*, p. 443. Stir the colors into the dioctyl adipate/tricresyl phosphate mixture. Grind the mass until it is homogeneous and add it to the previously prepared solution of nitrocellulose and camphor in ethylene glycol methyl ether. Add the remaining ingredients and stir until the mass is homogeneous. Pour immediately.

34. Keithler, *Drug Cosm. Ind.*, **80**, 308 (1957). Arochlor 5460 (Monsanto) is a chlorinated diphenyl. This formula is notable for the absence of nitrocellulose.

Even with careful selection of solvents it is not always possible to achieve a completely clear product immediately. Clouding can be removed by filtration or by allowing the cloud to settle. Filtration requires special equipment; clearing of highly viscous preparations by settling may take several weeks unless a centrifuge is used. The manufacture of nail lacquers presents certain difficulties because working with volatile solvents requires well-ventilated rooms and the high inflammability of nitrocellulose and the majority of solvents necessitates special safety measures. Small manufacturers of cosmetics therefore are often advised not to produce nail lacquers themselves but to use custom fillers.

## PREPARATIONS FOR MASKING SKIN IMPERFECTIONS AND SHININESS

With normal or intensified activity of sebaceous and sweat glands a thin lipid layer containing moisture forms on the skin. This is hardly noticeable unless it is exceptionally developed, at least under natural light, but under harsh electric light its distinct shininess becomes apparent, in particular on the nose, where lanugo hair breaks the smoothness of the skin surface least. This shininess is considered definitely unattractive, possibly because it is a symptom of all-too-natural skin functions.

The color of the skin also reflects physiological activities of the epidermal tissue and may even be an indication of a woman's general state of health. A red nose, possibly with some blood vessels delineated, strong, sharply defined red spots on the cheeks, a pale yellowish complexion, dark circles under the eyes—regardless of whether or not such signs are consciously observed—allow conclusions to be drawn about the constitution and way of life of the person concerned.

In addition, almost everybody has wrinkles and lines that are a sign of age or changing expressions and thus reflect the temperament; sometimes there are freckles, small birthmarks, enlarged follicle mouths ("pores"), acne pustules, scars of previous skin lesions, and so on. It is symptomatic of our attitude that a woman wishing to be considered attractive will cover up all such physiological irregularities of her appearance and in particular of her face and will show herself discreetly masked to the world.

This masking effect is achieved with face powders, foundation creams, and liquid makeup, and as an auxiliary, day creams.

### Face Powders

The main function of face powders is visual covering. For this reason they nearly always contain basic materials with the most effective masking properties: zinc oxide and titanium dioxide.

To judge the covering effect of a powder basic material we must know the refractive index not only of the dry substance but—even more important—the refractive index of this substance when it is in contact with water or fat. In an article that discusses various factors influencing the covering effect, Grady [25] points out that the covering effect of all powder ingredients decreases noticeably after contact with water or petrolatum and that zinc and titanium oxides are less strongly affected than all other common ingredients.

If the covering power of a powder is very high, it creates a "dead" or mask-like impression. Ordinarily women require only a delicate masking and the covering action need therefore be only enough to remove shininess, uneven coloring, or minor blemishes. Face powders for this reason are available in different grades, from light with little covering effect, to heavy or total covering.

Both zinc oxide and titanium dioxide are white. Since the purpose of face powders is not to give women a deathly pale appearance, they are tinted. The most widely used coloring materials for this purpose are iron oxides with yellow, red, or brown shades, and lakes with which all desired shades can be achieved. Water-soluble dyes are used only rarely, although they present no technical difficulties (by spraying the powder with an alcoholic dye solution); if perspiration loosened them from the powder, there might be the risk of an undesirable staining of the skin. In addition, water-soluble dyes are usually less resistant to light than lakes.

The action of powder ingredients in covering shininess is enhanced by substances such as colloidal kaolin, Cab-o-Sil, calcium, and magnesium carbonates, that absorb perspiration and sebum.

Some powder ingredients create a matting effect on the skin in yet another way: they adhere to the lanugo hairs and thereby accentuate them. The result is a velvety peachlike complexion which is most attractive. The user will judge a powder according to the frequency with which she has to touch up. This depends not only on the covering capacity and the absorbent effect but even more on adhesion to the skin. Substances that improve adhesion are, among others, zinc and magnesium stearates, undecanates, and laurates. These materials also facilitate application because they improve adhesion to the powder puff.

Some of the powder ingredients mentioned (in particular, colloidal kaolin, Cab-o-Sil, and calcium carbonate) feel dry on application: rubbing on the skin will cause some friction. Substances that contribute smoothness to the powder, such as talcum, zinc stearate, or similar metal salts, are therefore added to the blend. To lighten a powder which is too heavy and dense (which may happen with a high kaolin content) materials are added to fluff it. Cab-o-Sil and magnesium carbonate are particularly suitable for this purpose. The reader is referred to Chapter 4 for a more detailed discussion of powder ingredients and preparation methods.

**Loose Powders.** Except for a few newly introduced basic materials, formulations of face powders have hardly changed in the course of the last 35 years.

The following formulations appear in order of increasing covering effect:

|  | 35 | 36 | 37 | 38 | 39 | 40 |
|---|---|---|---|---|---|---|
| Zinc oxide | 5 | 15 | 20 | 24 | 19 | |
| Titanium dioxide | | | | | 4 | 20 |
| Kaolin | | | 10 | | | 30 |
| Cab-o-Sil | | | | | | 5 |
| Rice starch | 10 | 15 | 35 | | | |
| Precipitated chalk | | 15 | | 40 | | |
| Zinc stearate | 5 | 5 | | 6 | | |
| Magnesium stearate | | | | | 4 | 10 |
| Talcum | 80 | 50 | 25 | 30 | 65 | 30 |
| Magnesium carbonate | | | | | 5 | 5 |
| Strontium sulfate | | | 10 | | | |
| Coloring agents | q.s. | | | q.s. | 2 | q.s. |
| Perfume | q.s. | | | q.s. | 1 | 2 |

REMARKS

35. Harry, *Modern Cosmetocology*, 4th ed., p. 196.
36. Harry, *ibid.*, p. 197.
37. Janistyn, *Riechstoffe-Seifen-Kosmetika*, II, p. 220, according to Cerbelaud.
38. Harry, *op. cit.* p. 197.
39. Keithler, *The Formulation of Cosmetics and Cosmetic Specialties*, p. 119.
40. Rothemann, *Das grosse Rezeptbuch der Haut- und Körperpflegemittel*, 3rd ed., p. 680.

**Compact Powder.** Compact powder is dry powder pressed into cake form. Its composition is similar to that of loose powder, but its effect on the skin differs to a certain extent. The binders contained in compact powder give it increased adhesion. As a result of the pressing process, the average particle size is generally larger in compact than in loose powder; a pronounced coarsening of the grain is, of course, undesirable. Compact powder must adhere easily to the powder puff, and the cake must be sufficiently solid not to break under normal conditions of use.

Not all traditional powder constituents are suitable for compact powder. The basic raw material should have a certain binding effect. Rice starch, aluminum oxide, and kaolin as well as zinc stearate, barium and strontium sulfates have proved satisfactory in this connection.

Three methods of preparation for compact powder have been described in the literature.

In the *wet method* basic materials, colors, and binders are kneaded into a paste with water, pressed into molds, and slowly air dried [26]. At present this method is hardly ever employed because it is difficult to avoid cracks and other faults.

In *"dry" preparation* compacts are made by simple pressure of the dry mixture in special presses under strictly controlled conditions. Special binders are often incorporated; for example, a mixture of ammonia, stearic acid, and starch [27], stearic acid and starch [28], or a mixture of an emulsifying agent such as sodium stearate or triethanolamine stearate, with fats such as lanolin and cetyl alcohol [29]. Compact powders of this type are similar to pancake makeup. A variation of the dry method is *damp* preparation, in which the binder consists of aqueous mucilages or mucin-rich O/W emulsions. This is the most widely used method at present and is applicable to the following formulations:

| POWDER BLENDS | 41 | 42 | 43 | 44 |
|---|---|---|---|---|
| Zinc oxide | 9 | 16.7 | | |
| Titanium dioxide | | | 4 | 5 |
| Colloidal kaolin | 39 | 33.5 | 16.5 | |
| Rice starch | | | 4 | 10 |
| Zinc stearate | 6 | | 6 | |
| Magnesium stearate | | | | 8 |
| Barium sulfate | 40 | | | |
| Talcum | 6 | 33.3 | 60 | 39 |
| Magnesium carbonate | | 16.5 | 5 | 33.5 |
| Colors | q.s. | q.s. | 4.0 | 4.0 |
| Perfume | q.s. | q.s. | 0.5 | 0.5 |

REMARKS

41. Janistyn, *Riechstoffe-Seifen-Kosmetika*, II, p. 228. Mix 100 parts of powder with about 8 parts of binder (e.g., No. 45).

42. Janistyn, *op. cit.*, p. 229. An especially fine talcum grade is required. Proportion with binder as above.

43. Keithler, *The Formulation of Cosmetics and Cosmetic Specialties*, p. 141. Pour perfume oil over magnesium carbonate and leave for 24 hours. Then combine it with the other ingredients in a powder mixer, mix for about two hours, take a sample, grind it, and check for color, uniformity, and particle size. If everything is satisfactory, the powder itself will be ready for grinding. Mix 90 parts of powder with 10 parts of binder (No. 47) and prepare cakes by the wet or dry method.

44. Keithler, *op. cit.*, p. 139. The powder blend is prepared in the same way as No. 43 and then 93 parts mixed with 7 part of binder (No. 46) and pressed into cakes.

| BINDERS | 45 | 46 | 47 |
|---|---|---|---|
| Mineral oil | | | 2.0 |
| Lanolin | | | 3.0 |
| Cetyl alcohol | | | 4.0 |
| Triethanolamine lauryl sulfate | | | 1.0 |
| Gum tragacanth | 1.2 | | |
| Carboxymethylcellulose, low viscosity | | 1.0 | |
| Sodium alginate | | 0.5 | 1.0 |
| Alcohol | 5.0 | 2.0 | 4.0 |
| Water | 93.8 | 96.3 | 82.5 |
| Glycerol | | | 2.0 |
| Methyl-*p*-hydroxybenzoate | | 0.2 | |

REMARKS

45. Janistyn, *Riechstoffe-Seifen-Kosmetika*, II, p. 229. The proportion of vehicle is given as 1.0–1.5%.

46. Keithler, *The Formulation of Cosmetics and Cosmetic Specialties*, p. 140. Hot water (90°C), in which the preservative has been dissolved, is poured over the mucins wetted with alcohol; stir until they are completely dissolved.

47. Keithler, *op. cit.*, p. 141. The alginate used is "Sea-Kem," Type 4. Stir the solution of glycerol and triethanolamine lauryl sulfate in half the water (85°C) into the melt of lanolin, mineral oil, and cetyl alcohol (85°C). Dampen the mucins with alcohol, pour the remaining water (90°C) over them, and stir until the solution is smooth. This solution is then stirred into the other emulsified ingredients.

## Foundation Creams

Loose powders applied to untreated skin do not adhere well. Only a thin layer of powder is left on the skin and it does not stay there long. Adhesion of powders can be considerably improved by first treating the skin with a preparation on which the powder will remain much longer than on untreated skin.

These preparations are known under different names: day cream, vanishing cream, foundation cream. The different names emphasize the different aspects of the preparations. "Day creams" are used during the day in contrast to heavy night creams. "Foundation creams" serve as a base for powder or makeup. In "vanishing cream," the film left after application is very thin and hardly visible.

The requirements that these creams must meet (in addition to improving adhesion of the powder and providing a mat, certainly not glossy, effect on the skin) need hardly be specified because they are self-explanatory. They must not damage the skin, must have a suitable consistency (i.e., not too stiff, too soft, or too tacky), and must remain stable.

**Composition.** Usually these preparations are stearate creams. The composition of this type of emulsion has been discussed in Chapter 4. It may, of course, be varied extensively. Suitable additives provide stearate creams with skin-protecting properties (see Chapter 7); they can also be modified into genuine skin conditioners with emollient or depth effect or into cleansers of the "massage-cream" type. The composition of stearate creams intended for day-time use is usually very simple.

Mineral oil may be added to promote powder adhesion because it lends body to the film left on the skin. (A distinction is made in British and American formulations between light vanishing creams and heavier foundation creams with their stronger binding capacity for powder.) The low surface tension of isopropyl myristate, butyl stearate, and similar esters results in closer adhesion of the film and a softer feeling of the skin. Lanolin, cetyl alcohol, etc., are also often added to day creams; these additives provide emollient properties. With an increasing content of skin conditioning components day creams, which we have regarded as auxiliaries in decorative cosmetics, may develop into genuine skin-care products (see Chapter 8).

Some day creams are not based on stearic acid but on glycerol monostearate or diethylene glycol monostearate. Preparations of this kind are a little more glossy on the skin than stearate creams but hold powder firmly; they are particularly suited to women with dry skin.

Creams based on fatty alcohols or Lanette wax are sometimes discussed in the literature under "foundation creams." In our opinion they do not belong to this group but rather to skin conditioners.

We list only a few typical formulations from the wealth of literature on day creams:

| | 48 | 49 | 50 | 51 | 52 |
|---|---|---|---|---|---|
| Mineral oil | | | | | 1 |
| Butyl stearate | | | | 1.5 | |
| Spermaceti | 2 | | | | |
| Cetyl alcohol | | | | | 1 |
| Myristyl alcohol | | | | 2.5 | |
| Lanolin, anhydrous | | 4 | | 1.0 | 2 |
| Vitamin F (250,000 I.U./g) | | | | 0.2 | |
| Glycerol monostearate SE | | | | | 18 |
| Diethylene glycol stearate | | | 4 | | |
| Triple-pressed stearic acid | 20 | 25 | 20 | 20 | |
| Potassium hydroxide (100%) | 1.0 | | 0.33 | | |
| Sodium hydroxide (100%) | 0.133 | | 0.24 | | |
| Triethanolamine | | 1.35 | | | 1.58 |
| Isopropanolamine | | | 0.80 | | |
| Borax | | | | 0.3 | |
| Water | 71.867 | 60.65 | 69.63 | 65 | 76 |
| Glycerol | 5 | | | 10 | |
| Diethylene glycol monoethyl ether | | 9 | | | |
| Propylene glycol | | | 5 | | |
| Sorbitol | | | | | 2 |
| Perfume | q.s. | | q.s. | 0.5 | |
| Preservative | | | q.s. | | |

REMARKS

48. De Navarre, *The Chemistry and Manufacture of Cosmetics*, p. 250. Add the aqueous solution of alkali and glycerol (85°C) to the fat melt (85°C) with mechanical stirring. Allow the emulsion to cool, stirring occasionally to avoid crust formation at the surface. Leave the cream overnight and add perfume on the following day. Stir until the mass becomes much softer and pour cold. After a few days the cream will again become stiffer.

49. De Navarre, *op.cit.*, 252. The working method is the same as in 48. This cream is intended for dry skin, hence the high lanolin content. The high proportion of humectants (diethylene glycol monoethyl ether) prevents "rolling" of the cream during application; stearate creams always have this tendency on dry skin.

50. Harry, *Modern Cosmetocology*, 4th ed., p. 158. Stir the aqueous phase (75°C, including the isopropanolamine) into the melt of stearic acid and diethylene glycol stearate (75°C). Continue stirring until the mass has cooled to 45°C, add perfume, and let stand for 24–48 hours. Homogenize and fill.

51. Rothemann, *Das grosse Rezeptbuch der Haut- und Körperpflegemittel*, 3rd ed., p. 586. The fats are melted together at a temperature as low as possible and the aqueous solution of glycerol, triethanolamine, and borax (75°C) is added in a thin jet under constant stirring. Continue stirring until the cream is almost cool, add perfume, and fill.

52. Keithler, *The Formulation of Cosmetics and Cosmetic Specialties*, p. 65. All ingredients are heated together to 90°C. Stir until a uniform emulsion has formed.

## Foundation Makeup

As we have stated in the preceding sections, good makeup consists in treating the face first with a cream and then applying powder. There is only a small step from this practice to the use of foundation makeup (i.e., preparations that contain both powder and foundation). Foundation makeup in various forms, particularly liquid, has gained so much in popularity that in some countries it has replaced loose powder and vanishing creams altogether. The reasons are obvious: creams, particularly liquid creams, are more easily applied than powder and with them it is also much easier to obtain a smooth appearance. From the point of view of skin care foundation makeup, at least if it contains water, has certain disadvantages: the surfactants in the preparation cause pigments and lakes to penetrate the hair follicles and fine fissures of the epidermis (this is facilitated because they are rubbed into the skin rather than being dusted on as powder); if they are not completely removed they are much more likely to cause skin irritations than preparations that remain on the skin surface. This consideration, however, has not affected the popularity of foundation makeup. Various types are available at present. We discuss them individually.

**Anhydrous Foundation Makeup.** This product consists of a suspension of the basic materials of powder in a thixotropic fat/wax/oil mass. In this respect it resembles lipsticks but is much softer and must be formulated to leave only a very thin nonglossy film on the skin.

There are two types: soft, packed in jars or tubes, and firm, molded into sticks.

The most important powder ingredient in foundation makeup is titanium dioxide, which is generally preferred to zinc oxide. The amount of solids that can be added without making the preparation too hard or unstable is somewhat restricted. A good covering effect is obtained with much smaller quantities of titanium dioxide than of zinc oxide. In addition to white and reddish pigments (and possibly small amounts of lakes), small quantities of other powder ingredients may also be used.

In the following we give two formulations each for soft and solid (stick) anhydrous foundation makeup:

| | 53 Cream | 54 Cream | 55 Stick | 56 Stick |
|---|---|---|---|---|
| Paraffin wax (56–58°C M.P.) | 5.0 | | 7.7 | |
| Ozokerite (75–80°C M.P.) | 5.0 | | | |
| Carnauba wax | | 10 | | 14 |
| Beeswax | | | 2 | 4 |
| Paraffin oil, light | 23.5 | | 4.7 | 10 |
| Isopropyl myristate | | 49 | 20 | 37 |
| Petrolatum | 47.5 | | 12 | |
| Lanolin | 4.0 | | 0.6 | |
| Cetyl alcohol | | 1 | 12 | |
| Powder basic materials | 15.0 | 40 | 36 | 35 |
| Perfume | q.s. | | | q.s. |
| Antioxidants | | 0.15 | 0.1 | |

REMARKS

53. Fiedler in Sagarin, *Cosmetics: Science and Technology*, New York, 1957, p. 263. The basic powder materials consist of titanium dioxide, inorganic pigments (possibly with small additions of lakes), and talcum. Talcum serves as a diluent that maintains a uniform consistency in various grades of the makeup cream with varying pigment contents.

Certain pigments cannot be used in these preparations because they are not wetted by the fat. During production they would float to the surface in the liquid stage of preparation or form a sediment on the bottom.

*Procedure.* Mix the dry powders well, grind them several times until they are evenly dispersed, and add them to the melt of the other ingredients (70°C). Pass the cream through a colloid or roller mill and stir until cooled to 45°C, add perfume, and fill. If air has been entrapped during the incorporation of the powders, it can be removed by heating the mass to 70°C with slow agitation.

54. *The Use of Isopropyl Myristate in Cosmetics*, A. Boake Roberts & Co., London. The powder to be used may have the following composition:

| | Heavy | Light |
|---|---|---|
| Zinc oxide | 30 | 30 |
| Titanium dioxide | 12 | 6 |
| Kaolin | 25 | 25 |
| Magnesium stearate | 8 | 8 |
| Starch | 10 | 10 |
| Chalk, lightly precipitated | 20 | 20 |
| Magnesium carbonate | 2 | 2 |
| Talcum | 15 | 15 |
| Lakes | 1.5 | 0.66 |

The procedure follows 53. This cream is rather soft. To harden the product 60 parts instead of 40 pts of powder may be added.

55. The powder ingredients are zinc oxide (26 pts), titanium dioxide (7 pts), other pigments and lakes (3 pts). These proportions may be changed as required. Procedure follows 53.

56. Fiedler, *op. cit.*, p. 264. Procedure follows 53. Continuous stirring is essential to avoid separation of pigments from the liquid mass. A harder stick can be obtained by increasing beeswax or ozokerite portions. The stick should have a minimum diameter of ¾ in., since it breaks too easily otherwise. In addition, it should also fill its mold completely to avoid breaking.

**Solid Makeup Creams, O/W Type.** In principle these creams consist of a vanishing cream mixed with powder. Not every vanishing cream can arbitrarily be turned into a makeup cream, since the powder ingredients often cause instability of the emulsion by absorbing part of the fats or emulsifiers or by adsorbing at their surface.

According to their authors, the following formulations result in stable products:
57. Janistyn, *Riechstoffe-Seifen-Kosmetika*, II, p. 402.

| | |
|---|---|
| Butyl stearate | 1 |
| Stearic acid, triple pressed | 12 |
| Sorbitan monostearate | 2 |
| Polyoxyethylene sorbitan monostearate | 1 |
| Distilled water | 58 |
| Propylene glycol | 12.5 |
| Sorbitol liquid | 2 |
| Talcum, prime grade | 8 |
| Titanium dioxide, prime grade | 2 |
| Iron oxide, red | 1 |
| Perfume | 0.5 |
| Preservative | q.s. |

Emulsify at 90°C and add pigments wetted with water or propylene glycol to the emulsified mass. Perfume at 45°C and homogenize in an ointment or other suitable mill.

58. Rothemann, *Das grosse Rezeptbuch der Haut- und Körperpflegemittel*, 3rd ed., p. 689.

| | |
|---|---|
| Petrolatum, white, viscous | 4 |
| Paraffin oil | 3 |
| Eutanol G | 3 |
| Glycerol monostearate self-emulsifying | 20 |
| Distilled water | 70 |
| Titanium dioxide | 2 |
| Colloidal kaolin | 3 |
| Lakes and pigments | 1 |
| Perfume | 0.3 |

Either the pulverized colors are added during stirring through a fine mesh sieve and the completed cream is perfumed after cooling and then homogenized or passed through a pigment grinder or three-roller mill; or the lakes and pigments are separately ground with the petrolatum and homogenized and this mix is stirred into the still warm cream. The other powder ingredients (titanium dioxide and colloidal kaolin) may be sieved into the cream during stirring. Tubes are preferred to regular jars. Tin or aluminum jars are unsuitable.

**Liquid Makeup.** Since these products first appeared on the market they have gained exceptional popularity. Taken together with liquid emulsified rouges, they probably present the easiest method of applying good uniform makeup. The covering capacity of these preparations (and of makeup creams in general) is considerable and the masking effect usually more pronounced than with loose powders. Possible drawbacks of makeup creams have already been mentioned.

**Requirements of the Consumer.** The requirements that must be met can be divided into three groups: requirements regarding the product itself, its behavior during application, and the properties of the film left on the skin.

To start with the last, the covering effect must be neither too strong nor too light, and in order to obtain a correct balance, covering intensity and film thickness must be mutually adjusted. For extended stability of the makeup on the skin the film must have water-repellent properties, but it must not cover the skin so completely that it will prevent the exchange of vapor between it and the surrounding atmosphere. Finally the powder cream should also have some skin-conditioning properties or at least it must not be harmful to the skin.

As far as behavior during application is concerned, the product must be neither so viscous that it can not be poured out of the bottle easily nor have a viscosity so low that it runs off after application. Drying should not be so slow that the face will feel damp after application nor so rapid that even spreading is difficult.

In addition, the product must have good stability in the container. The powder ingredients must not form a permanent sediment at the bottom; the emulsion must not separate; the cream must not dry to a hard crust on the surface; it must not change color even after long storage; and it must be suitably preserved against bacterial decomposition and fungi.

Finally, liquid makeup must be available in various shades, if possible with various covering powers, and each grade must be uniform from batch to batch in color and covering intensity.

**Composition.** Since the composition of these preparations is rather complicated, we shall discuss one by one the purpose of each group of the normally used ingredients.

We need not enlarge on the purpose of *pigments* and *lakes*. Suspension of solids in products of this kind is not easy and their proportion must therefore be kept rather low; for this reason titanium dioxide with its excellent covering capacity is preferred as a white pigment. Staining of the skin itself, as is usual with lipsticks, is avoided in makeup; if the lips remain slightly red, it does not matter much, but it certainly would if this were to happen after removing makeup from the face.

**Oils** are an essential part of good makeup creams. They remain on the skin after the preparation has dried, as vehicle for the powder. Low-viscosity mineral oil and isopropyl myristate are often used, as are skin conditioners such as lanolin or cetyl alcohol which make the film on the skin slightly water permeable. The oil film ideally should not be too hydrophilic but rather slightly water-repellent so that the makeup will not be affected by perspiration. For this reason we do not think that the choice of polyethylene glycol waxes as film formers (e.g., formula 61) is a very happy one. Silicone oils might be useful here. The total content of film-forming fats is usually about as high as that of powder components. If it is too high, the film will look greasy; if it is too low, the powder will not adhere to the skin.

**Surfactants** have a double part to play in emulsified foundation makeup: they act simultaneously as emulsifiers for the fats and oils and as dispersing agents for the powders. To increase the stability of the dispersion-emulsion, thickening agents are always added to serve as auxiliary emulsifiers and to impart the desired consistency to the preparation. Bentonite has proved satisfactory in this connection, but other synthetic or natural organic thickening agents are also suitable.

Liquid foundation makeup usually contains humectants which serve several purposes simultaneously: they increase spreadability of the preparation on the skin and prevent too rapid drying during application and crust formation in the container.

Finally, these preparations obviously contain water (quantitatively the main ingredient), preservatives, and perfume.

59. Fiedler in Sagarin, *Cosmetics: Science and Technology*, New York, 1957, p. 267. Add the melt of stearic acid, propylene glycol monostearate, and mineral oil (75°C) in a thin jet with vigorous stirring to the aqueous solution of triethanolamine and preservative. When the emulsion has cooled to 55°C, stir in a finely pulverized mixture of sodium lauryl sulfate, bentonite, and the powder ingredients. Add perfume at 45°C and continue stirring until the cream has cooled to room temperature. Pass it through a colloid mill and let it mature for a few days. Avoid entrapping air during preparation by mounting the agitator completely under the surface of the mass and by avoiding too rapid stirring (about 80 rpm is recommended). An addition of antifoaming agents is helpful. Since the addition of dry powders usually introduces air into the mixture, subsequent stirring is required (50–80 rpm) until all air has been removed.

A variation of this method of manufacture consists in mixing 20% of the water with the

| | 59 | 60 | 61 |
|---|---|---|---|
| Mineral oil (70/80) | 15.0 | | |
| Isopropyl myristate | | 3.0 | |
| Petrolatum | | 2.0 | |
| Cetyl alcohol | | 4.0 | |
| Lanolin | | 3.0 | |
| Propylene glycol monostearate | 6.0 | | |
| Diethylene glycol stearate | | 4.0 | |
| Stearic acid, triple pressed | 2.5 | | |
| Sodium lauryl sulfate | 1.1 | | |
| Triethanolamine lauryl sulfate | | 1.0 | |
| Triethanolamine | 1.3 | | |
| Titanium dioxide | | 1.0 | 1.0 |
| Pigments and lakes | 11.0 | 8.0 | 7.0 |
| Talcum | | 10.0 | 8.0 |
| Kaolin | 5.2 | | |
| Magnesium carbonate | | 2.0 | |
| Calcium carbonate, precipitated | | | 3.0 |
| Water | 53.1 | 56.3 | 64.8 |
| Polyethylene glycol 4000 | | | 8.0 |
| Bentonite | 4.7 | | |
| Carboxymethylcellulose, high viscosity | | 1.0 | 1.5 |
| Glycerol | | | 4.0 |
| Propylene glycol | | 2.0 | |
| Alcohol | | 2.0 | |
| Perfume | q.s. | 0.5 | 0.5 |
| Methyl-*p*-hydroxybenzoate | 0.1 | 0.2 | 0.2 |
| | 100.0 | 100.0 | 98.0 |

bentonite and letting it stand until it has formed a gel; this gel is mixed into the aqueous phase before emulsification.

60. Keithler, *The Formulation of Cosmetics and Cosmetic Specialties*, p. 142. Wet carboxymethylcellulose with the alcohol, pour half the water (90°C) over it, and stir until a smooth gel has developed. Pour perfume over magnesium carbonate, let it stand for 24 hours, add the remaining powder ingredients, and mix 2–4 hours in a powder mixer. Work the powder thoroughly into the CMC solution (if necessary with a three-roller mill). Add the remaining water containing propylene glycol, triethanolamine, and preservative (80°C), stir in the powder dispersion and fill.

61. Keithler, *op. cit.*, p. 144. Heat the aqueous solution of glycerol and polyethylene glycol to 90°C, add the CMC dampened with alcohol, and stir until it is completely dissolved. Cool the solution and stir in the powder ingredients. Grind or pulverize the product and fill.

**Pancake Makeup.**  This is an interesting variety of foundation makeup. By appearance it can hardly be distinguished from compact powder, but according to its composition it is a dehydrated powder cream. British Patent 501,732 (U.S. Patent 2,101,843, 1937 is very similar) describes the composition as follows:

| | |
|---|---|
| Oils and fats | 0.8–24% |
| Water-soluble dispersing agents (triethanolamine soap, glycerol, or glycol derivatives) | 1–23% |
| Pigments and lakes | 12–50% |
| Fillers (basic powder materials) | 35–80% |

This preparation contains no water but it is still an O/W emulsion in application because it is applied to the skin with a moistened applicator. The emulsion formed on the applicator by the presence of emulsifying/dispersing agents leaves a covering film of excellent stability on the skin.

The following is a formulation for this type of preparation:
62. Fiedler in E. Sagarin, *Cosmetics: Science and Technology*, p. 269.

| | |
|---|---|
| Isopropyl myristate | 31.5 |
| Dry powders (titanium dioxide, pigment, talcum) | 35.5 |
| Ozokerite (80–88°C M.P.) | 17.5 |
| Cetyl alcohol | 2.5 |
| Sorbitan mono-oleate (Span 80, Atlas Chemical Co.) | 6.5 |
| Polyoxyethylene sorbitan mono-oleate (Tween 80, Atlas Chemical Co.) | 6.5 |
| Perfume | q.s. |

Melt all ingredients except the powder ingredients at a temperature as low as possible; then add the finely pulverized powders. Homogenize the mass in a colloidal mill or a three-roller mill. Heat to 55°C and stir slowly to remove the air. Pour into containers (not polystyrene or other plastic materials, since they are affected; metal pans are best) and allow to cool.

### Wrinkle Concealers

Some time ago a new type of wrinkle remover was put on the market. If this kind of lotion is thinly applied to the skin and allowed to dry, lines and wrinkles do actually disappear for a few hours. In spite of this effectiveness the sale of these preparations in the United States was prohibited soon after their introduction because of exaggerated and misleading advertising claims.

These preparations were mostly 5% preserved solutions of purified beef serum albumen (egg albumen in alcoholic solution according to U. S. Patent 2,043,657, Goncavora, and albumen from pig ovaries or placenta according to U. S. Patent 3,041,245, Keck and Tronnier, may also be used). Kligman and Papa [30] demonstrated in a clinical study that the effect of these preparations is purely superficial and mechanical: the invisible protein film contracts on drying, thereby stretching the skin which makes the wrinkles disappear.

## HAIRGROOMING AIDS

A neat appearance definitely includes well-groomed hair. However clean and carefully dressed a person may be, if the hair is untidy he or she will create a messy over-all impression. There is surely no need to argue the point—we are all agreed—from the men and women in Central Africa who rub colored butter or rancid coconut fat into their hair to the customers of elegant salons in the cities of the west who prefer somewhat more sophisticated preparations. The field of hairgrooming aids may be regarded as a microcosm of cosmetics: the preparations found here are based on varying principles, companion pieces to all types of skin preparation which were separately discussed in preceding chapters. Some hairgrooming aids are very similar to emollient preparations (Chapter 8) in composition and effect: they compensate for loss of water and fat in the hair shaft and thus restore natural suppleness and gloss. Other preparations contain, in addition to substances that fix the hair and make it lustrous, biological agents that affect the activity of the hair papillae or the antiseptic agents that have already been discussed in Chapter 9. Other types are particularly suitable as a protection against harmful effects of wind, sun, and water and may therefore be regarded as parallel in action to agents that protect the skin (Chapter 7). This may be only of theoretical value, however, since not much use is made in practice of brilliantines, hair oils, and hair creams as protective preparations. Others resemble setting lotions (Chapter 11): they soften the hair and fix it in the position in which it is dressed. There are preparations that have a purely decorative effect and serve only to hold the hair in position and give it luster. Finally there are lotions, pomades, and oils that are used because of the perfume they contain and may therefore be regarded as "olfactory decorative" preparations and some whose main purpose is a freshening up effect.

If we now discuss these preparations (except those that are biologically active and disinfectant) together and, inspite of their differing action, under the heading of "decorative," it is because of the current attitude toward the value and function of the hair. Although certain biological functions are attributed to the hair on the scalp, they are largely relegated to the background, compared with the decorative aspects. Baldness in men and very thin hair in women are primarily regarded as esthetic shortcomings, and for this reason all measures intended to influence the character and appearance of the hair must be regarded as decorative.

Many of the commercially available hairgrooming aids do not belong to just one of the categories mentioned but represent mixed types: for example, they may combine softening and glossy effects, or fixing and fragrant properties. It is therefore more practical to discuss these preparations not in order of their intended effect but according to their composition.

### Anhydrous Brilliantines, Pomades, and Hair Oils

Depending on their wax and oil content, these products are either hard (crystal or stick brilliantine), soft (brilliantine and pomades), or liquid (hair oils, liquid brilliantine). The original difference between brilliantine and pomade was their composition; brilliantine consisted mostly of mineral oils and waxes, pomades of animal and vegetable fats, and special active ingredients. Today there is no longer a sharp differentiation between them; the designations are almost synonymous.

These preparations adhere completely to the hair surface. If they are made of first-class raw materials, their reaction to scalp and hair is neutral. Their principal purpose is to hold the hair in the desired position and to make it lustrous.

They might actually be used as protective preparations against the effect of water and aqueous solutions but this is hardly ever done. Silverman [31] demonstrated that castor oil and lanolin increase the tear resistance of hair (water and alcohol diminish it), but this as well is hardly ever the purpose of using fat-containing hair preparations.

The ability of these preparations to hold the hair in place is based mostly on their cohesion (or their tackiness, less elegantly stated): the fat film surrounding the hair adheres to that surrounding other hairs and this keeps them together. In addition, the film surrounding each hair increases its weight and holds it down.

Still another factor may play a part: shampooing with certain synthetic preparations, and even combing, charge the hair electrostatically [32]. Since all hairs carry the same charge, each repulses the other, which makes the coiffure look ruffled. Brilliantine and hair oil achieve their effect by surrounding each hair with an insulating film which acts against the mutual repulsion.

The more viscous and tacky a preparation, the stronger its cohesion, hence its fixative effect; but tackiness also has disadvantages: it causes difficulty in spreading the preparation evenly through the hair. In addition, very tacky brilliantines attract dust and dirt. Preparations that are just tacky enough to hold the hair in the desired position (which depends on the character of the hair and the hair style) but no more are therefore preferred. Petrolatum, beeswax, animal fats, and certain oils (particularly castor oil and high-viscosity mineral oils) increase the cohesion of these preparations; mineral waxes, spermaceti, low-viscosity mineral oil, and fatty-acid esters, such as isopropyl myristate, decrease it.

Gloss depends on the microscopic characteristics of the surface, on the presence or absence of enevennesses on the order of magnitude of the wavelength of light, that is, 0.0001–0.001 mm; the smoother the surface, the glossier. The hair cuticle consists of minute scales placed like roof tiles; the surface is not microscopically smooth. Normally the hair surface is coated with a thin layer of natural fat secreted by the sebaceous glands of the scalp and has therefore a certain natural sheen. To enhance this or to restore it if it has been lost by the removal of fat or by soiling (dirt particles break the smooth surface of the fat film), brilliantine or hair oils may be used. These preparations make the hair lustrous by surrounding each of them with a smooth fat film. The gloss will be all the stronger, the less the fat is absorbed by the hair and the less it follows the outline of the hair surface; that is, the harder it is. For this reason mineral waxes give a better gloss than lanolin or beeswax, and high-viscosity mineral oils are better than those of low viscosity or isopropyl myristate.

In addition to the classical forms of solid brilliantine in sticks, soft brilliantine and pomades in tubes or jars, and hair oils in bottles, aerosol brilliantines have also become available, but they have not achieved much popularity because they are more expensive yet offer no particular advantages compared with the other types. Almost any hair oil may be turned into an aerosol preparation by filling 10–15 parts of the oil with 85–90 parts of the propellant (Freon 11/12) into suitable containers with spraying valves.

The following are formulations for traditional anhydrous hair preparations:

| | 63 | 64 | 65 | 66 | 67 | 68 | 69 |
|---|---|---|---|---|---|---|---|
| Ceresine | | | 18 | | | | |
| Astrolatum | | | | | 5 | | |
| Beeswax | | | | 5 | 5 | | |
| Spermaceti | | | | 4 | | | |
| Stearic acid | 21 | | | | | | |
| Magnesium stearate | | 10 | | | | | |
| Petrolatum | | | | 48 | | | |
| Paraffin oil | 79 | 89.59 | 30 | 80 | 10 | 75 | 55.5 |
| Isopropyl myristate | | | | | | 25 | |
| Isopropyl palmitate | | | | | | | 10 |
| Hydrogenated peanut oil | | | | | 50 | | |
| Hydrogenated lard | | | | | 30 | | |
| Castor oil | | | | | | | 21 |
| Olive oil | | | | | | | 13 |
| Lanolin, anhydrous | | | | 3 | | | |
| Dichlorophene (G-4) | | | | | | | 0.5 |
| Perfume oil | | 0.4 | 1 | 1 | | q.s. | |
| Color | | | | | | q.s. | |

REMARKS

None of the formulations listed prescribes antioxidants, but their addition is essential, particularly in preparations containing higher proportions of animal or vegetable fats and oils.

63. Crystal brilliantine. Winter, *Handbuch der gesamten Parfümerie und Kosmetik*, 4th ed. p. 500. To obtain an attractive crystallization effect, cooling must be very slow (by pouring into preheated containers). The specific weight of the liquid petrolatum should be 0.880–0.885.

64. Solid brilliantine. Swiss Patent 322,808 (1957). The mixture of mineral oil (s.g. 0.85–0.89) and metal soap is heated to 110–190°C until the mass is transparent. This is subjected to controlled cooling (within one hour the temperature should drop from 120 to 50°C) and the perfume is then added. The resultant mass is thixotropic.

65. Stick brilliantine. Winter, *op. cit.*, p. 501. Melt together with stirring, cool to 35°C, add perfume, and pour into molds.

66. Soft brilliantine. Chilson, *Modern Cosmetics*, 1st ed., 1934, p. 299. Melt the waxes in one container and heat the mineral oil in another to the same temperature. Mix the wax melt and oil thoroughly and add perfume at 45°C.

67. Soft brilliantine. Janistyn, *Riechstoffe, Seifen, Kosmetika*, II, p. 158.

68. Hair oil. *The Use of Isopropyl Myristate in Cosmetics*, A. Boake Roberts & Co., London.

69. Hair oil. Keithler, *The Formulation of Cosmetics and Cosmetic Specialties*, p. 243. The dichlorophene is dissolved in isopropyl palmitate; castor, olive, and mineral oil are then added in that order.

## Hair Creams (Water-in-Oil and Dual Emulsions)

The effect of these preparations is similar to that of the anhydrous products, but in application they have certain advantages so that in northwestern Europe and the United States they have largely replaced brilliantine, pomades, and hair oils. Even if higher proportions of high-viscosity substances are added, the presence of oil-soluble surfactants, which act not only as W/O emulsifiers but as wetting agents, facilitates easy distribution of these preparations in the hair. In addition, they are less tacky and fatty in themselves than the film they leave on the hair when dry. Their appearance is also more appealing than that of anhydrous products because they are white and not glassy-transparent.

One shortcoming of W/O emulsions, however, is their limited stability over long periods of time. The emulsions separate particularly with temperature fluctuations. The introduction of emulsifying agents such as sorbitan sesqui-oleate(Arlacel 83) has facilitated the preparation of emulsions of this type with satisfactory stability and even with comparatively high-water content and low viscosity.

In addition to pure W/O emulsions in which calcium or magnesium soaps are often used as emulsifiers, another type of preparation, dual emulsions (either on a beeswax/borax basis or with nonionic emulsifiers), has also become popular. Their behavior in the hair resembles that of pure W/O emulsions, but they invert to O/W emulsions in the presence of an excess of water and can then be washed off. In this way one of the disadvantages of brilliantines and pomades (fat-staining of clothes, cushions, etc.) has been overcome.

Although fats, oils, and waxes (particularly products of mineral origin) remain entirely on the surface of the hair, oil-soluble surfactants have a pronounced affinity with keratin and very probably penetrate into or under the cuticle. Lanolin, especially, is known to act in this way. It is doubtful, however, whether they also make the hair more manageable in the absence of water, which in preparations of this type hardly penetrates the hair.

| | 70 | 71 | 72 | 73 |
|---|---|---|---|---|
| Mineral oil | 40.60 | 37.5 | 37.5 | 30 |
| Silicone oil | | 1 | | |
| Isopropyl myristate | | | 9.5 | |
| Petrolatum | | 6 | | |
| Beeswax | 1.5 | 8 | 12.0 | 2 |
| Cetyl alcohol | | | 3 | |
| Lanolin | | 3 | | |
| Polyoxyethylene lanolin | | | | 2 |
| Oleic acid | 1.00 | | | |
| Stearic acid | | | 6 | |
| Calcium hydroxide | 0.07 | | | |
| Borax | | 0.5 | 1.4 | |
| Magnesium sulfate (25% in water) | 2.00 | | | |
| Sorbitan sesquioleate | | 3 | | 2 |
| Span 20 | | 1 | | |
| Tween 20 | | 2 | | |
| Span 60 | | | | 2 |
| Saccharose monopalmitate | | | | 2 |
| Water, distilled or deionized | 53.83 | 38 | 30.1 | 59.8 |
| Preservative | | q.s. | | 0.2 |
| Perfume oil | 1.00 | | | |

REMARKS

70. Harry, *Modern Cosmetocology* 4th ed., p. 479. W/O type. Calcium hydroxide is usually added in the form of limewater. This is stirred into the fat melt (70–75°C); then the magnesium sulfate solution is added and finally the perfume oil. Stir until cool.

71. Dual emulsion. "Questions and Answers," *Am. Perfumer*, January, 1957. Stir the aqueous borax solution containing the preservative (75°C) into the fat melt (70°C). Continue stirring until cool. Add perfume at 45°C.

72. Keithler, *The Formulation of Cosmetics and Cosmetic Specialties*, p. 240. Stir the aqueous borax solution (85°C) into the fat melt (85°C). Stir until cool. Add perfume at 50°C.

73. Osipow, Mara, and Snell, *Drug Cosmet. Ind.* **80,** 313 (1957). Stir the aqueous solution of saccharose monopalmitate (75°C) into the fat melt (75°C) in which the other emulsifying agents have also been dissolved. Stir until cool. The polyoxyethylene lanolin is "G-1441" of the Atlas Chemical Co.

## Hair Creams (Oil-in-Water Emulsions)

In many respects these preparations may be compared with the emollients discussed in Chapter 8. As in the corneal layer, flexibility of the hair also depends on the presence of a certain small amount of water in the tissue. In the hair this water is bound by substances such as urea, uric acid, keratin, glycogen, and lactic acid. In addition, the natural fat film surrounding each hair shaft also protects it from strong fluctuations in moisture content by at least delaying, if not preventing, penetration of water into, and evaporation from, the hair. Shampooing, and even more so dyeing, bleaching, and permanent waving, removes the protective film and then exposes the hair for periods of varying duration to alkaline solutions. These solutions, by penetrating the hair, remove the water-soluble water-binding substances and with them the capacity to retain the minimum amount of water required. The result is dry and brittle hair.

There are many similarities between dry skin and dry hair both as far as their causes and the means to combat them are concerned; but there are important differences also: the loss of water and water-binding substances in the skin is gradually restored from the deeper-lying layers; on the basis of present knowledge, however, it is believed that the hair shaft is no longer connected with living tissue and that regeneration is therefore impossible. If hair from which hygroscopic components have been leached out is to be protected from drying out, water must be supplied steadily from the outside. Dry skin is not only unesthetic by itself but also risks infection because the cracks may become seats of inflammation and irritation and affect the deeper layers. This, of course, does not apply to dry hair.

Oil-in-water emulsions may counteract this condition of the hair by supplying water to the hair shaft and surrounding it with a fat film that would prevent recurring evaporation. Usually these preparations also contain humectants, but they penetrate the hair only very slightly if at all; it is doubtful therefore whether they help to make the hair more supple. They may well increase the tackiness of the film on the hair and thereby assist in keeping it in place. On the other hand, they diminish the gloss. W/O creams also contain water, but it is enclosed in the fat phase and probably not accessible to the hairshaft.

The fat film left by O/W creams is much lighter than that left by W/O and anhydrous preparations; it is also less lustrous and less tacky and is soon washed off by rain or sweat. In spite of the slighter gloss-giving and hair-holding properties of these preparations, many consumers give them preference because they are less greasy and make the hair more supple.

REMARKS

74. *SÖFW*, **82,** 542 (1956). Melt stearic acid and lanolin together and add triethanolamine at the last moment. Add the previously prepared gum tragacanth mucilage (which also contains borax and the preservative methyl-*p*-hydroxybenzoate) into the saponified fat and

75. Keithler, *The Formulation of Cosmetics and Cosmetic Specialties*, p. 240. The aqueous polypropylene glycol solution (85°C) to which triethanolamine has been added in the last

| | 74 | 75 | 76 | 77 | 78 | 79 |
|---|---|---|---|---|---|---|
| Mineral oil | | 3 | | | | |
| Silicone oil, 100 cst | | | | | 5 | |
| Isopropyl palmitate | | 5 | | | | |
| Isopropyl myristate | | | | 25 | | |
| Lanolin | | 1.5 | | | | 1 |
| Cetyl alcohol | | 2 | | 1 | | |
| Propylene glycol monostearate SE | 1.5 | 3 | | | | 1 |
| Glycerol monostearate SE | | 2 | | 9 | 4 | |
| Polyethylene glycol (400) monostearate | | | | | 10 | 4 |
| Stearic acid | 15 | 4 | 5 | | | |
| Oleic acid | | 3 | | | | |
| Triethanolamine | 6 | 1.5 | 0.2 | | | |
| Potassium hydroxide 85% | | | 0.1 | | | |
| Borax | 0.75 | | | | | |
| Water, distilled or deionized | 76 | 71.8 | 69.7 | 62 | 81 | 91.64 |
| Polyethylene glycol 1500 | | | 12 | | | |
| Sodium alginate 2% | | | 4 | | | |
| Gum tragacanth powder | 0.9 | | | | | |
| Glycerol | | | | 3 | | |
| Diethylene glycol monoethyl ether (Carbitol) | | | 5 | | | |
| Propylene glycol | | 3 | 3 | | | 2 |
| Perfume oil | 0.4 | | q.s. | | | 0.36 |
| Preservative | 0.15 | 0.2 | q.s. | 0.1 | | |

minute, is stirred into the fat melt (85°C). Continue stirring until the mass has cooled to 50°C and add perfume.

76. Lehne in Sagarin, *Cosmetics: Science and Technology*, p. 572.

77. *The Use of Isopropyl Myristate in Cosmetics*, A. Boake Roberts & Co., London. Heat all ingredients together, with stirring to 85°C. Allow the mass to cool, stirring continuously.

78. Currie and Francisco, *Am. Perfumer*, December 1956. Mix 10 parts polyethylene glycol stearate and 4 parts of glycerol monostearate with 15 parts of water and heat to 80°C. Add silicone oil, with rapid mechanical stirring, and continue to stir while the remaining water is added and until the mass has cooled to about 50°C; pour at this temperature.

79. T. Ruemele, *SÖFW*, **84**, 37 (1958).

## Gum-Based Hair Dressings

After application these hair dressings dry to an entirely or almost entirely invisible elastic film that holds the hair firmly in position. It is a moot point whether the water contained in these preparations also softens the hair and helps to shape it in the same way as a water set (see Chapter 11). These preparations have no hair conditioning properties, nor do they impart gloss to the hair, but they are unexcelled in their capacity to hold curls and waves.

There is a choice of natural gums (tragacanth, karaya, alginate, and pectine) or synthetic mucins (Carbopol 934, polyvinylpyrrolidone, and polyvinyl alcohol). Plasticizers are often added to make the film more elastic: castor oil and mineral oil have been used for this purpose. According to Lehne [33], water-soluble or dispersible lanolin derivatives are suitable for this purpose. Humectants (glycerol, sorbitol, etc.) also help to prevent the film from becoming brittle and chipping off.

|  | 80 | 81 | 82 | 83 |
|---|---|---|---|---|
| Mineral oil, heavy |  |  |  | 1.0 |
| Cetiol V | 4 |  |  |  |
| Eutanol G | 3 |  |  |  |
| Beeswax, sunbleached | 2 |  |  |  |
| Glyceryl monostearate SE | 15 |  |  |  |
| Arnica flower extract | 4 |  |  |  |
| Alginate gel, high viscosity | 27 |  |  |  |
| Gum karaya powder, prime grade |  | 3 |  |  |
| Gum tragacanth powder |  |  |  | 1.0 |
| Quince seed mucilage |  | 20 |  |  |
| Ultra amylopectine, extra |  |  | 1 |  |
| Gelatin |  |  | 0.6 |  |
| Glycerol, white (28°Bé) | 5 | 1 | 2 | 4 |
| Ethyl alcohol |  | 3 |  |  |
| Isopropyl alcohol |  |  |  | 2.0 |
| Borax |  | 0.1 |  |  |
| Water, distilled or deionized | 40 | 72.9 | 96.4 | 91.0 |
| Perfume oil | 0.3 |  |  | q.s. |
| Color |  |  |  | q.s. |

REMARKS

None of the formulations given contains any preservative (the only exception is No. 81 which contains borax and even this is not sufficient for good preservation); for this type of product good preservation is essential because mucilages are susceptible to bacterial or fungus attacks which change their consistency and usually make them thin.

80. Rothemann, *Das grosse Rezeptbuch der Haut- und Körperpflegemittel*, 3rd ed., p. 452. This product represents a transition between O/W creams and gum-based preparations. The alginate mucilage is prepared according to the procedure described in No. 19, Chapter 11. The fats (including the arnica extract) are melted together at 65°C. A mixture of glycerol, alginate mucilage, and water (65°C) is stirred in in a thin jet. Perfume oil is added shortly before cooling.

81 and 82. Janistyn, *Riechstoffe-Seifen-Kosmetika*, II, p. 162.

83. Lehne in Sagarin, *Cosmetics: Science and Technology*, p. 567. Mix the powdered tragacanth with the alcohol, add the glycerol, perfume, and mineral oil, and finally all of the water. Stir until the gum tragacanth is completely dissolved, allow to stand for several hours, and strain. The appearance of the product can be improved by homogenizing it.

## Hair Lacquers

A detailed description of the composition and effect of modern hair lacquers is given by Harris [34].

The properties of hair lacquers are similar to those of gum-based preparations discussed in the preceding section; here as well film-forming substances are the main active ingredients. The difference is in application: hair lacquers are as a rule sprayed into the hair, and the solvent is not water but ethyl or isopropyl alcohol. The preparation therefore dries much faster but the hair-emollient effect of water (to the extent that it plays any part) is lost.

Preparations of this type, based on benzoin, styrax, or shellac solutions, have been known for many years but not widely used. Around 1950 two new inventions gave hair lacquers a new lease on life:

1. The introduction of polyvinylpyrrolidone, a water- and alcohol-soluble substance which, when dry, leaves a supple film with good adhesion to the hair but is removable by washing.

2. The technological refinement of aerosol containers (see Chapter 4), which made their use in cosmetic products possible. These new developments helped to make hair lacquers so popular within a few years that at present aerosol hair sprays are the most widely used aerosol cosmetics.

Some years ago reports that lung disorders could be caused by breathing hair sprays achieved world-wide attention. Subsequent critical tests could not confirm these reports. This matter is discussed in detail by Ludwig [35].

Soon after the introduction of polyvinylpyrrolidone it was found that this material also has certain shortcomings. The most important is its hygroscopicity: in high atmospheric humidity small water droplets precipitate in PVP-treated hair, making it dull and unattractive; in addition, the stability of permanent waves is also reduced. This disadvantage can be overcome at least in part, if a small quantity of shellac is used with the polyvinylpyrrolidone. A water-soluble synthetic resin containing natural rosin (e.g., Lanopal,

BASF) is also reported to improve the properties of the PVP film, according to Obrocki [36]. Additions of lanolin derivatives impart more gloss and elasticity to the film [37]. Silicones can have a beneficial effect on the feel of the hair, the duration of holding it in place, and occasionally also on its appearance [38].

Polyvinylpyrrolidone may be replaced by various other film-forming substances. Some formulations still contain only shellac. De Navarre [39] recommends a copolymer of polyvinylpyrrolidone and vinyl acetate; Philips [40], ethyl cellulose; Cohen [41], a dimethyl hydantoin formaldehyde polymer.

| | 84 | 85 | 86 | 87 |
|---|---|---|---|---|
| Isopropyl myristate | | | | 0.2 |
| Myristyl alcohol | | | | 0.2 |
| Lanolin, liquid | | 1.0 | | 0.2 |
| Lanogel (polyoxyethylene lanolin) | 6.0 | | | |
| Polyvinylpyrrolidone | 2.0 | 12.5 | 7.5 | |
| PVP vinyl acetate copolymer (50%) | | | | 8.0 |
| Dewaxed bleached shellac, dry | | 1.25 | | |
| Lanopal S | | | 0.75 | |
| Water, distilled | 91.8 | | | |
| Ethyl alcohol, anhydrous | | 84.25 | | 90.7 |
| Isopropyl alcohol, anhydrous | | | 90.00 | |
| Perfume oil | q.s. | 1.0 | 1.25 | 0.7 |
| Methyl p-hydroxybenzoate | 0.2 | | | |

REMARKS

84. Berger in Sagarin, *Cosmetics: Science and Technology*, p. 537. This product is not intended for aerosol containers but for glass or polyethylene spray bottles. Procedure: Dissolve the PVP in about half the water; dissolve the preservative in a small portion of boiling water, and the Lanogel in the remainder of the water by stirring slowly (64°C) into the melted Lanogel (63°). Add the preservative solution to the PVP solution and this mixture, when it has cooled, to the cooled Lanogel solution. Finally the perfume oil (water-soluble!) must be added.

85. *"Kinetic" Propellants Bulletin*, E. I. du Pont de Nemours. Twenty parts of this concentrate are mixed with 80 parts of Freon 11/12 (70:30). Freon may be replaced by an equivalent product (see Chapter 4). Unbleached shellac has given generally better results than bleached; it must, in any case, be dewaxed and dry.

86. Obocki, *SÖFW*, **83**, 663 (1957). Forty parts are filled with 60 parts of Freon 11/12 (50:50).

87. Lower and Cressy, *Drug Cosm. Ind.*, **81**, 450 (1957). A 50% solution in anhydrous ethyl alcohol of a copolymer of 60 mole % PVP and 40 mole % vinyl acetate should be used here; 30 parts of this concentrate are mixed with 70 parts Freon 11/12 (70:30).

## Alchohol-Based Hair Lotions

For a long time many people have been using hair lotions that consist merely of an alcoholic solution (possibly colored) of some perfume oil. These products do not hold the hair in shape, nor do they give it sheen or improve its suppleness. They are used because they have a pleasant odor and stimulate the scalp when rubbed in. Even if they cannot be counted as skin or hair conditioners (with the exception of a certain disinfectant effect which may be attributed to the alcohol in spite of its rapid evaporation), they certainly have their reasons for being. In addition to these products, there are others on the market whose cosmetic value has been improved by certain additives. The stimulating effect is increased by tincture of capsicum or arnica, quinine salts, and many other substances, and the antiseptic action, by disinfectants (hexachlorophene, o-phenylphenol, etc.). Quaternary ammonium salts are particularly valuable as disinfectant additives because they also serve to make the hair supple and reduce its electrostatic charge. Other substances may be added to increase the slight and fleeting foaming effect of alcoholic hair lotions (saponins, etc.), water- or alcohol-soluble waxlike substances (in particular, polyethylene glycols and their monofatty acid esters), which impart luster to the hair (similar to "genuine" waxes without being fatty) and hold it in place. Small quantities of fatty acid esters such as isopropyl myristate can be dissolved in 60–70% alcohol. Sometimes film-forming substances (gum tragacanth, CMC, etc.) are added. Higher proportions of these materials turn liquid hair lotions into solid fat-free gels.

The following are a few examples from the many possible formulations:

|  | 88 | 89 | 90 | 91 |
|---|---|---|---|---|
| Isopropyl palmitate |  |  | 6.0 |  |
| Polyethylene glycol (400) coconut fatty acid monoester |  |  |  | 2.0 |
| Propylene glycol monolaurate |  |  |  | 1.1 |
| Tween 20 |  |  | 3.0 |  |
| Butoxypolyoxy propylene glycol |  |  |  | 20 |
| β-Naphthol |  | 0.2 |  |  |
| Salicylic acid |  | 0.2 |  |  |
| o-Phenylphenol |  |  | 0.1 |  |
| Cetyl dimethyl benzyl ammonium chloride 50% |  |  |  | 1.0 |
| Capsicum tincture |  |  |  | 0.5 |
| Quillaja saponin | 0.11 |  |  |  |
| Alcohol 95% | 56.10 |  | 49.9 | 51.25 |
| Isopropyl alcohol |  | 49.6 |  |  |
| Water | 43.25 | 49.6 | 41.0 | 23.25 |
| Perfume oil | 0.54 |  | q.s. | 0.40 |
| Color | q.s. |  |  | q.s. |

REMARKS

88. Janistyn, *Riechstoffe-Seifen-Kosmetika*, II, p. 149. Eau de Portugal. The perfume used should be easily soluble. This preparation is colored a golden yellow.

89. Harry, *Modern Cosmetocology*, 4th ed., p. 387.

90. Keithler, *The Formulation of Cosmetics and Cosmetic Specialties*, p. 243. Dissolve the o-phenylphenol in alcohol; to this solution add a mixture of isopropyl palmitate and Tween 20 and then the water. Strain if required.

91. U. S. Patent 2,771,394.

## Two-Phase Lotions

Alcohol-based hair lotions have the disadvantage of having a rather strong drying effect on the scalp and hair. Whether this "defatting" actually amounts to a removal of scalp and hair fat or represents the removal of the water from only the top skin and hair layers (alcohol stronger than 50% has a dehydrating effect) is not clear. It is a fact, however, that people with dry scalps will increase this dryness if they use alcoholic lotions regularly; any tendency to dandruff will also be increased by these preparations as long as they contain no therapeutic additives.

It has been tried again and again to counteract this dehydrating effect by adding fats and at the same time to give the hair lotion control- and gloss-imparting properties. Fatty acid esters such as isopropyl palmitate may be added, but the dosage is restricted, for otherwise the solution would cloud. Castor oil, the only vegetable oil soluble in low alcohol concentrations, leaves an unpleasantly tacky film on the hair and is therefore not suitable for hair lotions, although it has been used on occasion. However, if castor oil is added, the alcohol concentration must be increased to about 80% instead of the normal 60–70%, which again strengthens the defatting effect.

The best way of adding considerable quantities of fats to alcoholic lotions is by creating two-phase products. In addition to the aqueous-alcoholic phase, they also contain an oil phase which forms a separate layer that floats on top or settles on the bottom. Shaking before use forms a simple coarse emulsion which enables the user to apply the oil and water-alcohol phases simultaneously in the correct proportions. It is not easy to prepare a good lotion of this kind: before shaking, both phases must be completely clear; in order to achieve this clarity, the selection of suitable color and perfume is essential. On the other hand, the surface tension between the two phases must be low enough to produce an emulsion that remains stable for at least as long as it takes to apply it. The surface tension may be reduced by adding surfactants (U. S. Patent 2,543,061, 1951).

The following formulations by Lehne (Sagarin, *Cosmetics: Science and Technology*, p. 564) should serve only as suggestions. It should certainly be possible to improve these

470 PREPARATIONS WITH SURFACE EFFECT

simple preparations with various additions:

|  | 92 | 93 | 94 |
|---|---|---|---|
| Mineral oil | 50 | | |
| Olive oil | | 8 | |
| Castor oil | | | 3 |
| Almond oil | | | 40 |
| Ethyl alcohol, 95% | 18 | 45 | 57 |
| Water | 32 | 47 | |
| Perfume and coloring | q.s. | q.s. | q.s. |

## REFERENCES

[1] *Am. Perfumer*, **36** (8), 50 (1936).

[2] *J. Allergy*, **12**, 135 (1940–1941).

[3] Daniels, *Drug Cosmet. Ind.*, **83**, 162 (1958).

[4] Janistyn, *Riechstoffe, Seifen, Kosmetika*, II, p. 221. Dr. Alfred Hüthig, Heidelberg, 1950.

[5] Kalish, *Drug Cosmet. Ind.*, **78**, 176 (1956).

[6] Hilfer, *Drug Cosmet. Ind.*, **80**, 450 (1957); Daniels, *ibid.*, **82**, 442 (1958).

[7] *J. Soc. cosmet. Chem.*, **16**, 105 (1965).

[8] *Schimmel Briefs*, **247**, (October 1955); Hoffmann, paper read at "Sepawa" Convention 1957; *SÖFW*, **83**, 729 (1957).

[9] *Kosmetik-Parf.-Drog.*, **4**, 86 (1957).

[10] Ruemele, *Kosmetik-Parf.-Drog.*, **4**, 3 (1957); Neumann, *J. Soc. cosmet. Chem.*, **8**, 44 (1957); *Parfum. Kosmet.*, **38**, 463 (1957).

[11] Jakovics, *Drug Cosmet. Ind.*, **80**, 316 (1957).

[12] *J. Soc. cosmet. Chem.*, **8**, 44 (1957).

[13] Keithler, *The Formulation of Cosmetics and Cosmetic Specialties*, p. 163. Drug and Cosmetic Industry, New York, 1956.

[14] *Schimmel Briefs*, **249** (1955).

[15] G. Achten, *Am. Perfumer*, **79** (9), 23 (1964).

[16] Sidi, *Verträglichkeit der Kosmetika*, German edition, p. 59.

[17] *Ibid.*, 59.

[18] *Parfum. Kosmet.*, **38**, 100 (1957).

[19] Kittel, *Celluloselacke;* Kraus, *Handbuch der Celluloselacke; Nitrocellulose Handbook*, Hercules Powder Co. Wilmington, Delaware, 1948.

[20] *Drug Cosmet. Ind.*, **80**, 308 (1957).

[21] Keithler, *Drug Cosmet. Ind.*, **80**, 308 (1957).

[22] French Patent 1,000,605; *Parfum. Kosmet.*, **38**, 650 (1957).

[23] *Parfum. Kosmet.*, **39**, 800 (1958).

[24] French Patent 1,000,605; *Parfum. Kosmet.*, **38**, 650 (1957).

[25] *J. Soc. cosmet. Chem.*, **1**, 17 (1947).

[26] Janistyn, *op. cit.*, II, 227.

[27] Winter, *Handbuch der gesamten Parfümerie und Kosmetik*, Springer, Vienna, 3rd ed., 1942, p. 547.

[28] Janistyn, *op. cit.*, II, 232.

[29] Harry, *Modern Cosmetocology*, 4th ed. p. 207. Leonard Hill, London, 1955.

[30] Kligman and Papa, *J. Soc. cosmet. Chem.*, **16**, 557 (1965).

[31] *Drug Cosmet. Ind.*, **90**, 292 (1962).

[32] Walker, *SÖFW*, **83**, 727 (1957).

[33] Sagarin, *Cosmetics: Science and Technology*, p. 566. Interscience, New York, 1957.

[34] *J. Soc. Cosmet. Chem.*, **14**, 469 (1963).

[35] *Parfum. Kosmet.*, **45**, 5 (1964).

[36] *SÖFW*, **83**, 663 (1957).

[37] Herzka, *Aerosol Report 2*, **119**, 150 (1963).

[38] Bishop, *Proc. Chem. Spec. Mfrs. Ass.*, **163**, 49.

[39] *Am. Perfumer* 31 (January 1957).

[40] *Drug Cosm. Ind.*, **75**, 30 (1954).

[41] *Drug Cosm. Ind.*, **81**, 304 (1957).

CHAPTER 11

# Decorative Preparations: Preparations with Lasting Effect

The decorative cosmetics that women use today consist mostly of coloring or matting preparations which may slightly stain the skin's top corneal layer. Occasionally more drastic measures are adopted: bleaching preparations degrade the pigments in the deeper skin layers or prevent pigment formation; peeling removes the top corneal layers. Of course, these procedures do not exhaust all possibilities of decorating the skin: dyes can be introduced into the epidermal tissue (tattooing) or scars can be produced arbitrarily. Western women, however, do not go so far.

It is quite common to deal more radically with the appendages of the skin, that is, the hair and nails, which are—justifiably or not—regarded as dead tissue: these tissues are regularly trimmed, the hair on various surfaces of the body is sometimes completely removed, and scalp hair is treated in such a way that it entirely changes color or shape for extended periods. In addition, hair and nails may be colored or the gloss heightened.

In the preceding chapter we discussed the preparations used to alter skin, hair, and nails superficially. In this chapter we discuss those preparations that are used to cause more lasting decorative changes. Logically, nonpermanent hair dyes should have been discussed in Chapter 10, but it seems more practical to include them with all other hair-dyeing preparations.

### HAIR DYES AND BLEACHES

Modern women, wishing to change the natural color of their hair, have three types of products at their disposal:

1. Temporary coloring that does not actually dye the hair but intensifies or brightens the natural shade. These tints usually last only until the next shampoo.

2. Permanent dyes that impart any desired shade to the hair. These dyes last for an almost unlimited period, but the dyed hair is gradually replaced by fresh growth.

3. Bleaching agents that make the color lighter; bleaches are occasionally used in conjunction with permanent or temporary coloring.

In the following section we discuss each type separately.

### Temporary Coloring

The most important representatives of this type are the so-called color rinses, most of which are marketed as dry powders. The powder consists of a crystalline organic acid (tartaric acid is preferable because it is less hygroscopic than most other crystalline acids), in which a solution of water-soluble synthetic dye is incorporated, or of a mixture of 0.5–2% dye in powder form and 98–99.5% crystalline acid. Before use the powder is dissolved in the prescribed quantity of hot water and the hair is rinsed with this solution until the solution has almost completely lost its color. Sometimes these preparations are sold in tablet or liquid form.

Color rinses are commercially available in all possible shades. They are mainly intended to give the hair a brighter and more vivid appearance after shampooing, or to "bring out the highlights." They are popular also for restoring coloring of hair that has faded from too much sun or permanent waving or for giving an attractive shade to graying hair that has yellowed and dulled. The colors of these rinses do not strongly adhere to healthy hair and are easily removed by shampooing.

If, however, the natural structure of the hair has been damaged by bleaching or permanent waving, the colors often adhere more strongly. The use of shampoos based on certain synthetic detergents may also cause stronger adhesion of the color. These rinses are often used at home without professional assistance. For this reason manufacturers of these preparations must supply complete directions for use with the recommendation that the rinse be tried first on a small strand of hair before treating the whole head. Preliminary tests to determine whether the user is allergic to one dye or another are hardly possible if the rinse is used at home.

A typical formula for an auburn rinse of this type is the following:
1. (F. E. Wall in E. Sagarin, *Cosmetics: Science and Technology*, p. 487):

| | |
|---|---|
| FD & C Orange No. 1 | 1.16 |
| FD & C Red No. 1 | 0.17 |
| D & C Violet No. 1 | 0.20 |
| Crystalline acid | 98.47 |
| | 100.00 |

Occasionally small quantities of water-soluble dyes are added to shampoos or setting lotions with the same intention of bringing out the highlights.

## Permanent Dyes

Color rinses are not sufficient if more than freshening up is required, that is, an actual change of color or the covering of gray hair. For this purpose dyes with better adherence or preferably those that even penetrate the hair shaft and thus produce much more intense shades are required: "permanent" dyes are needed.

A hair dye of this type must meet the following requirements:

If used correctly, it must not irritate the scalp, act as a sensitizer, damage the hair itself, or cause toxicity symptoms in the organism when the dye is applied only externally.

It should give the hair natural color and not affect gloss or suppleness.

The color must not change under the influence of sunlight, cold- or hot-wave solutions, shampoos, hair lacquer, brilliantines, hair creams, or alcoholic hair lotions.

A hair dye must never stain the scalp.

The dyeing process should be quick and simple.

The dye must never make subsequent permanent waving difficult or even impossible.

No one hair dye known today meets all of these requirements. For this reason, probably, numerous laboratories all over the world are engaged in intensive research in this particular field of cosmetics. Almost every month new patents appear, which often describe only small modifications of existing methods but occasionally present fundamentally new processes of dyeing. It is quite impossible to deal with all the new developments here particularly since their practical value cannot be predetermined. We limit ourselves to a general discussion of the three permanent dyeing methods that have been used on a large scale for many years: coloring with metal salts, vegetable extracts, and oxidation dyes.

**Dyeing with Metal Salts.**    Salts of lead, silver, copper, nickel, bismuth, cobalt, and manganese are used in products often erroneously described as "preparations to restore the natural color of hair." It was formerly assumed that sulfides formed by these salts with the sulfur of hair keratin were deposited in the hair shaft. Opinion today is rather that under the influence of light, air, and developer solutions insoluble oxides or sulfides are formed and are adsorbed on the surface of the hair shaft.

The advantage of these preparations is that their application is simple and that all shades from lightest blond to deepest black can be obtained with metallic dyes.

On the other hand, metallic dyes have a number of important drawbacks. Some of them, in particular lead colors, are toxic. The required coloring is obtained only after several treatments. Gray hair, for instance, gradually develops shades from yellow to brown and black if treated with lead acetate. Although the tints obtained with metallic salts are attractive when fresh, they often appear dusty with time. Permanent waving of hair dyed with metallic salts is often difficult and sometimes impossible. For these reasons metal colors have already lost much of their popularity and their use will probably continue to decline.

Space does not allow us to go into detail about the formulation of all the different types of metallic dye. We refer interested readers to the full discussion by Winter [1] and Janistyn [2] and give in the following merely a few formulas from Winter's book which may serve as examples:

2. BLOND

*Flask* 1           *Flask* 2

| Silver nitrate | 40 g | Pyrogallol | 20 g |
|---|---|---|---|
| Ammonia, 10% | 200 ml | Water | 1000 ml |
| Water | abt. 800 ml | | |

In Flask 1 ammonia is used in the amount required to dissolve the initially developing precipitation. The flasks containing the silver solution must be made of dark glass and be completely closed.

First apply solution 1, allow to dry, apply No. 2.

3. AUBURN

*Flask* 1           *Flask* 2

| Copper sulfate | 52 g | Pyrogallol | 18 g |
|---|---|---|---|
| Nitric acid, concentrated | 50 drops | Water | 850 ml |
| Water | 850 ml | | |

4. AUBURN

*Flask* 1           *Flask* 2

| Cobalt nitrate | 25 g | Potassium sulfide | 45 g |
|---|---|---|---|
| Nickel sulfide | 25 g | Alcohol | 500 g |
| Water | 350 g | Water | 500 g |

Silver salts are often used for coloring eyebrows and lashes. Pyrogallol, which is not recommended for use in the area of the eyes, is replaced here as a developer by sodium thiosulfate in solutions up to 5%. The solutions should be applied with a brush, first the thiosulfate solution, then after 2–3 minutes the silver salt solution.

**Vegetable Hair Colorings.** *Henna* is the most important ingredient of vegetable hair dyes. The word is arabic for the dried leaves and branches of the bush *Lawsonia alba* L. (also *Lawsonia inermis* L.). The substance responsible for the dying capacity of henna extract was isolated by Tommasi (1916) and identified as 2-hydroxy-1,4-naphthoquinone; the common name is Lawson.

Henna may be applied in various forms: in one it may be extracted with boiling water and poured several times over freshly washed hair. More permanent coloring is achieved by applying a paste made from henna powder and boiling water and leaving it on the hair until the desired shade is obtained. Finally, henna may also be mixed with shampoo, but it does not fully develop its effectiveness in this way since it works best in an acid environment. Henna extract is intensively red. The color left on the hair is orange red. However, this color appears only on white hair. Generally, a shade is obtained in which the natural color of the hair plays an important part. Combination of henna with other vegetable extracts or with metallic salt colors yields varying shades. Combining henna with a metallic salts improves its adhesion to the hair; the salts act as a precipitating agent and form stronger links with the hair keratin.

Even by itself henna has a strong affinity with hair keratin. For a long time it was not clear whether henna is adsorbed at the exterior of the hair shaft or actually penetrates it; today's opinion holds the former view. Henna (which is often unpleasant in application) also adheres strongly to the nails; women in Middle East and India dye their palms and soles with it as well.

Modern hair-coloring practice occasionally uses the extract of camomile flowers (*Anthemis nobilis*, Roman camomile, or *Matricaria chamomilla*, German or Hungarian camomile) which produces shades of golden yellow. Like henna, it may be used as a rinse, pack, or shampoo. It is often combined with henna; depending on the proportion of the extracts and the natural shade of the hair, golden blond to dark auburn can be obtained.

*Reng* (the powdered dried leaves of the bush *Indigofera argentea*) is also occasionally applied, mostly in combination with henna. It gives dark shades, for the active dye is indigo.

Formerly, bluewood and other wood extracts were used for hair-coloring preparations, but they have been replaced increasingly by oxidation dyes. The main advantage of vegetable extracts in hair coloring is their nontoxicity, their nonirritating effect on the scalp, and the infrequency of allergic reactions to them. Paradoxically, their main disadvantage is that the shades obtained with them appear less natural than those obtained with synthetic dyes. Henna, for example, tends to make the hair carroty to orange red. In addition, vegetable dyes seem to alter the structure of the hair keratin; after a time the hair becomes dry and brittle.

The range of shades can be increased by combining vegetable extracts with various salts. In this case, the advantage of nontoxicity and harmlessness is at least partly lost.

The following formulations will give the reader a general idea of the composition of the dyes based on vegetable extracts. A collection of more detailed formulations can be found in Winter [1] or Janistyn [2].

5. HENNA BLOND (Winter, *op. cit.*, p. 578)

Henna, 40 parts      Reng, 40 parts

The mixture is applied as a pack and left about 30 minutes. If left for an hour or two, brown shades are obtained.

6. Winter, *op. cit.*, p. 579.

| (a) Henna | 1 part | (b) Henna | 1 part |
|---|---|---|---|
| Reng | 0.3 part | Roman camomile | 0.5 part |
| Sumac | 0.3 part | Onion skin | 0.2 part |
| Walnut leaves | 0.3 part | | |
| Catechu | 0.3 part | | |

Each of these mixtures is ground and used according to requirements. The shades obtained are: mixture (a), black; 3 parts (a) and one part (b), brown; two parts each (a) and (b), dark blond; one part (a) and 3 parts (b), blond. Immediately before use 0.1% pyrogallol is added to each mixture. The mixture is then stirred into boiling soap water, heated for about 5 seconds, and applied hot to the hair. It is rinsed off after about 10–20 minutes. The presence of a triethanolamine soap is recommended in order to achieve a natural non-glossy shade.

7. MAHOGANY BROWN (Winter, *op. cit.*, p. 595)

| Henna powder | 400 g |
|---|---|
| Iron powder | 200 g |
| Cobalt nitrate | 40 g |
| Pyrogallol | 20 g |
| Borax | 20 g |
| Ammonium chloride | 20 g |

Powder and hot water are stirred to a creamy paste and applied to the well-degreased hair. After application the dyed hair is immediately covered with cotton and wrapped in a woolen cloth. Apply at 50–60°C for 15 minutes. Finally wash with abundant water and shampoo.

**Oxidation Dyes.** These dyes are steadily replacing vegetable and metallic colors in practice. They offer the possibility of creating a wide range of shades which are more natural in quality than those obtained with vegetable and metallic colors. (For their disadvantages, see p. 485.)

Oxidation dyes differ from the types already discussed by penetrating the hair shafts. This has been shown in an impressive series of photos by Preisinger and Dräger [3] which shows the microscopic picture of the dyeing process with oxidation dyes. The structure of the hair enables small molecules to penetrate the outer keratinic layers. Molecules of organic and inorganic dyes are too large to do so even if the hair keratin is swollen and loosened under the influence of water and alkalies [4]. Oxidation dyes contain substances such as *p*-phenylenediamine and *p*-aminophenol whose molecules are just small enough to penetrate hair keratin once it is loosened by water and alkalies; these substances are not actually dyes but may be transformed into dyes by treatment with oxidizing agents in an alkaline medium. The first stage of the reaction is the oxidation of the diamine or aminophenol to a quinone; this is followed by coupling three quinone molecules to one large molecule which, after further oxidation, develops into a dye with a strong affinity for hair keratin.

The principle of coloring with oxidation dyes is the introduction into the hair shaft of diamine or aminophenol (the base) and an oxidant (hydrogen peroxide or possibly molecular oxygen). The organic coupling reaction occurs within the hair shaft, and it is here that the actual dye develops. Finally, the excess oxidant and alkali are rinsed off.

A series of articles by Kass [5] is one of the few published accounts in which the composition of modern oxidation dyes is discussed in detail. Comprehensive descriptions are also given by Wall [6] and Mannheim [7].

According to Kass [5], the dye intermediates in modern oxidation dyes are variously substituted *o*- and *p*-phenylenediamines, aminophenols, and derivatives of these substances; *p*-phenylene and *p*-toluylenediamine are the most important basic ingredients for most dark and some blond shades. For many blond shades aminophenols are the most important bases; for red shades *p*-aminophenol and certain nitro derivatives are used. Some N-alkyl-*p*-phenylenediamines produce very attractive effects, but the substances of this group have a strong irritating action. N-alkylaminophenols are rarely used. Sulfonyl and nitrodiamines as well as nitroaminophenols were formerly important because of their low toxicity, but nowadays are used only as shading agents; they take much longer to act because with their large molecules they penetrate less easily into the hair.

More than 30 bases are in use at present, too many to discuss in detail. The interested reader is referred to Kass [5] and Wall [6].

Apart from the actual bases, modern hair dyes also contain color modifiers and stabilizers which by themselves have no coloring effect but combine in the coupling reaction with the bases and thus modify or stabilize the shade obtained. Substances used for this purpose are di- and trihydroxybenzene compositions, salicylic acid, and gallic acid in combination with *p*-phenylenediamine; *m*-phenylenediamine is also an important shading agent for *p*-phenylenediamine. It causes a deflection of the shades into blues and is therefore useful for silver blond, steel gray and similar colors.

The bases, of course, must be substances that are easily oxidized. It is undesirable, however, that oxidation occur during manufacture or storage because the dyes that would develop then have molecules too large to penetrate the hair shafts. For this reason oxidation dyes are generally manufactured and stored in a nitrogeneous atmosphere. In addition, antioxidants are added to the solutions in dosages that depend on the amount of oxidizable bases present.

The most widely used antioxidant in hair dyes is sodium sulfite; thioglycolic acid is also reported to be useful [8].

It follows from the foregoing that liquid oxidation dyes consist of an aqueous solution of bases, modifiers, and stabilizers, with an addition of antioxidants. Water as the only solvent does not yield clear solutions, however. *Auxiliary solvents* are therefore frequently added; that is, alcohols (e.g., ethyl or isopropyl alcohol) which tend to accelerate the effect of the dye on the hair or polyhydroxy compounds (propylene glycol, glycerol, sorbitol) which are said to inhibit the dyeing process.

Homogeneous solutions may also be obtained by adding *surfactants*. These solutions not only act as solubilizers for the bases but (as wetting agents) they accelerate the coloring of the hair and (as detergents) assist in rinsing out the unused chemicals after the dyeing process is finished. As mentioned by Wall [6], great care must be taken in selecting surfactants and determining their proper dosage; (some, e.g., alkyl aryl sulfonates) are easily absorbed by hair keratin and thus impede the dyeing process; others (e.g., Turkey red oils) may even remove the freshly applied color during subsequent shampooing. In the case of dosages of surfactants that are too high it may happen that the color will not adhere to the hair at all.

Only surfactants that are effective in an alkaline environment should be selected because oxidation dyes are always adjusted to the alkaline range, usually pH 9–10. Oxidation within this range is most satisfactory; furthermore the alkali promotes swelling of the keratin.

The most widely used alkali is *ammonia* because it softens the hair without damaging it; it has also been established that with ammonia at a given pH value a deeper color is obtained than if the identical pH has been produced by an addition of soda lye or other alkalies. (British Patent 712,451, 1954, covers the use of triethanolamine in combination with a polyhydroxyl compound and an ammonium salt as buffering agent at pH 7–9). Many dyes are sensitive to the prevailing pH, and a shift of only 0.5 units may affect the shade very noticeably. In the finished solutions, ready for application, ammonia should be present in a concentration not higher than 1%; an excess irritates the scalp.

So far we have discussed the solution of the base. When hair is colored with oxidation dyes, a second solution is used: that of the oxidizing agent. These two solutions are mixed shortly before the beginning of the dyeing process; 5–6% solutions of hydrogen peroxide have proved most satisfactory as oxidizing solutions. Stronger solutions act more rapidly but may easily cause serious skin lesions if improperly applied. A urea-hydrogen peroxide complex, a white solid substance containing about 35% hydrogen peroxide, is also often used. This complex is highly hygroscopic and becomes unstable when it has absorbed water. It is marketed in the form of tablets packed individually in water-impermeable envelopes; these tablets are dissolved in the prescribed amount of water for preparing an oxidizing solution.

Degradation of peroxide in contact with the dye should not occur too rapidly because it may result in an incomplete oxidation and consequently in wrong coloring, inadequate stability, or an irritation of the scalp. With well-formulated oxidation dyes the coloring process is completed after 50–60 minutes, with some peroxide left at the end. Oxidation occurs rapidly within the first 5–10 minutes after mixing the two solutions and slows down afterwards.

Commercially available solutions of peroxide always contain stabilizers because they are otherwise unstable and their oxidizing power decreases during storage. Suitable stabilizers, according to Weigel [9], are acetanilide, Komplexon III (a sequestering agent), and a mixture of acid potassium phosphate and phosphoric acid.

In addition to hydrogen peroxide and its urea complex, various perborates, bromates, or chlorites are used as oxidizing agents. Weigel [9] discusses the advantages and disadvantages of the various materials.

It is not easy to develop a really good formulation for oxidation dyes. Only very rarely can the desired shade be obtained with one base alone; usually it is necessary to use a combination of various bases, modifiers, and stabilizers. According to Kass, modern oxidation dyes often contain as many as 12 different bases. The effects of the individual ingredients are not additive because in the coupling reaction, which leads to the formation of the actual dyes, cross reactions among the bases may occur. The shade obtained always depends on the vehicle, its pH, the duration of the dyeing process, and the original color of the hair.

It is obvious that hair dying requires long practice and that chemists or companies that have developed good formulas are most reluctant to disclose them. This is the reason why the literature is so devoid of usable formulations for oxidation dyes.

Another factor adds yet a further complication: the shade not only depends on the formulation but also on the degree of purity of the bases used; often identically named products from different manufacturers result in different shades.

Oxidation dyes are marketed in various forms.

1. *Clear solutions.* The solvent is usually a mixture of water and alcohol (ethyl or isopropyl alcohol) which has been adjusted to the required pH with ammonia. The hair is first shampooed and treated with a hydrogen peroxide solution; then the base and oxidation solutions are mixed together and immediately applied to the hair. After completion of the dyeing process the hair is shampooed.

Clear colors are the oldest form of oxidation dyes. Many hairdressers perfer them because they permit constant observation of the dyeing process.

2. *Shampoo tints.* These tints contain larger quantities of surfactants and occasionally fats which are intended to protect the hair or restore the fat content. The base solution should not be too viscous to run out of the container, yet viscous enough to remain on the hair after being mixed with the peroxide solution.

3. *Cream dyes.* There is the same difference between cream and liquid dyes that occurs between cream and liquid shampoos. Since the development of the color is not easily distinguished on the hair, working with this type of preparation requires much practice in order to achieve good results.

Kass provides the following formulations, among others [10]:

|  | 8<br>Medium Brown | 9<br>Ash Blond | 10<br>Honey Blond |
|---|---|---|---|
| p-phenylenediamine | 2.00 | 0.50 | 0.20 |
| o-aminophenol | 0.20 | 0.10 | 0.13 |
| p-aminophenol |  | 0.10 |  |
| 4-nitro-1,2-diaminobenzene | 0.15 | 0.20 |  |
| p-methylaminophenol sulfate |  |  | 0.40 |
| p-aminodiphenylamine | 0.20 | 0.05 | 0.10 |
| 3,4-diaminoanisol |  | 0.025 |  |
| Resorcinol | 1.00 | 0.50 | 0.20 |
| Pyrogallol |  |  | 0.20 |
| Sodium sulfite |  | 0.30 | 0.20 |
| Borax |  |  | 0.40 |
| These mixtures of active ingredients are dissolved in |  |  |  |
| Ammonia (26°Bé = 29.4 wt% $NH_3$) | 10.0 |  |  |
| Isopropyl alcohol | 2.5 |  |  |
| Perfume | 0.5 |  |  |

The following emulsion (cold) is stirred slowly into this solution:

| | |
|---|---|
| Oleic acid | 35.00 |
| Polyoxyethylene sorbitan mono-oleate | 10.00 |
| Nonionic surfactant | 3.50 |
| Lanolin derivative, water-soluble | 1.75 |
| Lecithin | 1.25 |
| Chelating agent(s) | 0.25 |
| Water | abt. 33, to make |
| | 100 parts in total |

The pH of the finished product is adjusted with ammonia; for formula 8 it should be 9.2; for formula 9, 9.5, and for formula 10, 9.0.

Shortly before use these solutions should be mixed with an equal volume of 5% aqueous hydrogen peroxide solution. They are then brushed into the hair. The color develops within 15–40 minutes (usually 20–30 minutes). The process is finished by rinsing with water.

4. *Gel dyes.* To circumvent the disadvantage of not being able to observe the color development during treatment, oxidation dyes in gel form have been developed (Swiss Patent 308,685 of Kleinol A. G.) The following formula is given in this patent:

11. Prepare a mucilage from

> 2.4 parts cellulose ether and
> 87.6 parts water. Add
>
> 4.2 parts triethanolamine
> 2.4 parts ethylene glycol
> 2.4 parts ammonium tartrate
> 1.0 part paraffin sulfonate
> ___
> 100.0 parts

Heat 93.1 parts of this mixture to 50°C and add

> 0.6  parts *p*-toluylenediamine sulfate
> 0.05 parts *p*-aminophenolchlorohydrate
> 0.25 parts resorcinol dissolved in
> 6.0  parts ethyl alcohol
> ___
> 6.90

The pH of the finished product should be 8.7. Even without preliminary treatment this product is reported to impart a uniform dark color even if the hair does not "take" very easily.

5. *Dye crayons.* British Patent 749,045 (Indola N. V.) describes anhydrous crayons, dispersible in water, made of fatty acid alkanolamides, fatty

alcohols, and about 10% emulsifiers that contain the usual bases, an alkali (e.g., triethanolamine), and an antioxidant (e.g., sodium sulfite). The hair is treated first with hydrogen peroxide. The crayon is applied like oil chalk and after the required development period rinsed off with water.

Before any hair dye is marketed it must be thoroughly tested. It is not sufficient that the dye develops a satisfactory shade on healthy white hair; it must also be effective on hair that has undergone repeated permanent wave treatments and washed with strong alkaline soap or firmly adhering synthetic shampoos. In addition, the dye must not make the hair brittle or impede permanent waving.

Only when these tests have shown satisfactory results is there any point in checking on toxicity or irritating properties, and only when these conditions are negative may the product be marketed.

*Incompatibility to Oxidation Dyes.*   At the beginning of this section we spoke about the advantages of oxidation dyes compared with vegetable and metallic dyes. They also have an important drawback: incompatibility symptoms are relatively frequent.

There is an abundance of reports in the medical literature of the serious skin lesions and damage to general health that result from the use of oxidation dyes. These publications, however, should be examined critically if they are to be evaluated to their present significance. Oxidation dyes have been used for more than 60 years. Reports of damage in the first 30–35 years are hardly relevant today because the composition of the dyes, the purity of the basic materials, and practical application procedures have been considerably improved in the meantime. In addition, many reports in the literature are not based on personal observations of the authors but on the hearsay evidence of others. Studies during the last 15 years point to a lower incidence of incompatibility than might have been expected from the older literature, provided modern oxidation dyes are expertly applied to healthy subjects [11]. Nevertheless, it is advisable for the hairdresser to carry out a simple patch test before starting a dyeing treatment to determine whether the customer shows any symptoms of incompatibility. In France these tests are required by law.

The most widely used base has always been *p*-phenylenediamine, and for this reason it has generally been found that most incompatibility symptoms caused by hair dyes can be attributed to its presence. The fact that this material was so frequently mentioned led to the erroneous conclusion that it must be particularly harmful and several European countries (e.g., Germany and France) have prohibited its use. As a result, the manufacturers of hair dyes have in general replaced *p*-phenylenediamine with *p*-toluylenediamine. It is ironic that it is no less harmful [12]; in application it may even be more dangerous because it dyes less intensively than *p*-phenylenediamine and is therefore used in higher concentrations. As Sidi has mentioned, hairdressers believe that because *p*-phenylenediamine is prohibited, all products that do not contain it must be harmless and therefore they have become neglectful of certain precautions. Hopefully, the prohibition of *p*-phenylenediamine will eventually be rescinded and replaced with a more realistic regulation. Generally the dye base solution has a less harmful effect on the hair than the simultaneously applied oxidation solution. Strong oxidants cause certain irreversible reactions in the hair keratin which permanently and adversely affect the structure of the hair. Concentration and duration of the treatment with oxidizing solutions should therefore be limited as much as possible. Berth and Reese [13] have described a method of measuring damage to the hair by dyes and bleaches.

**Direct Hair Dyeing Methods [14].** New hair-dyeing procedures based on dyes resembling the bases in the oxidation dyes, without the need for an additional oxidation agent, have recently been developed. One method of so-called "direct dyeing" consists in the use of triaminophenols and their derivatives; these dyes may be developed to their final color under the influence of atmospheric oxygen alone.

Phototropic compounds, also recommended, are converted to a dye under the influence of sunlight; (salts of N,N'-diacetyl-4,4'-diaminostilbendisulfonic acid (2,2') are examples of such materials) [15].

Quaternary ammonium salts of the nitro compounds of *o*- and *p*-phenylenediamine are dyes themselves; they are strongly adsorbed on hair [16]. The same applies to complexes between anionic dyes and cationic surfactants which can be made water-soluble with the aid of nonionic solubilizers. Azobenzene derivatives also belong to this group; polyhydroxyazobenzene compounds are of special interest because they are capable of dying the hair even in the neutral or a weakly acidic range.

### Bleaches

Dyes can lighten dark hair to a certain extent, and metallic and oxidation dyes or camomile extract may be used for this purpose. It is impossible, however, to obtain a strong bleaching effect with this method; it is a well-known fact that it is much easier to color a light surface dark than to lighten a dark color. The most successful method of lightening dark hair is bleaching. This is not based on the application of a light shade but on the destruction of the dark pigment melanin. Oxidizing agents, preferably hydrogen peroxide, are used for this purpose. Weigel [17] discusses the advantages and disadvantages of this and the various other oxidation agents that may be considered.

To bleach gray hair completely, permanganate solutions have been recommended, but the application of these solutions is technically difficult and mistakes may cause serious damage to the hair [18]. For home use a 3–4% peroxide solution is usually recommended; for professional application, a 5–6% solution which acts much faster is generally used. Stronger solutions could seriously damage the hair. To avoid a decrease in strength during storage, hydrogen peroxide solutions must be stabilized with suitable substances, such as acetanilide or diluted acids. It is also advisable to add a sequestering agent to the solutions (see Chapter 5), since the presence of various metal ions promotes damage to the hair. Hair-conditioning substances such as cholesterol, water- or oil-soluble lanolin derivatives or fatty alcohols are also frequently added to hydrogen peroxide solutions [19].

Ammonia is added to the peroxide solution immediately before application. This accelerates the degradation of the peroxide, hence the oxidizing effect, and at the same time softens the hair. The alkaline peroxide solution is applied to the freshly washed hair with a cotton ball and is rinsed off with ample warm water whenever the desired bleaching has been obtained.

Bleached hair never regains its color; it is therefore sufficient to bleach only the freshly grown portions of hair in subsequent treatments. Repeated bleaching of the same hair must be avoided because it leads to damage and to a "dead" and strawlike look.

Occasionally the bleaching agent is not applied in liquid form but as a pack. These packs usually consist of magnesium carbonate mixed either with a solution of hydrogen peroxide and ammonia or equal parts of magnesium peroxide and sodium perborate. However, they have the disadvantage that the progress of bleaching cannot be observed.

**Brightening Rinses.** If no actual bleaching but merely a lightening of the hair is required, it can be achieved with a weakly acid peroxide solution (pH 4–4.5) [20]. In addition to hydrogen peroxide (about 3%), these solutions contain an organic acid, such as adipic, tartaric, or glutaminic acid (0.7–1.0%). Cationic substances, also frequently added (cetyldimethylbenzyl ammonium chloride or morpholine alkyl sulfate in 0.5–2.5% doses), are intended to have a certain regulating effect in the bleaching process. Sodium stannate or sodium pyrophosphate act as stabilizers. Such products may have the following composition:

| | | |
|---|---|---|
| 12. | Hydrogen peroxide, 3% | 97.1% |
| | Alkylethyl morpholine ethosulfate | 1.5% |
| | Adipic acid | 0.8% |
| | Sodium stannate | 0.6% |

**Combination of Bleaching and Dyeing.** It is impossible to obtain a platinum-blond shade by bleaching with hydrogen peroxide; the lightest color obtainable with simple bleaching is a yellow blond. To achieve the desired platinum a color rinse must be used to "neutralize" the yellow; a 0.001 % solution of methylene blue has proved to be suitable for this purpose [21]. It is essential that the hair be bleached as much as possible; otherwise, if too much yellow remains, the blue rinse will produce green!

If the natural hair color is to be replaced by a lighter shade with an oxidation dye, bleaching and dyeing may be combined. In any case, peroxide and ammonia are already required for use with oxidation dyes. If both substances are applied in higher concentrations than required for normal dyeing, a certain degree of bleaching will be obtained. This treatment takes experience because not all types of hair react in the same way and excessively high concentrations of peroxide and alkali may damage the hair or scalp.

If vegetable or metallic dyes are used, bleaching cannot be combined with the dyeing process but must be done beforehand.

### Dye Removers

Permanent hair colorings are formulated to be as stable as possible to all external influences and therefore are difficult to remove. According to Wall [22] the best and easiest way of removing color adhering to the hair shaft is a treatment with hot vegetable oils. First the hair is completely covered with oil; then it is heated. Wall recommends passing strands of hair through a heated iron (marcel or comb) and then rubbing it with a towel. Finally the hair is shampooed. The hot-oil treatment is even reported to be beneficial. Vegetable extracts and lead salt dyes can usually be removed by this method. Silver coloring adheres more strongly, and copper colors can be washed off only with difficulty. This kind of superficial treatment cannot reverse oxidation dyeing at all.

Instead of unprocessed vegetable dyes, sulfonated castor oil (Turkey red oil) may be used in shampoos of this kind. Turkey red oil has the advantage that various active ingredients can be incorporated; for example, salicylic acid (1–2%) to remove henna and metallic colors, hydrogen peroxide for bleaching oxidation dyes. Turkey red oil, however, must be applied with caution because it is capable of removing not only the artificial but also the natural color of the hair.

Artificial hair coloring is occasionally removed with aqueous solutions of certain chemicals. The most important are acid sodium thiosulfate solutions (5% sodium thiosulfate, 2% sulfuric acid, 93% water) for silver colors; acid sodium dithionate ($Na_2S_2O_4$) solutions for anilin and partial bleaching of oxidation dyes or color spots on the skin, and neutral or weakly ammoniacal solutions of sodium formaldehyde sulfoxylate ($NaSO_2CH_2OH$) which have a similar effect.

Hydrogen peroxide solutions (5–6%) may bleach light shades of oxidation dyes but have generally little effect on the dark shades. They must not be used on hair that has been treated with metallic dyes.

## SKIN-BLEACHING PREPARATIONS

As we saw in Chapter 10, one reason why women use powder is to cover irregularities of the complexion (freckles, red spots, scars, etc.) This covering, of course, is purely superficial, and the trouble can be attacked at the root by a peeling treatment or by using bleaching preparations.

Peeling treatments are rather drastic and hardly belong to cosmetics but to plastic surgery. We therefore limit ourselves to a discussion of bleaching preparations.

The active ingredient in most modern bleaching preparations is a mercury salt. The most widely used materials of this type are mercuric chloramide (mercury amide chloride, white precipitate, $HgNH_2Cl$), mercuric chloride ($HgCl_2$, sublimate), and mercurous chloride (calomel, $Hg_2Cl_2$). Red mercuric oxide and mercuric salicylate are also occasionally used. All of these compounds (with the exception of mercuric chloride) are insoluble in water, fats, and organic solvents and are incorporated in creams in fine dispersions. Mercuric chloride (sublimate) is soluble in water and alcohol and is mostly used in lotions.

Although mercury compounds are absorbed by the epidermal tissue to a certain extent and the resorption of higher proportions of mercury causes toxicity symptoms, creams containing insoluble mercury compounds in concentrations below 5% may be regarded as harmless, provided they are not applied to sore or broken skin or massaged into it. The indirect risk that the user may somehow swallow traces of the preparation seems to be greater [23]. Allergic reactions occur, but only infrequently [24].

The effect of mercuric salts is based on an inhibition of the enzymes which are responsible for the first stages of oxidation of tyrosine to melanin, the skin pigment. Existing melanin is not destroyed, but the formation of fresh pigment is impeded. In addition, sublimate has a peeling effect because it releases hydrochloric acid in the top skin layers, which attacks the corneum.

Bleaching creams based on mercury salts often contain bismuth subnitrate. The views on the role played by this additive are conflicting. Some experts think it increases the bleaching effect of the mercury salts; others say it decreases the probability of skin lesions caused by mercury salts. In the opinion of still others it has a peeling effect or is useful mainly as a whitener or clouding agent in bleaching preparations.

The monobenzyl ether of hydroquinone has been suggested as an active ingredient in cosmetic bleaching preparations [25]. This substance not only inhibits the formation of new melanin, it also destroys already developed melanin and is therefore particularly effective as a bleaching agent. On the other hand, it causes frequent allergic reactions [26] so that it must be handled with the requisite care. Hydroquinone monobenzyl ether has been used rarely, if at all, in commercial preparations.

Preparations containing hydrogen peroxide or certain metal peroxides (magnesium, zinc peroxide) also have been used as bleaches for many years. The mechanism of their action is not known.

The use of acid creams and lotions (generally based on lemon juice) as bleaches is also known. It is improbable, however, that such preparations have a bleaching effect. In any case, it has never been demonstrated clinically.

### ANHYDROUS AND WATER-IN-OIL CREAMS

|                                    | 13    | 14    |
|------------------------------------|-------|-------|
| Paraffin wax 59°C MP               | 4.5   |       |
| Ceresine                           | 3     |       |
| Beeswax                            | 7     |       |
| Spermaceti                         |       | 10    |
| Petrolatum                         | 54.5  | 40    |
| Absorption base                    |       | 20    |
| Mineral oil                        | 8     | 20    |
| Mercury chloramide                 | 5     |       |
| Bismuth subnitrate                 | 8     |       |
| Zinc oxide                         | 8     |       |
| Hydrogen peroxide (15–20 vol %)    |       | 8–10  |
| Perfume                            | q.s.  |       |

#### REMARKS

13. Ozier in Sagarin, *Cosmetics: Science and Technology*, p. 218. Interscience, New York, 1957. Waxes, petrolatum, and mineral oil are melted together and cooled to 45°C. Bismuth subnitrate, white sublimate, zinc oxide, and perfume oil are mixed in, and stirring is continued until the mixture is cool. The cream is then passed through an ointment mill and filled cold.

14. Janistyn, *Riechstoffe-Seifen-Kosmetika*, II, p. 372. Hüthig Verlag, Heidelberg. 1950, The hydrogen peroxide must be incorporated into the completely cooled mass. Traces of metallic salts and all impurities must be carefully avoided. *p*-Hydroxybenzoates or a small quantity of an acidic phosphate are used as preservatives.

OIL-IN-WATER CREAMS

|  | 15 | 16 | 17 |
|---|---|---|---|
| Mineral oil |  | 2.0 | 2.0 |
| Isopropyl palmitate | 2 |  |  |
| Cetyl alcohol | 2 |  | 4.0 |
| Stearyl alcohol |  |  | 4.0 |
| Lanolin | 2 |  |  |
| Glycerol monostearate SE (Tegacid) | 20 |  |  |
| Proplyene glycol monostearate SE |  | 3.5 |  |
| Diethylene glycol monostearate |  |  | 12.0 |
| Triple pressed stearic acid |  | 16.4 |  |
| Triethanolamine |  | 0.8 |  |
| Sodium lauryl sulfate |  | 1.5 |  |
| Triethanolamine lauryl sulfate |  |  | 1.3 |
| Mercury chloramide (white precip.) | 2.0 | 3.0 |  |
| Mercurious chloride (calomel) |  | 2.0 |  |
| Zinc peroxide |  |  | 6.0 |
| Water | 67 | 70.3 | 66.7 |
| Glycerol | 3 |  |  |
| Propylene glycol |  | 2.0 |  |
| Sorbitol |  |  | 4.0 |
| Perfume |  | q.s. |  |

REMARKS

15. Keithler, *The Formulation of Cosmetics and Cosmetic Specialties*, p. 99. Drug and Cosmetic Industry, New York, 1950. Add the aqueous phase (80°C) with stirring to the oil phase (80°C) and continue stirring until the mass has cooled to room temperature. Add the mercury salt and mill the mass until a smooth homogeneous cream is obtained.

16. Ozier, *op. cit.*, 219. Add the aqueous phase (70°C) to the oil melt (70°C) and stir. Stirring is continued to 44°C, when mercury salts and perfume are added. Before filling the cream must be milled.

17. Keithler, *op. cit.*, 100. The procedure is the same as in 15.

# PREPARATIONS THAT CHANGE THE CONFIGURATION OF THE HAIR

The custom of permanent waving might seem strange to a visitor from Mars: fashionable women all over the world submit their precious hair to a treatment that causes each hair to lose its original form; the purpose of the process is an adjustment to whatever fashion dictates is the current mode. They accept with equanimity the fact that the hair loses its gloss, suppleness, and to a large extent its "life." This attitude, however, is not new; women in ancient Egypt, Greece, and Rome did exactly the same, only their means were not quite so sophisticated as ours. Since we are not visitors from Mars, we will limit ourselves to a discussion of the physiological and technical aspects of permanent waving and the composition of the preparations used in this connection.

### Principle of Action

The form of the hair is determined by the structure of the cortex. As discussed in Chapter 1, this structure consists fundamentally of long parallel polypeptide chains connected by cross linkages. Normally the chains are folded and when dry cannot easily be stretched. If they are wet, they can be partly or wholly stretched to more than one and one half times their original length.

Permanent waving consists of the following stages [27]: first, the hair is thoroughly wetted; it is then rolled and the polypeptide chains extended with varying force. Some of the cross linkages are broken during the wetting process, others are maintained; rolling of the hair stretches the cross linkages and thus creates a tension that tends to pull the hair back into its original position. In the next stage most of the cross linkages are broken chemically and tension is thereby relaxed. Finally the cross linkages are restored in such a way that the hair is no longer strained in its new rolled form. Drying or cooling of the hair or removal of all chemicals fixes it in that form.

The process may best be visualized by imagining a rope ladder (Figure 11a). One of the vertical ropes is extended (b). This pulls the cross ropes out of their original position and tensions develop. The cross ropes are cut (c), thus relieving the tension, and finally the loose ends which lie opposite one another after one rope is stretched are tied (d). The result is a curved rope ladder, similar to waved hair.

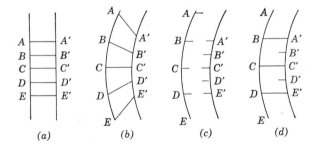

FIGURE 11    SCHEMATIC PRESENTATION OF A PERMANENT WAVE.

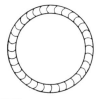

FIGURE 12   A CROSS SECTION OF HAIR WOUND AROUND A ROLLER.

We now discuss the individual stages of the permanent waving process:

1. *Differential stretching of the hair* (*changing the form*).   Understanding of the procedure used for this stage of the process is essential to the formulation of a good permanent-wave preparation. A detailed discussion can be found in Freytag's article on the subject [28].

As previously mentioned, the change in the configuration of the hair is based on a differentiated extension of the polypeptide chains in the cortex of each hair. When the hair is wound around a roller, the outside of each hair must be slightly longer than the inside in contact with the roller; the extension of the chains is therefore greater "outside" than "inside." The schematic illustration (Figure 12) demonstrates geometrically that the difference in the extension between inside and outside will be the greater, the smaller the diameter of the roller and the larger the diameter of the hair. Considering that hair will be more strongly waved, the greater the tension difference, important conclusions can be drawn for practical application.

Hair will be more strongly waved, the smaller the diameter of the roller around which it is wound. If the strands are wound in spirals, the diameter will remain the same for the whole length of the hair and it will be equally strongly waved for its total length. If the hair is wound around the roller like film on a spool, it will be more strongly waved at its ends than near the scalp because winding is always toward the head.

Thick hair (this does not refer to density of growth but to the diameter of each hair) will be more strongly waved than thin hair with equal treatment. (There may be other reasons as well.) [29a].

The character of the hair is an important factor that must be taken into consideration on applying a permanent wave. The time, for instance, needed for the solution to penetrate the cortex depends on the porosity of the hair cuticle. Hair weakened by bleaching, frequent permanent waving, or certain diseases generally takes up these solutions much more rapidly than healthy hair. Since damaged hair is particularly sensitive to the excessively strong effects of permanent-wave solutions and can be softened by relatively mild processes, special mild solutions are used.

Hairdressers often maintain that permanent waves applied during pregnancy or menstruation do not last long. If the behavior of the hair really depends on the physiology of the whole organism, this would, of course, be a weighty argument against the opinion that hair is "dead." No agreement has yet been reached on how much the hair shaft, that is, the so-called dead part of the hair, does indeed respond to processes in the organism.

A common cause of loose permanent waves is insufficient soaking of the hair with the wave solution. It is important for good wetting of the hair that it be first thoroughly washed.

In the hot-wave process softening of the hair and realignment occur almost simultaneously; the duration of the treatment depends on the temperature of the hair and its condition. In the cold process the realignment takes much longer than softening. The softening stage is completed when the cold-wave solution is rinsed off; realignment continues until the beginning of the neutralization process.

2. *Disruption of the cross linkages.* This stage of the process consists in breaking the cross linkages without at the same time degrading the polypeptide chains of the hair keratin, and in such a way that they can later be restored.

Four types of chemical linkage probably play a part in the connection between the parallel polypeptide chains in keratin (see Chapter 1): salt bridges, hydrogen bonds, disulfide groups, and, to a lesser extent, amide linkages. Salt bridges and hydrogen bonds can be broken by water alone. For this reason hair will swell when wet; it can be extended and is less resistant than when dry.

The hairdresser utilizes this condition by giving the hair the desired shaping while it is still wet and then letting it dry. In this process (the "water set") we again find the three stages of permanent waving: the dissolution of cross linkages in water, the rearrangement of the hair, and fixing it in the new form by drying. In this case the wave is not permanent because sooner or later the hair reverts to its original form. This is because not all of the cross linkages have been disrupted, and many (certainly amide and disulfide linkages) have been left in their original state. The "old" bridges cause a tension in the hair that pulls it back into its old form, particularly when it gets damp and the new salt and hydrogen bonds are loosened.

As discussed in Chapter 1, aqueous solutions break an increasingly large number of salt linkages, the further their pH value is removed from the isoelectric point of keratin (pH 4). For this reason alkaline solutions have a stronger swelling effect on hair than pure water. Theoretically it might be possible to obtain permanent waves with strongly alkaline solutions because these solutions (pH 11, 12) not only disrupt salt and hydrogen bonds but disulfide and amide linkages as well, but because they also break amide linkages they cannot be used in practice: the keratin chains (the "vertical ropes") consist of short fragments linked to one another by amide bonds, and the breaking of these bonds would lead to destruction of the hair fiber. The disulfide linkages can also be disrupted by weakly alkaline solutions, but only at high temperatures (above 100°C). Actually, the linkages are broken by steam. Many chemists have tried to determine the chemical reaction on which the disruption of disulfide linkages by steam is based, but no agreement has yet been reached [29b]. Since the amide linkages are largely preserved during the treatment of the hair with steam, this reaction is suitable for permanent waving and the hot-wave process is based on it.

Inorganic sulfites also attack the —S—S linkage of the disulfide bridges but not the CO—NH linkage of the polypeptide chains. The reaction between disulfides and sulfites is reversible and occurs in accordance with the formula

$$R—S—S—R + X_2SO_3 \rightleftharpoons R—S—X + R—S—SO_3X$$

where X is an alkaline metal and R, the remainder of the polypeptide chain. This reaction is also utilized in practice by adding sulfites to alkaline hot-wave solutions, thus facilitating more rapid softening of the hair.

The disulfide linkage can also be disrupted by reduction. Among the many reducing agents that have been suggested for this purpose, mercaptans and, in particular, thioglycolic acid have proved most satisfactory. The reduction can be expressed by the following formula

$$R—S—S—R + 2^-S—CH_2COO^-$$
Keratin  Thioglycolic acid (as dianion)

$$\rightleftharpoons R—S^- + {}^-S—R + {}^-OCC—CH_2—S—S—CH_2—CO^-$$
Reduced Keratin  Dithioglycolic acid (as dianion)

Even if this formula does not represent the actual reaction (it does not occur directly but through one or more intermediary stages) [30], several conclusions which have significance for the practice of cold waving may be drawn from it.

1. The reaction is reversible, which means that it does not proceed to completion so that at the end only reaction products and no reactants (initial products) are present. After a certain time the reaction reaches an equilibrium in which both reactants and reaction products are present (in this particular case both unreduced and reduced keratin). When equilibrium has been established, the concentration of the various products is subject to the law that the quotient

$$\frac{\text{product of the concentrations of all reaction products}}{\text{product of the concentrations of all reactants}}$$

is constant at a given temperature. In practice this means that if in an equilibrium reaction the concentration of one reactant product is increased the concentration of the other reactants will be correspondingly decreased when equilibrium is established. In the reaction under consideration it is therefore possible to lower the concentration of unreduced keratin present at the equilibrium stage by increasing the concentration of the thioglycolic acid anion (see below; this is called "shifting the equilibrium to the right"). On the other hand, the equilibrium can be "shifted to the left," that is, reduction is inhibited by adding one of the final products to the reaction mixture. U. S. Patents 2,719,813–5 (Procter & Gamble, 1955), which covers the addition of dithioglycolic acid to mitigate the action of the cold-wave solution, utilize this principle.

2. Here the more active reducing agent is not thioglycolic acid but its dianion. The formation of the dianion from thioglycolic acid under the influence of an alkali is also an equilibrium reaction represented by the formulas

$$HS—CH_2COOH + OH^- \rightleftharpoons HS—CH_2—COO^- + H_2O$$
$$HS—CH_2COO^- + OH^- \rightleftharpoons {}^-S—CH_2—COO^- + H_2O$$

The concentration of the thioglycolic acid dianion therefore depends on the initial concentration of thioglycolic acid as well as on the alkali concentration (the ruling pH). As shown by the formula on the preceding page, hair keratin is the more completely reduced the higher the concentration of thioglycolic acid dianion. For practical application this well-known fact results: the stronger the alkalinity of a cold-wave solution and the higher the content of thioglycolic acid concentration, the stronger its effect.

Thioglycolic acid has the following disadvantages as an active ingredient in cold-wave solutions:

1. It is toxic; for this reason the law in several countries prescribes maximum concentrations for cosmetic preparations.

2. It causes strong swelling which, with incorrect handling, may lead to splitting of the keratin fiber.

3. When the pH is too high, it has a depilatory effect and,

4. Finally, it has an unpleasant odor.

For these reasons the replacement of thioglycolic acid by several other mercaptic compounds has been suggested for use in cold-wave lotions: thiolactic acid [31], mercapto ethanol [32], 3-mercapto-1,2-propandiol (mercapto glycerol) [33], in particular, have attracted attention; Ruemele [34] mentions still other substitutes. Nevertheless, thioglycolic acid remains the most widely used reducing agent in cold-wave lotions. According to German patent application 1,009,765 (1957) [35], esters of mercapto carbonic acids with polyhydric alcohols or hydroxy acids [e.g., glycolmonothioglycolate, $HS—CH_2COOCH_2CH_2OH$, or lactic acid thioglycolate, $HS—CH_2COOCH(CH_3)COOH$] may also cause the rearrangement of the hair in an acid environment (pH 4–7) that will result in very good waves and eliminate the risk of skin irritation.

Several authors have reported on the hair-waving effect of 2,5-dimercapto adipic acid [36]. This acid is characterized by good stability, relatively slight odor, a mild action on the hair, but (in comparison to thioglycolic acid) a rather high price.

The search for suitable reducing agents for cold-wave lotions has not been limited to mercaptans. It is impossible to list all substances that have been recommended for this purpose, but we may mention here the use of titanium and zirconium compounds [37] and alkali borohydrides [38].

3. *The re-establishment of cross linkages.* In heat waving new cross linkages form under the effect of steam on the hair. What happens here chemically is not fully understood. The permanent wave is fixed by cooling: when the hair has reached body temperature, the cross linkages can no longer be rearranged. Special chemicals are not required for fixing heat-process waves.

More is known about chemical reactions in cold waving. We have here an oxidation combined with acidification. The disulfide linkages of keratin are disrupted by reduction and can be restored by oxidation:

$$\text{R—S—S—R} \xrightleftharpoons[\text{oxydation}]{\text{reduction}} \text{R—SH + HS—R}$$

The swelling of keratin (disruption of salt and hydrogen bridges) caused by alkaline solutions can be reversed by acid solutions, followed by drying. In practice this is not quite so simple. The joining of mercapto groups to a disulfide linkage presupposes that two disulfide groups occur within a suitable distance (we refer once again to the comparison with a rope ladder). This condition exists at some but not all places at which a disulfide linkage was broken. It may happen that mercapto groups are linked with amino groups of opposite side chains under formation of a —S—N bond. It may also happen that the mercapto groups that do not find suitable partners are oxidized to sulfuric or sulfonic acids. The oxidation agent may also attack established disulfide linkages and even disrupt them again under certain conditions. In any case, neutralization never completely restores the hair to its initial form, for a certain modification of the hair structure by permanent waving is unavoidable.

In the presence of certain catalysts oxidation may occur by air alone, but it is most commonly caused by aqueous solutions of suitable oxidizing agents. Mercapto groups may also be linked in nonoxidative processes, but the bonds formed would not be disulfide bonds. Formaldehyde may create a bridge between two mercapto groups [39].

$$\text{2R—SH + HCHO} \rightarrow \text{R—S—CH}_2\text{—R—S + H}_2\text{O}$$

Free amino groups at the ends of the side chains may be linked in a similar way (R—NH—CH$_2$—NH—R). In practice the reaction with formaldehyde and other nonoxidative reactions are not applied in hair waving.

*Tepid waving.* Two variations of cold and heat waving are frequently applied. In the first a weak cold-wave lotion is used and its effect accelerated by heating it to a maximum of 72°C. Neutralization is effected as in the cold-wave process. Compared with the traditional cold wave, this process has the advantage of being faster and reducing the luster of the hair to a lesser degree. It requires accurately titrated solutions, precise control of the temperature, and careful observation of the necessary period of treatment.

The second process is a variation of heat waving. A small amount of thio-glycolate is added to the developer lotion which facilitates the process considerably because lower temperatures are sufficient. Rinsing with an oxidizing lotion is not required.

## PREPARATIONS

### Waveset Preparations

Here water is the active ingredient that breaks the cross linkages at room temperature or with moderate heating. Water is not capable of disrupting the disulfide bridges; it merely breaks hydrogen and salt linkages. Hence there is only a limited swelling and softening of the hair; the hair is then arranged as desired, and setting is achieved by the evaporation of the water. Such waves do not last long because the amide and disulfide linkages remain in their initial position and the new hydrogen and salt bridges are soon loosened by moisture (from the atmosphere or perspiration). The setting effect can be improved by adding mucins to setting lotions (pectin, carrageen, alginates, etc.) or film-forming gums, either natural (karaya, tragacanth) or synthetic, which leave a thin film on the hair after the preparation has dried. This film, by mechanical resistance, keeps the hair for some time in the new arrangement. (The O/W hair-setting creams discussed in Chapter 10 are closely related to these setting lotions.)

Some suggested formulations or preparations of this type follow:

| 18. | | |
|---|---|---|
| | Apple pectin | 1.00 |
| | Citric acid | 0.50 |
| | Methyl-*p*-hydroxybenzoate | 0.17 |
| | Propyl-*p*-hydroxybenzoate | 0.08 |
| | Perfume oil | 0.01 |
| | Rose water, triple | 98.50 |
| | | 100.26 |

Rothemann, *Das grosse Rezeptbuch der Haut- Körperpflegemittel*, 3rd ed., p. 469. Apple pectin may be replaced by lemon pectin, and rose water by distilled water. The suggested perfume is rose.

Preservative and citric acid are dissolved in water (90°C). Sprinkle the pectin over the surface of the solution and stir thoroughly several times during the next few hours until it has dissolved without lumps. The preparation is poured into a bottle and shaken several times; finally perfume is added.

| 19. | Sodium carbonate, anhydrous | 3.0 |
|---|---|---|
| | Alginic acid, pure | 6.0 |
| | Preservative | 0.2 |
| | Rose water, triple | 100 |

Rothemann, *op. cit.*, p. 469.

Rose water may be replaced by distilled water or a mixture of 90 parts rose water, 5 parts glycerol (28° Bé), and 5 parts alcohol, 95%.

Sodium carbonate and preservative (sodium salt of methyl-*p*-hydroxybenzoate) are dissolved in water; the alginate is then sprinkled on the surface and stirred in. The preparation can be thickened by adding some calcium citrate.

Alginic acid may be replaced by commercial grades of alginates. The quantity varies according to the quality and must be determined in preliminary tests. In case sodium alginates are used, sodium carbonate may be omitted.

| 20. | Smyrna tragacanth | 1.5 |
|---|---|---|
| | Alcohol, 95% | 5.0 |
| | Glycerol, 28° Bé | 1.0 |
| | Castor oil | 2.0 |
| | Tincture of benzoin | 1.0 |
| | Rose water, triple | 90.0 |
| | Sodium salt of methyl-*p*-hydroxybenzoate | 0.2 |

Rothemann, *op. cit.*, p. 469. Gum tragacanth may be replaced by karaya which has the advantage of drying without visible residue; on the other hand, it occasionally produces allergic symptoms [40].

Gum tragacanth and alcohol are thoroughly mixed together, and glycerol, castor oil, and tincture of benzoin (omitted if a transparent solution is desired) are then added. The mass is thoroughly mixed once again and poured into a bottle. The water in which the preservative has been dissolved is added in one lot, and the mixture is shaken until a clear liquid free of lumps is obtained. Castor oil in this preparation makes the dry scaly film left by tragacanth less visible.

## Hot-Wave Preparations

The main ingredient (not only in terms of quantity) in these preparations is water which vaporizes when the hair is heated.

To promote disruption of the salt and hydrogen bridges and thus accelerate the treatment a base is always added to the lotions. Sodium and potassium hydroxide and carbonate as well as borax were once widely used for this purpose, but they have the disadvantage of fusing with the hair and combining with keratin to form a hard, brittle cuticle. For this reason they have been largely replaced in modern preparations by ammonia. Ammonia evaporates during the heating process and leaves no residue. Ammonia also has its drawbacks: the odor is unpleasant and the base tends to evaporate before the hair swelling is completed. Ammonia vapors may also give the hair a reddish tint. For some time hot-wave solutions have contained less volatile bases such as mono- or triethanolamine, or morpholine in combination with or in place of ammonia.

To initiate the disruption of the disulfide linkages sodium or potassium sulfite or the corresponding bisulfites are added to hot-wave solutions. The use of cyclic organic sulfonates, such as glycol sulfite or butadiene sulfonate, is covered by German Patent 952,469 (Chem. Werke Huels, 1956). Modern heat-wave solutions also often contain surfactants that promote rapid wetting of the hair and act as solubilizers of the perfume oil.

U. S. Patent 2,506,492 (1950) describes the addition of a sequestering agent that protects the solution from oxidation by inactivating the metal ions which have a catalytic effect (both sulfites and bisulfites are oxidation-sensitive).

The addition of fatting or conditioning agents has repeatedly been suggested for hot-wave solutions. Whether such substances (fatty alcohols, lecithin lanolin, etc.) have any value or whether they possibly limit the efficacy of the preparations has not yet been determined.

Some formulations for hot-wave preparations follow as an illustration:

|  | 21 | 22 | 23 | 24 |
|---|---|---|---|---|
| Ammonia (s.g. 0.910) | 1 | 5 |  |  |
| Monoethanolamine |  |  | 3 |  |
| Triisopropanolamine |  |  | 3 |  |
| Ammonium carbonate | 4 | 4 |  | 0.25 |
| Sodium carbonate |  |  |  | 0.45 |
| Potassium carbonate | 2 | 2 |  |  |
| Borax |  |  |  | 2.65 |
| Sodium hydroxide |  |  | 0.6 |  |
| Sodium sulfite | 10 | 10 | 3 |  |
| Tween 20 | 2.5 | 4 |  |  |
| Turkey red oil |  |  | 1.5 |  |
| Water, deionized or distilled | 80 | 74.5 | 88.9 | 90.65 |
| Perfume oil | 0.5 | 0.5 |  | 0.5 |

REMARKS

21, 22 and 23. Neumann, *SÖFW*, **83**, 276 (1957). 21 is a particularly mild; 23 is a strong solution.

24. Auch, *Soap, Perfum. Cosm.*, **10**, 43 (1937), Particularly good for dyed hair.

It must be borne in mind when formulating hot-wave solutions that a higher efficacy (increased alkali concentration) may have a deleterious effect on skin and hair but that under certain circumstances "hair conditioning" additives may have the same effect in practical application: using milder preparations requires a longer treatment period; this is not only inconvenient but it also increases the risk of damage to skin and hair. For this reason hair conditioners in heat-wave preparations are of value only if it can be shown that their presence does not necessitate longer periods of treatment which would obviate the beneficial effect. As far as we are aware, such evidence does not exist for these substances.

## Cold-Wave Preparations

In any discussion of cold-wave preparations the patent situation must be mentioned first. This field of cosmetics is almost entirely covered by a few patents, and the litigation that has developed around these preparations in several countries is a fascinating episode in the history of modern cosmetics [41]. A central part is taken by a patent registered by E. H. McDonough (or Sales Affiliates, Inc.) in several countries [42]. German Patent 948,186 covers "agents for the permanent change of form for hair on live subjects, containing or consisting of an aqueous alkaline solution of a substituted mercaptan with a pH over 7 and below 10, but preferably between 9.2 and 9.5." The substitution group of the mercaptan may be ionized or nonionized. The alkaline vehicle is a volatile base with a dissociation constant under $5 \times 10^{-3}$; the concentration of mercaptan is between 1 and 15%. This patent, however, has been fought in many countries and has been declared invalid in some.

As previously mentioned, the mercaptan used in most modern cold-wave preparations is thioglycolic acid. The concentration used depends on the intended strength of the solution and is usually between 4 and 8%. According to Korby [43], a cold-wave lotion produced by John H. Breck, one of the leading manufacturers in the United States, contained 6.83% thioglycolic acid for normal hair, 7.24% for hard-to-wave hair, and 4.07% for weakened hair.

In addition to thioglycolic acid, cold-wave solutions always contain an alkali. Nearly every conceivable base has been suggested for use in cold-wave solutions, but in practice only ammonia and monoethanolamine are important. Strong bases such as sodium or potassium hydroxide may be used only in very low concentrations (pH 9.5–10 must not be exceeded or thioglycolate will act as a depilatory!) and consequently their softening effect is inadequate. According to Heilingötter [44], triethanolamine should also be avoided.

Which of the two bases—monoethanolamine or ammonia—is preferable has been discussed repeatedly in the literature [45]. Whitman and Brooks [46] maintain that monoethanolamine is much less toxic than ammonia and far less irritating to the eye conjunctiva in dilute solutions; in addition, monoethanolamine thioglycolate irritates human skin less than ammonium thioglycolate. On the other hand, Draize and co-workers [47] found that monoethanolamine thioglycolate in animal tests (rabbits) penetrates the skin to a higher degree and therefore has a stronger toxic action in external applications than the ammonium salt. According to Fuhrmann [48], monoethanolamine thioglycolate has a stronger hair-softening effect which Heilingötter [45] attributes at least in part to the fact that ammonia evaporates during the waving process. This evaporation of ammonia is regarded as an advantage: it reduces the risk of tight waving (frizzing). In practice, ammonia has gained greater popularity in spite of its unpleasant odor and probably also because of its lower price, than monoethanolamine.

In addition to these main ingredients, other substances used are intended to promote the swelling of the hair or the disruption of the disulfide linkages. Urea or a low molecular alkyl derivative of urea should promote the swelling of the hair [49] so that lower concentrations of thioglycolate may be used. Ammonium salts of strong acids are supposed [50] to protect against over-waving because the pH value of preparations containing these salts drops below 7 during treatment which automatically discontinues the effect of thioglycolic acid. Ammonium carbonate and bicarbonate reportedly impart higher effectiveness to ammonium thioglycolate solutions [51].

We have already mentioned the use of disulfides to weaken the effect of cold-wave preparations. The relevant patent (U.S. 2,719,813) is interesting because an attempt is generally made to avoid the formation of disulfides in cold-wave solutions (which may occur spontaneously under the influence of atmospheric oxygen on the solution; the reaction proceeds according to the formula $2HS-CH_2COO^- + (O) \rightarrow {}^-OOC-CH_2S-S-CH_2COO^- + H_2O$) because this formation weakens them. For this purpose antioxidants are added to the solutions. The addition of sequestering agents which bind polyvalent metal ions is recommended because these ions catalytically accelerate air oxidation of the cold-wave solution in the container and because their presence in thioglycolate solutions may lead to hair damage.

U.S. Patent 2,564,722 is in exact opposition in regard to the addition of sequestering agents, since it covers the incorporation of traces of metal salts (in particular, manganese, copper, and iron) in cold-wave solutions. The purpose of these additives is the acceleration of air oxidation, not, however, in the container but after application to the hair. This prevents overwaving and makes subsequent use of an oxidized solution unnecessary: the thioglycolic acid is gradually oxidized to dithiodiglycolic acid, and the disulfide linkages disrupted by reduction are gradually restored.

Fatty substances are often emulsified in cold-wave solutions, either in order to impart a cloud to the solutions (a milky solution is regarded as more appealing than a clear one), to protect the hair, or to restore the fat that has been lost during the waving process. According to Leberl [52], silicone oils used either as additives to the lotion or for rinsing afterwards protect the hair from damage by cold-wave lotions [53].

It is not easy to obtain a stable emulsification of the fatty substances in the cold-wave solution because most emulsifiers are not effective in a strong alkaline solution with a high salt concentration or are decomposed by it. Nonionic emulsifiers that do not contain ester groups (e.g., fatty alcohol polyethylene glycol ether) are most suitable here. The addition of quaternary ammonium salts as hair conditioners has also been recommended.) Our general remarks regarding the value of hair conditioners in hot-wave preparations apply here as well.

Although nearly all modern cold-wave formulations are based on the same principle, a number of variations are still possible. These relate in general to the strength of the preparations: hard-to-wave hair requires stronger preparations than hair that has been weakened by many previous cold-wave treatments or bleaching. (Solutions for children's hair are especially strong!) As a rule, solutions used by hairdressers are stronger than those applied at home; the stronger the solution, the faster its action and the more accurate the timing required. A preparation recommended for home use must be formulated in such a way that there will be no damage if it is left on the hair 15–20 minutes too long. Additives that automatically inactivate these preparations after a prescribed time are of particular value for home use.

Another possibility of variation is the physical form of the preparation. It can be manufactured as a clear or cloudy, low- or high-viscosity solution—cream, gel, or powder. We discuss these individual forms briefly.

**Liquid Cold-Wave Preparations.** These preparations are used much more frequently than all other forms. From the point of view of formulation they are the simplest.

|                                              | 25   | 26  | 27   | 28   | 29    |
|----------------------------------------------|------|-----|------|------|-------|
| Thioglycolic acid, 100%                      | 6.9  | 7.0 | 7.5  | 4.2  | 6.43  |
| Monoethanolamine, 100%                       | 9.6  | 8.0 |      |      |       |
| Ammonia (35 wt %)                            |      | 2.0 | 5.1  | q.s. | 7.21  |
| Dimethylpolysiloxan (50 cp)                  |      |     | 2    |      |       |
| Polyethylene glycol (400) monostearate       |      |     | 1.5  |      |       |
| Ammonium sulfate                             |      |     |      | 6.6  |       |
| Urea                                         |      |     |      | 15.7 |       |
| Aerosol AY (sodium diamyl sulfosuccinate)    |      |     |      |      | 0.6   |
| Manganese chloride ($MgCl_2 \cdot 4H_2O$)    |      |     |      |      | 0.0720|
| Distilled water                              | 83.5 | 83  | 83.9 | 70   | 85.69 |

REMARKS

25 and 26. Ruemele. Use sufficient water to make 100 ml.

27. British Patent 753,241 (Unilever Ltd., 1956). First prepare an emulsion from Siloxan, emulsifier, and 6.5 parts water. Homogenize, add 60 parts water, then thioglycolic acid and ammonia, and finally enough water to make 100 g.

28. British Patent 723,917 (Gillette Co., 1955) Add enough ammonia to adjust the pH to 9.4 and water to make 100 g.

29. U. S. Patent 2,564,722.

A condensation product of a higher fatty acid with a quaternary ammonium compound (e.g., the distearyl amide of dihydroxyethylene triamine) may be used as thickening agent for liquid cold-wave preparations, according to French Patent 1,068,586 [54]. Higher dosages of these substances produce cream. According to British Patent 723,349, clouding can be obtained by adding 2–5% of the following mixture:

| | |
|---|---:|
| Low viscosity mineral oil (50/60) | 74 |
| Sulfonated castor oil | 5 |
| Diethylene glycololeate self-emulsifying* | 11 |
| Lanogene | 10 |
| | 100 |

British Patent 679,841 (1952) covers the use of chlorinated mineral oil in opacifying agents. The use of this oil permits the adjustment of the specific gravity of the oil phase to exactly or approximately 1, which avoids creaming, that is, the gradual floating of the oil droplets to the top of the solution.

**Cold-Wave Creams.** These creams are usually packed in tubes and, since they are hardly exposed to the air, they are protected against oxidation. It is also possible to incorporate considerable quantities of fatty substances into preparations of this type. However, it is certainly not easy to manufacture a cold-wave cream that meets all requirements: it must wet the hair well, it must be easy to wash off, it must not attack the tube material, and, in particular, it must have the stability that is hard to achieve with this type of formulation. Separation of the cream in the tube is most undesirable because it would mean that the active ingredient would come out before the fats, and the contents of the tube would produce a different result every time it was used.

*The use of the diethylene glycol ester for this purpose is surprising, since esters of this type are slowly hydrolized in cold-wave preparations. In addition to the other ingredients, the cold-wave solution should contain 1–2% of a fatty acid condensation product of the Maypon type.

**Cold-Wave Powders.** Powders have the advantage of easy packaging, but the salts must be carefully protected from moisture, for otherwise they would be inactivated on contact with the air. A formulation for such a preparation is described in U. S. Patent 2,751,327 [55].

| | | |
|---|---|---|
| 30. | Thioglycolic acid 95% | 20 |
| | Ammonium carbonate | 20 |
| | Sodium carbonate (soda) | 24 |
| | | 64 |

Thioglycolic acid and ammonium carbonate are mixed until no more carbon dioxide is liberated. Add soda and mix until the powder is free from lumps. Before use, about 15 g of this powder are dissolved in 100 cc water.

## Neutralizing Agents

After heat-waving, the hair, when cool, is usually rinsed with a weakly acid solution that may contain quaternary ammonium salts or emulsified fats. These rinses remove all chemicals from the hair and leave it smooth, supple, and lustrous.

Neutralizing agents play a much more important part in the cold-wave method, in particular when it is not based on air oxidation. Here they represent the third stage in permanent waving: the restoration of cross linkages. The alkaline thioglycolate solution leaves the hair swollen, and the disulfide linkages have to a large extent been reduced to sulfhydryl groups. The neutralizing lotions are intended to counteract swelling and to oxidize the isolated sulfhydryl groups back to disulfide linkages.

The active ingredients in these preparations are therefore (a) any weak acid (acetic, citric, or tartaric) and (b) an oxidizing agent. The following oxidants are preferred in practice: sodium or potassium bromate [56], sodium perborate, ammonium persulfate, sodium chlorate, and finally—the most widely used oxidant for this purpose—hydrogen peroxide. All the oxidants mentioned are marketed as aqueous solutions or in powder form, with the exception of hydrogen peroxide, which can, however, be brought into solid form as the urea-hydrogen peroxide complex. Advantages and disadvantages of the different oxidants are discussed by Weigel [57] and Ruemele [58].

## Determination of the Efficacy of Cold-Wave Preparations

Since the effect of a cold-wave solution depends largely on the characteristics of the hair, the hairdresser or, in the case of home use, the consumer herself must determine how the hair is affected by the solution and what period of treatment is necessary for the desired result. It is important, however, that the cosmetic chemist have a laboratory method at his disposal that will help him to predetermine the efficacy of his solutions. Such a method is described by Kirby [59]; but it would be beyond the scope of this study to enlarge on it here.

### Damage to Hair, Scalp, and Health by Permanent-Wave Preparations

According to Sidi [60], there are several different types of damage:

1. *Hair damage.* Damage to the hair can usually be attributed to the use or the faulty application of alkaline solutions that are too strong. Sidi also states that a correctly applied permanent wave need not damage the hair at all. Certain modifications of the hair, particularly after repeated treatments, are unavoidable.

H. Freytag [61] reports a method that permits the quantitative determination of the degradation of hair keratin by ammonium-thioglycolate-ammonia solutions. This method is based on extraction of the treated hair with diluted soda lye and determination of the loss in weight. Another method, described by Berth and Reese [62], is based on the fact that the extent of copper absorbed by the hair from a copper tetramine solution depends on the degree to which it has been damaged by dyeing, waving, or ultraviolet radiation [63].

2. *Scalp irritations.* These irritations are caused by strong alkaline reactions or the defatting effect of cold-wave preparations. They are usually benign and heal easily if treated with oils (e.g., almond oil) or mild disinfectants. Irritations of the eyelids and conjunctiva may also occur if the cold-wave preparations come in contact with face and eyes.

3. *Damage to the hands.* Hairdressers who work regularly with cold-wave preparations may have serious trouble [64]. It can be avoided by wearing rubber gloves, rinsing the hands with a neutralizing lotion after contact, and using a fat cream.

4. *Incompatibility Reactions.* These reactions are observed only rarely. Cross sensitizations, in which the alkalizing and defatting effect of cold-wave solutions promotes cases of dermatitis caused by other substances, are more frequent.

5. *Damage to General Health* [65]. This damage has not been observed in healthy subjects and only occasionally in women in a poor state of health in general, or with a special disposition to anaemia.

In his survey of the relevant literature Böss [66] comes to the conclusion that permanent-wave lotions based on thioglycolate and correctly applied to healthy subjects cannot be regarded as harmful.

## COSMETICS USED IN THE REMOVAL OF HAIR

After changing the color and the form of the hair, the third drastic decorative modification is depilation.

Thousands of years ago Egyptian dancers and courtiers already knew how to remove hair growth on arms and legs; men probably started shaving even longer ago than that. Most civilized people and some primitive tribes have the urge to remove hair from certain parts of the body. This may be symptomatic of man's drive to suppress his animal side and to permit his hair to grow how and where he wants it and not according to nature.

Nowadays women in Western countries use depilatories to remove hair from armpits, arms, legs, and, if necessary, the face. Men partly or totally remove only the facial hair.

## Methods

Different methods of removing visible hair can be imagined. Fine hair can be made "invisible" by bleaching. Coarser hair may be removed by the purely *mechanical* means of cutting it at the skin surface or pulling it out by the root. It can be decomposed either by *chemical* or *physical* means by attacking (surface measures) the hairshaft or, more drastically, hairshaft and hair root and even the hair papilla. Finally *biological* measures that might affect the physiological processes in the hair papillae and cause loss of hair can be visualized.

Among methods known today shaving, plucking with tweezers, or tearing out with a wax preparation (epilation) can be regarded as purely mechanical methods. Undesirable hair was once removed by abrasion in which the skin surface was rubbed with pumice stone. This method is probably merely of historical interest. Certain other abrading methods are still being used in salons, however [67]. Present-day mechanical methods have the advantage that they do not attack the surrounding skin tissue too strongly. Even regular daily use does not cause skin lesions; these measures may be carried out even with sensitive, diseased, or damaged skin if proper care is taken. A disadvantage of these methods is that they are comparatively inconvenient. Plucking or pulling the hair is unpleasant. Shaving carries the risk of cutting and must be repeated rather frequently because the hair is cut only just above the skin surface.

Destruction of the hair by chemical means is the purpose of a number of preparations discussed in the next section. These preparations are convenient to apply, for they destroy the hair on the level of the skin surface (i.e., somewhat deeper than with shaving) and, if applied correctly, do not normally damage the skin. They must not, however, be applied too often or on areas of the skin that have somehow been weakened or damaged. Nor are they suitable for use on tender facial skin.

Among physical depilatory methods we must mention electrolysis and diathermy in particular. In both a needle is introduced into the hair follicle and an electric current passed through it (in electrolysis, a weak direct current, in diathermy, a high-frequency alternating current). If applied correctly, the hair is destroyed without the surrounding skin tissue being affected, and it does not grow again because the hair papilla has also been destroyed. It is a disadvantage of these methods that they take a long time (each hair must be treated individually and subsequent treatments are required because it is almost impossible to destroy all hair papillae at once), and that only experienced specialists can carry them out. For this reason these methods are used only to remove facial hair of women.

Hair removal by X rays is not acceptable because it entails too much risk of skin damage and because it is not advisable to expose the body more than absolutely necessary to these rays.

No good biological methods for hair removal are known today. Internal administration or external application of thallium salts may cause loss of hair, but this method is completely unsuitable for cosmetic purposes because thallium salts may become highly dangerous to the whole organism. The depilatory effect caused by them is not limited to definite areas of the body but may extend to all hirsute parts. Depilatories containing enzymes that specifically degrade hair keratin as active ingredients are theoretically interesting but have not yet found practical application. U. S. Patent 2,988,487 [68] describes such preparations. The keratinase contained in them is derived from *streptomyces fradiae*.

Harry [69] mentions a report by Ritter and Carter [70] according to which certain polymers of chlorobutadiene cause temporary loss of hair in experimental animals, and apparently also in humans, in which the hair loosens from the root but no change is observable on the hair itself. In a report by Flesch [71] it is also stated that squalene and certain other unsaturated fat-soluble substances cause temporary loss of hair in experimental animals. An ideal depilatory might perhaps be developed on this basis.

## PREPARATIONS

We now discuss the preparations used in chemical depilation as well as some auxiliaries in physical hair removal (epilation and shaving).

### Chemical Depilatories

These depilatories act by degrading the hair keratin. As we have already shown, keratin is sensitive to the influence of strongly alkaline aqueous solutions and reducing agents; it is therefore not difficult to degrade it chemically. The difficulty in formulating depilatories is the necessity to degrade the hair keratin without affecting the keratin of the corneum. No preparations that attack the hair keratin and leave the skin completely unaffected are known, but it has been found that products that combine a strong reducing effect with a strong alkaline reaction (i.e., attack on both fronts) degrade the hair in so short a time that the skin is hardly affected. (It is interesting to compare depilatories with nail-outicle softeners that are supposed to soften the skin keratin without attacking the nail keratin, which is closely related to hair keratin. Strongly alkaline preparations which contain no reducing agents are used here).

An active ingredient in a depilatory should not only attack hair keratin more rapidly than skin keratin but it must also be nontoxic and cause allergic reactions only in rare instances. It should act as quickly as possible (this also depends on its concentration and the alkalinity of the preparation) and should have no unpleasant odor nor develop one during use.

**Active Ingredients.** Inorganic sulfides must be mentioned first. *Sodium sulfide* has a strong depilatory effect (a 2% aqueous solution (pH 12) can easily degrade hair in 6–7 minutes [72]), but it has so strong an effect on skin keratin as well that it must be used with great caution, if at all. (A 2% alcoholic solution of sodium sulfide has no alkaline reaction because hydrolysis of the sulfide is not possible; it also has no depilatory action.) *Barium sulfide* cannot be recommended because of its high toxicity, but it is still mentioned in some formulations in modern literature. *Calcium sulfide* is less toxic but also less effective. The alkaline reaction of *magnesium sulfide* is too weak to be effective, and *zinc sulfide* is not sufficiently soluble. *Strontium sulfide* is more suitable for use in depilatories [73] than any other inorganic sulfide. Preparations with a high content of strontium sulfide (25–50%) soften the hair to such an extent in 3–4 minutes that it can be removed easily by light rubbing. Preparations with about 15% strontium sulfide require 5–7 minutes. The treatment period also depends on the alkalinity of the preparation; the optimum pH value is about pH 12. Here the action is rapid and there is almost no skin irritation in the short treatment period.

As salts of a weak acid, all sulfides are subject to hydrolysis in the presence of water, according to the following formulas (we are taking sodium sulfide as an example):

$$Na_2S + H_2O \rightleftharpoons NaHS + Na^+ + OH^-$$

$$NaHS + H_2O \rightleftharpoons H_2S + Na^+ + OH^-$$

We may conclude from these formulas and the general rule for equilibrium reactions that aqueous solutions of sulfides will always have a strong alkaline reaction that, in particular, when water is in excess of sulfide, hydrolysis in these solutions will result in unpleasantly odorous hydrogen sulfide, and that hydrolysis will be suppressed if alkali is added to the solution.

The same applies to strontium sulfide: it is partially hydrolyzed in aqueous media and hydrogen sulfide develops. As long as there is only a little water present and the pH value is above 11, hydrogen sulfide will develop only slightly and the odor will be less obtrusive. On the other hand, a strong repulsive odor occurs if a preparation based on an inorganic sulfide is rinsed off with water after application. For this reason the preparation should as far as possible be scraped off with a wooden spatula (and certainly not be flushed down the sink!) The remainder is then removed with a dilute solution of a zinc salt from which no hydrogen sulfide will develop but only a poorly soluble, hence odorless, zinc sulfide.

Another disadvantage of strontium sulfide in aqueous preparations is the formation of hard granules during extended storage caused by the poor water solubility of the strontium hydroxide developed through hydrolysis.

In the patent literature of the years 1930–1945 the use of *stannites* and, in particular, *sodium stannite* ($NaH_3SnO_3$) as active ingredients in depilatories is frequently mentioned. In the presence of water these salts have a strong reducing and alkaline effect; compared with sulfides, they have the advantage of being odorless. Their application, however, is made difficult by their poor stability in the presence of water. Although patents mention a variety of stabilizers for stannite preparations, they have not been able to establish themselves in practice.

Nowadays the most widely used active ingredients in depilatories are *mercaptans*, especially *thioglycolic acid*. The substance used for hair waving at pH 9–9.5 has a depilatory effect in a stronger alkaline environment. Thioglycolic acid may not be completely odorless but its odor is much less obtrusive than that of hydrogen sulfide. In addition, thioglycolic acid and its salt retain an almost unlimited stability even in aqueous preparations as long as they are protected against oxidation. Although thioglycolic acid is not nontoxic, its toxicity does not carry any risks if the preparation is handled and applied correctly. With correct formulation, depilatories can be prepared on the basis of thioglycolic acid which act within 5–15 minutes without any damage to normal skin.

According to Barry, the concentration of thioglycolic acid should lie between 2 and 4% [74]; lower concentrations act too slowly, higher ones not more rapidly. The alkali concentration should be adjusted to provide sufficient alkali to convert the thioglycolic acid completely into the dianion, but leaving a small excess to give the desired pH (usually 12–12.5). Alkali hydroxides (sodium, potassium hydroxide; a French patent covers the use of lithium salts of thioglycolic acid, $\alpha$ and $\beta$ mercaptopropionic acids, and mercapto carbonic acids in depilatories) may be used as bases, but earth alkali hydroxides are more suitable because of their limited solubility. Calcium hydroxide is particularly good and widely used because only very little free hydroxide, in excess of the amount required for the formation of the thioglycolic acid dianion, goes into solution. For this reason the alkalinity will never be strong enough to cause skin irritations within a short period. The undissolved calcium hydroxide present serves as an alkali reserve: when part of the dissolved base is neutralized, it is automatically compensated by undissolved hydroxide going into solution. Combinations of calcium hydroxide and more highly soluble hydroxides may also be used in proportions of 2 moles of soluble base per each mole of thioglycolic acid, with calcium hydroxide added as the alkali reserve.

In addition to thioglycolic acid, other organic sulfides have also been suggested for depilatories. Morelle [75] recommends the *strontium salt of thiolactic acid* which is less toxic than calcium thioglycolate and reportedly more effective, if considerably more expensive. Morelle has made an interesting observation to the effect that calcium thiolactate has almost no depilatory action even at pH 12.5. In his opinion the significance of the cation in these preparations is much greater than generally assumed. Evans and McDonough have patented the use of $\alpha$ and $\beta$ isomers of *thioglycerol* and a number of other mercaptans in depilatories [76].

Chemical depilatories are marketed as powders, liquid preparations, and pastes with or without fats.

Regardless of the active ingredients used and the form in which the preparation is marketed, every depilatory must meet certain general requirements. It must be easy to apply to the skin (possibly after mixing with water) and must have good adhesion. The depilatory must wet the hair; for this purpose alkali- and electrolyte-resistant surfactants are often added.

Morelle strongly objects [77] to the use of surfactants in depilatories because they float the active ingredient into the hair follicles and promote the penetration of the keratin-degrading substance into deeper skin layers. The result is unavoidable lesions. Whether this is correct depends on the way these ingredients penetrate the skin: transfollicularly or transepidermally. To our knowledge this has not been established.

The depilatory must not dry on the skin before it has served its purpose because all keratin-degrading substances are effective only in the presence of water. The preparation must also be clearly visible on the skin so that the areas on which it has already been applied or removed are obvious.

Finally, it should be easy to remove after treatment by scraping or washing.

In addition to active ingredients and water, depilatories also contain the following basic materials:

*Surfactants* to emulsify any fats used in the formulation, to promote wetting of the hair, and to assist in washing off the preparations.

*Mucins* to give the preparation the required consistency and assist in the dispersion of any solids used.

*Humectants* (glycerol, propylene glycol) to prevent quick drying on the skin.

*Inert powders* that provide the required consistency, also prevent quick drying on the skin, and make the film easily visible.

*Polyethylene glycols* that form a film on the skin which is easy to wash off.

*Fats* that are supposed to have a skin-protecting or conditioning effect and occasionally disinfectants, used prophylactically to prevent infection on the skin, which is somewhat weakened after the treatment.

*Astringents* are sometimes added, as well as substances that act as *local anaesthetics* (menthol, etc.)

## Powders

Powders are the simplest to manufacture. In preparations based on organic sulfides they are preferred because no hydrolysis of the sulfide can occur before application if the preparations are packed in airtight containers; storage stability is therefore very good. A disadvantage is the impossibility of incorporating humectants and mucins and the fact that they are not ready for use but must first be mixed with the requisite amount of water.

|  | 31 | 32 | 33 |
|---|---|---|---|
| Strontium sulfide, prime grade | 50 | 30 | |
| Calcium sulfide | | 20 | |
| Calcium thioglycolate | | | 18.6 |
| Calcium hydroxide | | | 6.2 |
| Sodium lauryl sulfate | | | 0.6 |
| Zinc oxide | 25 | | |
| Powdered starch | 20 | 30 | |
| Calcium carbonate, precipitated | 5 | | 74.6 |
| Talcum | | 17 | |
| Alum, powdered | | 3 | |

REMARKS

31. Rothemann, *Das grosse Rezeptbuch der Haut- und Körperflegemittel*, 3rd ed., p. 414. The ingredients are thoroughly mixed with a porcelain or wooden spatula in an earthenware container (contact with iron or other metal must be strictly avoided). Perfuming is impossible; perfume compositions are decomposed during storage. For application the powder is mixed with just enough water to produce a thick paste which can just about be spread. It is applied with a wooden spatula on the skin area to be depilated. After 5–7 minutes, when the paste has dried, it is scraped off and then washed off with ample water (to reduce the odor of hydrogen sulfide; instead of water, a scented aqueous solution of

zinc acetate may also be used); this should be followed by rinsing with acidified water, treatment with cold cream, and dusting with a mild baby or wound powder. This product may be poured into 50-g packs in strong impermeable cartons which are sealed with insulating tape and preferably wrapped in plastic foil.

32. Janistyn, *Riechstoffe, Seifen, Kosmetika*, II, p. 178.
33. Hansel, *Parfum. Kosmet.*, **34**, 413 (1953).

## Liquid Depilatories

Liquid depilatories are less popular than pastes and powders. In most cases the active ingredient is potassium or sodium sulfide; because of their strong skin-irritating action, they must be used with great caution.

|  | 34 | 35 | 36 |
|---|---|---|---|
| Sodium sulfide | 8 | | |
| Potassium sulfide | | 10.0 | |
| Calcium thioglycolate | | | 8 |
| Ammonia | | | q.s. |
| Turkey red oil | 1 | | |
| Polyethylene glycol 6000 | | | 4 |
| Carboxymethylcellulose, low viscosity | | 0.3 | |
| Sorbitol liquid | 10 | | |
| Propylene glycol | | 11.5 | 11 |
| Menthol | | 0.2 | |
| Alcohol | | 4.0 | 6 |
| Water | 81 | 73.0 | 70 |
| Perfume | | 1.0 | 1 |

REMARKS

34. Janistyn, *Riechstoffe, Seifen, Kosmetika*, II, p. 177.
35. Keithler, *The Formulation of Cosmetics and Cosmetic Specialties*, p. 253. Wet CMC with alcohol, add a little water, and stir until a smooth solution has developed. Add to this mixture a solution of potassium sulfide in the remaining water. Add propylene glycol and stir until the mixture is homogeneous. Finally add the perfume oil in which the menthol has been dissolved.
36. Keithler, *op. cit.*, 254. Mix water, calcium thioglycolate, and propylene glycol. Stir in polyethylene glycol and finally the perfume oil dissolved in the alcohol. When the mixture is clear, ammonia should slowly be added until the pH of the solution is 13.4 (*Author's note:* This is an extremely strong preparation; on the other hand, the film thickness of liquid preparations is much less than of pastes.)

## Pastes

This form is by far the most popular among chemical depilatories.

| | 37 | 38 | 39 | 40 | 41 | 42 |
|---|---|---|---|---|---|---|
| Strontium sulfide | 28 | 40.00 | 15 | | | |
| Calcium thioglycolate trihydrate | | | | 6 | 6.0 | |
| Thioglycerol | | | | | | 3.16 |
| Triethanolamine | | 12.50 | | | | |
| Calcium hydroxide | | | | | 1.5 | |
| Calcium oxide | | | | | | 2.44 |
| Strontium hydroxide Sr(OH)$_2$ · 8H$_2$O | | | | | | 10.20 |
| Triethanolamine oleate | | | 1 | | | |
| Sodium lauryl sulfate | | | | | 0.5 | |
| Petrolatum, white, viscous | | | 2 | | | |
| Lanolin, anhydrous | | | 1 | | | |
| Cetyl alcohol | | | | | 4.5 | |
| Polyethylene glycol 6000 | | | | 9 | | |
| Starch | 10 | 4.00 | | | | |
| Gum tragacanth | | 1.50 | | | | |
| Methylcellulose | | | 3 | | | 2.24 |
| Alginate | | | | 2 | | |
| Sodium silicate solution (37 wt %) | | | | | 3.5 | |
| Glycerol | 6 | 12.50 | 5 | 10 | | |
| Talcum | 42 | | | | | |
| Magnesium carbonate | | 1.25 | 2.5 | | | |
| Calcium carbonate, light | | | | | 21.0 | |
| Zinc oxide | | 4.00 | | 20 | | |
| Titanium dioxide | | | 5 | | | |
| Colloidal kaolin | | | | | | 20.80 |
| 8-oxyquinoline sulfate | | 0.025 | | | | |
| Menthol | | 0.15 | | | | |
| Ethyl alcohol | | | | 5 | | |
| Water, distilled or deionized | 13 | 23.55 | 65.5 | 47 | 62.5 | 62.00 |
| Perfume oil | 1 | | 1 | 1 | 0.5 | 0.16 |

REMARKS

37. Keithler, *The Formulation of Cosmetics and Cosmetic Specialties*, p. 257. Mix the strontium sulfide with glycerol and water, add the mixture of talcum and starch slowly until a smooth paste results, add perfume, and fill.

38. German Patent 965,920 (1957). The addition of 8-oxyquinoline sulfate prevents skin irritation.

39. Rothemann, *Das grosse Rezeptbuch der Haut- und Körperpflegemittel*, 3rd ed., p. 416. Boiling water (with 0.25% methyl-*p*-hydroxybenzoate as a preservative) is poured over the methylcellulose. Stir and allow the mucilage to cool; then stir it in a mortar with a strained mixture of strontium sulfide, magnesium carbonate, and titanium dioxide. At the same time add the separately prepared mixture of the other ingredients. Pour into pure tin tubes. Application and removal of the paste follows No. 31.

40. Keithler, *op. cit.*, p. 256. Moisten the alginate (Sea-Kem Type 11, Seaplant Chemical Co.) with alcohol, add half the water (85°C), and stir until a smooth mucilage has formed. Dissolve the polyethylene glycol in the remaining water (heat if required), stir in the glycerol and, finally, the calcium thioglycolate into the cooled solution. Stir until everything is dissolved and then stir in the cooled alginate mucilage. Continue stirring until the mass is smooth, add the perfume oil, stir for another 10 minutes, and fill immediately.

41. Barry in E. Sagarin, *Cosmetics: Science and Technology*, p. 471. To make 100 g add the melted cetyl alcohol to the solution of sodium lauryl sulfate (0.45 g) and sodium silicate in 15.5 g water (65°C) and stir until the mass has cooled to form an emulsion (A). In a separate vessel mix the calcium carbonate with 36 g of hot water, add emulsion A and stir for 30 minutes at 40°C. In a third vessel make a suspension of calcium thioglycolate and calcium hydroxide in 11 g of water containing 0.05 g of sodium lauryl sulfate and add this suspension to the previously prepared mixture; continue stirring at 40°C. Add the perfume oil and stir for another 30 minutes. Add water if necessary. The product must be roller-milled to be free from gritty crystals or entrapped air. Pour the cream into waxlined lead tubes when cooled to room temperature.

42. British Patent 593,438.

## Preparations for Mechanical Hair Removal

**Adhesive Compositions.** One method of removing quantities of hair simultaneously consists in applying a preparation that on drying or solidifying forms a tough film in which the individual hairs are firmly embedded. When this film is pulled off, the hair is also removed. This method can be painful and may cause inflammations; it is, however, simple and effective and retains some popularity.

The preparations used for this purpose are either wax-rosin mixtures which are applied hot (liquid or soft) and soon solidify to a hard mass or solutions of a film-forming substance; for example, nitrocellulose.

The following formulations are taken from Janistyn, *Riechstoffe, Seifen, Kosmetika*, II, p. 184:

43. Epilatory Wax

| | |
|---|---|
| Gum Elemi | 40 |
| Benzoin | 10 |
| Rosin, light | 8 |
| Styrax resinoid | 2 |
| Beeswax | 10 |
| Diachylon plaster | 30 |
| | 100 |

44. Collodion Preparation

| | |
|---|---:|
| Collodion solution | 80 |
| Castor oil | 5 |
| Turpentine | 5 |
| Tincture of iodine 5% | 2 |
| Alcohol 95% | 8 |
| | 100 |

U. S. Patent 2,067,909 covers the use of a latex solution for this purpose.

**Shaving Preparations.**   These preparations must be divided into those used before shaving and those intended for use after shaving. Preparations used before shaving again consist of two groups which we discuss separately because they must meet widely differing requirements: accessories for shaving with a straight razor or a safety blade and preshave preparations for electric shaving.

PREPARATIONS FOR SHAVING WITH A RAZOR OR BLADE [78].   It is no doubt possible to shave with a blade or razor without the assistance of cosmetic preparations but it is certainly not convenient. Dry keratin is a hard substance through which a blade can pass only with difficulty under conditions in which real force cannot be safely applied. The hard keratin would also soon dull the blade. Many hairs escape the blade by flattening down and therefore the same skin area must be gone over several times for a smooth shave. The skin becomes scraped and irritated, and since the whole process of shaving is rough it is often impossible to avoid cutting oneself. Shaving would be considerably facilitated if the resistant external layer of the stubble could be softened.

As already discussed, keratin can be softened by water alone. Mowery demonstrated this in experiments [79] by pressing a blade against a taut hair and accurately measuring the force required to cut it at different degrees of moisture. His results were confirmed and extended by Habicht [80]. Mimra [81] also reports on the part played by the swelling of the hair in shaving. As a shaving auxiliary, water has certain drawbacks: it cannot properly wet the hair and it evaporates before real swelling of the hair has occurred.

These deficiencies of water can be overcome by the use of shaving soaps and creams; but we must not forget that water is still the principal ingredient. Shaving preparations support the action of water by promoting the wetting of the hair by their content of wetting agents, by causing faster swelling of the keratin by their alkaline reaction, and by preventing rapid evaporation of the water by their content of humectants and water-impermeable substances. These products also help (particularly the lathering preparations) to hold the hair erect so that it cannot easily escape the blade, and have a lubricating effect that permits the blade to glide smoothly over the skin.

It might be obvious to add other hair-softening substances to shaving preparations, particularly reducing agents, but since the whole shaving process lasts only 5 to 10 minutes and shaving starts immediately after lathering such additions would be useful only if they acted very fast. No reducing agents have yet been found, however, that act so rapidly that they would make shaving easier and that are stable, have no unpleasant odor, and do not damage the skin even with daily use. The preparations discussed here can be divided into three groups: shaving soaps (solid and creams), brushless shaving creams, and aerosol preparations.

SHAVING SOAPS.   The first step is lathering. Here a concentrated aqueous solution of soap, supported by the mechanical action of the brush, acts on the beard. This step resembles normal washing; the fat film that normally surrounds each hair is removed, and the hairs are wetted with an alkaline soap solution which initiates swelling and softening. The dense lather covers the beard, prevents the evaporation of the water (this would lead to rehardening of the keratin), and holds the hairs erect until they are cut. In addition, the soap solution on the skin makes it smooth and the razor can glide over it more easily. The consumer demands a rich, soft, and fine lather that develops quickly and remains on the skin without drying for at least 5 minutes. Soap should be easy to rub on the skin or a cream should be easy to spread. Shaving soaps are marketed in three types: solid cakes (molded), sticks (milled), or creams. Since powdered and liquid shaving soaps have almost no significance any more, we shall not discuss them.

Whereas toilet soaps are pure sodium soaps, shaving soaps are mostly potassium soaps, with a smaller proportion of sodium soap. Potassium soaps are more suitable for the purpose intended because they are more readily soluble in water and become effective more quickly. They also produce a finer, denser lather than sodium soaps. Potassium soaps of lauric acid and lower fatty acids lather strongly but the foam is coarse and not very stable. Fatty acids with 8–12 carbon atoms also have an irritating effect and should therefore not be present in shaving soaps in large amounts. Palmitic and stearic acid produce a fine stable lather but it is not abundant. The best lather seems to develop from myristic acid with small additions of higher and possibly also lower fatty acids. Just like toilet soaps, shaving soaps can be produced by saponification of neutral fats, by neutralization of suitable fatty acids, or by a combination of these reactions. In the saponification of neutral fats glycerol develops at the same time; if the starting material is a pure fatty acid, glycerol must be added. The glycerol content of solid shaving soaps is around 5–10 % and somewhat higher for shaving creams.

Superfatting agents are often added to shaving soaps because they make the lather softer and creamier and also have a beneficial effect on the skin.

Superfatting agents are, among others, mineral oil, petrolatum, free fatty acids, fatty alcohols, polyoxyethylene glycols, and lanolin. Occasionally shaving soaps contain disinfectants and other active ingredients. The most difficult manufacturing problem with shaving creams is to give them the correct consistency which must remain stable over a wide temperature range. Creams of this type tend to thicken at elevated temperatures and must be observed over extended periods at varying temperatures before they can be considered for marketing. Absence or presence of certain salts (potassium chloride, or borax) strongly affects the consistency of these creams. Slight changes in formulation or even changing the source of supply of certain raw materials may have a considerable effect on the consistency or the storage life of a cream.

A few formulations from the literature follow:

45. Solid shaving soap (Janistyn, *Riechstoffe, Seifen, Kosmetika*, II, p. 94).

| | |
|---|---|
| Coconut oil, prime (S. V. 256) | 20 kilos |
| Beef tallow (S. V. 196) | 80 |
| Caustic potash, 40Bé (39%) | 27.5 |
| Caustic soda, 40°Bé (35%) | 21.2 |

The saponification value of the fat constituent and the caustic potash content in the lye must be determined. The free alkali content in the completed soap should not exceed 0.1%.

The fat mixture is melted in a soap kettle and slowly mixed with the lye mixture at a temperature not exceeding 50°C. Stirring is continued until the mass thickens. Add perfume and preservative (150 g of sodium thiosulfate, pure, dissolved in 200–300 ml of water). The mass is then poured into wooden molds lined with unbleached cotton cloth. These are well covered and allowed to stand. Unpack after two days, allow to cool, cut into bars, dry, and pack.

46. Shaving soap in bars, milled (Janistyn, *op. cit.*, 96).

| | |
|---|---|
| Saponification stearic acid, prime | 80 kilos |
| Coconut oil, prime | 20 |
| Caustic potash, 38°Bé (36%) | 36 |
| Caustic soda, 38°Bé (32%) | 19 |
| Water | 2 |
| Sodium dioxystearate, 50% | 1 |
| Sorbitol liquid, light | 2 |
| Glycerol 28°Bé, pharmaceutical grade | 1–2 |

The iodine value of the stearic acid used should be below 4.

About 75 kilos of stearic acid and the coconut oil are melted together and filtered into a soap kettle (75°C). The mixture of pure iron-free lye is combined with water, glycerol, and sodium dioxystearate, heated slightly, and stirred slowly into the fat mixture. Spontaneous heating develops, and external heating should be stopped. The rising of the soap mass in the kettle can be arrested by spraying with cold water. When the lye has been stirred in, agitation is continued for a short period with careful heating; the kettle is then covered and left to stand for 1–2 hours. The temperature of the soap should not drop below 80°C during this period. Stir once again and add the remainder of the melted stearic acid and sorbitol liquid. After another hour test the soap: free alkali should be present only in traces. If larger amounts are present, the requisite quantity of stearic acid is added or neutralization is effected with Turkey red oil. The free fatty acid content must not exceed 0.5%. Subsequently the mass is poured into wooden molds and stored for 10–14 days before further processing. The blocks are cut, shaved, carefully dried, mixed with perfume, milled, and molded. The soap must be pure white and neither too dry nor too tacky. It must run off the roller in coherent bands. The temperature of the extruder head should not exceed 25°C.

47. Shaving cream (Keithler, *The Formulation of Cosmetics and Cosmetic Specialties*, p. 287).

| | |
|---|---|
| Stearic acid | 33.10 |
| Coconut fatty acids | 9.12 |
| Propylene glycol | 8.40 |
| Glycerol | 11.01 |
| Potassium hydroxide | 7.13 |
| Sodium hydroxide | 0.86 |
| Borax | 0.59 |
| Hexachlorophene | 0.25 |
| Menthol | 0.21 |
| Perfume oil | 0.91 |
| Water | 28.42 |
| | 100.00 |

Heat the stearic acid, coconut fatty acids, and hexachlorophene together to 75–80°C in a suitable vessel. Heat the water, glycerol, propylene glycol, potassium, sodium hydroxide, and borax to the same temperature in a second vessel and add the solution to the fat melt with slow agitation. After the solution has been stirred in, agitation is continued for 30 minutes at 75–80°C; the soap mass is then checked analytically to determine whether saponification is complete and the desired alkali excess is present. If everything is in order, the mass is left to cool to room temperature; stir every five minutes for about two minutes. Perfume, in which menthol has been dissolved, is stirred into the cooled cream, which is left to mature for one to two weeks and then filled.

BRUSHLESS SHAVING CREAMS. With brushless shaving preparations the first step in routine shaving, that is, lathering, is omitted. It is therefore essential that before using one of these creams the face be thoroughly washed with warm water and soap. This washing causes the necessary defatting and softening of the hair. The task of the shaving cream is then to prevent the keratin from drying and hardening, to keep the beard erect and to facilitate the movement of the blade over the skin.

Nearly all brushless shaving creams are more or less superfatted stearate creams (occasionally the stearic acid is partly replaced by myristic acid). The emulsifying agent is usually triethanolamine, but sometimes nonionic or other emulsifiers are used. Creams of this type have the advantage of being easily rinsed off the face and blade, but even if they remain on the face, they do not give it a greasy look.

Varying additives have been used in brushless creams. Mineral oils and petrolatum are supposed to promote lubricity. Mention is sometimes made in the literature that such additives retard the drying of the cream on the skin; however, it is difficult to see how they can do this. It may well be that these substances prevent quick hardening of the hair, even if the cream dries, by leaving a water-impermeable film around each water-soaked hair. Emollients such as lanolin and cetyl alcohol may be used here in larger quantities than in regular shaving creams in which the demand for a rich lather restricts the use of fats. Brushless shaving creams also often contain humectants, glycerol, or sorbitol. It is also said of these substances that they delay the drying of the cream on the skin, but this has not been substantiated.

If a substance can bind a certain amount of water when it is in contact with atmospheric humidity, it does not necessarily follow that it can also delay the evaporation of water from a solution within the first few minutes (which is what actually matters in shaving). Griffin, Behrens, and Cross [82] did determine a delay in water evaporation caused by these substances but their tests extended over many hours. According to Guest [83], glycerol did not affect the softening of the hair during shaving in a test carried out according to Mowery's method.

Although their effectiveness in retarding drying may be doubtful, glycerol and Sorbitol are often useful in other ways. They give shaving creams their required smoothness, soft consistency, and easy spreadability; they also help to leave the skin smooth and soft after shaving.

Natural and synthetic mucins (gum tragacanth, alginates, polyvinyl-pyrrolidone, and methylcellulose) are also useful additives. They thicken the cream, and make it smooth, facilitate application and spreading, promote lubricity, and may also act as humectants. The film of cream on the skin is given more substance by polyoxyethylene glycols which also help to make it easier to rinse off.

In addition to the required emulsifiers, these creams sometimes contain other surfactants (sodium lauryl sulfate or Turkey red oil). The main purpose of these additives is probably to facilitate the rinsing of the blades. Occasionally borax, metaphosphates, or other alkaline salts are added to promote softening of the hair. A slight excess of triethanolamine acts in a similar way. Good preservation, prevention of oxidation, and suitable perfuming are as important in these creams as in all other cosmetic preparations.

Some formulations follow:

| | 48 | 49 | 50 | 51 | 52 |
|---|---|---|---|---|---|
| Paraffin oil, prime grade | 8.7 | 3.0 | | | |
| Petrolatum | | | | | 8.0 |
| Olive oil | | | 5 | | |
| Acetoglyceride L/C | | | 5 | | |
| Cetyl alcohol | 2.2 | | | | |
| Lanolin, anhydrous | 2.2 | | | | |
| Stearic acid, prime grade | 19.6 | 12.5 | 32 | 12.6 | 20.0 |
| Oleic acid | | | | | 2.0 |
| Propylene glycol monostearate SE | | 3.5 | | | |
| Glyceryl monostearate | | | | | 4.0 |
| Sorbitan monostearate (Span 60) | | | | | 3.1 |
| Polyoxyethylene sorbitan monostearate (Tween 60) | | | | | 2.2 |
| Triethanolamine | 1.3 | 1.5 | 2 | 1.0 | |
| Potassium hydroxide (85%) | | | 0.6 | 0.52 | 0.7 |
| Borax powder | 0.2 | | | | |
| Water, distilled | 54.5 | 77.5 | 44 | 60.6 | 44.7 |
| Polyoxyethylene glycol 1500 | | | | 15.1 | |
| Sodium alginate | | | | 1.18 | |
| Glycerol | 10.9 | 2.0 | 8 | | 9.5 |
| Propylene glycol | | | | 4.0 | |
| Diethylene glycol monoethyl ether | | | | 5.0 | |
| Perfume oil | 0.4 | q.s. | q.s. | q.s. | 0.3 |
| Preservative | | | 0.1 | | |

REMARKS

48. Rothemann, *Das grosse Rezeptbuch der Haut- und Körperpflegemittel*, 3rd ed., p. 754. The aqueous solution of glycerol, triethanolamine, and borax (80°C) is stirred into the fat melt (about 75°C) in a thin jet. Slow stirring is continued until the mass has almost cooled. The perfume oil then is stirred in carefully, and the cream is left to stand overnight in an earthenware vessel. It is stirred once again next day and immediately filled into tubes with wide nozzles. Enameled iron vessels, and chrome or Monel metal kettles are suitable containers for manufacture.

49. De Navarre, *The Chemistry and Manufacture of Cosmetics*, p. 436. Pour the aqueous solution of triethanolamine and glycerol (70°C) into the hot fat melt, stirring continuously. After emulsification stir occasionally to avoid crust formation. Add the perfume at 45°C, mix once again on the following day, and fill. (*Author's note:* It is interesting to compare this

procedure with the preceding one. The ingredients are similar but the ratio alkali: stearic acid differs considerably, as does the glycerol content.)

50. Newman, *J. Soc. cosmet. Chem.*, **8**, 44 (1957). The aqueous solution of glycerol, alkali, and preservative (75°C) is stirred into the fat melt (75°C). Stirring is continued until the cream has formed, and the perfume is added after cooling. The cream is left overnight, stirred once again for 20 minutes, and filled.

51. Harry, *Modern Cosmetocology*, 4th ed., p. 525. Dissolve the potassium hydroxide (0.52 parts) in water (0.65 parts) and then add the triethanolamine. Stir this mixture into the melt of stearic acid and polyoxyethylene wax (70°C). Add the alginate and the remaining water (70°C), the propylene glycol, and part of the Carbitol (diethylene glycol monoethyl ether). The perfume oil, dissolved in the remaining Carbitol, is stirred in at 50°C. Fill at 45°C.

52. Keithler, *The Formulation of Cosmetics and Cosmetic Specialties*, p. 276. The procedure is the same as for 49. The nonionic emulsifiers are added to the fat melt.


AEROSOL SHAVING CREAMS. The composition of aerosol shaving creams is similar to that of brushless creams. Another point both types have in common is the fact that they are not worked into a lather on the face, but simply spread over the skin, which must therefore be washed first with soap and water. Aerosol creams combine many of the advantages of both types already discussed: quick and easy application, with no lathering, and abundant foam.

U. S. Patent 2,655,480 [84] is important in this connection; many formulations and procedures discussed in the literature are covered by its claims. A good survey of the factors affecting the properties of aerosol shaving creams appears in Carter and Truax [85]. Liu [86] provides a theoretical analysis of the behavior of shaving lather on the skin. Some examples follow.


REMARKS

53. Keithler, *The Formulation of Cosmetics and Cosmetic Specialties*, p. 268. Add the aqueous solution of triethanolamine lauryl sulfate and propylene glycol, to which triethanolamine has been added at the last moment (85°C), to the fat melt (85°C), which also contains nonionic emulsifiers. Stir until a cream has formed and allow to cool to 45°C, stirring occasionally. Add the perfume oil. The concentrate is packed in an aerosol container (with a foam valve) in one of the following proportions: 90% concentrate, 10% Freon 12/114 (50:50) or 92% concentrate, 8% Freon 12/114 (60:40).

54. di Giacomo, *Am. Perfumer.*, May 1957, p. 45. Aerosol containers are filled with 90 parts concentrate and 10 parts Freon 12/114 (40:60). (*Author's note:* Consider the higher alkalinity of this product compared with No. 53).

55. Bergwein, *Parfum. Kosmet.*, **37**, 71 (1956). Aerosol containers are filled with 90 parts concentrate and 10 parts Freon 12/114 (40:60). (*Author's note:* This product resembles a lathering shaving cream in composition.)

| | 53 | 54 | 55 |
|---|---|---|---|
| Mineral oil | 4 | | |
| Petrolatum | 10 | | |
| Cetyl alcohol | 2 | 0.5 | |
| Lanolin, anhydrous | | 0.8 | |
| Stearic acid | 10.5 | 6 | 8.1 |
| Myristic acid | | 2 | |
| Coconut fatty acids | | | 8.1 |
| Span 60 | 2 | | |
| Tween 60 | 1 | | |
| Tween 80 | | 5 | |
| Tween 20 | | 5 | |
| Soap, neutral | | 1 | |
| Triethanolamine lauryl sulfate (60% active ingredients) | 4 | | 4.5 |
| Triethanolamine | 1 | 4 | |
| Borax | | 0.1 | |
| Potassium hydroxide (85%) | | | 2.3 |
| Water | 62.2 | 71.1 | 68.9 |
| Glycerol | | | 7.2 |
| Propylene glycol | 3 | | |
| Sorbitol liquid | | 3.5 | |
| Perfume oil | 0.3 | 0.1 | |

**Pre-electric Shave Preparations.** Since the end of World War II many men in Western countries have discarded the traditional methods of shaving in favor of the electric shaver. The main reason for the success of this method is its somewhat greater speed and convenience. It can be done any time, anywhere (e.g., in bed or in the car), and fully clothed, since there is no need for preliminary washing, soaping, and subsequent rinsing. This provides two considerations which must not be neglected in developing a pre-electric shave preparation:

1. Although it is very hard to shave with a blade without the help of a cosmetic preparation, it is easy with an electric razor. For this reason few men who use electric shavers will also use a preshave preparation unless some revolutionary products are developed.
2. Preparations will be successful only if they are not greasy, unpleasant, or time consuming in application.

For electric shaving it is not particularly important to soften the hair first (the impact of the electric blades is sufficient to cut through the stiffest beard), but the hair must be erect and not stick to the skin. The skin must be taut but smooth enough for the razor to glide over it.

Products intended to prepare the skin and hair for electric shaving are commercially available in various forms. Advantages and disadvantages of the different forms have been discussed in the literature by Jason [87] and Uexküll [88].

POWDERS. If the skin is covered with perspiration and a thick film of skin fat, the stubbles will not remain erect but will stick to the skin and therefore cannot be easily attacked by the electric razor. Moreover, moist skin is soft and shaving may cause lesions and irritations. Powders with a good lubricating effect and absorbent drying properties facilitate shaving and reduce the strain on the skin. By incorporating suitable additives these powders can be given astringent or disinfectant properties.

The powder should be tinted so that it is hardly visible on the face. It is important that it should contain no gritty particles that might damage the blades of the razor. Loose powders are inconvenient for men to use: they are too easily spilled. Only a stick powder which can be rubbed over the face shortly before shaving will have any chance of success.

How such sticks are made can be seen in the following suggestions:

56. Bell in Sagarin, *Cosmetics: Science and Technology*, p. 441.

| | | |
|---|---|---|
| (a) | Zinc stearate | 5.0 |
| | Light magnesium carbonate | 2.0 |
| | Iron oxide pigments | q.s. |
| | Perfume | q.s. |
| | Talcum to make | 98.5 |
| (b) | Veegum | 1.5 |
| | Water | 30 |

PROCEDURE. Mix perfume oil and magnesium carbonate thoroughly, add zinc stearate and pigments when the perfume has been completely adsorbed, and disperse the whole in the talcum. Stir the Veegum rapidly into the water until smooth. Add (b) to (a) and more water if required to obtain a fluid paste. Pour into molds, dry until hard, and then completely oven-dry the sticks.

57. H. Goldschmidt, *Am. Perf.*, **65** (6), 44 (June 1955).

| | |
|---|---|
| Calcium sulfate | 40 |
| Magnesium oxide | 10 |
| Talcum | 49.5 |
| Aluminum chloride | 0.5 |
| Perfume and pigments | q.s. |

The powder is worked into a paste with the requisite amount of water, poured into molds, and dried.

The procedure described for these two formulations is identical with the "wet" method used for compact powder (see Chapter 10). Powder sticks which can be prepared according to the moist process require less water. The dry method in which the powder is pressed into a stick under high pressure is also possible [89]. This type of stick is treated on the outside with a solution of polyvinyl chloride or polyvinyl acetate which dries to a tough film and prevents crumbling or cracking.

CREAMS. The literature describes liquid as well as solid emulsions which soften the beard and supply fat to the skin. Several of these preparations are available. Most of them are supposed to be applied the night before; and the residue of the cream is removed just before shaving. Since these creams are somewhat tacky and make the shaving procedure more complicated, we do not think it very likely that they will achieve much popularity.

ALCOHOLIC LOTIONS. These lotions, like powders, cause the hair stubble to be more erect and the skin to become taut and dry; they also have a tonic effect. Various active ingredients may be used: astringents help to stiffen the hair and tauten the skin. (If weak acids are used for an astringent effect, it should be borne in mind that the lower the pH of the preparation, the more the metal of the razor will be attacked. Disinfectants help to prevent infections that might develop during shaving.

Menthol and camphor have a cooling effect on the skin; azulene (in concentrations of about 0.025%) counteracts minor inflammations. Glycerol is added to promote smooth gliding of the razor over the skin, but if it is used in sufficiently high concentrations to produce a good lubricating effect it may coat the razor blades and leave them sticky. Isopropyl myristate or a similar ester would be preferable. A solution of these substances in concentrated alcohol, with a correct adjustment of the fatty acid esters (about 15–25%; the optimum dosage depends on the type of ester used), can ease shaving considerably [90].

Among the following formulations [91] No. 58 represents the type just described, No. 59 is an astringent product.

| 58. | Isopropyl myristate | 20 |
| | Alcohol 96% | 80 |
| | Disinfectant | q.s. |
| | Perfume oil | q.s. |
| 59. | Zinc phenol sulfate | 1 |
| | Hamamelis water | 40 |
| | Alcohol 96% | 40 |
| | Water | 19 |
| | Menthol | traces |

The literature also describes lotions without alcohol, but they lack the tonic effect so desirable in a shaving lotion.

GELS.  These have the advantage of being easy to use, and can be packed in tubes.

Berghausen [92] describes an acid gel based on alcohol. It dries to a smooth film and is reported to contain one ingredient that raises goose pimples, so that the hair can be cut deeply at the root, and some growth-retarding agents.

**Aftershave Preparations.**  Perfect shaving cuts the beard close to the skin surface without affecting the skin itself. Unfortunately there is no perfect

### SHAVING LOTIONS

|  | 60 | 61 | 62 | 63 |
|---|---|---|---|---|
| Alcohol, 96% | 40.00 | 32.6 | 15 | 22.0 |
| Isopropyl alcohol C.P. |  |  | 15 |  |
| Water | 59.72 | 40 | 65 | 74.9 |
| Quaternary ammonium salt (25%) | 0.25 |  |  |  |
| Oxyquinoline sulfate |  |  |  | 0.4 |
| Birch extract |  | 10 |  |  |
| Aluminum acetate |  | 10 |  |  |
| Alum |  |  | 1 |  |
| Zinc phenol sulfate |  |  | 0.1 |  |
| Lactic acid (80%) |  | 1 |  |  |
| Menthol | 0.005 |  |  |  |
| Spirit of camphor |  |  | 1.9 |  |
| Benzocain | 0.025 |  |  |  |
| Glycerol |  |  | 2 |  |
| Sorbitol |  |  |  | 1 |
| Propylene glycol |  |  |  | 1 |
| Perfume oil |  | 0.5 |  | 0.3 |
| Anilin dye (2%) |  |  |  | 0.3 |

REMARKS

60. *Schimmel Briefs*, **190**, (January 1951).

61. Rothemann, *Das grosse Rezeptbuch der Haut- und Körperpflegemittel*, 3rd ed., p. 578. Mix the alcoholic solution of the perfume oil and the aqueous solution of lactic acid, add birch extract and aluminum acetate, and filter the solution on the following day.

62. Janistyn, *Riechstoffe-Seifen-Kosmetika*, II, p. 187. The completed mixture should be cooled to about 0°C and filtered. Contact with iron should be avoided, since it causes discoloration in the presence of zinc phenol sulfate.

63. Keithler, *The Formulation of Cosmetics and Cosmetic Specialties*, p. 324. Dissolve sorbitol, propylene glycol, and the pigment in water, menthol and oxyquinoline sulfate in alcohol. Mix the two solutions, add perfume oil, allow to mature, and filter.

shaving method. How the skin is affected depends on many different factors (e.g., the condition of the skin and hair, the shaving technique, the sharpness of the blade or the construction of the electric razor, and the shaving accessories used), but a certain amount of irritation can never be completely avoided. The top layers of the corneum are scraped off, particularly around the mouths of the hair follicles, and shaving with a blade usually causes minute, mostly nonbleeding, cuts. Wherever the skin has been damaged foreign matter and bacteria may penetrate, and these spots become seats of irritation or infection. If shaving soap or cream is used (brushless shaving creams usually have only a weak alkaline reaction), the skin is alkalized, which further promotes the development of infection, and is deprived of fat, with unfavorable consequences for men with dry skin. Another result of scraping the epidermis is the well-known burning feeling.

Aftershave preparations are intended to relieve the objective as well as subjective undesired side-effects of shaving. This purpose can be met adequately by a 50% solution of ethyl alcohol to which a suitable fragrance has been added. It has a cooling and refreshing effect and is slightly astringent and disinfecting, to which the perfume contributes, as shown by Theile and Pease [93] and Mazurella [94]. Usually, however, special astringent and disinfecting agents are incorporated; menthol and camphor strengthen the cooling effect. Small additions of glycerol, sorbitol, or polyethylene glycols give the skin a soft, smooth feeling.

Next to shaving lotions, sticks based on alcohol are also very popular. They resemble lotions in composition and effect but also contain a stearate soap as the gelling agent.

64. Aftershave stick lotion. Bell in Sagarin, *Cosmetics: Science and Technology*, p. 450.

| | |
|---|---|
| Ethyl alcohol, 95%, specially denatured | 80.5 |
| Water, demineralized | 5.0 |
| Sodium stearate | 6.0 |
| Glycerol | 4.0 |
| Propylene glycol | 3.0 |
| Perfume oil | 1.4 |
| Menthol | 0.1 |

PROCEDURE.    Place all ingredients, except the perfume oil, in a closed, stainless-steel or glass-lined, steam-jacketed kettle fitted with an agitator and a water-cooled condenser. Heat with stirring and, when the temperature reaches about 55°C, add the perfume oil. Continue heating to reflux temperature and stir until completely dissolved. Adjust temperature to 71–74°C and pour into molds. Color, if desired, is added by dissolving it in the water of the formulation.

*Shaving powders* contain astringent and often disinfecting ingredients as well. Since they accelerate water evaporation from a moist skin, they also have a certain cooling effect and cover any reddening that might have been caused by shaving. With their absorbent properties they may also have a drying and firming effect.

*Creams*, which act as emollients, have also been marketed for use after shaving. Since they are not particularly refreshing, they have not achieved any great popularity.

SHAVING POWDERS

| | 65 | 66 | 67 | 68 |
|---|---|---|---|---|
| Alum, finest powder | | | 0.5 | |
| Aluminum stearate | | | | 5 |
| Zinc undecanate | | | | 10 |
| Boric acid | 2.5 | | 2 | |
| Zinc stearate | | 3.5 | | |
| Magnesium stearate | 3.4 | | | |
| Zinc myristate | | | 4 | |
| Colloidal kaolin | | | 10 | 25 |
| Silicic acid, superfine | | | 10 | |
| Zinc oxide | | | | 5 |
| Titanium dioxide | | 3.0 | | |
| Talcum | 54.5 | 68.0 | 70 | 30 |
| Magnesium carbonate | 35.0 | | | |
| Calcium carbonate, precipitated | | 25.0 | | 20 |
| Perfume oil | 0.6 | 0.5 | 0.5 | |
| Pigments | 0.3 | 0.3 | 1 | |

REMARKS

65 and 66. Keithler, *The Formulation of Cosmetics and Cosmetic Specialties*, p. 126.
67 and 68. Janistyn, *Riechstoffe-Seifen-Kosmetika*, II, p. 234.

## REFERENCES

[1] Winter, *Handbuch der ges. Parfümerie und Kosmetik*, Springer Verlag, Vienna, 3rd ed. 1941, pp. 580–596.
[2] Janistyn, *Riechstoffe-Seifen-Kosmetika*, II, p. 439 et seq. Dr. Alfred Hüthig, Heidelberg, 1950.
[3] *SÖFW*, **83**, 301 (1957).
[4] Holmes, *J. Soc. cosmet. Chem.*, **15**, 595 (1964).
[5] *Am. Perfumer*, **69** (1), 25; (2), 34; (3), 47 (1956).

[6] Sagarin, *Cosmetics, Science and Technology*, Interscience, New York, 1957, Chapter XXI, F. E. Wall.

[7] Mannheim, *Soap. Perfum. Cosm.*, **35**, 611, 713 (1962).

[8] Schneller, U. S. Patent 2,610,941 (1952).

[9] *SÖFW*, **83**, 133 (1957).

[10] *Am. Perfumer*, **68** (3), 47 (1956).

[11] Schwartz and Barban, *Archs. Derm. Syph.*, **66**, 223 (1952); Reiss, Gahgygler, and Lustig, *J. Allergy*, **28**, 131 (1957).

[12] Sidi, *Verträglichkeit der Kosmetika*, Hüthig, Heidelberg, 1959, p. 17.

[13] *J. Soc. Cosmet. Chem.*, **15**, 659 (1964).

[14] Tobler, *Kosmetic-Parf.-Drog.*, **11**, 167 (1964).

[15] Austrian Patent 237,805 (Farbenfabrik Wolfen).

[16] French Patent 1,355,110 (N. V. Ind. Ond., W. H. Braskamp).

[17] *SÖFW*, **83**, 133 (1957).

[18] Wall in Sagarin, *op. cit.*, p. 484.

[19] Conrad and Mentecki, *J. Soc. cosmet. Chem.*, **13**, 362 (1962).

[20] *Schimmel Briefs*, **255** (1956).

[21] Harry, *Modern Cosmetocology*, Leonard Hill, London, 1955, 4th ed., p. 498.

[22] Sagarin, *op. cit.*, p. 525.

[23] Gibbs, Shank, Pont, and Hansman, *Archs. Derm. Syph.*, **44**, 862 (1941).

[24] Harry, *Cosmetic Materials*, Leonard Hill, London, 1948, p. 31.

[25] Lerner and Fitzpatrick, *J. Am. med. Ass.*, **152**, 577 (1955).

[26] Denton, Lerner, and Fitzpatrick, *J. invest. Derm.*, **18**, 119 (1952).

[27] Astbury in Saville, *The Hair and Scalp*, 4th ed., Williams and Williams, Baltimore, 1952, p. 65 et seq.

[28] H. Freytag, *J. Soc. cosmet. Chem.*, **15**, 667 (1964).

[29a] Stoves, *Perfum. essent. Oil. Rec.*, **34**, 232 (1952).

[29b] Schöberl et al., *Biochem. Z.*, **317**, 174 (1944); Rosenthal and Oster, *J. Soc. cosmet. Chem.*, **5**, 286 (1954).

[30] Bersin and Stendel, *Ber. dt. chem. Ges.*, **71**, 1015 (1938).

[31] J. Morelle, *Industrie Parfum.*, **7**, 201 (1952); French Patent 1,031,538.

[32] J. Morelle, *Industrie Parfum.*, **5**, 173 (1950).

[33] J. Morelle, French Patent 984,231; *Archs. Derm. Syph.*, **198**, 274 (1954).

[34] *Perfum. essent. Oil Rec.*, **46**, 410 (1955).

[35] Chem. Fabrik Sulfonchemie, in *Parfum. Kosmet.*, **38**, 666 (1957).

[36] Santoianni and Rothman, *J. invest. Derm.*, **37**, 489 (1961); Finkelstein, Hsiung, and DeMytt, *J. Soc. cosmet. Chem.*, **13**, 253 (1962); Walker, *Drug Cosmet. Ind.*, **92**, 709 (1963).

[37] British Patent 745,179 (1956); *SÖFW*, **83**, 62 (1957).

[38] U. S. Patent 2,766,760 (1956) and British Patent 766,585 (1956); Weigel, *Parfum Kosmet.*, **37**, 532 (1957).

[39] Stoves, *Trans. Faraday Soc.*, **39**, 294 (1943).

[40] Frigley, *J. Am. med. Ass.*, **123**, 747 (1940).

[41] G.T.H., *Kosmetik-Parf.-Drog.*, **3**, 68, 124 (1956); **5**, 30 (1958).

[42] German Patent 948,186 (1956); *SÖFW*, **82**, 577 (1956); U. S. Patents 2,577,710 and 2,577,711; British Patent 589,956; Australian Patent 117,071; French Patent 983,334; Austrian Patent 176,301; Swiss Patent 241,113.

[43] *SÖFW*, **83**, 341 (1957).

[44] *Parfum. Kosmet.*, **38**, 204 (1957).

[45] Heilingötter, *Parfum. Kosmet.*, **38**, 204 (1957).

[46] *Drug Cosmet. Ind.*, **79**, 326 (1956).

[47] Meeting Scientific Section Toilet Goods Association, May 9, 1957.

[48] *Melliand Text Ber.*, 1025 (1953).

[49] U. S. Patent 2,717,288 (1955); British Patent 723,917; German Patent Application 1,011,581 (1957), The Gillette Co.

[50] U. S. Patent 2,613,965 (1953).

[51] U. S. Patent 2,708,940.

[52] *Kosmetik-Parf.-Drog.*, **4**, 85 (1957).

[53] British Patent 753,241 (1956).

[54] *Schimmel Briefs*, **253**, (1956).

[55] *Schimmel Briefs*, **244** (1955); *Parfum. Kosmet.*, **36**, 506 (1955).

[56] *Ibid.*

[57] *SÖFW*, **83**, 133 (1957).

[58] *SÖFW*, **83**, 695 (1957).

[59] *SÖFW*, **83**, 341 (1957).

[60] Sidi, *Hautverträglichkeit der Kosmetika*, p. 38 et seq.

[61] *Aesth. Med.*, **11**, 278 (1962); *Parfum. Kosmet.*, **43**, 201 (1962).

[62] *J. Soc. cosmet. Chem.*, **15**, 659 (1964).

[63] Schulte, Meinek, and Hobl, *Parfum. Kosmet.*, **45**, 87 (1964); Gerthsen and Gohlke, *Parfum. Kosmet.*, **45**, 277 (1964).

[64] Bauer, *SÖFW*, **82**, 269 (1956); Burckhardt, *J. med. Kosmet.* 259 (1953–1954).

[65] Schulte, Meinek, and Hobl, *Parfum. Kosmet.*, **45**, 153 (1964).

[66] *SÖFW*, **78**, 107 (1953).

[67] Volk and Winter, *Lexikon der kosmetischen Praxis*, Springer-Verlag, Vienna, 1936, p. 108.

[68] Walker, *Drug Cosmet. Ind.*, **92**, 563 (1963).

[69] Harry, *op. cit.*, 571.

[70] *J. ind. Hyg.*, **30**, 192 (1948).

[71] *J. Soc. cosmet. Chem.*, **3**, 2 (1952).

[72] J. Morelle, *Industrie Parfum.*, **11**, 176 (1956).

[73] Atkins, *Perfum. essent. Oil Rec.*, 231 (1947).

[74] Sagarin, *op. cit.*, 469.

[75] *Industrie Parfum.*, **11**, 176 (1956).

[76] French Patent 844,529 (1940); British Patent 521,240 (1940), and 593,438 (1945).

[77] *Industrie Parfum.*, **11**, 176 (1956).

[78] Bhaktavizian, Mescon, and Maltoltsy, *Arch. Derm.*, **88**, 874 (1963).

[79] *Text. Res. J.*, **24**, 711 (1954).

[80] Habicht, *Fette Seifen, Anstrichmittel*, **61**, 985 (1959); **62**, 101 (1960).

[81] *Kosmetika* (Prague), **2**, 3 (1946); *Parfum. Kosmet.*, **34**, 86 (1953); **44**, 153 (1963).

[82] *J. Soc. cosmet. Chem.*, **3**, 5 (1952).

[83] Sagarin, *op. cit.*, 424.

[84] Spitzer, Reich, and Fine, U. S. Patent 2,655,480 1953.

[85] *Proc. scient. Sect.*, Toilet Goods Ass., **35**, 37 (1961).

[86] *Archs. Biochim. Cosm.*, 6 (51), 12 (1962).

[87] *J. med. Kosmet.* 142 (1956).

[88] *SÖFW*, **81**, 487 (1955).

[89] Bell in Sagarin, *op. cit.*, 442.

[90] von Uexküll, *SÖFW*, **81**, 487 (1955).

[91] Harry, *op. cit.*, 535.

[92] *SÖFW*, **81**, 646 (1957).

[93] *J. Soc. cosmet. Chem.*, **15**, 745 (1964).

[94] Mazurella, *Am. Perfumer*, **77** (1), 67 (1962).

# CHAPTER 12

# Preparations for Enjoyment

So far this book has dealt with protective and decorative preparations, with auxiliaries in hygiene, and with depth-effect preparations. A number of cosmetics, however, do not easily fall into any of these categories but must have a certain value or appeal because they are widely used. We have only to consider colognes and other toilet waters, dusting powders used after bathing, certain hair lotions that are really nothing but solutions of perfume, and bath oils and bath salts. Why are they used?

These preparations could be fitted into the categories discussed so far, and we have done so in most cases: hair lotions have a disinfectant effect because of their alcohol content; body powders accelerate the evaporation of the last water traces after washing and provide some protection to the softened skin against chafing; certain bath preparations, by softening the water, make soap more effective and thus become auxiliaries in hygiene. However, this classification does not really do justice to the character of these products. The consumer would use hair and shaving lotions even if they had no disinfectant effect; nobody used dusting powder because he is afraid that the softened skin might be chafed by his clothes, and bath salts that do not act as water softeners are just as popular as those that do.

The reason why the consumer uses these products can therefore not lie in their measurable effectiveness.

It is noteworthy that in all products mentioned fragrance plays an important part. Should they therefore, like perfume itself, be regarded as olfactory decorative preparations. This does not apply either, because a decorative preparation must be noticeable to others after application; the products we have just mentioned generally are not. On the contrary: if bath salts or shaving lotions smell too strong too long after application, many consumers will reject them. What is required is a momentarily refreshing effect and some stimulation. All of these preparations have this in common: the main purpose of using them is the immediate effect on the consumer—a vitalizing action. They give us a feeling of freshness and good grooming, and nobody needs to know that we have used them.

Here we discuss one aspect of cosmetic preparations that so far we have hardly considered: the psychological effect on the user. If it is important that a woman *look* clean, well groomed, or stylish, it is just as important that she *feel* clean, well groomed, or stylish.

Some observers consider this aspect to be so important that they regard cosmetics as belonging ultimately to the field of psychotherapeutics [1].

Every cosmetic product therefore acts in three ways: on the environment, on the body of the user, and on the user's psyche.

With decorative preparations the effect on the environment (at least directly) is the main purpose; with skin conditioners it is the effect on the skin, and with tonic preparations the psychological effect is dominant. On no account should any cosmetic preparation have a negative effect in any of the three directions.

A decorative preparation should not be harmful to the skin, nor should a skin conditioner adversely affect the appearance of the user. (This is the difference between cosmetic and therapeutical skin care: a medical preparation will be accepted even if it has an unpleasant odor or looks unattractive on the skin; a cosmetic preparation, never). If at all possible, all cosmetics should be pleasant to use so that the consumer can enjoy them even during application. (There are some regrettable exceptions here (e.g., cold-wave preparations), and even they are being made more attractive by scenting them).

It is very difficult, however, to draw the line at which the agreeable sensation of using hair lotions, dusting powders, etc., stops being incidental and becomes the main purpose. For this reason we have discussed most preparations used primarily for the user's enjoyment, in preceding chapters with other preparations they resemble. There is just one group of products for which enjoyment is clearly the main reason for being: bath preparations. Even if some bath salts soften the water and some bath oils prevent the formation of a calcium soap ring around the tub, the main purpose is always their pleasant scent and possibly their rich, soft foam.

## BATH PREPARATIONS

We shall not discuss preparations based on dried therapeutical herbs or their extracts: they border on medical practice. We refer the interested reader to the relevant chapter in Rothemann, *Das grosse Rezeptbuch der Haut- und Körperpflegemittel* [2], and also to Bergwein [3]. Among the other bath preparations, salts, tablets, and oils are important.

### Bath Salts

These products consist of an inorganic salt, or a mixture of various inorganic salts, which are scented and colored. Among the many salts used as a base for these preparations the following are probably the most important:

*Common Salt.* (rocksalt, sodium chloride, NaCl). This product forms attractive crystals that are stable, however, only when the salt is free of magnesium chloride; otherwise they soon lose their shape. It is easily soluble in water but has no softening effect and reduces the lathering of soap.

*Sodium Sesquicarbonate.* ($Na_2CO_3 \cdot NaHCO_3 \cdot 2H_2O$). This is available in the form of fine crystal-needles; it is easily soluble in water, softens it, and is used extensively, particularly in the United States.

*Sodium Carbonate.* The most suitable form is anhydrous sodium carbonate or calcined soda, $Na_2CO_3$, which is a fine powder, not hygroscopic and not easily soluble in water. It is inexpensive, has a good storage stability, and is an efficient water softener. $Na_2CO_3 \cdot H_2O$, which is not hygroscopic and hard to dissolve, is also used occasionally. Soda ($Na_2CO_3 \cdot 10H_2O$) forms attractive, easily soluble crystals but they tend to soften during extended storage, particularly in warm temperatures.

*Sodium Thiosulfate* ($Na_2S_2O_3 \cdot 5H_2O$). This forms beautiful easily soluble crystals. If used in large quantities, the bath water and the skin may develop a slightly unpleasant odor.

*Borax* ($Na_2B_4O_7 \cdot 10H_2O$). Borax forms small even crystals; it has a mild alkaline reaction and can easily be colored. It is not hygroscopic, but it is hard to dissolve in water.

*Disodium Phosphate* ($Na_2HPO_4 \cdot 12H_2O$) is a good softener and not hygroscopic, but it clouds the bath water. Disodium pyrophosphate and trisodium phosphate are also occasionally recommended for bath salts, but the latter is too strongly alkaline to be advisable.

The salts mentioned above are the basis for bath salts but perfume oil is the principal active ingredient.

Fresh scents (pine, lavender, citrus or floral) are generally preferred, but even heavier fragrances are also used. It is a moot point whether the effect of the perfume is purely psychological or whether the physiological action of the perfume materials also plays a part [4]. Perfume oil is usually sprayed on to the salt crystals in solution.

Water-soluble alkali-resistant dyes used to color bath salts can be applied in two ways: by spraying the crystals with a dye solution or by adding the colorant(s) to the concentrated salt solution from which the crystals are made by slow evaporation.

The following procedures illustrate the preparation of bath salts.

1. Rothemann, *Das grosse Rezeptbuch der Haut- und Körperpflegemittel*, 3rd ed, p. 658. A sodium chloride solution in water which has been colored with basic dyes is boiled down to 43°Bé and allowed to cool. The crystals are sprayed with a solution of the perfume oil. A hot sodium thiosulfate solution should be thickened in a similar way to 46°Bé, and a disodium phosphate solution, to 21°Bé. (Rothemann insists on essential oils only for the perfume, but in my opinion his suspicion of synthetic fragrances is not justified. Innumerable perfume compositions are made with synthetic fragrances which are just as harmless to the skin as the mildest natural perfumes.)

2. Keithler, *The Formulation of Cosmetics and Cosmetic Specialties*, p. 396.

| | |
|---|---|
| Sodium sesquicarbonate | 98.5 |
| Perfume oil | 1.0 |
| Dye 2% | 0.5 |

Perfume and dye solution are sprayed over the crystals in a mixing drum. Mix thoroughly (about 45 minutes) and fill.

3. Rothemann, *op. cit.*, p. 659.

| | |
|---|---|
| Sodium chloride, pure, medium fine | 98 |
| Sodium sulfate, dehydrated | 2 |
| Uranin, 5% in alcohol | 2 |
| Carbitol | 4 |
| Perfume oil | 4 |

Mix the salts thoroughly and spread them out. The mixture containing the color solution, perfume oil, and Carbitol is evenly sprayed over the salts with an atomizer and then mixed in a mixer, once again spread out, and repacked on the following day. (In my opinion the use of hygroscopic Carbitol is not advisable.) The preparation is suitably packaged in wide-neck glasses with cut stoppers, plexiglass, or other plastic containers and cartons with airtight cellophane wraps (contents about 250 ml). The direction "store in a cool and dry place" should not be omitted on any package.

## Bath Tablets

In addition to finely ground salts, perfume oil, and color, these tablets contain a substance that prevents them from developing into a rocklike block that is hard to dissolve. Bath tablets often contain a crystalline organic acid (e.g., tartaric or citric acid) in addition to sodium carbonate, sesquicarbonate, or bicarbonate. As soon as they are placed in water carbon dioxide develops with an effervescent effect. The tablets rapidly decompose and dissolve. If they also contain a foam-forming substance (e.g., sodium lauryl sulfate), the carbon dioxide gas helps in foam formation. Bath tablets also often contain a salt that releases oxygen in water (e.g., sodium perborate or hydrogen peroxide-urea complex). The oxygen is supposed to have a beneficial and refreshing effect on the skin. If these tablets are not stored completely dry, the perfume oil is soon destroyed by the oxidizing substances.

4. H. Jankowitz, *SÖFW*, **82**, 694 (1956).

| Sodium carbonate, anhydrous | 82.5 |
|---|---|
| Starch | 10.0 |
| Perfume oil | 5.0 |
| Tincture of benzoin | 2.25 |
| Fluorescine | 0.25 |

Perfume oil, benzoin, and color are mixed with the sodium carbonate. This is strained through a coarse sieve, starch is added, and the mixture is strained again and compressed.

5. Rothemann, *op. cit.*, p. 664. Effervescent bath tablets.

| Sodium bicarbonate powder | 25 |
|---|---|
| Wheat- or cornstarch powder | 30 |
| Colloidal kaolin | 17.5 |
| Tartaric acid powder | 15 |
| Boric acid powder | 5 |
| Perfume oil | 5 |
| Sodium cholate | 1.5 |
| Malic or citric pectin | 1 |
| Uranin | 0.15 |

The essential oils are mixed with the colloidal kaolin. The sodium cholate (intended to retard the effervescent effect) and the pectin (which promotes the decomposition of the tablets) are carefully mixed.

The sodium bicarbonate is sprayed with a 5% solution of the uranin and left to dry at max. 50°C. When it is completely dry, half the starch is added and well mixed in.

Acids and perfume oil are mixed separately and the remainder of the starch added. Finally everything is mixed together for 20 minutes and pressed into tablets of about 40 g each which are wrapped into metal or plastic foil.

6. Rothemann, *op. cit.*, p. 664.

| Sodium perborate | 65.0 |
|---|---|
| Wheat- or cornstarch powder | 31.5 |
| Manganese sulfate | 1.5 |
| Potassium bitartrate | 2.0 |

The sodium perborate contains about 10% active oxygen. The manganese sulfate acts as a catalyst in the release of oxygen, and the bitartrate stabilizes the dry tablets.

PROCEDURE. The perborate is mixed with 20 g powdered starch, the manganese sulfate with 5 g starch, and the bitartrate with 6.5 g starch. The three separately prepared mixtures are then combined, thoroughly mixed in a mixer, and immediately pressed into tablets.

## Bubble Bath Powders

In addition to the usual bath salt ingredients, these powders contain large amounts of strongly foaming surfactants in powder form.

7. Keithler, *op. cit.*, p. 398.

| | |
|---|---|
| Sodium sesquicarbonate | 20 |
| Sodium lauryl sulfate, pdr | 18 |
| Sodium bicarbonate | 30 |
| Citric acid | 29 |
| Borax | 2 |
| Perfume oil | 1 |
| Color | q.s. |

8. *Ibid.* p. 399.

| | |
|---|---|
| Sodium lauryl sulfoacetate | 69 |
| Saponin | 15 |
| Tetrasodium pyrophosphate | 15 |
| Perfume oil | 1 |
| Color | q.s. |

Various types of liquid bath preparation are available commercially. Apart from consistency, they differ from bath salts in their higher perfume content.

## Bath Oils

Because they are insoluble in water, bath oils spread as a thin layer on top of the bath water. To promote this spreading effect they often contain oil-soluble surfactants. Bath oils are adsorbed on the skin (surfactants, if present, help them to penetrate the topmost layers) and make it smooth and supple and keep it from drying out. Haensch and Blaich [5] found that 4 ml/10 l of bath water are sufficient to deposit an oil film on the skin that remains even after washing with soap and can still be observed three hours after the bath.

The perfume in these oils pleasantly pervades the air in the bathroom and traces cling to the skin. These preparations, however, do not actually help in the cleansing process. On the contrary: they inhibit the lathering of soap and remain as a thin film, that is hard to remove from the tub after the water has run off. Bath oils are marketed in bottles, foil or plastic pouches, and gelatin capsules.

9. Keithler, *op. cit.*, p. 400.

| | |
|---|---|
| Mineral oil | 46.5 |
| Isopropyl myristate | 17.5 |
| Triethyl citrate | 15.0 |
| Sulfated olive oil | 15.0 |
| Perfume oil | 6.0 |
| Color | q.s. |

10. Haensch and Blaich [6].

| | |
|---|---|
| Peanut oil | 90 |
| Cremophor O | 10 |

Mix all ingredients and filter if required.

## Solutions of Perfume Oils in Solubilizers

Perfume oils dissolved in solubilizers are easily dispersed in water. The perfume does not develop so fully as that in insoluble bath oils, but these preparations have the advantage of not remaining in the bathtub when the water has run out and of preventing the formation of a ring. They also have a certain foaming effect.

The solubilizers used are mostly Tween 20 (Atlas, polyoxyethylene sorbitan monolaurate) and sulfonated castor oil (Turkey red oil). To make the preparation less viscous, water or Carbitol (diethylene glycol monomethyl ether) are added.

| | |
|---|---|
| 11. Perfume oil | 15 |
| Tween 20 | 85 |

Both ingredients are mixed at room temperature. Any amount of water or Carbitol may be added without clouding the mixture.

12. Rothemann, *Das grosse Rezeptbuch der Haut- und Körperpflegemittel*, 3rd ed., p. 655

| | |
|---|---|
| Turkey red oil, anhydrous, neutralized (80–85%) | 80 |
| Perfume oil | 20 |
| Uranin | 0.15 |

Solutions of perfume oil in Carbitol have also been described as bath oils in the literature, but in my opinion they are not suitable because the perfume oil precipitates in the bath water, causes clouding, and accumulates in large drops which are harmful if they adhere to the skin or get into the eyes.

## Bubble Bath Oils

Bubble bath oils contain strongly foaming surfactants and occasionally foam stabilizers. The rich foam that develops when these preparations are used is their main purpose, apart from the scenting of the bath water and bathroom. Kalish [7] mentions fatty acid alkylolamides, fatty alcohol sulfates, alkyl aryl sulfonates, polyoxyethylene alkyl phenols, and alkyl polyoxyethylene sulfates as possible ingredients. The foaming effect of fatty alcohol sulfates and alkyl aryl sulfonates is inhibited by hard water but can be protected by the addition of phosphates or other water softeners to the bath oil.

The following is an example of such a product [8]:

| | |
|---|---|
| 13. Triethanolamine lauryl sulfate (50%) | 30 |
| Lauric acid diethanolamide | 10 |
| Water, perfume oil, and color | 60 |

## Bath Milks

Bath milks are oil-in-water emulsions in which the oil phase consists almost entirely of perfume oil. They disperse in water with hardly any clouding.

These products are similar in effect to solubilized bath oils but less expensive to prepare.

14. Rothemann, *op. cit.*, p. 651.

| | |
|---|---|
| Perfume oil | 10 |
| Sodium lauryl sulfate | 9 |
| Water, distilled | 81 |
| Uranin (5% in alcohol) | 2 |

Dissolve the lauryl sulfate in water by heating and add the other ingredients after cooling.

## REFERENCES

[1] H. Freytag, *Fette Seifen*, **55**, 174 (1953); *Kosmetik-Parf.-Drog.*, 3/4, 33 (1955).

[2] Rothemann, *Das grosse Rezeptbuch der Haut- und Körperpflegemittel*, Hüthig Verlag, 3rd ed., Heidelberg, 1962.

[3] Bergwein, *Parfum. Kosmet.*, **39**, 199 (1958).

[4] Müeller, *Die physiologischen und pharmakologischen Wirkungen der ätherischen Oele, Riechstoffe und verwandten Produkte*, Hüthig Verlag, 2nd ed., Heidelberg, 1950.

[5] *Fette, Seifen, Anstrichmittel* **64**, 854 (1962).

[6] *Ibid.*

[7] *Drug Cosmet, Ind.*, **79**, 36 (1956).

[8] *Am. Perfumer*, **71**, 35 (March 1956).

# Postscript
# Perfuming and Coloring
# Cosmetic Preparations

I have quite deliberately omitted saying anything in this book about the composition of the perfumes used in various cosmetic preparations. Formulating perfumes and fragrances is a matter for the perfumer, not the cosmetic chemist. Since he constantly receives samples of various fragrances and regularly comes across articles on perfumery in the literature, it is quite natural for the cosmetic chemist to begin taking an interest in the field and possibly even trying to create his own perfumes for his products. However, perfumery and cosmetics do not belong together in the sense that every expert in cosmetics must also be a perfumer.

Obviously every company that produces cosmetics must have somebody who understands something about fragrances. According to Jellinek [1], this is the actual "perfumer." The man responsible for creating the perfume is called by Jellinek a "perfume composer." Every cosmetic manufacturer has an important task in regard to fragrances: from the wealth of samples offered on all sides he must select the perfume that will be most suitable for his product or he must know what kind of fragrance will be the most suitable so that he can have one "custom made."

The selection of a suitable scent for a newly developed product is being left more and more to the consumer, by running consumer tests. This procedure does not, of course, eliminate the perfumer's function because, after all, somebody must select from the thousands of perfumes available those that are to be submitted to the consumer.

In this section we consider a few points important in the selection of a fragrance or a type of perfume for a definite cosmetic product. Adding a fragrance to the product has first of all the purpose of making its use pleasant for the consumer. Possibly existing unpleasant odors of the raw materials must be masked. What is actually considered pleasant, depends, of course, on

538

the product and the type of user for whom it is intended. One thing is certain, the perfume largely influences the acceptance of a cosmetic. We illustrate this point with a comment from a study by Powers [2]:

"A recent market test showed clearly that fragrance is most important in the selection of a product. When the fragrance of a shampoo which had been judged the poorest of a group in a consumer test was improved, the same product was placed first in a new test although all other properties remained unchanged. In the new test, the consumers stated that the shampoo, with the improved fragrance, was easier to rinse out, foamed better, and left the hair more lustrous and glossy."

This statement not only demonstrates that the consumer prefers a pleasantly perfumed product to one less so, it also points to the remarkable fact that the fragrance of a product and its perceived quality are closely and even *inseparably* linked.

The consumer does not regard a cosmetic product with a professional eye. The manufacturer is aware of the various raw materials that have gone into the end product, which he regards as the result of the manufacturing process; for better or worse he cannot do otherwise. The consumer does not think of raw materials and manufacturing processes. She sees a cosmetic product the way it appears on the market, as an entity, an organic whole as, for example, an apple is an entity. The manufacturer sees the perfume oil as something added when the product is almost completed, something that may be substituted without in any way affecting the product itself. The consumer regards the fragrance of a product as an intrinsic part of the whole, belonging as much to its character as color or smoothness of the skin belong to the apple. Therefore the consumer judges unconsciously that a pleasantly perfumed product must be good and a less pleasant one inferior; in any case, she will feel this way as long as she is not convinced of the opposite by other properties of the preparation. With consistency and color, fragrance belongs to the few aspects of a cosmetic preparation that can be judged by the consumer immediately and before use and which establish in her eyes the standard of the product. An unscented cold cream is a fatty paste; the same cream, discretely scented, becomes a fine cosmetic. A cheaply perfumed toilet soap is a modest utilitarian product; the same soap, elaborately perfumed and correspondingly packaged, becomes a luxury.

Some important conclusions may be drawn from the fact that consumers regard cosmetic products as inseparable wholes.

First of all we come to this rule: the more difficult it is to judge the actual efficacy of the cosmetic, the more important its fragrance. After all, we evaluate every object on the basis of the properties we are able to observe immediately: a stone according to its color, its smoothness, hardness, and weight; a person according to his face, voice, clothing, and movements. The same goes for cosmetics.

We can, for example, observe the color, transparency, and viscosity of a shampoo when it is still in the bottle. During use we register foaming capacity and fragrance and judge the shampoo on the strength of these properties, although they have nothing to do with its real function: the removal of soil. Toothpastes are judged similarly when consistency and taste largely determine success. With lipsticks and brilliantines it is much easier to judge performance because the effect of these preparations is superficial and directly visible. Perfuming plays a much smaller part in their evaluation.

Another basic rule is that it is not only the quality of the fragrance that is important but whether the type chosen is in harmony with the purpose of the product, its characteristics and presentation. The fragrance must be in harmony with the image of the product in the mind of the consumer. A product with a cleansing action should never be heavily perfumed; a sophisticated makeup should not smell naïvely of roses. A revolutionary new product, publicized as such, should have a novel and out of the ordinary fragrance. A preparation that emphasizes the content of plant extracts should have a herb scent and not some exotic composition. Products that accent their biological bases (vitamins, hormones, or organic extracts) must be discretely perfumed—just enough to mask the odor of the basic vehicle. These considerations are discussed in greater detail by Jellinek [3].

If fragrance and cosmetic are to blend into a harmonious whole, correct dosage and fixation corresponding to the character of the product are also essential. If the proportion is too low, the fragrance will not develop sufficiently; if it is too high, it will be obtrusive and disturbing. It should also be noticeable only as long as the consumer wishes. In most cases this means that the scent will have disappeared a short time after application. The length of lingering depends not only on the composition but on its dosage in the cosmetic product; the higher the dosage, the longer the life of the fragrance. If a hand cream, a hair lacquer, or a sunscreen preparation can still be distinctly discerned about 30 minutes after application it is generally not acceptable. A lingering fragrance is desirable only for certain decorative preparations (face powders or hair lotions).

These considerations are so important that I should describe the following as the basic rule for the perfuming of cosmetic products: "The fragrance of cosmetic products must have a meaningful relationship with their purpose and image. It must blend to a harmonious entity with the name, the package, the appearance, and the expected effect of the product." This rule may sound self-evident but is all too often neglected. Occasionally certain "unharmoniously perfumed" products even enjoy a certain popularity but it is usually only temporary and hardly ever lasts longer than a few years. Among the famous cosmetic products that have maintained a leading position in the market over the years every one is a textbook example of a successful harmonious perfuming.

Because of the importance of imparting to a product a fragrance that will appeal to the consumer, many manufacturers are trying to enlist the public in making a selection. Large firms carry out consumer tests; the smaller ones that cannot afford them often help themselves by selecting a type of fragrance that has been proved successful in a well-known brand of the same kind. The argument behind this runs as follows: "The public likes buying Cream X, hence it likes the fragrance. If my product has a similar fragrance, I will also be successful." Sometimes this may apply, but not always. What has been overlooked is that consumers regard cosmetics as unified entities. The result is not only that people tend to regard a pleasantly scented product as generally high grade but the reverse as well: once it has been established (possibly by wide publicity coupled with tasteful presentation of the product) that a preparation is good, everything including the perfume will be approved. However, if the same or a similar fragrance is used for a product that is not equally well presented and publicized, it is often found that the perfume alone does not particularly appeal to the public's taste. Generally speaking, the flair of a cosmetic chemist working with a perfumer and knowing his market will be a better guideline than the sales figures of well-known brands.

In order to find a fragrance that has a meaningful relationship with a producer's purpose and will harmonize with its image, the perfumer must develop an understanding of the meaning of specific fragrances to the consumer; he will have to know the kind of message the fragrance conveys. To get this understanding the perfumer has relied traditionally on three sources of information: introspection (what message does this fragrance convey to me?) observation of market performance (what kinds of fragrances are successful in what products?), and an awareness of certain chemical-psychological relationships (phenolic odorants occur in smoke, hence connote danger; citrus oils smell refreshing, for they are associated with highly acid fruits; fatty aldehydes and indol are related to components of bodily excretions hence have erogenous meanings). To these three sources of understanding, a fourth can now be added: the direct questioning of consumers. There are many difficulties in this procedure because the average consumer is far from eloquent about fragrances and rarely is consciously aware of their values. However, testing techniques have been developed that make an assessment of consumer tastes possible [4]. In time, these techniques may well become important tools for the perfumer.

Our discussion of fragrance in cosmetics has dealt so far only with the psychological effect on the user. We must not overlook the physiological effects. The negative physiological rule is well known: the perfumed product must not irritate normal skin. Allergic reactions of hypersensitive persons can never be completely excluded, but they can be avoided to a large extent by eliminating the use of compounds containing ingredients that cause frequent reactions.

From the dermatological point of view every perfume is a burden on the cosmetic product; it can never have a beneficial effect on the skin and at best it is harmless. The situation is not improved by the fact that many of the standard perfume aromatics and essential oils can rapidly penetrate the corneum into the deeper skin layers [5]. It is not correct that essential oils, being natural products, are more skin compatible than synthetic fragrances, even if this opinion is still found in the literature. The demand has often been made in dermatological and cosmetic circles that only those fragrances that demonstrably do not harm the skin should be used for cosmetic perfuming. Although this demand, if extended to all cosmetic products, seems unnecessarily harsh, the following conditions should still be observed:

1. Cosmetic preparations that leave the perfume oil in contact with the skin for any length of time (skin creams, in particular) should contain perfume compositions described by the manufacturers as "dermatologically harmless," "cream perfume," etc.
2. The perfume content in all cosmetic products, but in particular in skin creams, should be as low as possible. To achieve this objective, pure odorless basic materials should be used and the perfume compositions should be as concentrated as possible. (The solvents used in perfumery are no more skin compatible than the fragrances, and since they do not contribute to the olfactory effect they represent a deadweight in cosmetic preparations.) Perfume dosages above 0.3% should be employed in cosmetics only in exceptional cases.
3. The finished product should, before it is marketed, be submitted to a patch test on a few hundred subjects.

A few technical requirements must also be met by every cosmetic product:

The fragrance must not affect the appearance or consistency of the finished product. Clear preparations (oils, aqueous or alcoholic lotions, clear shampoos, etc.) must not be clouded; light products (in particular, creams and light-colored soaps) must not be discolored; colored products must not be bleached; powders must not be made tacky.

The fragrance must not affect the stability of the product. Cases have been described in which the fragrance has caused the separation of an emulsion or promoted rancidity in an oil-rich product. These cases are very rare, however, and can be avoided by correct formulation of the emulsions and adequate preservation.

The fragrance must remain stable within the maximum period elapsing between preparation and use and under the conditions prevailing during storage. Some preparations, particularly strongly alkaline or acid products and those that contain oxidizing or reducing substances, impose heavy demands on the perfume composition. It is the task of the perfumer to create compositions that will meet these requirements.

It is important in any case, particularly with "risky" products, to conduct thorough storage tests with the finished preparations. These tests can be accelerated by conducting them at elevated temperatures, but the results so obtained are not always reliable.

The physiological effect of a fragrance may not be restricted to the negative nonirritation of the epidermal tissue. It is said of many essential oils and isolated and synthetic aromatics that they are able to cause positive effects on the whole organism, particularly the nervous system. A detailed discussion of the physiological properties of fragrances is given by Müller [6]. Some Italian scientists have also dealt with the so-called aroma therapy [7]. Even if only minute quantities of perfume are contained in cosmetic products, a certain physiological effect cannot be ruled out.

It is difficult to determine where the psychological effect of perfume ends and the physiological action begins. When we say that lemon oil is "refreshing," lavender oil, "mild," eugenol, "stimulating," and methyl anthranylate, "narcotic," it is not easy to tell whether these effects are psychological or physiological. We can match a basic physiological action with a psychological rule: the physiological effect of a perfume oil must be in harmony with the intended action of the cosmetic.

Coloring plays a similar but less important part than perfuming. It contributes less in classifying the product on first acquaintance as "good" or "bad" but even so it is important to the general appearance of the preparation. A white or green sandalwood soap is just not right, and many uncolored hair and shaving lotions resemble pure water too closely to appeal to the user.

From the dermatological point of view colors, just as fragrances, are a burden on the product. They should therefore be used as sparingly as possible [8].

The most important law in perfuming cosmetic products may also be expressed as follows: "Consider carefully the effect you expect of the fragrance in your product. Search until you have found one that actually meets your demands." In this form the rule applies not only to the selection of a perfume but to every ingredient of a cosmetic preparation. The less what others have said and done is uncritically accepted, the sharper one's own aim is focused, the more patiently the raw materials are selected and compositions developed, the more original and successful the newly created cosmetic preparation will be.

# REFERENCES

[1] *Parfum. Kosmet.*, **32,** 252 (1951).

[2] *Drug Cosm. Ind.*, **79,** 850 (1956).

[3] Jellinek, *Die psychologischen Grundlagen der Parfümerie*, Hüthig Verlag, 2nd ed., Heidelberg, 1965, p. 177 et seq.

[4] Jellinek, *J. Soc. cosmet. Chem.*, **18,** 755 (1967).

[5] Valette, *Kosmetik Parf.-Drog.*, **4,** 23 (1957).

[6] Müller, *Die physiologischen und pharmakologischen Wirkungen der ätherischen Oele, Riechstoffe und verwandten Produkte*, 2nd ed., Hüthig Verlag, Heidelberg, 1950.

[7] Thomas, *Parfum. Kosmet.*, **37,** 766 (1956).

[8] G. Everts (ed.), *Färbemittel zum Anfärben kosmetischer Präparate, Parfum. Kosmet.*, **43,** 387 (1961).

# Incompatibilities

Acids and:
  Agar 150
  Esters 53, 63
  Gelatin 150
  Lecithin 63
  Penicillin 82
  Polyvinyl alcohol 151
  Proteins/protein degradation products
    163, 150
  Soaps 53, 62
  Sodium alzinate 151
  Vinyl chloride 182
Alkali and:
  Ammonium compounds (quaternary)
    63
  Esters 53, 63
  Lecithin 63
  Penicillin 82
  Polyvinyl alcohol 151
  Protein degradation products 63
  Sapamines 245
  Sodium alginate 151
  Sorbic acid 85
Alkyl aryl sulfonates and Calcium salts
  244
Aluminum and Ethyl alcohol 187
  Isopropyl alcohol 187
Ammonium compounds, quaternary,
  and:
  Alkali 63
  Anionic surfactants 65

Ammonium compounds (*cont.*)
  Calcium salts 92
  Cellulose 92
  Glass 92
  Iron salts 92
  Kaolin 82, 92
  Magnesium salts 92
  Phospholipids 92
  Proteins 92
  Talcum 82, 92
Antibiotics and:
  acids 82
  bases 82
  oxidizing agents 82
  surfactants 96
Borax and:
  Glycerol 146, 155
  Sorbitol 146
Boric acid and:
  Glycerol 85
  Sorbitol 85
Calcium salts and:
  Ammonium compounds (quaternary)
    92
  Alkyl aryl sulfonates 244
  Soaps 52, 213, 242
Carbonates and methyl cellulose 150
Carbopol and:
  Electrolytes 150, 152
  Phenols 102

Carboxymethylcellulose and Metal ions, polyvalent   149, 151

Cellulose and ammonium compounds (quaternary)   92

Detergents and Lanolin   117, 221

Electrolytes and:
  Carbopol   150, 152
  Polyvinyl alcohol   151
  Soaps   53
  Sodium alginate   151

Esters and:
  Acids   53, 63
  Alkali   53, 63

Ethyl Alcohol and:
  Aluminum   187
  Sodium alginate   151

Fats and copper, iron, and heavy metal ions   126, 359

Formaldehyde and proteins   103

Freon II and Water   151

Gelatin and:
  Acids   150
  Gum arabic   150
  Gum tragacanth   150
  Tannins   150

Glass and ammonium compounds (quaternary)   92

Glycerol and Borax   146, 155

Gum arabic and:
  Gelatin   105
  Lead salts   150

Gum Karaya and Borax

Gum Tragacanth and:
  Gelatin   150
  Gum arabic   151
  Phenols   102

Hydrogen peroxide and unsaturated compounds   62

p-Hydroxybenzoates see Phenols

Iodine and unsaturated compounds   62

Iron salts and:
  Ammonium compounds (quaternary)   92
  Fats (oils)   126, 142, 359
  Phenols   142
  Triethanolamine   142

Kaolin and Ammonium compounds (quaternary)   89, 92

Lanolin and detergents   117, 221
  Soap   117

Lead salts and:
  Carboxymethylcellulose   149, 151
  Gum arabic   150

Lecithin and Acids, Alkali   63

Magnesium salts and:
  Ammonium compounds (quaternary)   92
  Soaps   52, 154, 213

Mercury salts and:
  Mercapto compounds   96

Metal ions, polyvalent and:
  Carboxymethyl cellulose   149
  Soaps   65, 154

Methylcellulose and:
  Phenols   102, 148
  Phosphates   150
  Silicates   149
  Tannins   150

Oleic acid and:
  Iodine   65
  Hydrogen peroxide   65

Oleyl alcohol and sodium cetyl sulfate   52

Oxidizing agents and:
  Antibiotics   82
  Unsaturated compounds   65

Pectines see Proteins

Penicillin and:
  Acids, alkali 82
  Lanolin 395
  Lard 395
  Oxidizing agents 82
  Petrolatum 395
Phenols and:
  Carbopol 102
  Gum Tragacanth 102
  Iron salts 142
  Methyl cellulose 102, 148
  Polyoxyethylene compounds 86, 101, 102, 165
  Polyvinyl pyrrolidone 102
  Proteins/protein degradation products 86
  Surfactants (non-ionic) 86, 159, 298
  Unsaturated acids 86
Phosphates and methyl cellulose 150
Phospholipids and ammonium compounds (quaternary) 92
Polyoxyethylene compounds and Phenols 86, 101, 102, 165
  Acid 151
  Alkali 151
Polyvinyl alcohol and Electrolytes
Polyvinylpyrrolidone and phenols 102
Potassium chlorate and Organic substances 271
Proteins/protein degradation products and:
  Alkali 63
  Electrolytes 64
  Phenols 86, 396
  Surfactants (ionic) 91
Quaternary ammonium salts see Ammonium Salts, quaternary
Quince seed mucilage and Acids 151
Sapamines and Alkali 245

Silicates and Methylcellulose 149
Soaps and
  Acids 53, 62, 154
  Calcium salts 52, 154, 213, 242
  Electrolytes 53
  Heavy metal ions 65, 154
  Magnesium salts 52, 154, 213
  Mercury salts 65
  Sodium lauryl sulfate 65
  Sodium lactate 145
Sodium alginate and:
  Alkali 151
  Electrolytes 151
  Ethyl alcohol 151
Sodium cetyl sulfate and Oleyl alcohol 52
Sodium lactate and Soaps 145
Sodium lauryl sulfate and Soaps 65
Sorbic acid and Alkali 85
Sorbitol and Borax 146
Stearates see Soaps
Surfactants and Bacteracin 96
Surfactants, anionic and Quaternary ammonium salts 64, 65
Surfactants, ionic, and Proteins 91
Surfactants, non-ionic, and Phenols 86, 159, 298
Talcum and Ammonium compounds (quaternary) 92
Tannins (see also Phenols) and:
  Gelatin 150
  Methylcellulose 150
Trichloromonofluoromethane and water 181
Triethanolamine and iron salts 142
Vinyl chloride and Acids 182
Water 182

# Author Index

Achten, 437, 470
Adam, 60
Adams, 12, 30
Agarwala, 349
Ainsworth, 411, 412
Alexander, 23, 31, 73
Ali, 349
Allen, 380
Alvarez, 350
Andersen, 245, 285
Andersen, D. C., 74
Andersen, D. L., 106
Anderson, 107, 199
Anglin, 349
Anson, 212
Appeldorn, 357
Appy, 24, 31
Ardin, 383, 410, 437
Astbury, 17, 20, 30, 31, 527
Atkins, 528, 570
Auch, 167, 199, 209, 498
Avalle, 392

Babayan, 74
Babicka, 98, 107
Baer, 106
Bailey, 65, 98, 107
Baird, 59
Baker, 106, 294
Ball, 106
Barail, 117, 273, 294, 303, 310, 396, 397
Barban, 527
Barker, 200
Barmak, 349
Barnett, 196, 285, 357
Barr, 103
Barry, 513
Batdorf, 198
Battista, 282, 285
Bauer, 287, 324, 528, 567
Beal, 105

Beam, 107, 138
Beaver, 106
Bech, 96
Becher, 73, 138, 198
Bechtold, 95, 106
Behrens, 143, 146
Bell, 522, 529
Benedikt, 390
Benk, 19
Benson, 198
Berger, 199, 467
Bergeron, 349
Berghausen, 524
Bergwein, 181, 194, 196, 284, 314, 316, 334, 350, 436, 521, 531, 537
Bersin, 527
Berth, 484, 504
Bever, 349
Bhaktavizian, 528
Bien, 304
Biermann, 308
Bigi, 391, 411
Birman, 273, 286, 294, 310
Bishop, 471
Bjorksten, 366
Blakistone, 350
Blackman, 275
Blaich, 535
Blanck, 55, 73
Blancy, 349
Blank, 11, 30, 79, 284, 309, 310, 352, 354, 364, 412
Bloch, 14, 30, 36, 81
Blum, 324
Blumenthal, 222
Bober, 284
Boehme, 101
Boelke, 438
Bolle, 91, 102
Böss, 504
Bossina, 181

549

Botwright , 92, 93
Bouchardy, 65, 199
Bourgeois, 105
Bowers, 309
Brambilla, 391
Braus, 266, 270
Brews, 199
Brigon, 412
Brocklehurst, 310
Bromley, 48
Brooke, 350
Brooks, 499
Brown, A. S., 106
Brown, C. S., 411
Brudevold, 274
Brühl, 19
Brun, 291, 292
Brune, 107, 129
Bryce, 198, 250, 286
Buettner, 11, 30, 364
Bullied, 286
Burckhardt, 13, 30, 284, 528
Bureau, 390, 411
Burger, 411
Burler, 399
Burmeister, 212
Burrell, 107, 132
Burtenshaw, 30
Bussius, 30
Butenandt, 393

Cahn, 96, 106, 294
Calandra, 285
Calvery, 93
Cameron, 385, 410
Cantor, 106, 127
Carrel, 391
Carrié, 210, 219, 320
Carrière, 55, 73
Carroll, 98
Carson, 398, 411
Carter, 506, 520
Cellis, 381
Cerutti, 310
Cessna, 146
Chapman, 130
Charpy, 409
Chavkin, 73
Chilson, 268, 296, 344, 461
Chodat, 91
Chong, 198
Christensen, 331
Christian, 293, 309
Chun, 147, 198
Clarkson, 45
Clausen, 106
Cleney, 74
Cohen, 269, 467
Cohh, J. A., 107
Cohn, R. M., 179
Colbert, 196
Cole, 199, 416
Collins, 309

Conley, 200
Conn, 197, 199
Conrad, 529
Conrad, L. J., 118, 196, 256, 314, 317, 334,
    361, 362
Cook, 198
Cooper, 107
Cosgrove, 107
Cressy, 467
Cross, 143, 146
Cumming, 322
Currie, 122, 316, 317, 337, 349, 464
Curtis, 199
Curwen, 349
Cutter, 91
Cyr, 196
Czetsch-Lindenwald, 73, 104, 105, 110, 196,
    200, 213, 284, 287, 319, 320, 322, 349,
    364, 410, 411

Daley, 293
Danielisova, 411
Daniels, 339, 470
Darvichian, 47
Daute, 138
Davidow, 29, 31
Davidsohn, 45
Davies, 287
Davies, J. T., 39, 73, 74
Davies, R. E., 149, 198
Davis, 81
Dawes, 309, 310
Day, 275
Deakers, 104
Deem, 30
De Jong, 284
De Mytt, 529
De Navarre, 65, 96, 98, 102, 103, 107, 114,
    126, 129, 139, 146, 147, 196, 197, 198,
    199, 228, 231, 232, 283, 285, 287, 309,
    334, 335, 339, 342, 349, 350, 356, 363,
    364, 416, 449, 467, 519
Denton, 527
Desai, 177, 200
Dethier, 350
De Vries, 47
Dietrich, 196
di Giacomo, 193, 302, 521
Dijkstra, 256
Dittmar, 199
Dobson, 308
Dodds, 410
Dohr-Lux, 27, 31
Doisy, 380
Domagk, 106
Dowling, 409
Downing, 322
Dräger, 478
Draize, 105, 237, 285, 350, 500
Draves, 45, 74
Dreyling, 347
Dubrow, 74

Ecker, 96
Edman, 196
Edwards, 211, 213, 216
Ehlers, 219
Ehrhardt, 278, 279
Eibel, 120
Eisman, 107
Ekbom, 197
Eller, 399, 400
Elson, 106
Emery, 211, 213, 216
Epstein, 287
Ernst, 121, 314, 317, 362
Erwin, 293
Eschbach, 390
Escoda, 349, 409
Evans, 197, 509
Everett, 349
Everts, 544
Ewing, 149, 199

Fahlberg, 105
Fassbender, 385
Faust, 74
Fayard, 391
Felletschin, 74
Fenske, 264, 278, 287, 328
Ferguson, 294
Ferrati, 201
Fiedler, H. P., 105, 308, 411
Fiedler, J. G., 451, 452, 455, 456
Figley, 147, 198
Filatov, 392
Findlay, 350, 398
Fine, 529
Finholt, 197
Finkelstein, 527
Finlayson, 366
Fischer, 46
Fiser, 30, 411
Fisher, 102, 105, 344, 350
Fisk, 199
Fitzpatrick, F. B., 527
Fitzpatrick, T. B., 30, 349
Flesch, 4, 11, 29, 30, 349, 352, 356, 364,
    366, 367, 370, 375, 405, 409, 411, 413
    506
Foresman, 201
Forscher, 274
Fosdick, 274, 275
Fox, 11, 30, 145, 198, 353, 356
Francis, 198
Francisco, 316, 317, 337, 464
Franz, 224, 225, 226, 235, 285
Franzke, 376
Fredell, 303
Freese, 74, 106, 245, 285
French, 350
Fretzdorff, 196, 356
Freytag, 491, 504, 527, 537
Friedrich, 24, 31
Frigley, 527
Fuhrmann, 500

Fulton, 190, 201
Furia, 106

Gahygler, 527
Galli, 391, 411
Galloway, 104, 107
Gans, 46
Gardenhje, 96
Garrett, 107
Gartmann, 349
Gates, 15, 30
Gathen, von zur, 146, 198
Gaul, 353
Gaunt, 24, 285
Gee, 310
Gemmel, 106
Genzsch, 200
Gergle, 122, 197, 346
Gerhard, 375, 383, 405, 410
Gerthsen, 528
Gibbs, 527
Giese, 331
Glanzmann, 409
Glasenapp, 19
Glendenning, 412
Glick, 30, 352
Gohlke, C., 19, 73
Gohlke, H., 400, 528
Goldhamer, 398, 411
Goldman, 349, 409, 413
Goldschmiedt, 12, 30, 522
Goldzieher, 380, 400, 405, 409
Goncavora, 457
Götte, 74, 210, 211
Gould, 412
Govett, 309
Grady, 169, 349, 444
Grandel, 410
Gregory, 197
Greither, 219, 284
Gribou, 387
Griesemer, 6, 412
Griffin, 38, 58, 62, 143, 144, 146, 198, 199
Grimmer, 410
Gross, 412
Gross, 401
Grover, 412
Gruskin, 272, 309
Gsell, 409
Guba, 8, 30
Guignon, 8, 30
Gump, 86, 105

Haas, 179
Habicht, 514, 529
Haensch, 535
Hafer, 287, 294, 310
Hain, 349
Haldwick, 287
Hamilton, 410
Hans, 175
Hansel, 511
Hansmann, 527, 548

Hanusch, 385
Harber, 366
Harnisch, 262, 273
Harper, 241, 285
Harris, 74, 399, 412, 468
Harry, 13, 24, 30, 31, 105, 106, 136, 139,
    153, 154, 170, 196, 198, 199, 200, 223,
    228, 230, 234, 253, 254, 256, 257, 266,
    269, 271, 285, 286, 287, 305, 306, 310,
    322, 335, 347, 348, 349, 367, 397, 408,
    409, 412, 413, 425, 426, 436, 445, 449,
    462, 469, 471, 506, 520, 527, 528, 529
Hart, 93
Hartley, 73
Hass, 201
Hausam, 105
Heald, 228, 403, 412
Hecht, 416
Heilingötter, 499, 500, 528
Heimann, 197
Helbring, 171
Helfer, 200
Heller, 196, 356
Helton, 293
Heman-Ackah, 107
Herberholz, 266, 270
Hermann, 6, 287
Herrmann, 309
Herzka, 176, 196, 471
Hess, 274
Heu, 87, 105
Hewitt, 8, 30
Hexter, 106
Heymann, 287
Hilfer, 470
Hill, 196
Hjorth, 105
Hobl, 528
Hoch, 86, 105, 285, 286
Hoff, 6
Hoffmann, B., 182, 200
Hoffmann, H., 74, 105, 285, 470
Hofmann, 262
Holden, 350
Holm, 197
Holmann, 410
Holmes, 526
Holt, 98
Holtkamp, 276
Honisch, 194, 201, 239
Hopf, 189, 212, 291, 303, 310
Hopkins, 318
Hopp, 167, 197, 342
Hoppe-Seyler's, 196
Hornby, 350
Hsiung, 526
Hunter, 106
Hurley, 290, 310
Husa, 107

Idson, 29, 31
Ikai, 295, 354, 364
Imbrie, 349

Ippen, 366

Jacobi, 210
Jacobsen, 88, 105
Jaconia, 107
Jadassohn, 30
Jaffé, 404
Jager, 61, 212, 219, 354, 364
Jakovics, 470
Janecke, 197
Janistyn, 73, 114, 134, 139, 147, 196, 197,
    198, 199, 209, 219, 230, 235, 236, 254,
    266, 277, 283, 285, 286, 287, 300, 306,
    308, 314, 331, 338, 342, 343, 344, 347,
    349, 386, 406, 407, 408, 410, 420, 422,
    424, 445, 447, 452, 461, 466, 469, 470,
    471, 475, 488, 511, 513, 516, 524, 526
Janku, 387, 411
Janowitz, 361, 410, 534
Jansion, 412
Jason, 522
Jellinek, 287, 309, 538, 540, 544
Jenkins, 274, 286, 287
Johnson, 105, 187, 200
Jones, 101, 129, 142, 213, 284
Joslin, 147, 198
Juon, 406, 409

Kaden, 91
Kalish, 199, 200, 293, 297, 298, 300, 470, 536
Kalz, 399, 412
Kanig, 73, 177, 179, 200
Kantorowitz, 273, 287, 294, 310
Kärcher, 320
Kashara, 376, 399
Kass, 478, 480, 481
Kaufmann, 74
Kawashima, 376, 399
Kay, 285
Keck, 457
Keddie, 106
Keenan, 222
Keithler, 139, 209, 229, 230, 231, 234, 251,
    253, 254, 256, 266, 277, 280, 283, 297,
    298, 306, 308, 317, 319, 322, 337, 342,
    343, 344, 345, 347, 348, 360, 361, 364,
    421, 422, 423, 425, 426, 427, 428, 436,
    439, 443, 445, 447, 450, 455, 456, 461,
    462, 464, 469, 470, 489, 511, 512, 513,
    517, 520, 521, 524, 526, 533, 535
Keller, 309
Kelley, 105, 237, 285
Kellner, 310
Kempe, 201
Kerschbaumer, 411
Kesel, 274
Khawas, 200
Killian, 88, 105, 290, 291, 303, 310
Killingsworth, 114
Kimmig, 374, 375
King, 287
Kinmont, 24, 31
Kirby, 412, 499, 504

Kittel, 472
Klarmann, 106, 296, 297, 299, 300, 309,
    331, 339, 349, 350, 380, 409
Klave, 349
Klawik, 287
Klein, 386, 406
Kleine-Nathrop, 57, 73, 127, 196, 199
Kleinschmitt, 284
Klema, 198
Klempson-Jones, 198
Kligman, 6, 30, 290, 309, 381, 412, 457, 471
Klim, 128, 197
Kluczka, 286
Kludas, 390, 411
Klussmann, 339
Knight, 105
Knowles, 260, 286
Köhler, 404
Konzales, 295
Kostenbauer, 102
Kowalczyk, 213
Krajkemann, 107
Kral, 349
Kraul, 387
Kraus, 470
Kritchevsky, 246
Krögler, 411
Kroll, 286
Kröper, 213
Krs, 30, 411
Kruse, 412
Kübler, 180
Kumer, 366, 409, 412
Kummerow, 128, 197
Kuno, 310
Kuntscher, 410
Kunzmann, 198
Kuramoto, 198
Kvicalova, 411

Lach, 102
Laden, 356, 364, 367
Lamanna, 107
Lammers, 286
Lane, 284
Lang, 399
Lange, 106
Lasser, 349
Lauffer, 155, 199
Lawrence, 95, 106
Lea, 129
Leberl, 121, 432, 436, 501
Lebeuf, 409
Lehman, 74
Lehmann, 306
Lehne, 464, 465, 466, 469
Leideritz, 200
Leifer, 308
Lemaire, 106
Lemon, 106
Lennon, 286
Lenstra, 284
Leonhardi, 19
Lerea, 73

Lerner, 349, 527
Lessenich, 200
Lesser, 223, 235, 317
Levenstein, 380, 401
Levy, 74, 199
Lhoest, 91
Lietz, 27, 31, 51, 73, 154, 156, 157, 198, 199
Lindgren, 107
Linn, 378
Linser, 404
Lips, 130
Little, 274
Liu, 520
Lloyd, 58
Lodi, 384, 385, 402, 410
Loeser, 199
Loewenthal, 309
Lohmann, 285
Lomber, 412
Lorenz, 142, 213
Lotz, 320
Lower, 157, 196, 199, 342, 467
Luckiesh, 199, 328, 349
Lück, 105
Ludwig, 466
Lustig, 19, 527
Luzuy, 394
Lychalk, 200
Lyon, 212

MacBain, 41
McCabe, 346
McCords, 219
McDonough, 196, 200, 509
McFarlane, 130
McGrea, 93
Macht, 412
McNamara, 84, 105
McSweeney, 285
Maguire, 412
Malette, 107
Maltoltsy, 528
Manly, 287
Manneck, 29, 285
Mannheim, 478, 527
Mannheimer, 74, 285
Manuila, 291, 292
Mantegazza, 383
Mantsavinos, 309
Mara, 269, 462
Marchionini, 12, 13, 21, 30, 31, 218, 310
Marcussen, 29, 31
Martin, 147, 198, 237, 285
Masch, 328
Matson, 412
Mayhew, 74
Mazurella, 96, 525, 531
Mead, 287
Mecca, 360, 410
Mecham, 284
Meier, 409
Meigs, 291, 303
Meinek, 528

Meinhard, 74
Meinhof, 95, 106
Mellon, 142
Memmesheimer, 110
Mentecki, 527
Mescon, 528
Messer, 12, 30
Meyer, 196
Meyer, E., 309
Meyer, F. O. W., 167, 170
Meyer, G., 105
Meyer-Rohn, 309
Mezikofski, 106
Michelfelder, 30
Michell, 107
Miescher, 411
Miles, 47, 48
Miller, 106, 262, 274, 286, 287
Milling, 74
Mimra, 514
Mina, 191, 200
Minford, 200
Mirimanoff, 65, 102, 107, 199
Mitchell, 309, 409
Modde, 73
Molin, 31
Moncrieff, 310
Montagna, 308
Montgomery, 294
Moreland, 309, 310
Morelle, 107, 509, 527, 528
Morgan, 46
Morris, 189, 200
Most, 106
Motiuk, 118, 196, 256, 334, 361
Muehler, 275
Müller, 537, 543, 544
Mumford, 199
Münch, 411
Mutimer, 196

Nabokov, 346
Nachtigall, 294
Nebergall, 275
Needleman, 275
Neidig, 107
Neis, 207, 283
Nelson, 284
Netherton, 199
Neu, 106
Neuhaus, 216, 219
Neumann, 405, 410, 411, 470, 498
Newman, 196, 520
Nichols, 290, 310
Niederl, 93
Nikolowski, 376, 409
Nitta, 354, 364
Nobile, 199
Nowak, 97, 98, 103, 104, 105, 106, 107, 196, 317

Obrocki, 467
Ochoa, 30
Oesch, 409

Ohlmann, 146
Ohmart, 322
Oppenheim, 25
Orelup, 349
Osipow, 145, 198, 199, 269, 462
Ostendorf, 197
Oster, 527
Ottenstein, 295
Owen, 95, 106
Ozier, 488, 489

Pantaleoni, 256
Panzarella, 290
Papa, 457, 471
Paroulkova, 30, 411
Parsons, 139
Passedouet, 74, 101
Patel, 102
Pathak, 349
Patterson, 254
Pease, 83, 105, 525
Peck, 13, 14, 30, 308, 352, 409
Pemberton, 409
Perdok, 275, 287
Perry, 51, 73
Pertsch, 171
Pescatore, 117, 396, 397
Peters, 350
Peterson, 198
Petzold, 197
Peukert, 213
Pfeifer, 105
Phillips, 265, 467
Pichlmayr, 443
Pichon, 39, 73
Pickthall, 136, 200
Pijvan, 346
Pillsbury, 310
Pincus, 263
Pinson, 470
Pirillä, 96
Pisha, 309
Plaxco, 107
Plein, 317
Pochi, 381
Pokorny, 130, 197
Polano, 133, 334
Polite, 149, 199
Politzer, 309
Pont, 527
Powell, 310
Powers, 11, 30, 145, 198, 237, 244, 253, 285, 287, 353, 356, 539
Preisinger, 478
Profand, 196
Puls, 107

Quisero, 29, 31

Raab, 30
Radike, 275
Rahn, 107
Rajka, 196
Ramsay, 212

Randenbrock, 30
Randoin, 372
Rappaport, 374
Rawling, 106
Read, 303
Reese, 484, 504
Reich, 529
Reichel, 91
Reimers, 349
Rein, 7, 10, 11, 30, 354, 396, 397, 398
Reiss, 381, 527, 543
Reller, 308
Rembolt, 395
Renaud, 134, 198
Rhodes, 62
Richardson, 291, 303
Rideal, 82
Riegelman, 39, 73
Rieger, 11, 30
Rieth, 105
Riffin, 196
Rihava, 412
Riley, 349
Ritter, 506
Rivera, 391
Roberts, 406
Robinson, 289, 309
Roccheggiani, 375
Roehm, 146
Roelcke, 91
Rogers, 95
Roia, 105, 367
Root, 177, 186, 194, 200, 302
Rosenberg, 295
Rosenblum, 105
Rosenfeld, 308
Rosenthal, 106, 287
Rosenthal, N. A., 527
Rosenwald, 197
Ross, 47, 48
Ross-Miles, 47, 48
Roth, 201
Rothemann, 114, 134, 139, 162, 196, 197,
    199, 200, 229, 252, 253.256.257,268.269,
    283, 285, 286, 308, 317, 334, 336, 338,
    342, 344, 360, 361, 363, 367, 374, 391,
    394, 401, 402, 403, 408, 409, 411, 422,
    423, 425, 426, 427, 436, 445, 450, 452,
    466, 497, 510, 513, 519, 524, 531, 533,
    534, 536, 537
Rothman, 4, 8, 14, 23, 29, 30, 110, 397,
    409, 412, 413, 527
Rovesti, 199, 383, 384, 385, 391, 393, 402,
    410, 411
Rowley, 274
Rowson, 149, 198
Royce, 197
Rubenkönig, 29, 31
Rubin, 293
Rubino, 309
Rubisz-Brzezinska, 410
Ruckebusch, 30, 411
Ruehs, 386, 406
Ruemele, 436, 464, 470, 494, 502, 503

Ruf, 210, 213, 267, 284
Russell, 86, 105, 285, 286
Ruys, 197
Ryan, 200

Sabalitschka, 105
Sabetay, 111
Sagarin, 30, 401, 410, 412, 451, 455, 456,
    464, 466, 467, 469, 471, 473, 488, 513,
    522, 527, 528, 529
Salfeld, 409
Sanders, 246
Sanders, H. L., 47
Sanders, P. A., 73
Santioanni, 30, 527
Santon, 74
Sarkany, 105
Sasko, 411
Satanove, 411
Saunders, 200, 201
Saville, 30, 527
Schaaf, 110, 196, 401
Schade, 21, 31
Schädel, 219
Schlaf, 30, 33
Schmidt, 394, 410, 411
Schmidt-La Baume, 73, 105, 110, 154, 156,
    157, 196, 198, 199, 200, 213, 284, 320,
    322, 349, 364, 410, 411
Schneider, 85, 101, 120, 197, 211, 219, 386,
    410, 412
Schneller, 527
Schöberl, 527
Schoch, 110
Schofield, 198
Scholz, 285
Schönherr, 30
Schoonhover, 278, 287
Schopping, 31
Schramm, 106
Schulte, 528
Schulz, 24, 31
Schulze, 339, 349
Schuster, 74, 269, 285
Schwartz, 223, 284
Schwartz, A. M., 260, 286, 319
Schwartz, B. S., 105
Schwartz, L., 527
Schwarz, 51, 73
Schwarz, T. W., 199
Schwob, 389
Scott, 399, 412
Seastone, 105
Secard, 199
Seidenberg, 106, 310
Senft, 197
Seyfert, 46
Sfiras, 127, 158, 197, 198, 199
Shackelford, 149, 199
Shank, 527
Shanks, 256, 302
Shapiro, 30
Shappirio, 11, 30, 352, 364, 410
Shappiro, 410

Shaw, 12, 30
Shehaden, 290, 309
Shelanski, 106
Shelley, 96, 290, 294, 310
Shelmire, 356, 360
Shepherd, 377, 378
Sherman, 399, 412
Shohl, 286
Shumard, 106
Sidi, 24, 25, 27, 31, 111, 285, 358, 364, 416, 437, 470, 504, 527, 528
Siebert, 121
Siess, 411
Silson, 410
Silverman, 310, 458
Simmonite, 55
Sisley, 196
Sivadjian, 310
Sluis, 31, 316
Smart, 250, 286
Smiljanic, 30
Smith, 30, 366
Snell, 221, 269, 285, 462
Sobel, 374, 375
Sollmann, 199
Sommer, 198
Sonder, 278, 287
Spanlangova, 30, 411
Speakman, 31
Spector, 385, 410
Spitzer, 528
Spoor, 352, 364, 381
Stambovsky, 339
Steigleder, 30
Stein, 91
Steinbach, 105
Stejskal, 196
Stendel, 527
Sterba, 411
Stoklosa, 322
Stolz, 95
Stonehill, 81
Stoughton, 412
Stoves, 17, 31, 527
Strakosch, 412
Strauss, 381
Stüpel, 210, 219, 283, 284
Stürmer, 199
Sugden, 198
Sugie, 354, 364
Sulzberger, 117, 292, 293, 298, 309, 310, 349, 416
Svampa, 199
Swan, 105
Swanson, 220, 284
Sweralow, 30
Szakall, 7, 13, 30, 210, 211, 214, 215, 218, 283
Szczesniak, 399, 412
Szent-György, 372

Tainter, 265, 267, 286, 287
Takahashi, 302, 310
Taplin, 105

Tarnoff, 95, 106
Tassoff, 11, 30
Tate, 382
Tawashi, 200
Taylor, 199, 328, 349
Tekenbroek, 278, 279
Thaczuk, 74
Theile, 83, 105, 525
Thewlis, 287
Thomas, 107, 387, 409, 544
Thomson, 286
Thorvik, 197
Thurmon, 295, 300
Tice, 103
Tillman, 198
Tobler, 527
Todd, 197
Tommasi, 476
Torok, 200
Tornow, 31
Trabaud, 349
Traub, 88, 106
Treon, 285
Trolle-Lassen, 105
Tronnier, 30, 313, 339, 348, 357, 390, 411, 457
Truax, 198, 506
Trutey, 198
Tschakert, 146, 198, 244
Tuura, 105
Tzanck, 24, 31

Uexküll, 522, 529
Ullmann, 199
Underwood, 353
Urbantschitsch, 287

Valentine, 256
Valette, 396, 411, 412, 544
Vandenbelt, 349
Van der Minne, 139, 198
Vanderwyk, 105, 367
Van Huysen, 265
Van Scott, 212
van Steenis, 273, 287, 294, 310
Varma, 107
Velde, 67
Velon, 144, 198
Vermeer, 284
Villela, 375
Vinson, 106
Vischer, 309
Viucze, 196
Vogt, 129
Volk, 197, 528
Volker, 287
Volterra, 411
Vonkennell, 29, 31, 196
Vossnacker, 286
Vyhnanek, 196

Wada, 302, 310
Waddans, 222
Wagener, 411

Wagner, 410
Walker, 82, 286, 386, 471, 527, 528
Wall, 473, 478, 479, 486, 527
Wallenius, 96
Walter, 86, 105
Wazeter, 105
Weber, 19, 219, 293, 349
Webster, 200
Weed, 96
Wegemann, 8, 30
Weigel, 480, 484, 503, 527
Weinberg, 105
Weis, 375
Weiss, 292
Weitkamp, 30
Weitzel, 196, 356, 411
Wellendorf, 117, 196
Westcott, 272, 294, 309
Weybrecht, 366
Wheatley, 5, 29
Whitesell, 350
Whitman, 499
Wiame, 105
Wilkins, 107
Wilkinson, 106
Willems, J. B., 283, 285, 286
Williams, 107, 527
Wilmsmann, 216, 430, 487

Wilson, 91
Wilson, K., 139, 397, 412
Winkler, 6, 120, 196
Winter, 197, 348, 422, 460, 471, 475, 477, 526, 528
Wiskemann, 338-
Wode, 130, 197
Wohnlich, 211
Wolff, 74, 199, 399, 400
Woods, H. J., 20, 31
Woods, O. R., 107
Woodward, 93
Wright, 264, 274, 278, 286, 287, 412

Yashuda, 375
Yeomans, 190, 201

Zander, 286
Zenisek, 12, 30, 324, 349, 388, 389, 395, 411
Zentmayer, 90, 106
Zimmermann, 338
Zita, 387, 411
Zorn, 387
Zuckermann, 412
Zuntz, 404
Zupko, 290
Zussmann, H. W., 106
Zussmann, W., 241, 253
Zwickley, 105

# Subject Index

Abietic acid glycol esters, 442
Abrasives, 264
Absorption bases, 134, 488
Acanthosis test, 29
Acetanilide, 480, 485
Acetic acid, as neutralizing agent, 503
  as sequestering agent, 259
  in shampoos, 252
Aceto fats, 116; *see also* Acetoglycerides
*Acetoglyceride L/C*, 519
Acetoglycerides, 433, 435; *see also* Aceto
      Fats
Acetone, in nail lacquers, 440, 441, 442
  in nail lacquer removers, 282, 283
  in protective preparations, 318
Acetophenone, 331
Acetylcholine, 393
N-Acetyl-N-(l-cyanocyclohexyl)-alkyl-
      amine, 346
Acid mantle, 12, 135
Acids, as disinfectants, 84
  in toothpastes, 275
*Actamer*, 88, 95, 301
Active ingredients, complexes of, 387
  penetration capacity of, 399
*Adeps lanae*, anhydrous, *see* Lanolin,
      anhydrous
  in mascara, 426
  in preparations with depth effect, 402
  in rouges, 421
Adipic acid, 485
Aerosil, 226; *see also* Cab-o-sil
Aerosol AY, 501
Aerosol OT, 244; *see also* Sodium dioctyl
      sulfosuccinate
Aerosol plasters, 28
Aerosol preparations, 171

advantages and disadvantages, 172
containers, 186ff., 466
corrosion, 195
corrosion prevention, 189
deodorants, 300
effectiveness, 188
filling, 193
foam emulsion, oil-in-water, 176
  water-in-oil, 177
formulation, 188
hair lacquers, 466
history, 171
non-emulsified, 174
powders, 179
preparation, 193
production costs, 190
propellant mixtures, 184
propellants, 177, 179ff.
protective caps, 188
raw materials, 179
safety, 189
shaving creams, 520
shelf life, 195
solvents, 185
spray emulsion, oil-in-water, 177
  water-in-oil, 177
spraying speed, 194
spray pattern, 190
  testing of, 194
stability, 188
storage tests, 195
sunscreens, 333
testing, 194
three-phase, 174
two-phase, 173
ultra-low pressure, 191
valves, 188

weight loss, 195
After-shave preparations, 524
Alcohols, low molecular, in preparations
	without oil, 161
	as preservatives, 103
	see also Ethyl alcohol; Isopropyl alcohol;
	Propyl alcohol; etc.
Aldehydes, determination of, 129
Aleurones, 392
Alginate, in depilatories, 512
	in hair dressings, 465
Alginates, in dentifrices, 277
	in shaving creams, 518
	as thickening agents, 147
	in tooth powders, 266
Algofrenes, 183
Alkalization, 210
Alkalonamides, see Alkylolamides
Alkannin, 417
N-Alkyl-β-aminopropionates, 249; see also
	Deriphats
Alkyl aryl sulfonates, 249, 258
	in hair dyes, 479
	in rinses, 258
	in solid detergents, 222, 223
Alkyl dimethyl benzyl ammonium chlor-
	ide, 296
Alkyl ethyl morpholine ethosulfate, 485
Alkylolamide/fatty acid condensation
	products, 260
Alkylolamides, 242
Alkylolamine/fatty acid condensation
	products, 249; see also Alkyl-
	olamides
Alkyl phenols, 86
N-Alkyl-p-phenylenediamines, 478
Alkyl polyether sulfates, 243
Alkyl polyoxyethylene sulfates, 536
Alkyl sulfates, 243, 249
Allantoin, 359, 386
Allergy, 25, 26
	to dyes, 416
Almond Oil, in emollients, 359, 361
	in hair lotions, 470
	in hand lotions and jellies, 363
	in preparations with depth effect, 401
Alum, 291
	in deodorants, 305
	in depilatories, 510
	in shaving lotions, 524
	in shaving powders, 526
Alumina hydrates, 419
Aluminum acetate, in deodorants, 291
	in shaving lotions, 524
Aluminum alcoholate chloride, 291
Aluminum chloride, in deodorants, 291, 296
	in shaving preparations, 522
Aluminum chlorohydrate, 299, 301, 302;

	see also Aluminum hydroxy-
	chloride
Aluminum formate, 291
Aluminum hydrosilicate, 167, 168
Aluminum hydroxide, 419
Aluminum hydroxychloride, 291, 302; see
	also Aluminum chlorohydrate
Aluminum lactate, 291
Aluminum oxide, 446
Aluminum palmitate, 189
Aluminum phenolsulfate, 291, 296, 299
Aluminum phosphate, 419
Aluminum salts, 291
Aluminum silicates, 418
Aluminum stearate, 125
	in shaving powders, 526
Aluminum sulfamate, 291, 299
Aluminum sulfate, 291, 296, 299
Amaranth, 418
Amerchol L, 101
	in protective preparations, 314, 316
	in shampoos, 255
Amido sulfonic acids, 275
Amino acid derivatives, 274
Amino acids, in preparations with depth
	effect, 383
	in skin, 19
	in skin fat, 4
	structure of, 19, 20
p-Aminobenzoic acid, in hair lotions, 406
	in sunscreens, 337
p-Aminobenzoic acid ester, 331
β-Amino ethyl alcohol, 406
Aminoglycol, 155, 233
2-Amino-2-methylpropanol-1, 253
p-Aminophenol, 128, 478, 481
p-Aminophenolchlorohydrate, 482
Aminophenols, 478
p-Aminophenylamine, 481
Aminosulfuric acid ester, 70; see also
	Trilon A
Amino triacetic acid, 259
Ammonia, in cold-wave preparations, 499,
	501
	in depilatories, 511
	in hair dyes, 475, 479
	in hot-wave preparations, 498
	in powders, 446
Ammonium bicarbonate, 500
Ammonium carbonate, in cold-wave prep-
	arations, 500, 503
	in hot-wave preparations, 498
Ammonium chloride, in hair colorings, 477
	in shampoos, 252
Ammonium lauryl sulfate, 255
Ammonium persulfate, 503
Ammonium salts, 273
	quaternary, 37

in biological hair lotions, 404
in cold-wave preparations, 503
in deodorants, 293
in hair dyes, 481, 486
in hair lotions, 470
in shaving lotions, 526
in toothpastes, 272
Ammonium stearate, 235
Ammonium sulfate, 501
Ammonium tartrate, 482
Ammonium thioglycolate, 500
Amyl acetate, in nail lacquer, 440, 441
in nail lacquer removers, 283
Amyl alcohol, 282
Amyl-*m*-cresol, 100
*p*-tert-Amyl phenol, 100
Amyl salicylid, 331
Anabin sulfate, 346
Androstenediol, 370
Anhydrous creams, composition of, 108
Anhydrous products, preparation of, 132
Aniline dyes, 417
*Anobial*, 90
Anthranylic acid esters, 331
Antibiotics as disinfectants, 96
Anticholinergic drugs, 290
Antihistamines, 325
Antioxidants, 108, 125, 128
in hair oils, 460
increase of effect, 128
in lipsticks, 434, 435
in oil-in-water emulsions, 142
Antiperspirants, 288
principle of effectiveness, 290
*see also* Deodorants
Antiseptic agents, 362
Apple pectin, 496
Arachidonic acid, 377
Archil powder, 407
*Arctons*, 183
*Arlacel C*, in hand cleansers, 223
in rouges, 423
*see also* Sorbitan sesquiolate
*Arlacel 80*, 302
*Arlacel 83*, 136
in skin cleansers, 228
Arnica, tincture of, 468
Arnica flower extract, 465
*Arochlors*, 439, 442
Aryl alkyl sulfonates, 536
Ascorbic acid, 128; *see also* Vitamin C
*Aspergillus*, 98
Astringents, 510
Astrolatum, 113
in brilliantines, 460
in protective preparations, 314
*Atlas G-1442*, 255
*Atlas G-1612*, *see* Polyoxyethylene oxy-

propylene stearate
Avocado oil, 389
in emollients, 359
in preparations with depth effect, 401
Azo dyes, 430
Azorubin extra, 418
Azulene, 387, 523

Baby oils, 340
*Bacillus subtilis*, 78
Bacitracin, 96
Bacteria, 75
in cosmetic preparations, 98
gram-negative, 77
gram-positive, 77
Baldness, 366
Balsam peru, tincture of, 406
Barium chloride, 419
phosphate, 419
sulfate, in lakes, 419
in powders, 446
in solid detergents, 221
sulfide, 507
Barrier cream, 313
Basal cells (*stratum basale*), 6, 7, 9
Base, functions of, in preparations with
depth effect, 394
Bath milks, 536
oils, 535
preparations, 531
salts, 531
tablets, 533
Beef tallow, 516
Beeswax, 134
in bleaching creams, 488
in brilliantine, 460
in cleansing creams, 228
in cleansing emulsions, 229
in cold creams, 231
in deodorants, 299
in emollients, 359
as emulsifying agent, 134
in epilatories, 513
in eyebrow pencils, 428
in eye shadow, 425
in foundation makeup, 451
in hair creams, 462
in hair dressings, 465
in lipsticks, 431, 435
in mascara, 426
in preparations with depth effect, 402
in protective preparations, 314, 316, 318,
322
in rouges, 421, 423
in solid detergents, 222
in sunscreens, 335
Beeswax/borax reaction, 135
emulsifier system, 230

Bentonite, 124
  in foundations, 455
  in powders, 169
  in solid detergents, 221
  as thickening agent, 149
Benzidine test, 130
Benzocain, 524
Benzoic acid, 98
  in face lotions, 209
  in mouthwashes, 308
  in toothpastes, 272
Benzoic tincture, 308
Benzoin, in epilatories, 513
  in hair lacquers, 466
  in nail lacquers, 439
  in protective preparations, 318
  tincture of, 534
Benzyl acetophenone, 331
2-Benzyl-4-chlorophenol, 90
N-Benzylethylene diamine triacetic acid,
    259
Benzyl-p-hydroxybenzoate, 99
Benzyl lactate, 345, 347
Benzyl salicylate, 331
Betaine, 385
  in hair lotions, 406
Bialeurones, 392
Bicarbonate, 276
Binders in compact powders, 447
Biostimulines, 392
Birch extract, 524
Birch lotion, 408
Bismuth carbonate, 419
  subnitrate, 487, 488
"Blackheads," 6; see also Comedones
Bleaches, hair, 484
  skin, 487
Bleaching and dying, combination of, 485
Bleaching creams, 488
Bolus, 420
Borax, in bath salts, 532
  in bubble bath powders, 535
  in cold creams, 231
  in emollients, 359
  in foundation creams, 449
  in hair colorings, 477
  in hair creams, 462, 464
  in hair dressings, 465
  in hair dyes, 481
  in hot-wave preparations, 497
  in preparations with depth effect, 402
  in protective preparations, 314
  in rouges, 423
  in shampoos, 257
  in shaving creams, 517, 518, 519, 521
Boric acid, in bath tablets, 534
  in body powders, 343
  in deodorants, 300, 305

  as disinfectant, 85
  in face lotions, 209
  in hand lotions/jellies, 363
  in protective preparations, 314
  in rolling creams, 235
  in shaving powders, 526
Boric acid solutions, preservation of, 102
Bradosol, 93
Brightening rinses, 487
Brij 30, 316
Brij 35, 316
Brilliantines, 458
Bubble bath oils, 536
Bubble bath powders, 534
Burdock roots, tincture of, 408
n-Butane, 182
1,2,4-Butanetriol, 157
Butoxypolyoxypropylene glycol, 468
Butyl acetate, in nail lacquers, 440, 442
  in nail lacquer removers, 283
n-Butyl acetate, 441
Butyl alcohol, 440, 441
p-tert-Butyl-m-cresol, 100
Butyl-p-hydroxybenzoate, 99, 232, 359
Butyl stearate, in foundation creams, 448,
    449
  in lipsticks, 432
  in makeup creams, 452
  in nail lacquers, 439
  in nail lacquer removers, 283
N-n-Butyl-3-phenylsalicylamide, 90
Butylated hydroxyanisole (BHA), 128
Butylated hydroxytoluene (BHT), 128
Butylmesityl oxalate, 345

Cab-o-Sil, 149
  in baby powders, 344
  in face powders, 444, 445
  in hand cleansing pastes, 226
  in powders, 170
Cadmium sulfide, 403, 419
Calcium carbonate, in baby powders, 344
  in body powders, 343
  in deodorants, 300
  in face powders, 444
  in foundation makeup, 455
  in powders, 170
  precipitated, 510, 512
  in shaving powders, 526
  see also Chalk; precipitated
Calcium citrate, with alginates, 148
  in hand lotions/jellies, 363
Calcium gluconate, 148
Calcium hydroxide, in depilatories, 500,
    510, 512
  in hair creams, 462
Calcium phosphate, see Dicalcium phos-

phate; tricalcium phosphate
Calcium salt dispersing agents, 247
Calcium salts, with alginates, 148
  effect on shampoos, 258
Calcium salts of higher fatty acids, *see*
  Calcium soaps, precipitation of
Calcium soaps, precipitation of, 213
Calcium stearate, 125
Calcium sulfate, in shaving preparations,
  522
  in tooth powders, 265, 266
Calcium sulfide, 507, 510
Calcium thioglycolate, 510, 511
  trihydrate, 512
Calculus, 261; *see also* Tartar
Calculus-loosening agents, 275
Calgon, 220
Calomel, *see* Mercurious chloride
Camomile flowers, 476, 477
Camphor, in nail lacquers, 439, 442
  in shaving preparations, 523, 525
  spirit of, 524
Candelilla wax, 431, 435
Cantharidin, 386, 405
Capsicin, 386, 405
Capsicum, tincture of, 408, 470
Captan, 95
Carbitol, 163, 535, 538; *see also* Diethylene
  glycol monoethyl ether
Carbon black, *see* Lampblack
Carbon dioxide, as aerosol propellant, 179,
  184
  in toothpastes, 276
Carbopol C-940, 152, 268
2-Carboxyethyl amino acetic acid, 259
Carboxymethylcellulose, in compact
  powders, 447
  in depilatories, 511
  in foundation makeup, 455
  in mascara, 426
  in O/W emulsions, 148
  in rolling creams, 235
  in soaps, 219
  *see also* Sodium, carboxymethylcellulose;
  CMC
Carcinogenic effect, 110, 323
Caries, 261
Carmine nacarate, 435
Carnauba wax, in eyebrow pencils, 428
  in foundation makeup, 451
  in lipsticks, 435
  in mascara, 426
  in rouges, 421
  in solid detergents, 221
Carotene, 399, 402
Carrageenan, 337
Casein, 222, 322
Castor oil, 215

  in epilatories, 514
  in hair lotions, 408, 470
  in hair oil, 460
  in lipsticks, 430, 431, 435
  in mascara, 426, 427
  in nail lacquers, 439
  in nail lacquer removers, 283
  in protective preparations, 314, 318
  semi-hydrogenated, 423
  in shampoos, 251
  sulfated, 252, 253, 536; *see also* Turkey
  red oil
Catechu, 477
Caustic potash, 516; *see also* Potassium
  hydroxide
Caustic soda, 516; *see also* Sodium
  hydroxide
Cavity, oral, microorganisms of, 270
  physiology of, 260
*Ceeprin*, 93; *see also* Cetyl pyridinium
  chloride
Cellulose acetate, 439
Cellulose acetobutyrate, 347, 439
Cellulose ethers, in hair dyes, 482
  in hand cleansing powders, 225
  in protective preparations, 319
  in solid detergents, 221
  *see also* Ethyl cellulose; Methylcellulose
Ceresine, 113
  in bleaching creams, 488
  in brilliantines, 460
  in cleansing creams, 228
  in cleansing emulsions, 229
  in emollients, 359
  in lipsticks, 431, 435
  in protective preparations, 314
  in rouges, 421
  in sunscreens, 333
Cerium salts, 293
Cetaceum, *see* Spermaceti
*Cetavlon*, 93
Cetiol V, in cleansing creams, 228
  in emollients, 361
  in hair dressings, 465
  in preparations with depth effect, 401,
  402
  in protective preparations, 316
  in skin lubricants, 341
Cetostearyl alcohol, 401; *see also* Lanette
  wax O
Cetyl alcohol, in bleaching creams, 489
  in cleansing creams, 228
  in cleansing emulsions, 229
  in compact powders, 447
  in deodorants, 297, 299
  in emollients, 356, 358, 359, 361
  in eyebrow pencils, 428
  in eye shadow, 425

in foundation creams, 448, 449
in foundation makeup, 451, 455
in hair creams, 462, 464
in lipsticks, 433, 435
in makeup creams, 454
in mascara, 426
in pancake makeup, 455
in powders, 446
in preparations with depth effect, 401
in protective preparations, 314, 316, 322
in rouges, 421, 423
in shampoos, 253, 255
in shaving creams, 518, 519, 521
in skin cleansers, 233
in skin lubricants, 341
in solid detergents, 221
in sunscreens, 335
as thickening agent, 146
Cetyldimethylbenzylbenzyl ammonium
    chloride, 470, 487
Cetyl palmitate, 117, 119, 131, 396
Cetyl pyridinium chloride, 36; see also
    Ceeprin
Cetyl triethylammonium bromide, 308
Chalk, ground, abrasive effect of 279
    precipitated, abrasive effect of, 279
    in deodorants, 305
    in face powders, 445
    in foundation makeup, 451
    in toothpastes, 268
    in tooth powders, 265, 266
    see also Calcium carbonate
Chelates, 220
Chelating agents, 484
Chloramin, 300
Chlorethene, 186
Chlorocavracol (4-chloro-3-isopropyl-6-
    methyl phenol), 100
Chlorocresol, in emollients, 361
    in protective preparations, 322
p-Chloro-m-cresol, 100
p-Chlorophenol-2-glyceryl ether, 100
Chlorophyll, 294
Chlorophyllins, 272
Chlorotetracyclin, 294
Chlorothymol (4-chloro-3-isopropyl-5-
    methyl phenol), 100
p-Chloro-m-xylenol, 100
"Chloroxylenol" (CMX), 100
Cholesterol, 36, 52
    in eyebrow pencils, 428
    in eye shadow, 424
    in hair bleaches, 485
    in hair lotions, 404, 408
    in lipsticks, 435
    in rouges, 421
    in sebum, 5
    in skin fat, 4

in sunscreens, 335
Choline, 5, 385, 406
Cinchona bark, tincture of, 407
Citric acid, in bath tablets, 533
    in bubble bath powders, 535
    as neutralizing agent, 505
    in protective preparations, 319
    as sequestering agent, 259
    in shampoos, 253
    in wavesets, 496
Citric pectin, 534
Cleansing creams, 227, 228, 230
    liquefying, 227
Cleansing effect, 60
    determination of, 61
Cleansing preparations, 205
    rolling creams, 235
    solid, 234
Clove blossom, tincture of, 408
CMC, in hair lotions, 468
    in tooth powders, 268
    see also Carboxymethylcellulose
Coal tar dyes, 419
Cobalt compounds, 419
Cobalt nitrate, 475, 477
Cocoa butter, in eyebrow pencils, 428
    in eye shadow, 424
    in lipsticks, 433, 435
    in mascara, 426
    in skin lubricants, 341
Coconut oil, in shampoos, 251
    in shaving soaps, 516
    in sunscreens, 333
Coconut oil fatty acids, 251
    in shampoos, 256
    in shaving creams, 517, 519
Coconut oil fatty acid monoethanolamine,
    252, 253
Coconut soap, 257
Cod-liver oil, 389
Coenzyme A, 406
Coenzymes, 383
Cold creams, 134, 140, 360
    as skin cleansers, 230
Cold-wave creams, 502
    lotions, 494, 501
    powders, 503
    preparations, 499
        efficacy of, 503
    process, 22, 499, 501
Collodion solution, 514
Colloids, protective, 51
Coloring agents, in cosmetics, 416, 538
    in face powders, 445
    in lipsticks, 430, 433, 435
    in nail lacquers, 444
Color modifiers, 478
    rinses, 437

solvents, 435
Colts foot, tincture of, 408
Comedones, 110, 374; *see also* "Black-
    heads"
Complexes, cosmetic, 387
Conditioners, 260
Conditioning agents, 248
Contact dermatitis, 29
Contamination, microbiological of cos-
    metics, 97
Copal, 439
Copper sulfate, 475
Corium, 6, 9, 366, 397, 428
Corneal layer, 5, 11, 17, 397, 430; *see also*
    *Stratum corneum*
Cornification, 4, 8
Cornstarch, in bath tablets, 534
    in body powders, 343
    in deodorants, 300
    in rolling creams, 235
*Cosbiol, see* Perhydrosqualene
Cottonseed oil, 341
Coumarone indene polymers, 440
Crayons, *see* Eyebrow pencils and crayons
Cream dyes, 481
Cream rouges, 423
Creams, anhydrous, 108
    anti-wrinkle, 400
    based on fatty alcohol sulfate, 156
    based on glyceryl monostearate, 157
    coloring of, 418
    hormone, 400
    nongreasy, 131
    preservation of, 103
    protective, 132
    rolling, 235
    thixotropic, 131
    vanishing, 448
*Cremophores,* 158
*Cremophor FM,* 134
Cross linkages, disruption of, 492
    re-establishment of, 495
Cross sensitization, 27
Cutis, 6
Cyclohexane, 441
Cyclohexylacetoacetate, 345
Cysteine, 384
Cystine, 21, 384, 404

Damar, 439
Dandruff, 366
Day creams, 448
Decorative preparations, *see also* individual
    headings
*Deltol,* 116; *see also* Isopropyl myristate
Dentifrices, consistency of, 280
    evaluation of, 278
    flavoring of, 278

liquid, 277
    polishing effect of, 279
    shelf-life control of, 280
    toothpastes, 267
    tooth powders, 263
Denture cleaners, 280
Deodorants, 288
    active ingredients, 291
    aerosol preparations, 300, 301
    body, 288
    compatibility, with fabric, 304
        with skin, 303
    creams, 298, 299
    effectiveness of, 290, 302
    evaluation of, 302
    foot, 305
    jellies, 300
    liquids, 295, 296
    mouth, 306; *see also* Mouthwashes
    powders, 300
    shelf life, 304
    sticks, 297
Deodorizing agents, 272
Depilatories, chemical, 506
    liquid, 511
    methods, 505
    powders, 510
Depth effect, 396
    preparations with, 365, 400
Deriphats, 94, 245
*Dermis,* 6; *see also* Corium
*Dermolanes,* 219
Detergents, in shampoos, anionic, 239, 242
    amphoteric, 240, 245
    cationic, 240, 244
    nonionic, 240, 246
    solid, 221, 222
    table of properties, 239, 240, 241
Diachylon plaster, 513
N,N-Dialkylamides, 346
3,4-Diaminoanisol, 481
Diathermy, 505
Diatomaceous earth, 221, 224; *see also*
    Kieselgur
Dibutyl malate, 345
Dibutyl phthalate, 283, 439, 442
Dicalcium phosphate, abrasive effect of, 279
    in toothpastes, 268
    in tooth powders, 265
Dichlorodifluoromethane (Freon 12), 180
Dichlorophene, 88
    in deodorants, 305
    in hair oil, 460
Dichlorotetrafluoroethane (Freon 114), 181
Dichloro-*m*-xylenol-2.4-dichloro-3,5-di-
    methylphenol, 88, 100
Diethylene glycol butyl benzyl ether, 345
    monobenzyl ether, 345

monobutyl ether, 345, 347
monoethyl ether, in foundation creams,
    450
  in hair creams, 464
  as humectant, 142
  in nail lacquers, 440, 441
  in nail lacquer removers, 283
  in shaving creams, 519
  see also Carbitol
monomethyl ether, 442
mono-oleate, 357
monophenyl ether, 345
monostearate, in bleaching creams, 489
  in emollients, 361
  in protective preparations, 316
  stearate, 449, 455
Diethyl ether, 443
  malate, 345, 347
  stilbestrol, 405; see also Stilbestrol
  m-toluamide, 346
Diglycol laurate, 233
  stearate, 427
Dihydric alcohols, 432
Dihydrobenzene, 478
Dihydrochromans, 128
Dihydroquercetine, 128
Diisobutyl ketone, 440
Diisoeugenol, 128
Diisopropyltartrate, 345
Diluents, in nail lacquers, 440
2,5-Dimercapto adipic acid, 495
Dimethyl hydrantoin formaldehyde poly-
    mer, 467
Dimethyl phthalate, 345, 347
Dimethylpolysiloxan, 501
Dimethylsulfoxide, 440
Dioctyl adipate, 439
Dioxane, 223
Dioxine, 96
Dioxyacetone, 326
Dioxyphenylalanine (dopa), 15
Diphenylamine, 128
Diphenyls, chlorinated, 439
  hydrated, 346
Dipropylene glycol, in deodorants, 301
  in sunscreens, 337
Dipropylene glycol salicylate, 337
Disinfectants, in biological hair lotions, 404
  characteristics of, 81
  concentration of, 81
  in deodorants, 294
  determination of effect, 82
  principle of effectiveness, 80
  selection of, 83
  significance of, 80
Disoium ethylene diaminetetra acetate, 251
Disodium phosphate, in bath salts, 532, 533
  in hand cleansing powders, 226

Dispersing action, determination of, 59
Dispersing effect, 58
Distearyl amide of dihydroethylene tri-
    amine, 502
Disulfides, 500
"Dove," 218, 220
Draves Test, 45
Drug extracts, 307
"Dulgon," 220
Duponol C, 91, 223; see also Sodium lauryl
    sulfate
Duponol WA, 45
Dye crayons, 482
Dyes, affinity to skin and hair, 417
  for bath salts, 532
  natural, soluble, 417
  oil-soluble, 417
  solubility of, 417
  synthetic, 417
  toxicity, 417
  water-soluble, 417
Dyestuffs, properties of, 418

Earth colors, see Pigments, natural
Eau de Quinine, 407
Edema, 28, 324
Egg powder, 257
  yolk, 255
E Grandelat, 400, 401, 402
Electro CF, 183
Electrolysis, 505
Elements, inorganic, penetration capacity
    of, 399
Elemi, 439
  in epilatories, 513
Emcol 14,
  in aerosols, 186
  in deodorants, 302
Emcol IL (isopropyl laurate), 116
Emcol IP, 116; see also Isopropyl pal-
    mitate
Emollients, 351, 355
  anhydrous creams, 359
  dual emulsions, 359
  fat-based preparations, 358
  glycerol-based preparations, 361
  in preparations without oil, 163
  physiological principles, 351
  in shaving creams, 518
  W/O emulsions, 359
Empicol LZ, 257
Ems salt, 276
Emulgin M-8, 401
Emulsifiers, see Emulsifying agents
Emulsifying action, determination of, 57
Emulsifying agents, in aerosols, 186
  anionic, for O/W emulsions, 153
  auxiliary, 50

concentration of, 160
nonionic, in cold-wave solutions, 501
  incompatability with phenols, 102
  for O/W emulsions, 158
precipitation of, 52
in W/O emulsions, 133
see also Surfactants
Emulsifying effect, 48
Emulsions, classification of type, macro-
    scopic methods, 56
  miscroscopic methods, 55
  cleansing, dual, 230; see also Cold
    creams
  O/W, 233
    comparison of types, 140
    dual, 138
      preparation, 140
      as protection against aqueous solu-
        tions, 313
    form, origin, stability, 49
    W/O, 229
  oil-in-water (O/W), 141
    formulation, 159
    insoluble solids in, 159
    preparation, 160
    as protective preparations, 315, 316
    viscosity of aqueous phase, 146
  separation of, 52
    complete (breaking), 52
    partial (creaming), 54
  water-in-oil (W/O), 133
    as protection against aqueous solu-
      tions, 313
Enamel (of teeth), 260
Enzyme inhibitors, 294
Enzymes, 383, 400
Eosine dyes, 416
  in lipsticks, 435
  in rouges, 421, 423
Epidermin, 391, 401, 402
Epidermis, 6, 7
Epilation, 505
Epilatories, 513; see also Hair, removal of,
    mechanical
Epoxy esters, 440
Equisetum, tincture of, 408
Erythema, 28, 169, 324, 390
Erythrosine, 424
Erythrosine J, 418
Essential oils, in mouthwashes, 308
  penetration capacity of, 399
Ester ethers, 72
Esters, synthetic, 119
Estradio, 380
  in hair lotions, 405
  in scalp disorders, 370
Estradiol monobenzoate, 405
Estriol, 380

Estrogen creams, 382
Estrogens, effectiveness of, 380
  in hair lotions, 405
  in preparations with depth effect, 401
Estrone, 380
  in scalp disorders, 370
Ethanolamine, see Monoethanolamine
o-Ethoxy-N,N-diethylbenzamide, 346
Ethyl acetate,
  in nail lacquer removers, 282, 283
  in nail lacquers, 441, 442
Ethyl alcohol, in after-shave preparations,
    525
  in deodorants, 299, 301
  in depilatories, 512
  as disinfectant, 84
  in face lotions, 209
  in fat-free preparations, 162
  in hair dressings, 465
  in hair dyes, 479
  in hair lacquers, 466
  in hair lotions, 470
  in hand cleansers, 226
  in insect repellents, 347
  in nail lacquer removers, 283
  in nail lacquers, 441, 442
  in protective preparations, 318
  in rouges, 424
  in sunscreens, 337
  in toothpastes, 268
Ethyl-p-aminobenzoate, 331
Ethyl butyrate, 282
Ethyl cellulose, in hair lacquers, 467
  in insect repellents, 347
  in nail lacquers, 439
  in protective preparations, 318
  see also Cellulose ethers
Ethyl-p-dimethylaminobenzoate, 331
Ethylene diamine N-benzyl-triacetic acid,
    259
Ethylene glycol, 145
  in hair dyes, 482
Ethylene glycol diacetate, 283
Ethylene glycol lauryl ether, 440
Ethylene glycol monoethyl ether, 283
Ethylene glycol monoeugenol ether, 345
Ethylene glycol monomethyl ether, 442
Ethylene glycol monophenyl ether, 345
Ethylene glycol monosalicylate, 337
Ethylene glycol monostearate, 252, 255
Ethyl gallate, 128
2-Ethylhexandiol-1,3, 337, 345, 347
2-Ethylhexylsalicylate, 333
Ethyl-p-hydroxybenzoate, 99
Ethyl lactate, 441
Ethyl polyglycol acetate, 408
Ethyl stearate, 341
Eucalyptol, 308

Eugenol, 543
*Eutanol G,* in eye shadow, 425
  in hair dressings, 465
  in lipsticks, 435
  in makeup creams, 452
  in preparations with depth effect, 401
  in rouges, 421
Extracts, animal organ, 389
  botanical, 407
  from germinal plants, 391
  of pharmaceutical herbs, 394
*Extrapon S birch,* 408
*Extrapon VC,* 401
Eyebrow pencils and crayons, 427
Eye shadow, 424

Face lotions, 207, 209
Fats, 108
  in depilatories, 510
  hydrogenated, 115
Fatting agents, 282
Fatty acid alkanolamides, 482; *see also*
        Fatty acid alkylolamides
Fatty acid alkylolamides, in bubble bath
        oils, 536
  in lipsticks, 430, 432
Fatty acid condensation products, 214
Fatty acid monoethanolamine, 435
Fatty acids, metal salts of, 136
  in O/W emulsions, 142
  polyunsaturated, penetration capacity of,
        399
    in preparations with depth effect, 376
  salts of, 37
  in skin fat, 4
  unsaturated, in emollients, 356
Fatty alcohols, 108, 119
  in emollients, 358
  as emulsifying agents, 134
  in hair dyes, 482, 485
  in oils and anhydrous creams, 119
  in O/W emulsions, 141
  in shaving soaps, 516
Fatty alcohol sulfates, in bubble bath oils,
        536
  in hand cleansing pastes, 225
  in protective preparations, 316
  salts of, 37
Fillers, inert, 125
  mechanically active, 224
Film formers, 439
  in O/W emulsions, 152
  in preparations without oil, 164
*Filtrosol A,* 333
*Filtrosol B,* 337
Finishing agents, 249
Fissan colloid, 168, 171
Florentine lake, 419

*Fluilan,* 360
Fluorescine, 534
Fluorides, 274
Fluorocortisones, 325
Foam builders, 249
Foaming effect, 46
  determination of, 47
Follicle, *see* Hair, follicles
Foragynol, 380, 401
Formic acid, 386
Foundation creams, 448, 440
  makeup, 450, 454
Fragrances, 538
Freckles, 487
Free fatty acids, 516
Freon 11 (trichloromonofluoromethane),
        181
Freon 12 (dichlorodifluoromethane), 180
Freon 114 (dichlorotetrafluoroethane), 181
Freons, 183, 301
  in deodorants, 301
  in sunscreens, 333, 337
  *see also* Propellants
Frigens, *see* Freons
Fruit juices, 362
  condensed, 393
Fungi, 76
  in cosmetic preparations, 98
Furfuryl alcohol, 430

G-4, *see* Dichlorophene
G-11, *see* Hexachlorophene
G-2160, 277
Gallic acid, 478
Gelatin, in hair dressings, 465
  in hand lotions/jellies, 363
  in protective preparations, 319
  in sunscreens, 337
  as thickening agent, 149
Gel hair dyes, 482
Gels, inorganic, 149
Genetron 101, 333
Genetrons, 183; *see also* Freons; Propellants
Gingivitis, 262
Gingivosis, 262
Gloves, invisible, 317, 318; *see also* Protec-
        tive preparations
Glutamic acid, 487
Glycerol, in after-shave preparations, 524,
        525
  in bleaching creams, 489
  in compact powders, 447
  in detifrices, 277
  in deodorants, 296, 297
  in depilatories, 510, 512
  in emollients, 357, 361
  in face lotions, 209
  in foundation creams, 449

in foundation makeup, 455
in hair creams, 464
in hair dressings, 465
in hair dyes, 479
in hair lotions, 407
in hand cleansers, 223
in hand jellies, 363
in hand lotions, 363
as humectant, 143
in insect repellents, 347
in preparations with depth effect, 401, 402
in protective preparations, 314, 316, 319, 322
in rolling creams, 235
in rouges, 423
in shampoos, 253
in shaving soaps, 515, 516, 517, 518, 519, 521
in skin cleansers, 233
as skin-smoothing agent, 145
in sunscreens, 337
in toothpastes, 268
Glycerol jellies, preservation of, 102
Glycerol monostearate, see Glyceryl monostearate
Glyceryl-p-amino benzoate, 333, 337
Glyceryl monolaurate, 253, 255
Glyceryl monolaurate monosulfate, 253
Glyceryl monomyristate, 316
Glyceryl mono-oleate, 357
Glyceryl monostearate, in bleaching creams, 489
in deodorants, 299, 302
in emollients, 358, 359, 361, 362
in eye shadow, 425
in foundation creams, 449
in hair creams, 463
in hair dressings, 465
in hand lotions/jellies, 363
in insect repellents, 347
in lipsticks, 435
in makeup creams, 452
in mascara, 426
in O/W emulsions, 141
in protective preparations, 316
in rinses, 260
in rouges, 421, 423
in shampoos, 255
in shaving creams, 519
in shaving lotions, 523, 524
in skin cleansers, 229
in solid detergents, 221
Glycerylmonosulfate monofatty acid esters, sodium salts of, 216, 220
Glycol ethers, 440, 442
Glycolmonothioglycolate, 494
Glycol sulfite, 498

Gramicidin, 96, 294
Guanidine carbonate, 220
Gums as thickening agents, 147
in fat-free preparations, 163
Gum tragacanth, see Tragacanth

Hair, anatomy of, 17
bleaches, 472, 484
cleansing of, 236
color and gloss of, 18
coloring, temporary, 473
colorings, vegetable, 476, 477
creams, 461, 462, 464
dressings, gum-based, 465
dyeing, direct method, 484
dye removers, 486
dyes, 472
oxidation, 477
permanent, 474
temporary, 473
follicle mouths, 6, 321, 374
follicles, 6, 10, 17, 19, 170, 213, 396ff., 422, 450
Hairgrooming aids, 457
growth, 18
lacquers, 465, 466
loss of, 367
lotions, alcohol-based, 407, 408, 468
biological, 403, 408
two-phase, 469, 470
Hair oils, 458
preparations, anhydrous, 460
removal of, 504
mechanical, 513; see also Shaving preparations
methods, 505
preparations, 506
see also Depilatories; Epilatories
rinses, 258
Hamamelis water, 209, 523; see also Witch hazel
Hand cleansers, 223, 225, 226
Hand lotions and jellies, 363
Hemoglobin proteolysate, 385
Henna, 476, 477
Hexachlorophene, 87ff.
in deodorants, 297, 301
in shaving creams, 517
in skin lubricants, 341
Hexahydrophthalic acid diethyl ester, 345
Hexane triol, 319
Hexestrol, 380
Hexyl resorcinol, 408
Higher fatty acids, salts of, as emulsifying agents for W/O emulsions, 136
Histamine, 386
HLB (Hydrophilic/lipophilic balance, 38, 154

Homoentyl anthranylate, 331
Honey, in emollients, 362
  in hand lotions/jellies, 363
  as humectant, 143
Hormo-Fruit Extracts, 391
Hormones, in hair lotions, 405
  penetration capacity of, 399
  in preparations with depth effect,
    379
  in scalp disorders, 370
*Hostaphats,* 120
*Hostapons,* 214
Hot-wave preparations, 497ff.
  process, 497, 498
Humectants, in depilatories, 510
  in foundation makeup, 454
  in O/W emulsions, 143
  in shaving creams, 518
*Hyamine 10 X,* 93
*Hyamine 1622,* 93
*Hyamine 2389,* 92, 93
Hydrocarbons, halogenated, as pro-
    pellants, 180, 182
  as propellants, 182
Hydrogen peroxide, in bleaching
    creams, 488
  in cold-wave neutralizing solutions,
    503
  in hair bleaches, 484, 485
  in hair dyes, 478, 480
  in rinses, 485
Hydrocortisone acetate, penetration
    capacity of, 399
Hydrocortisones, 325
Hydrophilic-lipophilic balance, *see*
    HLB
Hydroquinone monobenzyl ether,
    487
Hydroregulatory system, 10
*p*-Hydroxybenzoic acid esters, 98ff.;
    *see also* Butyl-*p*-hydroxy-
    benzoate; Ethyl-*p*-hydroxy-
    benzoate; Methyl-*p*-hydroxy-
    benzoate; Propyl-*p*-hydroxy-
    benzoate
Hygroscopicity, dynamic, 143, 145
  effect of emollients on, 356
  equilibrium, 143, 145
Hypodermis, 6, 10

*Igepon A,* 243; *see also* Sodium
    lauryl isoethionate
*Igepal CA* 630, 223
*Igepon T,* 220, 242, 257; *see also*
    Sodium oleyl taurate
Imidazol compounds, *see* Miranols
Indalon, 345, 346, 347
Indanthrene blue, 419

Indigotin, 418
Insect repellents, 345ff.
  evaluation of, 348
  perfuming of, 348
Interfacial films, 43; *see also* Surface film
Intolerance, *see* Allergy
Iodine, 400
  complexes, 94
  tincture of, 94, 514
Iodophores, 98; *see also* Iodine, com-
    plexes
Ion concentration, effect of, 64
Ion exchange resins, in dentifrices, 276
  in deodorants, 295
Iris, tincture of, 308
Iron oxide, red, 452
Iron oxide pigments, 522
Iron powder, 477
Irritants, 386ff.
  in biological hair lotions, 405
  in preparations with depth effect, 386
  primary, 25, 26
Irritaion, primary, 28; *see also* Reaction,
    toxic
Isoamyl salicylate, 331
Isobutane, 184
Isobutyl-*p*-aminobenzoate, 337
Isobutyl stearate, 283
Isoelectric point, 21, 492
*Isolan,* 425, 435
Isolinoleic acid ester, 402, 408
Isopropanolamine, 449
Isopropyl alcohol, in deodorants, 301
  in face lotions, 209
  in hair dressings, 465
  in hair dyes, 479, 481
  in hair lacquers, 466, 467
  in hair lotions, 408, 468
  in insect repellents, 347
  in shaving lotions, 524
  in sunscreens, 337
Isopropyl laurate, 116
Isopropyl myristate, 116
  in bath oils, 535
  in cold creams, 231
  in deodorants, 297, 301
  in emollients, 359
  in eye shadow, 425
  in foundation creams, 448
  in foundation makeup, 451, 455
  in hair creams, 462, 464
  in hair lacquers, 467
  in hair lotions, 468
  in hair oils, 460
  in lipsticks, 432, 435
  in makeup creams, 454
  in nail lacquer removers, 283
  in pancake makeup, 455

in preparations with depth effect, 401
in rouges, 421, 423
in shaving lotions, 523
in skin lubricants, 341
in sunscreens, 333
*see also* Deltol
Isopropyl palmitate, 116
in bleaching creams, 489
in cleansing creams, 228
in emollients, 357, 361
in hair creams, 464
in hair lotions, 468
in hair oils, 460
in insect repellents, 347
in lipsticks, 432
in protective preparations, 315, 316
in rouges, 421
in skin lubricants, 341
in suncreens, 333, 335
Isothymol, 100
Isotrons, *see* Freons; Propellants

Japan wax, synthetic, 316
Jellies, 165, 224, 333, 336, 337, 362, 363, 465
Juices, fruit and vegetable, condensed, 393

Kaolin, 124
colloidal, in baby powders, 344
in body powders, 343
in deodorants, 300
in depilatories, 512
in face powders, 444, 445, 446
in makeup creams, 452
in powders, 169
in shaving powders, 526
in toothpastes, 268
in face masks, 165
in face powders, 446
in foundation makeup, 451, 455
in lakes, 419
in powders, 168
in protective preparations, 323
in solid detergents, 221
Karaya, 465
Karlsbad salt, 276
Keratin, 4ff., 17ff., 117, 211, 259, 386, 430
affinity with henna, 476
chemistry of, 19ff., 494ff.
reaction, to shampoos, 259ff.
to shaving soaps, 515
to soap solutions, 211ff.
structure of, 22ff.
Keratin hydrolisates, 404, 407
Keratinization, 8, 374
effect of hormones on, 379

Keratohyalin, 14, 16
Kerosene, 223
Ketones, 440
Kieselgur (diatomaceous earth), in deodorants, 305
in powders, 170
*Komplexon III*, 480; *see also* Sequestering agents
Kreis Test, 129

Labilin, 167, 385
Lactic acid, as humectant, 145
in protective preparations, 316
as sequestering agent, 259
in shampoos, 252
in shaving lotions, 524
thioglycolate, 494
Lakes, 419
in eyeshadow, 425
in foundation makeup, 451, 454
in lipsticks, 430, 435
in makeup creams, 452
in rouges, 421, 423
Lampblack, in eyebrow pencils, 428
in mascara, 426, 427
Lanette creams, 157, 360, 401
Lanette wax D, 119
Lanette waxes, in emollients, 358, 362
Lanette wax K, 119
Lanette wax, N, 156
in emollients, 361
in lipsticks, 435
in O/W emulsions, 141
in preparations with depth effect, 401, 402
Lanette wax O, 435
Lanette wax S, 322
Lanogel (polyoxyethylene lanolin), 467
Lanogene, 301
Lanolin, 116ff.
acetylated, 118
in emollients, 361
in shampoos, 255
in sunscreens, 333
anhydrous, 116
in emollients, 357, 359
in preparations with depth effect, 401
in shaving creams, 520, 522
in rouges, 423
*see also Adeps lanae,* anhydrous
in baby powders, 344
in bleaching creams, 489
in brilliantines, 459
in cold creams, 231
as conditioner in rinses, 260
in emollients, 358
as emulsifying agent, 134
in eyebrow pencils, 428
in eyeshadows, 425

in foundation creams, 448, 449
in foundation makeup, 451, 454
in hair creams, 462, 463
in hand cleansers, 223
hydrogenated, 314
in lipsticks, 433, 435
liquid, 118, 359
in makeup creams, 454
in mascara, 427
in nail lacquer removers, 283
in powders, 446, 447
in preparations with depth effect, 402
in protective preparations, 316, 318, 322
in rolling creams, 235
in rouges, 421
in shampoos, 252, 255
in shaving soaps, 516, 518, 519, 520
in skin cleansers, 229
in skin lubricants, 341
in solid detergents, 222
in sunscreens, 335
Lanolin absorption bases, 433
Lanolin alcohols, acetylated, 36; see also
    Wool fat alcohols
Lanolin derivatives, in hair dyes, 482, 485
    in hair lacquers, 467
Lanolin oil, 357
Lanopal, 466
Lanopal S, 467
Lanthanium salts, 293
Lantrol, 333
Lanugo hair, 6, 16, 170, 443
Lard, hydrogenated, in brilliantines, 460
    in skin lubricants, 341
Lauric acid, 250, 515
Lauric acid diethanolamide, 536
Lauryl pyridinium-5-mercaptobenzothiazol,
    93, 126; see also Vancide, 126
Lavender oil, 543
Lecithin, 120
    in hair dyes, 482
    in hair lotions, 408
    in preparations with depth effect, 402
    in shampoos, 253
    in solid detergents, 221
Lemon juice, 362, 488
Lemon oil, 543
Linoleic acid, 377
Linolenic acid, 377
Linseed oil, 215
Lip makeup, 428ff.
    cream, 437
    liquid, 437
Lipsticks, 429, 435
    flavoring of, 434
    perfuming of, 434
    preservation of, 102
    thixotropic, 431

Lithium salts of thioglycolic acid, 508
Lithium stearate, 168
Lycopodium, 344
Lyophilization, 389

Magnesium aluminum silicate, see Veegum
Magnesium carbonate, abrasive effect of, 279
    in baby powders, 344
    in body powders, 343
    in deodorants, 300, 305
    in depilatories, 512
    in face powders, 444, 445
    in foundation makeup, 451, 455
    in lakes, 419
    for perfume solubilization, 208
    in powders, 170, 446
    in rouges, 420
    in shaving powders, 522, 526
    in toothpastes, 268
Magnesium hydroxide, 268
Magnesium oxide, abrasive effect of, 279
    in preshave preparations, 522
Magnesium palmitate, 139
Magnesium peroxide, 271, 485
Magnesium silicate, 268
Magnesium stearate, 125
    in baby powders, 344
    in body powders, 343
    in brilliantines, 460
    in deodorants, 300
    in face powders, 444, 445, 446
    in foundation makeup, 451
    in insect repellents, 347
    in powders, 168
    in shampoos, 255
    in shaving powders, 526
Magnesium sulfate, in hair creams, 462
    in preparations with depth effect, 401
    in skin cleansers, 229
Magnesium sulfide, 507
Magnesium undecanate, 168
Makeup, creams, 452
    liquid, 453
    sticks, coloring of, 418
Malic acid, 259
Mandelkleie, 235
Manganese chloride, 501
Manganese oxides, 418
Manganese sulfate, 534
Marshmallow, 147
Mascara, 425
    anhydrous creams, 426
    cake, 425, 426
    emulsified creams, 427
    liquid, 427
Massage creams, 345
Mastic, 318
Maypons, 214, 242; see also Protein-fatty

acid condensation products
*Medialanes,* 242; *see also* Sarcosides; Sodium
lauryl sarcoside
Melanin, 15, 16, 324ff., 384, 487
biosynthesis of, 14
Melanoid, 15
Menthol, 305
in depilatories, 511, 512
in face lotions, 209
in mouthwashes, 308
in shaving creams, 517, 523, 525
Menthyl anthranylate, 331, 333
Menthyl salicylate, 331, 333
Mercaptans, 508
Mercapto carbonic acids, in depilatories, 509
in permanent wave preparations, 497
Mercapto ethanol, 494
3-Mercapto-1,2-propandiol, 494
Mercuric chloramide, 487, 488, 489
Mercuric chloride, 487
Mercuric salicylate, 487
Mercurious chloride (calomel), 487, 489
Metal peroxides as bleaches, 488
Metal salts, in face powders, 444
in hair dyes, 474, 475
Metaphosphates, 518
Metasilicates, 225
Methacrylates, 439
8-Methoxypsoralane, 326
*p*-Methylaminophenol sulfate, 481
Methyl anthranylate, 543
Methylcellulose, in dentifrices, 277
in depilatories, 512
in hand cleansing powders, 226
in protective preparations, 322
in rolling creams, 235
in shampoos, 255
in shaving creams, 518
in solid detergents, 222
in sunscreens, 337
as thickening agent, 148
*see also* Cellulose ethers
Methylcellulose carboxylic acid, *see* Carboxymethylcellulose; CMC
Methylene blue, 485
Methylene chloride, 182, 442
Methyl ethyl ketone, 441, 442
Methylhexaline, 225
Methyl-*p*-hydroxybenzoate, 99
in foundation makeup, 455
in hair lacquers, 467
in powders, 447
in toothpastes, 268
in wavesets, 496
Methyl isobutyl ketone, 283
Methyl salicylate, 308
*β*-Methyl umbelliferone, 335
Micelle colloids, 41

Micelle formation, 41ff., 45, 48
Microflora of cosmetic preparations, 98
Mineral oil, in bath oils, 535
in bleaching creams, 488, 489
in cleansing creams, 228
in cleansing emulsions, 229
in deodorants, 299
in emollients, 357, 359
in foundation creams, 448, 449
in foundation makeup, 455
in hair creams, 462, 464
in hair dressings, 465
in hair lotions, 470
in makeup creams, 454
in powders, 447
in protective preparations, 322
in shampoos, 253
in shaving creams, 518
in shaving soaps, 516, 521
in skin lubricants, 341
in sunscreens, 333, 337
in toothpastes, 268
*see also* Paraffin oil
Mineral oils, in oils and anhydrous creams,
108
Mineral waxes, in brilliantines, 459
in oils and anhydrous creams, 108
*see also* Paraffin wax
*Miranols,* 94
*Miranol SM concentrate,* 246
Moisturizers, 358
Moisturizing creams, 358
Molds, 75ff.
Monobenzyl ether, 345
of hydroquinone, 487
Monoethanolamine, in cold-wave prepara-
tions, 499, 501
in hot-wave preparations, 498
in shampoos, 251
Monoethanolamine thioglycolate, 500
Morpholine, 498
Morpholine alkyl sulfate, 485
Morpholinium compounds, 69, 93
Mouthwashes, 306
disinfectants for, 307
flavors for, 307
Mucins, in depilatories, 510
in emollients, 362
preservation of, 102
vegetable, as thickening agents, 147
Myristic acid, 515, 517, 521
Myristyl alcohol, in foundation creams, 449
in hair lacquers, 467
Myrrh, tincture of, 308
*Myrj,* 52
*Myvacet 5-00,* 116
*Myvacet 9-40,* 116

*Nacconol NRSF,* 223
Nail lacquer, 437, 438, 442
Nail lacquer removers, 282ff.
  preparation, 282
Nails, anatomy and physiology of, 437ff.
  cleansing of, 281
Naphthol blue-black, 418
Naphthol derivatives, 346
Naphthol sulfonic acids, 331
$\beta$-Naphthol, 47
2-Naphthol-6-sulfonic acid, 331
Neatsfoot oil, 341
Neomycin, 294
Neutralizing agents, 503
Nickel sulfide, 475
Nicotinic acid benzyl ester, 405
Nicotinic acid derivatives, 375
Nicotylamide, 375
Night creams, 359ff.
Nigrosine, 426
Nipa, 48; *see* Ethyl gallate
Nipagins, in emollients, 361
  in hand lotions/jellies, 363
  *see also* Butyl-*p*-hydroxybenzoate; Methyl-
    *p*-hydroxybenzoate; Propyl-*p*-hy-
    drobenzoate
Nitric acid, 475
Nitroaminophenols, 478
Nitrocellulose, 439, 440
4-Nitro-1,2-diaminobemzene, 481
Nitrophenylenediamines, 478
Nitrogen as aerosol propellant, 178, 184
"Nobecutan," 318
Nor-dihydroguaiaretic acid (NDGA), 128
Normolactol, 209
Nucleic acids, 407

Ochre, 418
Octylene glycol, 252
Oil-in-water (O/W) emulsions, 50, 141, 233
  emulsifying agents for, 152
  preservation of, 142
  raw materials, for aqueous phase, 142
    for oil phase, 141
  viscosity of aqueous phase, 146
Oil red XO, 418
Oils, anhydrous, composition of, 130
  animal, 108, 114
  hydrogenated vegetable, 433
  in makeup creams, 454
  mineral, 108
  natural, 108
  sulfonated, 215
  vegetable, in emollients, 358
    in oils and anhydrous creams, 114
    in soap shampoos, 250
  vitamin-rich, 389
Oleates, HLB values of, 154

Oleic acid, in emollients, 359, 361
  in hair creams, 462, 464
  in hair dyes, 482
  in mascara, 426
  in protective preparations, 316
  in shampoos, 251
  in shaving creams, 519
  in sunscreeens, 335
Oleic alcohol, 283
Oleyl alcohol, in emollients, 361
  in lipsticks, 433, 435
  in shampoos, 252
Oleylsarcosinate, 357
Olive oil, 215
  in emollients, 359
  in hair lacquer removers, 283
  in hair lotions, 470
  in hair oil, 460
  in preparations with depth effect, 402
  in shampoos, 251, 253
  in shaving creams, 519
  in skin lubricants, 341
  in sunscreens, 333
  sulfated, in bath oils, 535; *see also* Turkey
    red oil
Onion skin, 477
Opacifying agents, 254
Orange I, 418
Orange blossom water, 209
"Orbacid," 171
Orthosilicates, 122
Oxidation dyes, 477, 481
  incompatibility to, 483
Oxidation-reduction balance, 212
Oxidizing agents, in hair dyes, 478, 480
  as neutralizers, 503
Oxidizing solutions, 480
8-Oxyquinoline, 90
8-Oxyquinoline benzoate, 100
8-Oxyquinoline sulfate, 5
  in baby powders, 344
  in depilatories, 512
  in shaving lotions, 524
  in skin lubricants, 341
Ozokerite, 113
  in cleansing creams, 228
  in cold creams, 231
  in eyebrow pencils, 428
  in foundation makeup, 451
  in lipsticks, 431, 435
  in pancake makeup, 455

Palmitic acid, 5, 153, 515
Palmkernel oil, hydrogenated, 435
Pancake makeup, 446, 455
Panthenol, in hair lotions, 406
  penetration capacity of, 399
Pantothenic acid, in hair lotions, 406

in scalp disorders, 375
Papain, 384
Papillary layer, 6
"Parabens," 98; *see also* p-Hydroxybenaoic
    acid esters
Parachlorometacresol, 100
Paradentosis, 262
Paraffin hydrocarbons, 109, 110ff.
    carcinogenic effect of, 110
Paraffin oil, in brilliantines and hair oils,
    460
    in cold creams, 231
    in eyebrow pencils, 428
    in foundation makeup, 451
    in lipsticks, 432, 435
    in makeup creams, 452
    in protective preparations, 314, 316
    in rouges, 421, 423
    in shaving creams, 519
    in skin cleansers, 233
Paraffin sulfonate, 482
Paraffin wax, 113
    in bleaching creams, 488
    in cold creams, 231
    in deodorants, 299
    in emollients, 359
    in eyebrow pencils, 428
    in foundation makeup, 451
    in lipsticks, 435
    in mascara, 426
    in preparations with depth effect, 401
    in protective preparations, 322
    in rolling creams, 235
    in solid detergents, 221
Pastes, 132, 161
    hand-washing, 225
Patch test, 28, 213ff.
Peachkernel oil, 341
Peanut oil, hydrogenated in brilliantines,
    460
    in skin cleansers, 233
    in sunscreens, 335
    in protective preparations, 314
Pectin, 534
Peeling, 206, 487
Penetration capacity, 399
Pentachlorophenol, 90
Pentoses, 4
Peptides, peptones, in preparations with
    depth effect, 383
Perfume, physiological action, 543
    psychological effect, 543
Perfume aromatics, penetration capacity of,
    399
Perfume oils in bath oils, 536
Perfuming of cosmetic preparations, 538
Perhydrosqualene, 115
Permanent waving, 489

preparation, 496
principle, 490
Permanganate solutions, 485
Peroxides, determination of, 130
Perspiration, *see* Sweat
Petrolatum, 108
    as barrier cream, 313
    in bleaching creams, 488
    in brilliantines, 460
    in cleansing creams, 228
    in cleansing emulsions, 229
    in cold creams, 230
    in emollients, 357
    in eyebrow pencils, 428
    in eye shadow, 425
    in foundation makeup, 451, 455
    in hair creams, 462
    in lipsticks, 433, 435
    in makeup creams, 452
    in mascara, 426
    in oils and anhydrous creams, 108
    in O/W emulsions, 230
    in preparations with depth effect, 401
    in protective preparations, 314, 322
    in rouges, 421, 423
    in shaving soaps, 516, 518, 519, 521
    in skin lubricants, 341
    in sunscreens, 335
Petroleum ether, 441
Phemerol, 93
Phenol, in deodorants, 305
    in protective preparations, 322
Phenolphthaleine, 347
Phenols, as disinfectants, 86
    in hair lotions, 403, 406
    penetration capacity of, 399
    as preservatives, 98
    properties of, 98
    soap, 87
    in sunscreens, 331
    in toothpastes, 271
    value, 82
Phenylenediamine dyes, 416
Phenylenediamines, 478
p-Phenylenediamine, 478
Phenyl-p-hydroxybenzoate, 99
Phenylmurcuric, salts, 96
o-Phenylphenol, 99, 468
Phenyl salicylate, 331
Phloxine, 307
Phospholipids, 108
    in oils and anhydrous creams, 120
    in skin fat, 4
Phosphoric acid ester, synthetic, 120
Photodermatitis, 26
Phthaloyl phenylalanine, 275
Pigments, natural, 418
    synthetic, 419

Pilocarpine, 405
Piperonyl vutoxide, 345
*Pityroxporum ovale,* 78, 404
Placenta extract, 389ff.
  liquid, 400, 401
Plaque, 261
Plasticizers, 439
*Pluronics,* 71
*Polawax,* 316
Pollen, 393
Polyacrylates, 149, 224, 318, 440
Polyacrylic acid, 296
Polyester resins, 440
Polyethylene glycol 1500, 519
Polyethylene glycol 6000, 511, 512
Polyethylene glycols, in aftershave prepara-
      tions, 525
  in deodorants, 305
  in depilatories, 510
  for derivatives, *see* specific polyoxyethy-
      lene, for example, Polyoxyethy-
      lene alkyl phenols
  in emollients, 362
  as film formers, 152, 164ff.
  in foundation makeup, 455
  in hair creams, 464
  in hair lotions, 468
  in hand cleansers, 223
  as humectants, 142, 145
  hygroscopicity of, 145
  in insect repellents, 347
  in lipsticks, 430
  in protective preparations, 322
  in shaving creams, 516, 517
  properties of, 164
Polyethylene glycol waxes, 454; *see also*
      Polyox resins
Polyfibron, *see* Cellulose ethers
Polyhydric alcohols, fatty acid esters of
      as emulsifying agents, 134, 136,
      141
Polyisobutylene resin, 440
Polymethyl methacrylate, 442
Polyox resins, 152; *see also* Polyethylene
      glycol waxes
Polyoxyethylene alkyl phenols, in bath oils,
      536
  in shampoos, 251
  *see also Igepal,* 630
Polyoxyethylene coconut fatty acid mono-
      ester, 468
Polyoxyethylene distearate, in emollients,
      361
  in mascara, 427
  in shampoos, 252, 255
Polyoxyethylene lanolin, 462, 467; *see also*
      Lanogel
Polyoxyethylene mono-oleate, 38

Polyoxyethylene monostearate, 299, 357,
      501
Polyoxyethylene oleyl ether, 357
Polyoxyethylene oxypropylene stearate,
      299
Polyoxyethylene sorbitan monolaurate
      (Tween 20), 240, 357, 536
Polyoxyethylene sorbitan mono-oleate
      (Tween 80), in hair dyes, 482
  in pancake makeup, 455
Polyoxyethylene sorbitan monopalmitate,
      *see* Tween 40
Polyoxyethylene sorbitan monostearate
      (Tween 60, 61), in makeup
      creams, 452
  in shaving creams, 519
Polypeptides, 4
Polyphosphates, 220
  in hand cleansing powders, 225
Polypropylene glycols, 142, 145, 299
Polypropyl methacrylate, 442
Polystyrene, 440
Polyunsaturated fatty acids, cosmetic sig-
      nificance of, 378
Polyvinyl acetate, 440, 442
Polyvinyl alcohol, in protective prepara-
      tions, 319
  in shampoos, 255
  as thickening agent, 149
Polyvinyl pyrrolidone, in hair lacquers, 466,
      467
  in shaving creams, 518
  as thickening agent, 149
Polyvinyl pyrrolidone-vinyl acetate copoly-
      mer, 301, 467
*Polyvitamin Concentrate L,* 391
Pomades, 460
Pores 17, 168; *see also* Hair, follicle mouths
Potassium bitartrate, 534
Potassium bromate, 503
Potassium carbonate, in hand cleansing pow-
      der, 226
  in hot-wave preparations, 497, 498
  in shampoos, 251
Potassium chlorate, 271
Potassium hydroxide, in deodorants, 297
  in foundation creams, 449
  in hair creams, 464
  in hot-wave preparations, 497
  in insect repellents, 347
  in protective preparations, 316
  in shampoos, 251, 255
  in shaving creams, 517, 519, 520
  *see also* Caustic potash
Potassium metaphosphate, 226
Potassium oleate, 226
Potassium soaps, 515
Potassium sulfide, in depilatories, 511

in hair dyes, 475
Potassium sulfite, 498
Powders, 166
  absorbency, 169
  adhesion, 168
  aerosol, 179
  baby, 85, 169, 343, 344
  binders for, 446
  body, 85, 169, 343
  coloring of, 418
  compact, preparation methods of, 446
  covering power, 168
  deodorant, 300
  face, 169, 444, 445
  foot, 169
  hand cleansing, 225, 226
  inert, in depilatories, 510
  preparation, 171
  protective, 343
  raw materials, 166
  slip, 167
  softness, 167
  "Praecutan", 216
Pre-electric shave preparations, 52ff.
  alcoholic lotions, 523
  creams, 523
  gels, 523
  powders, 522
Pregnenolone, in preparations with depth
      effect, 400
  in scalp disorders, 370
Preservatives, 108
  concentration of, 102
  irritation and sensitization caused by, 105
  in lipsticks, 434
  in oils and anhydrous creams, 130
  in O/W emulsions, 142
  in shampoos, 250
  solubility of, 103
  in W/O emulsions, 136
Products, anhydrous, preparation of, 132
Products without oil, preparation of, 166
Progallin A, see Ethyl gallate
Progallin P, see Propyl gallate
Promelanin, 325
n-Propane, 184
Propellant mixtures, 184
Propellants, in deodorants, 301
  halogenated hydrocarbons, 180
  hydrocarbons, 182
  inorganic, 177, 184
  properties of, 183
Propyl alcohol, 84
Propylene glycol,
  in bleaching creams, 489
  in deodorants, 296, 297, 299
  in depilatories, 510, 511
  in emollients, 357, 361

in face lotions, 209
in foundation creams, 449
in foundation makeup, 455
in hair creams, 464
in hair dyes, 479
as humectant, 142, 145
in lipsticks, 429
in makeup creams, 452
in protective preparations, 316, 321
in rouges, 423, 424
in shampoos, 251, 255
in shaving creams, 517, 519, 521
in shaving lotions, 524, 525
in sunscreens, 337
in toothpastes, 268
Propylene glycol monolaurate, 468
  monomyristate, 316
  monostearate, in bleaching creams, 489
    in foundation makeup, 455
    in hair creams, 464
    in insect repellents, 347
    in shaving creams, 519
    in sunscreens, 335
  ricinoleate, in nail lacquer removers, 283
    in sunscreens, 335
Propyl gallate, 128
Propyl-p-hydroxybenzoate, 99, 496
Prostearin, 235, 236
Protective preparations, 311ff.
  alcoholic lotions, 317
  anhydrous, 313
  against aqueous solutions, 312, 313
  against chemical agents, 311
  against dry soils, 320
  insect repellents, 345
  invisible gloves, 317, 318
  massage creams, 340, 345
  against mechanical stress, 340
  against organic solutions and solvents, 318
  O/W emulsions, 315
  powders, 343
  skin oils and fats, 341
  testing of, 320
  against ultraviolet radiation, 323
  W/O and dual emulsions, 313
Proteinases, 383
Protein-fatty acid condensation products,
      214
  in shampoos, 253, 255
  in skin cleansers, water-based, 213
  see also Maypons
Protein hydrolysates, in hair lotions, 405
  in preparations with depth effect, 384,
      401
Proteins, 383
  in skin, 19
Proteus vulgaris, 78
Pseudomonas, 78

Purines, 4
PVP-VA, *see* Polyvinylpyrrolidone vinyl
　　acetate copolymer
Pyrethrum extract, 346
Pyridinium salts, 70
Pyrogallol, 386
　in hair colorings, 477
　in hair dyes, 475, 481
Pyrogallol monoacetate, 386

Quartz, ground 224
Quillaja saponin, 468
Quince seed mucilage, in hair dressings, 465
　in hand lotions/jellies, 313
Quinine, 405, 468
Quinine oleate, 337
　salts, in hair lotions, 406
　in sunscreens, 331
Quinizarin green SS, 418

Radiation, effect on absorption, 331
　ultraviolet, protection against, 323
Radio isotopes, 396
Rancidity, causes, 125
　determination, 129
　ketone, 125
　meaning, 125
　oxidative, 125
　prevention, 126
Rare earths, salts of, 293
Rays, ultraviolet, effect on epidermal tis-
　　sue, 324
　physiological effect of, 323
Reaction, toxic, 25; *see also* Irritation,
　　primary
Redox potential, 21, 212
Rein's barrier, 7, 297, 298
Renex, 20, 223
Reng, 476, 477
Resin, cation exchange, 299
Resins, 439
　ion exchange, 295, 299
Resorcinol, in hair dyes, 481, 482
　in hair lotions, 408
　in mouthwashes, 308
Resorption, 396ff.
　transepidermal, 397, 398
　transfollicular, 397, 398
Reticular layer, 6
Rhatany, tincture of, 308
Ribonuclease, 383
Rice starch, in body powders, 343
　in face powders, 445, 446
Ricinoleic acid, 363
Rideal-Walker Test, 82
Rinses, 258ff.
*Roccal,* 93
*Rohagit,* 219

Rose water, in face lotions, 209
　in hair lotions, 408
　in rouges, 424
　in wavesets, 496
Rosin, 513
Ross-Miles Test, 47, 48
Rouges, 420, 421
　anhydrous creams, 420
　compact, 420
　emulsified creams, 422
　liquid, 424
　loose, 420
Royal Jelly, 393, 400

"S-7," 88
"S-54," 386
Saccharin sodium, in dentifrices, 277
　in mouthwashes, 308
　in toothpastes, 268
Saccharose monofatty acid esters, 159
Saccharose monopalmitate, in hair creams,
　　462
　in toothpastes, 268
Safflower oil fatty acid monoglyceride, 357
Saffron, 307
　tincture of, 407
Salicylic acid, 98
　in deodorants, 300
　in hair dyes, 478
　in hair lotions, 407, 468
　penetration capacity of, 399
　in toothpastes, 272
Salicylic acid esters, 331
Salts, alkaline, 225
　aluminum, 291
　common, in bath salts, 532
　　penetration capacity of, 399
　　in toothpastes, 276
　inorganic, 225
　organic, 221
　phenylmercuric, 96
Santomerse D, 223
Sapamine citrate, 253
Sapamines, 244
Saponin, in bath powders, 535
　in hair lotions, 407
Sarcosides, 220, 242
*Sarcosyl NL,* 242
*Sarzins,* 78
Satol, in eyebrow pencils, 428
　in lipsticks, 435
Scabies, 94
Scalp, disorders in physiology of, 366
　irritations, 504
Sebaceous glands, 5, 16, 354, 366, 379,
　　397, 443, 459
Sebacic acid diethyl ester, 435
*Seborrhoea,* 94, 366, 386, 404

*capillittii,* 18
*oleosa,* 367
*sica,* 367
Sebum, composition of, 5ff.; *see also*
　　Sebaceous glands
Selenium compounds, 403
Sensitizers, 25
Sequestering agents, in hot-wave prepara-
　　tions, 498
　in shampoos, 247, 248, 256, 257
　stability of, 259
　in toothpastes, 276
Sequestrants, *see* Sequestering agents
Sequestren No. 3, 253
Sesame oil, in emollients, 359
　in sunscreens, 333, 335, 337
Shampoos, 236ff.
　based on fatty alcohol sulfates, 252
　discoloration of, 97
　dry, 256, 257
　liquids, clear, 247
　opaque creams, 254
　properties of, 241
　soap, 250, 251
　special, 258
　tints, 481
　transparent creams, 256
Shaving creams, 517ff.
　aerosol, 520
　brushless, 518
Shaving powders, 526
Shaving preparations, 514ff.
Shaving soaps, 515, 516
Shellac, 164
　in hair lacquers, 466, 467
　in nail lacquers, 439
Silica gel, 344
Silicic acid, in powders, 170
　in shaving powders, 526
Silicone oils, 108, 120
　in cold-wave lotions, 501
　in deodorants, 301
　in emollients, 357
　in hair creams, 462, 464
　in hair lacquers, 467
　in lipsticks, 435
　in makeup creams, 454
　in oils and anydrous creams, 120
　in protective preparations, 314, 316, 317
　solubility of, 122, 123
　in sunscreens, 331, 333, 337
　viscosity of, 122
Silicone salicylates, 331
Silicone waxes, 108, 120
Silver nitrate, 475
Silver salts, 475
*Sipon ES,* 243; *see also* Sodium polyoxy-
　　ethylene lauryl sulfate

*Sipon LS,* 256
*Sipon LT/6,* 253
Skin, acid mantle of, 12, 79
　anatomy of, 4ff.
　bleaches, 487
　breathing of, 12
　care of brittle, dry, flaky, 402
　chemistry of, 19ff.
　cleansing of, 206ff.
　　heavily soiled, 224
　color of, 14
　compatibility, with cosmetic preparations,
　　24
　　determination of, 27
　deeper layers, 6
　defense methods of, 79
　degeneration of, 365
　dry, anatomic picture of, 354
　exterior appearance of, 14
　fat, 4, 5, 207, 227, 522
　　composition of, 5
　flabby, 400
　flora, 77ff.
　hydroregulatory system, 10, 353ff.
　imperfections of, 443
　lubricants, 341
　luster of, 16
　microbiology of surface, 77
　physiology of, 10
　reaction to soap, 210ff.
　relief, 16, 323
　senescence and degeneration of, 365
　shininess of, 443
　stimulation of flabby, 400
　surface, 4ff.
Skin cleansers, 230, 231
　detergent based jellies, 223
　dual emulsions, 230
　face lotions, 207
　oil based, 226
　O/W emulsions, 233
　soapless, solid, 220
　solid, 234
　surfactant based, 217
　water based, 206
　　for heavily soiled, 224
　　for normal use, 217
　W/O emulsions, 229
Skin oils and fats, 341
Soap, 67, 351
　adsorption of, to skin keratin, 212
　in dentifrices, 266
　and phenols, 66ff.
　in shampoos, 257; *see also* Shampoos
　toilet, 217ff.
Soaps, 63, 91
　additives for, 218
　calcium precipitation, 213

dental, 276
in face lotions, 209
of higher fatty acids, 42
improved, 218
phenolic, 87
as skin cleansers, water based, 210ff.
shaving, *see* Shaving soaps
Soda, 226; *see also* Sodium carbonate
Sodium alginate, in compact powders, 447
in deodorants, 297
in hair creams, 463
in hand lotions/jellies, 363
in protective preparations, 322
in shampoos, 253
in shaving creams, 519
in tooth powders, 266
Sodium alkyl aryl sulfonate, 239, 244
Sodium alkyl benzene sulfonate, 253
Sodium alkyl sulfates, 216; *see also* Cetyl
    alcohol; Fatty alcohols; Oleyl al-
    cohol; Stearyl alcohol
Sodium alum, 209; *see also* Sodium
    aluminum sulfate
Sodium aluminum chlorohydroxy lactate,
    291, 297
Sodium aluminum sulfate, 300; *see also*
    Sodium alum
Sodium amyl pectin glycolate, 170; *see also*
    Ultra amylopectin
Sodium bicarbonate, in bath powders, 535
in bath tablets, 533, 534
Sodium bromate, 503
Sodium carbonate,
    in bath salts, 532
    in bath tablets, 533, 534
    in cold-wave preparations, 503
    in hot-wave preparations, 497, 498
    in shampoos, 257
    in solid detergents, 222
    *see also* Soda
Sodium carboxymethylcellulose, in hand
    cleansers, 223
    in protective preparations, 319
    as thickening agent, 148
    *see also* Carboxymethylcellulose; CMC
Sodium cetyl sulfate, in shampoos, 252
    in solid detergents, 222
Sodium chlorate, 503
Sodium chloride, 532, 533; *see also* Salts,
    common
Sodium cholate, 408, 534
Sodium cuprum chlorophyllin, 277
Sodium dehydroacetate, 277
Sodium diamyl sulfosuccinate, *see* Aerosol
    AY
Sodium dioctyl sulfosuccinate ("Aerosol
    OT"), 42, 45, 69, 239, 244
Sodium dioxystearate, 516

Sodium fatty alcohol sulfate, in hand
    cleansing powder, 226
in shampoos, 255
Sodium formaldehyde sulfoxylate, 486
Sodium hydroxide, 153, 154
    in foundation creams, 449
    in hot-wave preparations, 497, 498
    in protective preparations, 322
    in shampoos, 251, 255
    in shaving creams, 517
    *see also,* Caustic soda
Sodium hypochlorite, 281
Sodium iodide, 292
Sodium ixopropyl naphthalene sulfonate, 36
Sodium lactate, 143, 145
Sodium laurate, 68
Sodium-N-lauroyl sarcosinate, 274, 277
Sodium lauryl β-aminopropionate, 240; *see
    also* Deriphats
Sodium lauryl isoethionate (Igepon A), 243
Sodium lauryl sarcoside, 266; *see also*
    Sodium-N-lauroyl sarcosinate
Sodium lauryl sulfate, 52
    in bath oils, 537
    in bath powders, 535
    in bath tablets, 533
    in bleaching creams, 489
    in deodorants, 299
    in depilatories, 510, 522
    in emollients, 359
    in foundation makeup, 455
    in protective preparations, 316
    in shampoos, 237, 243, 252, 255, 256,
        257
    in shaving creams, 518
    in solid detergents, 222
    in toothpastes, 268
    in tooth powders, 266
Sodium lauryl sulfoacetate, 277
Sodium lauryl sulfosuccinate, 535
Sodium metaphosphate, 266
Sodium metasilicate, 266; *see also* Sodium
    waterglass
Sodium myristyl sulfate, 215, 277
Sodium oleate, 38, 226
Sodium oleyl methyl aminoethyl sulfonate,
    243
Sodium oleyl sulfate, 252
Sodium oleyl taurate, 239; *see also Igepon T*
Sodium oxystearyl sulfate, 216
Sodium perborate, in bath tablets, 533, 534
    as neutralizing agent, 503
    in toothpastes, 271
Sodium persulfate, 271
Sodium polyacrylate, 319
Sodium polyoxyethylene lauryl sulfate, 239
Sodium polyphosphate, 226
Sodium pyrophosphate, 485

Sodium sesquicarbonate, 532, 533, 535
Sodium silicate, in depilatories, 512
  in solid detergents, 222
Sodium stannate, 485
Sodium stannite, 508
Sodium stearate, 52
  in aftershave lotions, 525
  in deodorants, 297
  as emulsifying agent in O/W emulsions, 154
  in insect repellents, 347
  as opacifying agent in shampoos, 254
  in powders, 446
  in protective preparations, 319
Sodium stearyl sulfate, 141
Sodium sulfate, 533
Sodium sulfide, 507, 511
Sodium sulfite, in hair dyes, 479, 481
  in hot-wave preparations, 498
Sodium sulfacetamide, 403
Sodium sulforicinoleate, 276; see also Turkey red oil
Sodium tetrapolyphosphate, 225
Sodium thiosulfate, as antioxidant, 128
  in bath salts, 532, 533
  as dye remover, 486
Sodium waterglass, 319
Sodium zirconium lactate, 296, 300
Soils, dry, protection against, 320, 321
Solids, dispersed in oils and anhdrous creams, 124
  suspended in preparations without oil, 165
Solprotex Hydro, 337
Solubilizers, 163, 165, 342; see also Solubilizing agents
Solubilizing agents, effect, 48
  in face lotion perfumes, 208
  see also Surfactants
Solutions, aqueous, protection against, 312
  organic, protection against, 318, 319
Solvents, in aerosol preparations, 185
  auxiliary, 479
  lacquer, evaporation rates of, 441
  in nail lacquer removers, 282
  in nail lacquers, 440
  in shampoos, 248
Sorbic acid, 85, 103
Sorbitan monolaurate, 240; see also Span 20
Sorbitan mono-oleate, in pancake makeup, 455
  in preparations with depth effect, 400
  see also Span 80
Sorbitan monopalmitate, 236; see also Span 40
Sorbitan monostearate, in makeup creams, 452
  in shaving creams, 519
  see also Span 60

Sorbitan sesquioleate, in emollients, 357
  in hair creams, 461, 462
  in rouges, 423
  see also Arlacel, 83
Sorbitol, in aftershave lotions, 524, 525
  in bleaching creams, 489
  in foundation creams, 449
  in hair dyes, 479
  as humectant, 142, 145
  in nail lacquers, 442
  in shaving creams, 517
  in protective preparations, 314
Sorbitol liquid,
  in dentifrices, 277
  in depilatories, 511
  in emollients, 361
  in hand lotions/jellies, 363
  in makeup creams, 452
  in preparations with depth effect, 401, 402
  in protective preparations, 316, 319, 321
  in rouges, 423
  in shaving soaps, 516, 521
  in skin cleansers, 229
  in sunscreens, 335, 337
Sorel cement, 221
N-Soy-N-ethyl morpholinium ethosulfate, 240
Soy lecithin, 222
Span 20, 462; see also Sorbitan mono-laurate
Span 40, 235; see also Sorbitan mono-palmitate
Span 60, in hair creams, 462
  in O/W emulsions, 141
  in protective preparations, 322
  in shaving creams, 521
  in sunscreens, 335
  see also Sorbitan monostearate
Span 80, 455;
  in insect repellents, 347
  in mascara, 427
  see also Sorbitan mono-oleate
Spans, 134, 158
  in aerosols, 186
  in shampoos, 237
Spermaceti, 116
  in bleaching creams, 488
  in brilliantines, 460
  in cleansing creams, 228
  in cleansing emulsions, 229
  in cold creams, 231
  in deodorants, 299
  in emollients, 359
  in eye shadow, 425
  in foundation creams, 449
  in lipsticks, 431, 435
  in mascara, 426

in preparations with depth effect, 402
in protective preparations, 314, 316
in rouges, 421
Squalene, in emollients, 357
in sebum, 5
Stabilizers, 51
in hair dyes, 478, 480
in rinses, 485
Stannites, 507
*Staphylococci*, 77, 270
Starch, 125
in bath tablets, 534
in depilatories, 510, 512
in foundation makeup, 451
in powders, 170, 446
in solid detergents, 221
Starch glycolate, 319
solutions, preservation of, 102
Stearate creams, 146, 153ff., 160, 161, 316,
321, 401, 448ff., 464, 517
Stearic acid, 52
in brilliantines, 460
in cleansing creams, 228
in deodorants, 297, 299
in emollients, 361
as emulsifying agent in O/W emulsions,
153, 155
in foundation creams, 449
in foundation makeup, 455
in hair creams, 462, 464
in hand lotions/jellies, 363
in insect repellents, 347
in lipsticks, 435
in makeup creams, 452
in mascara, 426
in powders, 446
in preparations with depth effect, 401,
402
in protective preparations, 314, 316, 319,
322
in rouges, 421, 423
in shampoos, 255
in shaving creams, 515, 517, 519, 521
in shaving soaps, 516
in skin cleansers, 233
in solid detergents, 221
in sunscreens, 335
Stearyl alcohol, in bleaching creams, 489
in emollients, 359, 361
in lipsticks, 433
in mascara, 427
in protective preparations, 322
in skin cleansers, 233
in solid detergents, 221
Sterols, 108, 119
as emulsifying agents in W/O emulsions,
134
in oils and anhydrous creams, 119

Sticks, cologne, 161, 164
deodorant, 161, 164, 297ff.
insect repellent, 348
powder, 525
Stilbestrol, 370, 380
*Stratum basale,* 6; *see also* Basal cells
*Stratum corneum,* 4, 6; *see also* Corneal layer
degreasing of, 35
dehydration of, 352
*Stratum cylindricum, see Stratum basale*
*Stratum germinativum,* 6, 7
*Stratum granulosum,* 6, 7
*Stratum lucidum,* 6
*Stratum spinosum,* 6, 7
*Streptococci,* 78, 270
Streptomycin, 96
Stress, mechanical, protection against, 340
Strontium hydroxide, 512
Strontium sulfate, 445, 446
Strontium sulfide, 507ff., 510, 511, 512
Strontium thiolactate, 509
Styrax, 466, 513
*Subcutis,* 6
Sugar, penetration capacity of, 399
Sulfated oils, *see* Turkey red oils
Sulfides, 507
Sulfonamide-formaldehyde resin, 439
Sulfonamides, 94, 95
Sulfonic acids, 430
Sulfonic acid salts, 37
Sulfonylphenylenediamines, 478
Sulfopon OK, 226
Sulfur, colloidal, 215, 400
in hair lotions, 403, 407
in preparations with depth effect, 386
in shampoos, 258
Sulfur compounds as disinfectants, 94ff., 407
Sulfuric acid, 215, 486
Sumac, 477
Sunburn preventives, *see* sunscreens
Sunscreens, 325, 333
active ingredients, 326
anhydrous preparations, 332
emulsions, 334, 335
evaluation of, 338
greaseless preparations, 336, 337
liquid oils, 332
perfuming of, 340
principle of effectiveness, 325
Superfatting agents, 218, 515
Surface active agents, *see* Surfactants
Surface effect, preparations with, 414
Surface film, 43
Surface tension, reduction of, 40
Surfactants, anionic, 68, 69, 91, 216ff.
amphoteric, 70, 93, 216ff.
in bath oils, 535, 536
cationic, 69, 91

in deodorants, 293
in skin cleansers, water based, 216ff.
chemical classification, 66ff.
cleansing effect, 60ff.
deactivation of preservatives bactericidrs, 65
in depilatories, 509
as disinfectants, 90ff.
in disinfectants, 90
dispersing effect, 58ff.
emulsifying effect, 48ff.
  determination, 57
in face lotions, 209
foaming effect, 46ff.
general structure, 33
in hair dyes, 479
incompatibility between, 64
irritating and sensitizing effect of, 65
in lipsticks, 434
in makeup creams, 454
metal corrosion caused by, 65
nonionic, 71, 91, 216ff.
nonpolar groups of, 36
polar groups of, 37
principle of effectiveness, 33
in shampoos, 237
in skin cleansers, 209, 216ff.
solubilizing effect, 48
in tooth powders, 265
wetting effect, 44ff.
Sweat, composition of, 289
physiology of, 288
Sweat glands, 16, 288ff., 303, 305, 354, 366, 397, 443

Talcum, 124
in baby powders, 344
in body powders, 343
in deodorants, 300, 305
in depilatories, 510, 512
in face powders, 445
in foundation makeup, 451, 455
in powders, 167, 466
in pre-electric shave preparations, 522
in protective preparations, 314, 319, 322
in rouges, 420
in shave powders, 526
in solid detergents, 221
in tooth powders, 265
Tannic acid, 159, 208, 331, 419
incompatibility with polyoxyethylene compounds, 159
Tartar, 261; see also Calculus
Tartaric acid, in bath tablets, 533, 534
in deodorants, 301
in hair colorings, 473
as neutralizing agent, 503
in rinses, 485

as sequestering agent, 259
Tartrazing, 418
"Teepol," 244
Teeth, anatomy of, 260
cleansing of, 260ff.; see also Dentifrices; Toothpastes; Tooth powders
Tellurium oxide, 403
Tepid waving, 495
Tergitols, 244
Terra di Siena, 418
Testosterone, 370
Tetracetylorthosilicate, 122
Tetrahydrofurfurly alcohol, 432
Tetrahydrofurfuryl lactate, 345
Tetrahydrofurfuryl oleate, 345
Tetrahydrofurfuryl stearate, 435
Tetramethylthiuramide sulfide (TMTD), 95
Tetrasodium ethylene diamine tetra acetate, 251
Tetrasodium pyrophosphate, 535
in shampoos, 251, 257
Tetrasodium silicate, 226
Texapon CS, 225
Texapon Extract A, 226
Thickening agents, 146ff.
in preparations without oil, 163
properties of, 150, 151
in shampoos, 248
Thioglycerol, 509, 512
Thioglycolic acid, 493
in cold-wave preparations, 499, 501, 503
in depilatories, 508
in hair dyes, 481
Thiolactic acid, 494
Thiourea, 128
Thixtropy, 131, 227, 421, 431, 450
Thymol, in deodorants, 305
in hair lotions, 407
in mouthwashes, 308
Titanium dioxide, 124
in deodorants, 299
in depilatories, 512
in eye shadow, 425
in face powders, 444, 445
in foundation makeup, 450, 451, 455
in lakes, 419
in lipsticks, 433, 435
in makeup creams, 452
in powders, 168, 446
in protective preparations, 319
in rouges, 421
in shaving powders, 526
in tooth powders, 266
$\alpha$-Tocopherol, 128
$\beta$-Tocopherol, 128
Toluene, 442
$p$-Toluylenediamine, 478
sulfate, 482

Toothpastes, 267ff.
  preservation of, 102
Tooth powders, 263, 264ff., 266
Tragacanth, in compact powders, 447
  in dentifrices, 277
  in depilatories, 512
  in hair creams, 463
  in hair dressings, 465
  in hair lotions, 468
  in hand lotions/jellies, 363
  in protective preparations, 316
  in shaving creams, 518
  in toothpastes, 268
  in tooth powders, 266
Trephones, 391
Triacetin, (glyceryl triacetate), 85
Tricalcium phosphate, abrasive effect of, 279
  in toothpastes, 268
  in tooth powders, 266
Trichloroethylene, in hand cleansers, 266
  in rolling creams, 235
N-Trichloromethyl thio-4-cyclohexene-1-2,
    dicarboximide, 95; see also Vancide,
    89
Trichloromonofluoromethane (Freon 11),
    181
Tricresyl phosphate, 439, 442
Triethanolamine, as antioxidant, 128
  in bleaching creams, 489
  in emollients, 359, 361
  in foundation creams, 449
  in foundation makeup, 455
  in hair creams, 464
  in hair dyes, 479, 482
  in hand lotions/jellies, 363
  in hot-wave preparations, 498
  in mascara, 426
  in preparations with depth effect, 401, 402
  in protective preparations, 314, 316, 322
  in rouges, 423
  in shampoos, 251, 255, 256
  in shaving creams, 517, 519, 521
  in skin cleansers, 233
  in solid detergents, 222
  in sunscreens, 335
Triethanolamine alginate, 319
Triethanolamine alkyl aryl sulfonate, 244
Triethanolamine cholate, 408
Triethanolamine lauryl sulfate, in bath oils,
    536
  in bleaching creams, 489
  in compact powders, 447
  in emollients, 361
  in foundation makeup, 455
  in insect repellents, 347
  in mascara, 427
  in mouthwashes, 308
  in protective preparations, 322

  in rouges, 423
  in shampoos, 243, 252, 255, 256
  in skin cleansers, 229, 233
  in shaving creams, 521
Triethanolamine β-methyl umbelliferone ace-
    tate, 337
Triethanolamine oleate, 36
  in depilatories, 512
  in shampoos, 252
Triethanolamine ricinoleate, 361
Triethanolamine stearate, in eye shadow, 425
  in mascara, 426
  in powders, 446
Triethyl citrate, in bath oils, 535
  in nail lacquers, 439, 442
Triglycerides, 5
Trihydroxybenzene compounds, 478
Triisopropanolamine, 155
  in hot-wave preparations, 498
  in mascara, 426
Trilon A, 257
Trioleine, 357
Trisodium phosphate, 226
Trypsin, 384
Tubes, swelling of, 97
Turkey red oil, 215
  in deodorants, 299
  in depilatories, 511
  as dye remover, 486
  in hair dyes, 479
  in hot-wave preparations, 498
  in shampoos, 244
  in shaving soaps, 517, 518
  in skin cleansers, 229
Turpentine, 514
Turtle oil, 370
Tween 20, in bath oils, 536
  in dentifrices, 277
  in face lotions, 208
  in hair creams, 462
  in hair lotions, 468
  in hot-wave preparations, 498
  in shaving creams, 521
  as solubilizer, 165
  see also Polyoxyethylene sorbitan mono-
    laurate
Tween 40, 235; see also Polyoxyethylene
    sorbitan monopalmitate
Tween 60, in protective preparations, 322
  in shaving creams, 521
  in sunscreens, 335
  see also Polyoxyethylene sorbitan mono-
    stearate
Tween 61, 314; see also Polyoxyethylene
    sorbitan monostearate
Tween 80, 455
  in deodorants, 302
  in hand cleansers, 223

in shaving creams, 521
    see also Polyoxyethylene sorbitan mono-
        oleate
Tween 85, 223
Tweens, 158
    in aerosols, 186
    in insect repellents, 347
    in shampoos, 237
Tyrosin, 15, 384

Ultra amylopectine, in hair dressings, 465
    in powders, 170
Ultramarine, 426
Ultraviolet radiation, carcinogenic effect of,
        323
    protection against, see Protective prepara-
        tions
Ultraviolet rays, effect of, on epidermal
        tissue, 324
    physiological effect of, 223
"Ultrawet," 223
Umber, 418
Uranin, 533, 534, 537
Urea, in cold-wave preparations, 500, 501
    in deodorants, 269, 299
Urea derivatives, 439
Urea-hydrogene peroxide, 480
    peroxide, 281
Urocaninic acid, 324

Valves for aerosols, 188
Vancide 30, 95
Vancide 89, 95
Vancide 126, 93
Vanishing cream, 448
Veegum, 149
    in pre-electric shave preparations, 522
    in shampoos, 255
Vegetable extracts, astringent effect,of, 208
Vegetable juices, 393
Vegetable oils, as dye removers, 486
"Vel Beauty Bar," 220
Vinyl chloride, 182
Vinyl chloride-vinyl acetate copolymer, 442
Vinylmethyl ether maleic anhydride polymer,
        223
Vinyl resins, 439
Vitamin A, 132, 370, 374ff., 389, 391, 394
    effect of deficiency on skin and hair, 374
Vitamin B, 370, 375ff., 389, 391, 394, 406
Vitamin C, 376, 394, 399
Vitamin D, 132, 323, 376, 389, 399
Vitamin E, as antioxidant, 128
    in preparations with depth effect, 376ff.,
        389, 391, 402
    see also α-Yocopherol; β-Tocopherol
Vitamin F, 370, 376ff., 389
    in baby powders, 344

effect of definiency on skin, 378
    in foundation creams, 439
    in preparations with depth effect, 376ff.
    in skin lubricants, 341
    in sunscreens, 333
    see also Polyunsaturated fatty acids, cos-
        metic significance of
Vitamin K, 379, 399
Vitamin oil, 389, 402
Vitamins, penetration capacity of, 399
    in preparations with depth effect, 372ff.
    in scalp disorders, 370, 372

Walnut leaves, 477
Water-in-oil (W/O) emulsions, compositions
        of, 133
    emulsifying agents for, 133
    raw materials, of aqueous phase, 133
        of oil phase, 133
Waveset preparations, 496
Wax, microcrystalline, 359; see also Astro-
        latum
Waxes, animal, 108
    macrocrystalline, 114
    microcrystalline, 114
    mineral, 108, 113
    in O/W emulsions, 141
    in oils and anhydrous creams, 116, 119
    synthetic, 108, 109
    vegetable, 108
Wax-rosin mixture, 513
Wetting effect, 44ff.
    determination of, 45
    see also Surfactants
Wheat germ oil, 389
Wheatstarch, in bath tablets, 534
    in body powders, 343
White oils, 113
White pigments, see Titanium dioxide; Zinc
        oxide
Witch hazel see, Hamamelis Water
Wood extracts, 476
Wool fat alcohols, 118
    acetylated, 118
    in emollients, 358
    as emulsifying agents in W/O emulsions,
        134
Wool fat sterols, 118
Wool wax, in lipsticks, 435
    in preparations with depth effect, 402
    see also Wool fat alcohols
Wool wax alcohols, 361
Wrinkle concealers, 457

Xylene, 441

Yeast, brewers, 391
Yeasts, 76, 98

Yellow AB, 418

Zephyrol, 93
Zinc carbonate, 124
Zinc dimethyl dithiocarbonate (DMDTC),
 95
Zinc hydroxide, 124
Zinc myristate, 526
Zinc oxide, 124, 419
 in baby powders, 344
 in bleaching creams, 488
 in deodorants, 300, 305
 in depilatories, 510, 512
 in eye shadows, 425
 in face powders, 444, 445
 in foundation makeup, 451
 in lakes, 419
 in powders, 168, 446
 in protective preparations, 314

 in shaving powders, 526
Zinc peroxide, 489
Zinc phenol sulfate, 124, 209
 in shaving lotions, 523, 524
Zinc salts, 125
Zinc stearate, in baby powders, 344
 in body powders, 343
 in deodorants, 300, 305
 in face powders, 444, 445, 446
 in insect repellents, 347
 as opacifying agent in shampoos, 255
 in powders, 168, 446
 in pre-electric shave preparations, 522
 in protective preparations, 322
 in rouges, 420
 in shaving powders, 526
Zinc sulfide, 507
Zinc undecanate, in powders, 168
 in shaving powders, 526